D1246296

Health and Healing in
Eighteenth-Century Germany

The Johns Hopkins University Studies
in Historical and Political Science

114th Series (1996)

1.

Antwerp in the Age of Reformation:
Underground Protestantism in a Commercial Metropolis, 1550–1577
by Guido Marnef

2.

The World of the Paris Café:
Sociability among the French Working Class, 1789–1914
by W. Scott Haine

3.

A Provincial Elite in Early Modern Tuscany:
Family and Power in the Creation of the State
by Giovanna Benadusi

4.

Health and Healing in Eighteenth-Century Germany
by Mary Lindemann

MARY LINDEMANN

Health &
Healing in
Eighteenth-
Century
Germany

The Johns Hopkins University Press
BALTIMORE AND LONDON

This book has been brought to publication with the generous
assistance of the National Endowment for the Humanities.

© 1996 *The Johns Hopkins University Press*
All rights reserved. Published 1996
Printed in the United States of America on acid-free paper
05 04 03 02 01 00 99 98 97 96   5 4 3 2 1

The Johns Hopkins University Press
2715 North Charles Street
Baltimore, Maryland 21218–4319
The Johns Hopkins Press Ltd., London

Library of Congress Cataloging-in-Publication Data
will be found at the end of this book.
A catalog record for this book is available from the British Library.

For Michael

C O N T E N T S

List of Illustrations and Maps ix

Acknowledgments xi

Introduction 3

C H A P T E R I
Medicine, State, and Society 22

C H A P T E R 2
The Physici 72

C H A P T E R 3
*Quacks, Bread-Thieves, and Interlopers; Friends,
Neighbors, and Kin* 144

C H A P T E R 4
Illness and Society 236

C H A P T E R 5
Choices and Meanings 289

Conclusion 369

List of Abbreviations 375
Notes 379
Bibliography 459
Index 489

Illustrations

Title page, *Stolpertus, ein junger Arzt am Krankenbette*	78
"Der Oculist"	152
Duke August's handwriting before his cataract operation	154
Duke August's handwriting after his cataract operation	155
"Der Wundarzt"	183
"Der Bader"	184
A mastectomy procedure	344
A "quack" dressed in Turkish garb	360

Maps

North Germany in 1648	2
Braunschweig-Wolfenbüttel	28
Wolfenbüttel and surroundings	86
Königslutter am Elm	122
Hehlen	254
Schöppenstedt	282

ACKNOWLEDGMENTS

It is always pleasant to acknowledge the support received while research-
ing and writing a book. Numerous institutions provided me with financial
and other assistance. First among these was the Herzog August Bibliothek
in Wolfenbüttel, which granted me a postdoctoral research fellowship for
1980–82. This fellowship allowed me to work in the superb holdings of
the library, as well as to do extensive archival research in the Niedersächsisches Staatsarchiv-Wolfenbüttel and the Stadtarchiv Braunschweig.
The German Academic Exchange (DAAD) sponsored further work in
these sources in summer 1983, and an IREX/Fulbright Hays Grant during summer 1985 allowed me to spend three months in what was then
the German Democratic Republic doing comparative research at the
Franckesche Stiftungen in Halle and Zentrales Staatsarchiv-Dienststelle
Merseburg. Two Faculty Development Grants from Carnegie Mellon
University in summer 1988 and summer 1992, course relief in spring 1989,
and an NEH Travel to Collections Grant allowed me to make short return
trips to Wolfenbüttel. During those months, I expanded my research
in the Stadtarchiv Helmstedt, Stadtarchiv Königslutter, and Ratsarchiv
Hornburg, as well as doing more work in the Wolfenbüttel and Braunschweig archives. Other time for research and writing in 1989 and 1990
was generously covered by a NIH–National Library of Medicine Pre-
Publication Grant (Grant LM 04949). A very early draft of Chapter 3,
"Quacks, Bread-Thieves, and Interlopers; Friends, Neighbors, and Kin,"
was worked out while I was a Fellow at the Shelby Cullom Davis Center
for Historical Studies (Princeton University) during fall 1985. I spent
seven months in London in 1994, enjoying the very "welcoming" hospitality of the Wellcome Institute for the History of Medicine. The Wellcome provided me with an office and computer support, and there I
produced the final draft of this book. I simply cannot think of a more
physically comfortable and intellectually stimulating place to work.

Many people at all of these institutions made my professional life productive and my personal life enjoyable. While I cannot possibly thank
everyone to whom I owe a debt, I must single out for special mention the

following: Sabine Solf, Paul Raabe, Christian Hogrefe, and Gotthard Frühsorge at the Herzog August Bibliothek; Dieter Matthes, my *Betreuer*, and the helpful staff of the reading room at the Staatsarchiv-Wolfenbüttel; various members of the staff in Braunschweig's Stadtarchiv; Eva Mühl and Jürgen Storz at the Franckesche Stiftungen, as well as Wolfram Kaiser and Arina Völker of the Institute for the History of Medicine, Martin Luther University, in Halle; Meta Kronke, archivist at the Staatsarchiv in Merseburg; Heinz Röhr, archivist, and Wilfred Kraus in Königslutter; Hans-Eberhard Müller in Helmstedt; Hermann Himmler in Hornburg; and Bill Bynum, Roy Porter, Andrew Wear, and Sally Bragg at the Wellcome.

I owe a whole series of debts, intellectual and personal, to many others. I must first thank Peter Albrecht, whose own knowledge of the ins and outs of the history of Braunschweig-Wolfenbüttel is unrivaled. He was the perfect guide and prevented me from making many stupid mistakes. He also read more than half of the manuscript while on "vacation" in the United States and gave me a place to stay in Braunschweig on several occasions. I also must thank my friends and intellectual companions Tom Broman and Mimi Wessling. Their own work on academic medicine and on medicine and government informed this study in several ways. Tom also volunteered to read the manuscript and offered helpful criticism at several points. Here, too, I want to thank Jill and Jochen Bepler. They were my best friends during those early years in Wolfenbüttel when this book was but a gleam in my eye. They must have wondered whether I would ever pull it all together. They have remained friends ever since and only grow dearer with time and, alas, distance. I owe many other people many debts and hope they will understand if I list them without further comment: Andrew Barnes, Steven Beaudoin, Natalie Zemon Davis, Herrick Chapman, Lizabeth Cohen, Wendy Goldman, Gina Hames, Donna Harsch, Franklin Kopitzsch, Katherine Lynch, Guido Ruggiero, Kris Ruggiero, Donna Schroth, Peter Stearns, Jan Steinberg, and Ursula Stephan.

Jacqueline Wehmueller, my editor at the Johns Hopkins University Press, showed great interest in, and enthusiasm for, this work at a very early stage in its development. She and the Johns Hopkins University Press have been delightful to work with, and I can only wish that every author would have so gratifying an experience. Here, too, I wish to thank Jodie Minor, who helped me proofread the manuscript before it was submitted to the Press and did her normal, efficient job, and my colleague David Miller, director of the Center for Historical Information Systems and Analysis of the Department of History, Carnegie Mellon University, Margaret Miller, and Ian Brown for creating the computer-generated maps in this volume (all of which are based on maps from the Niedersächsisches Landesverwaltungsamts–Landesvermessung, Hannover). The Interlibrary Loan departments at Hunt Library, Carnegie Mellon University, and Bird Library, Syracuse, helped me track down obscure materials, and Sue Collins of the Hunt Library cheerfully pursued arcane references.

A note of thanks is due to the several publishers who have permitted me to reprint here parts of articles that originally appeared in other places: to Editions Rodopi (Jill Kohl and Mary Lindemann, "Augustus in tenebris," in *Barocker Lust-Spiegel: Studien zur Literatur des Barock. Festschrift für Blake Lee Spahr*, ed. Martin Bircher, Jörg-Ulrich Fechner, and Gerd Hillem, 187–204 [1984], and my "The Enlightenment Encountered: The German Physicus and His World, 1750–1820," in *Medicine in the Enlightenment*, ed. Roy Porter, 181–97 [1995]); to New York University Press (Mary Lindemann, "Confessions of an Archive Junkie," in *Theory, Method, and Practice in Social and Cultural History*, ed. Peter Karsten and John Modell, 152–80 [1992]); to Routledge (Mary Lindemann, "Professionals? Sisters? Rivals? Midwives in Braunschweig, 1750–1820," in *The Art of Midwifery*, ed. Hilary Marland, 176–91 [1993]); and to Max Niemeyer Verlag GmbH (Mary Lindemann, "'Aufklärung' and the Health of the People: 'Volksschriften' and Medical Advice in Braunschweig-Wolfenbüttel, 1756–1803," in *Das Volk als Objekt obrigkeitlichen Handelns*, ed. Rudolf Vierhaus, 101–20 [1992]).

The final debt of gratitude that must be paid is that to my husband, Michael Miller. I really have no idea what to say to convey the depth of my feelings, so let it suffice to admit that I cannot imagine history or life without him.

Health and Healing in
Eighteenth-Century Germany

Baltic Sea

Denmark

Duchy of
Braunschweig-
Lüneburg

Electorate of Brandenburg

Braunschweig -
Wolfenbüttel

Electorate of Saxony

Duchy of
Hannover

Landgraviate
of Hesse-Kassel

North Germany in 1648

Introduction

In May 1747, Georg Spangenberg, an obscure physician practicing in a remote corner of Braunschweig-Wolfenbüttel, penned a long report to the ducal Collegium medicum (Board of Health). After thanking the Collegium for advice he had received about three serious cases that had occurred in his practice that March, he surveyed medical conditions in his district of Walkenried:

An apothecary once lived in Walkenried [but no longer does]; about half an hour from here, in the town of Ellrich, are two apothecaries; there are two more in the town of Bleichrode, about three hours distant; and one [living] about two miles away in Nordhausen. The apothecary shops in Bleichrode and Nordhausen are in good condition; the shop in Ellrich is, however, [only] just adequately maintained. The drugs I use routinely I order from the New Apothecary in Nordhausen. Those medicines that require no special apparatus [to make], I concoct myself; prescriptions, however, I write sometimes for one, sometimes for another apothecary, depending on which is closer to my patients. . . .

At present, only one surgeon, Siegfried Nezel by name, lives in the Walkenried district, in the village of Zorge. He was examined by Physicus Blumen in Blankenburg, and sworn in . . . [and] since that time everyone has seemed quite satisfied with his performance. He visits his patients diligently and willingly, his fees are very moderate, he attempts no treatments without asking for further information and instruction, and, in difficult cases, when [for example] an operation becomes necessary . . . he always consults another, [more] experienced surgeon in Nordhausen or elsewhere, [calling him in] to perform such operations, while he pays close attention in order to learn what he does not know.

As to midwifery, the situation is very unsatisfactory. The three villages [in my district]—Zorge, Wiede, and Hohegeiss—are large and populous. Each village holds about two hundred families, yet each has only a single midwife. When she is ill, or when, as often happens, two women go into labor simultaneously, then the mothers must turn to other women . . . to assist them [in childbed]. According to local custom, each [lying-in] woman may choose any matron as her midwife; the authorities only insist that she pay the regular midwife the [normal] fee of six groschen. No one is ever denied the right to select any woman she pleases as midwife. This principle is sound insofar as it provides the [regular] midwife with an adequate income, but the public [as a whole] suffers. Previously, I supervised the midwives in Walkenried . . . yet am no longer asked to do so. Frau Neuhofer has acted as midwife for several years now [in Zorge?], without being either examined or sworn in; [and] I can do nothing to remedy such [disorders] because Amtmann [Magistrate] Heiland completely shuts me out [of affairs and does not allow me] to busy myself with the tasks generally incumbent on a physicus. [Thus] for some years now I have had to let everything take its own course. [At first] I believed that Heiland would eventually see the light and put the common good above all other considerations . . . [but this has not happened].

I took the liberty, then, to denounce the midwife in Zorge officially for her brutal treatment of a birthing woman; she sought to force her into labor too soon and even tried to pull [the child] out of her. For my "audacity," the ecclesiastical court reprimanded me harshly, fully without cause and quite contrary to any sense of justice.

Because I am allowed knowledge of nothing going on around here and am permitted to attend to nothing, the entire medical situation in Walkenried, since Heiland has become Amtmann, has fallen into the worst possible disarray. Twenty years ago, I received a gracious concession [from the privy council] . . . to practice medicine here, and from the very beginning [of my residence] and until the previous Amtmann Mattenberg died, I executed all the official duties of a physicus, conducted the *visa reperta* [on corpses] and [inspected] all severely wounded persons, tested the abilities of *operateurs* before they . . . cut for the stone, or repaired hernias, or couched cataracts, and I supervised all such operations personally. Whenever workers at one of the ducal . . . mines or foundries fell ill or suffered injury, I treated them without charge, even journeying to them at my own expense. When dysentery, or *febres maligna, purpure et petectia* raged, as often happens here, I went in person to visit all patients without distinction, and assisted many of the needy among them, and even gave them medications free of all charge. For all these and [many] similar services, I have never received a penny's worth of salary or in *accidentzen*, except for an annual grant of six cords of firewood and nine shocks of grain, and [as a result] performed these tasks completely without recompense and merely in hope of future preferment. I do not even enjoy the freedom [from taxes] granted to the surgeon [here] . . . but rather

must pay all contributions and levies, [provide] all services, and [even] hire someone to do corvée for me. For eighteen years I was allowed to pasture my few animals [on communal meadows] without fee. [But] in the past two years, through
the instigation of a certain someone [Heiland], I have been sharply warned that if
I wish to enjoy this right in the future, I must request special authorization . . .
from the ducal treasury. In the Geröder districts, about three hours' journey from
here, I have held the office of physicus for eighteen years. In 1743, His Royal
Highness the king of Prussia named me as adjunct-physicus for the County of
Hohenstein. . . . [A] dispensation granted me by the king of Prussia has permitted
me to reside in Walkenried, almost in the middle [of the various areas entrusted
to me], only one hour away from the city of Sachsa, and scarcely one-half hour
distant from Ellrich. Thus I can attend to my duties in Hohenstein . . . and there
as well as in Geröder . . . every aspect of public health is in perfect order. In
Walkenried, however, . . . everything is going to the dogs because I have not been
appointed physicus and Heiland opposes me. All kinds of people have settled
here, who were not tolerated in Hohenstein and were driven from there. [These],
however, wander freely around in Walkenried, cajoling the inhabitants into unnecessary treatments and depriving them of both their money and their health. A
tanner's apprentice named Prümann, who was banished from Hohenstein because of his medicating, dwells in the village of Wiede without fear; he has
cheated many people out of their money and their health. A baptized Jew, who
calls himself Christian Fridrich and was born in Dessau, was found out in Hohenstein and was sentenced to the workhouse in Halberstadt because he violated
the Royal [Prussian] Medical Ordinance. Now he practices unhindered in Walkenried. Eight days ago, he treated the mining clerk Fischer, who was consumptive, and in all probability caused his death. [But] last year Amtmann Heiland
himself asked Fridrich's help [for an illness], [an action] that prejudices and
affronts all [proper] physicians, and engenders feelings of trust in persons [like
Fridrich] throughout the population. [Such consultation] clearly transgresses . . .
the ducal Medical Ordinance. A vagrant, who pretends to be an *operateur*, and
goes by the name of Winsil, attempted to couch the cataract of Gürze Kylingen
in Hohegeiss. With Heiland's permission, and in the presence of the local pastor
Schlegel and the village headman Grimme, he so badly botched the operation
that the vitreous humor of both eyeballs welled forth to about the size of a pea.
Kylingen, whom a skilled oculist could probably have helped, now stumbles
about stone blind. . . .

In January of this year, a journeyman blacksmith and Catholic convert from
Quedlinburg took up lodgings in Hohegeiss and Zorge and, posing as a priest,
sought to cure many people with all sorts of superstitious nonsense, by blessings
and by the laying on of consecrated vestments; he also promised to exorcise evil
spirits. . . . Pastor Colditz in Zorge wrote to Heiland about one of the parish
paupers who had taken ill, requesting that Heiland instruct me—according to the

provisions of the ducal regulations on poor relief—to assist the man with essential medicines. Heiland responded that such [aid] had to be requested, not from me, but from the district physicus in Blankenburg, who lives five miles [from Zorge], and the medicines must be procured from him. About three years ago, a man from Hohegeiss . . . was discovered dead on the road to Zorge. [The body] was only perfunctorily viewed by the military surgeon [feldsher] who, finding no wounds [on it], allowed the body to be buried without any further investigation. Similar deeds that contravene the Medical Ordinance occur daily, and the public has to suffer under them, [and] I must hold my tongue, no matter what, because I am not a regularly appointed physicus and must fear the fierce enmity [Heiland bears] against me. . . .

Over sixty years ago, Nicolaus Kästner was physicus here; almost forty years ago [c. 1707], Dr. Meder [became physicus]. Although he enjoyed a handsome salary, [Meder] found himself unable to make a go of it. He left and went to Zorge, where he later became city and district physicus. From then on, and until I arrived in 1727 . . . there was no physician here. The reason why Meder could not remain—the great poverty of the inhabitants—still exists. In Walkenried, there are approximately 700 to 750 large families . . . who have no farmland, and who are also not artisans. [They] work either as day laborers, wood choppers, sharecroppers, miners, stokers, smiths, or the like. [And for] all of these, on the day they do not work, they also do not eat, and [they] often are not able to come up with four groschen to save their lives. Among these poor people, many are chronically ill. For every one [of them] that can afford medicines, there are two or three that I must treat for free. . . . This makes it impossible for a physician to earn his bread here or for an apothecary to make a living. What I obtain from my practice outside [of Walkenried] in the Brandenburg jurisdictions and in Geröder and then only [by undertaking] long and wearying journeys, I am forced to spend and throw away again [here] in Walkenried.[1]

Spangenberg's report is only one of thousands of "stories" preserved in the archives. This book uses such stories to marry up three often estranged historical traditions: the history of mentalities, *Alltagsgeschichte*, and *Strukturgeschichte*.[2] On one hand, the materials lend themselves beautifully to an exploration of the unknown individuals in history, and toward what German scholars have baptized *Alltagsgeschichte*, or the "history of everyday life."[3] On the other hand (and without seeking to advance extravagant claims for the representativeness of my sources), these stories of individuals acting converge in ways that permit broader generalizations about social and economic structures (*Strukturgeschichte*), as well as offering insights into the coalescence of early modern mentalities. The underlying methodological problem is, how do we move from stories of individuals acting to a crafting of larger analyses of society and mentality? What does a report like Spangenberg's really tell us? Why are these stories central to our understanding of the medical worlds of early modern Europe and to the larger history of late seventeenth- and eighteenth-century Germany?

Perhaps it is most expedient to suggest what these materials *cannot* reveal. The "truth" of the relations between Spangenberg and Amtmann Heiland eludes us. We cannot verify Spangenberg's charges against Heiland, and Heiland's motives and actions are likewise forever lost in a documentary black hole. Likewise, Spangenberg's claims—the basis for his conflict with the midwives, the validity of his contentions about the "miserable conditions" in his area, his own occupational and economic position—remain unsupported by other testimony.

Another sort of truth is present, however, and it is of a kind extremely valuable to historians. That truth nests in the terms of the debate and in the language of the report. Even aspects of the narrative that may well be "fictional" are revelatory. Spangenberg chose his words, framed his arguments, and marshaled his evidence in ways calculated, consciously or unconsciously, to render his points believable and comprehensible and to win a favorable hearing for his tale.[4] I examine all the stories presented here, all the tales recounted, from this perspective, and not merely with a view to determining "objective" facts. As William Sewell reminds us in his work on "the language of labor" in France, such materials, when taken as "a set of interrelated texts," offer valuable insights into how people perceived the world around them, and perhaps even divulge how they constructed (and expressed) their own distinctive realities. Likewise, such readings question "the ontological priority of economic events," suggesting a certain independence for culture and for mentalities that is not chiefly molded by socioeconomic structures.[5]

Nor should we worry excessively about the fragmentary nature of Spangenberg's report; that he subsequently disappears from the archival record, and that nothing at all illuminates the reaction of the Collegium medicum to the feud between the doctor and the Amtmann should not bother us unduly. Such shards are in the nature of the materials archives yield up to us. What matters is that stories like this one constitute the essence of cultural history. Taken together, they deepen our understanding of how people envisioned their social, political, economic, and cultural milieux: they reveal to us how people in the past saw their positions in their world; how they related to others, to government, to disease, to their own physicality, and to their environment.

For example, Spangenberg's portrayal of himself as a hard-working, altruistic, long-suffering, much-maligned soul is perhaps accurate and perhaps not. His perception of what his position should be, what he was "due" in life from his government and his community, cannot, however, be denied. As one who had exercised the office of physicus (a state-appointed and -salaried medical officer of health), he felt entitled to the rights and privileges of the position. His own actions, not the title or official sanction, were what counted for him. One suspects that he hoped to sell himself as physicus to the Collegium medicum. He based his claim neither merely on his humanitarianism and spirit of sacrifice to the public good nor on his learning alone, but most forcefully on his needs. The picture Spangenberg draws of the problems a physician encountered in wringing a living from poverty-stricken districts is a poignant one and not totally exaggerated. He advances his right to a legitimate livelihood, a livelihood that will, moreover, allow him to fulfill his duties as subject and citizen—among them, paying taxes. He speaks a language measured and shaped to please the Collegium medicum. To what extent he actually internalized the values he expounded is impossible to determine. Yet remember what he says: I carried out the forensic duties of a physicus; I attended ducal employees free of charge; I visited rich and poor alike when "dysentery, or *febres maligna, purpure et petectia* raged"; I treated the destitute at my own expense; and for all this, I enjoyed "not a penny's worth" of salary or perquisites.

For years Spangenberg had dutifully answered the calls of charity and conscience. He had built for the future—*in spem futuri*—but also anticipated fair returns on that investment, returns he ultimately expected the government to secure for him. In his report, he plays on the good will of the Collegium medicum and voices a general feeling that the state bears a moral obligation to provide sustenance for "good and faithful" servants like himself. He trots out the language of *bonum publicum* to appeal to a government caught up in cameralist and mercantilist webs of concern for economic progress and populationism. Those he denounces—the tanner's apprentice, the journeyman, and their ilk—have flouted medical legislation, while defrauding the "people" and, secondarily, doing irreparable damage to their health. Spangenberg conjures up common religious prejudices to reinforce his arguments. Two of the people he attacks are condemned not merely for their "bad cures" but equally for their aberrant beliefs: one is a "baptized Jew," the other, a "Catholic convert," whose superstitious malarkey is just as damnable.

Similarly prominent in this account is Spangenberg's perception of his hierarchical relationship with other practitioners. His ordering seems, however, to have little relation to an incipient sense of a modern professional identity; instead, it apparently springs from an older corporatism, akin to that of the guilds.[6] The surgeon Siegfried Nezel basks in Spangenberg's favor, but not because he has demonstrated special talents; Spangenberg portrays him as an adequate surgeon and a humble man. Nezel's virtues are those of diligence and worthiness, of modesty and deference. Nezel exhibits the decorum and spirit of cooperation Spangenberg misses in his tempestuous dealings with Heiland. Apparently, Spangenberg's association with Heiland's predecessor in office, the Amtmann Mattenberg, had proceeded in a more harmonious and cordial manner. When Mattenberg died, this agreeable modus vivendi vanished.

It is necessary, here, to tune out the historical background noise, to move beyond the cacophony of personality clashes and personal dislikes. Although we have only Spangenberg's version, the terms of his quarrel with Heiland are evident. The tension developed in the course of several confrontations: over Spangenberg's right to enjoy the favors he had secured under Heiland's predecessor; over who was authorized to grant concessions to practice medicine, to examine surgeons, and to appoint midwives; in short, over the exercise of power in a local setting. Spangenberg stood on shaky terrain. Heiland was incontestably an agent of central government, whereas Spangenberg's position derived from usage, from the tacit agreement or the mutual sympathy that had sprung up between him and Mattenberg. He lacked official authority. In Spangenberg's mind, however, custom justifies his prerogatives. He argues that he, not Heiland, has best adhered to the government's wishes and laws; in seeking to lay a more solid new foundation for his position in the community, so that it will no longer be predicated solely on custom and service, he repeatedly emphasizes the bonum publicum.

Spangenberg's account thus tells us much about the man who filed the report, and about the cast of characters who peopled the medical worlds of the late seventeenth and eighteenth centuries. Yet it gives only a partial picture. Spangenberg leaves other actors waiting in the wings. Among those he ignores are the patients, who appear only as slow-witted victims of frauds and humbugs. Nor does Spangenberg say much about the dubious types, the quacks, such as the "baptized Jew," whom he accuses Amtmann Heiland of shielding.

The account of a physicus from another district confronts these issues squarely and introduces the quacks and the patients who fill out this historical tableau vivant. In 1761, Physicus Jacob Müller of Seesen wrote to the Collegium medicum to excuse his laxity in reporting on mortality and morbidity in his district:[7]

The reason why rests partly in the distance between Seesen and the [other] areas entrusted to me, [and] partly in audacious, unrestrained, and totally forbidden, yet up to now totally invincible, quackery. The *Amt* [district] of Harzburg lies four miles away and like Amt Langelsheim (two miles from Seesen) is located very near to Goslar [in Hannover]. I have never seen a patient from Harzburg in my ten years here, and I rarely treat one person a year from Langelsheim. Only seldom do people come over to me from Amt Lutter am Barenberge, because most of the villages lie nearer to Bockenum and Salzgitter. Of the [many] villages belonging to my district, only Herrhausen, Engelade, Bornumhausen, and Klein-Rhüden are less than a mile away [from Seesen]. From these few villages, a patient occasionally consults me, [while] the inhabitants of the "lower" villages— Bornum, Mahlum, Jerze, Schlewecke, and Volkersheim—go to Bockenum, as each village is only half an hour distant [from there].

Practitioners everywhere in Braunschweig-Wolfenbüttel and [in territories] bordering [the duchy] frustrate my every opportunity . . . of discovering anything, far less anything reliable, about the state of medical affairs in these [more distant] parts of my district. As long as these meddlers go uncontrolled, their forbidden activities render the accomplishment of the goals set by our splendid medical and sanitary organizations totally impossible. Regimental surgeons, surgeons, bathmasters, apothecaries, schoolmasters, executioners, shepherds, cobblers, old wives, and similar such people . . . to whom no medical practice is entrusted, still ply their trade, against the intentions of our Gracious Duke, against the rulings of the Collegium medicum for the protection of proper physicians, and to the detriment of the health and the purses of [the duke's] subjects. At the same time . . . they rob me of the opportunity to execute my duties conscientiously, and *per praxie* expand my knowledge, and to gain esteem in my métier. [They also] steal my bread in such an unscrupulous manner that I suffer not only the most grievous damage but also see that as a result . . . I shall soon have to pawn or sell my [few] possessions in order to get by.

As in Spangenberg's account, questions of livelihood dominate Müller's report. But Müller identifies the sources of the problem: those who practice medicine "illicitly"—the "quacks"—and, implicitly, those who consult them—"average" patients. In doing so, he forces us to think about these people as well.

The eighteenth-century *philosophes* projected no clearer image than that of the oafish, willful peasant or common man.[8] "The people" were simple, superstitious, and ignorant, but also sly, conniving, and deceitful: patsies and fools who preferred quacks to licensed healers and who scorned the ministrations of physicians, even when these were provided free. Every physicus in Braunschweig-Wolfenbüttel (and probably elsewhere) sounds this note; it is the almost ubiquitous theme of every writer who discusses health conditions and their improvement in the eighteenth century. "Superstition" is the villain, and would-be reformers employ elaborate metaphors to depict its pernicious, pervasive influence: "The tree [of superstition] stands firm on its roots, and the people lounge in indolent ease under its poison-dripping boughs."[9] Superstition, however, lurks everywhere: "Respectable burghers are too ashamed to admit any belief in witchcraft; [yet] superstition and prejudice sit as deeply in them as in the common mob. . . . A charlatan, a down-at-the-heels cobbler, an herb peddler, old hags, unscrupulous apothecaries are more prized by the common and the refined man [alike]. . . . than the most skilled and conscientious physician."[10] For those in the ranks of the "enlightened," from philosophes to the members of the Collegium medicum sitting in Braunschweig, to the physicians scattered across the duchy, ignorance alloyed to superstition constructed massive barriers to enlightenment, as well as blocking the improvement of material conditions, including health.[11]

Similar themes run through most of the reports on the "Causes of the Increase and Decrease of the Inhabitants" that ended up in the archives of the Collegium medicum. Physicus Scheibner in the small town of Schöningen noted among the inhabitants a deep-seated, unshakable fatalism, linked to an equally obdurate belief in magical causes of disease and thaumaturgic cures. "Most [peasants]," he continued, "believe that a person suffering from a chronic malady is hexed, and that he should find someone who . . . promises he can . . . 'deafen' the curse."[12]

How widespread these "superstitious practices" were is almost impossible to document. We are notoriously ill-informed about such things as the amulets slipped between the wedding-night sheets of young couples to ensure fertility, the newborn puppies slit open and pressed still squirming to the heads of epileptics to draw out their maddening ill-humors, and the small knives placed under the beds of lying-in women to "cut" the pain. The archives are silent as to the popularity of these remedies, and whether people actually put much stock in them. And it is also well to remember that many such customs were not simply hoary "folk-superstitions," but had once been weapons in the medical armamentarium of academic physicians.

The fact that philosophes and physicians, government officials and pastors alike tilted at the windmills of superstition cannot be construed as prima facie evidence that superstition ran rampant. Although some historians have all too readily accepted and perpetuated notions of fatalism and invariably superstitious responses to illness,[13] the tendency to regard "the people," and peasants in particular, as uniquely benighted has waned markedly over the past decade or so. Unwillingness to consult physicians, once labeled "stupidity" or "ignorance" by generations of progress-minded physicians and medical historians, has recently (especially under the influence of anthropological perspectives) been more sympathetically and more intelligently evaluated as "logical" and "goal-oriented," if different from the "official" logic of the bourgeoisie.[14] What has seldom been questioned, however, is the view that physicians were rarely consulted—indeed, were regarded as almost alien beings by the vast majority of Europeans before the twentieth century. In a major work on medicine in eighteenth-century France, for instance, Matthew Ramsey has argued that "two centuries ago most Frenchmen and Frenchwomen saw 'healers' as familiar figures and doctors as exotic ones."[15]

There has likewise been a tendency among historians to assume that folk and "fringe" healers, as well as surgeons and apothecaries, filled untenanted niches as general practitioners to "the people" who did not want physicians, could not afford them, or simply had no recourse to them. A 1979 article by Charles Webster and Margaret Pelling set the tone by insisting that any examination of medical practice in early modern times that ignored nonphysician practitioners was hopelessly incomplete. The fashion since then has been to stress the significance and prevalence of these "other" practitioners.[16] New terms, none of them fully satisfactory, such as *the fringe*, *popular healers*, and *alternative healers*, have arisen to characterize them, while the word *quack* has been rejected as pejorative and, increasingly, as reflecting a "privileged discourse" of elites.[17] Licensed practitioners other than physicians have thus often been seen as a sort of medical corps for nonelites; in this view, apothecaries, surgeons, and midwives were the "general practitioners" of the common folk.[18]

Many historians have, however, come to doubt facile distinctions between "popular" and "elite" medicine, and between "popular" and "elite" responses to disease. Sabine Sander, for example, has demonstrated that surgeons in eighteenth-century Württemberg by no means served only as "physicians to the poor," but drew a good portion of their clientele from the respected and moneyed members of their communities.[19] Moreover, if such a split truly separated "popular" from "elite" healers, how do we explain the frequency of stories such as that of the smallholder and cottager Conrad Böckel, whose wife developed "hard swellings on both breasts from suckling her child"? First, Böckel brought in a Dr. Heym, whose medicines failed to work. Then, "because all the surgeons seemed too expensive," he turned to a paperhanger named Johann Busch, who cured his wife in four weeks, "without cutting," by the application of poultices.[20]

Despite Physicus Müller's complaint about how loath the common folk were to consult physicians, people certainly did go to physicians, and even to him. In 1767, Amt Seesen conducted an investigation of the "quackery" of the executioner Schwartze. One of Schwartze's patients, a man suffering from consumption, testified that "[he] had indeed conferred with Schwartze, [but] as Schwartze was unable to help, he sent to Dr. Müller for medicines; thereafter he consulted with the cowherd in [the village of] Liebenberg, and now Dr. Streuberg in Goslar is treating him."[21] This patient saw not one but two doctors, albeit in between meetings with a hangman and a cowherd.

Roy Porter has suggested that such serial or simultaneous consultations were common in the medical marketplace of eighteenth-century England, where a precocious consumer economy encouraged an increase in the number of those offering goods and services—including medicines and treatments—for sale.[22] The concept of a "medical marketplace" has been repeatedly invoked to discuss—or even explain—the process of medical decision making, as well as to illustrate the wide assortment of practitioners available.[23] As long as the concept of medical marketing is not reduced to a mere criterion of cost, it offers insight into the problem of medical decision making and effectively portrays the early modern profusion of practitioners. Especially in the late eighteenth century, the market was glutted; far from being devoid of health care, even rural areas swarmed with medical practitioners. In addition, the concept of marketing moves medical history nearer to the historical mainstream by linking it to current debates on bigger historical issues, such as the birth of a consumer society. One cannot, however, ignore the important role a sense of moral economy played in the haggling that went on in the medical bazaar.[24] Expense was hardly the only variable in the calculations that led to the selection of a healer: a notion of "moral cost accounting" counted for as much. Money might be freely disbursed for medicines, or for an operation, but medical advice itself was apparently transformed into a commodity more gradually. Medical counsel continued to be either a part of the assistance one normally expected from neighbors and friends or was regarded as a gift extended with no anticipation of immediate material or monetary recompense.[25] Furthermore, as we shall see, people often, sometimes quite vigorously, asserted their right to shop around for a healer. One might also question whether this truly represented an embryonic consumer mentality in action rather than the persistence of habitual conceptions of home doctoring, neighborliness, and communal networking expressed with fiercer adamancy in the face of novel possibilities and changed circumstances. These are some of the larger questions about German and European history this book raises.

"Quackery," therefore, is the point where the stories of Physicus Spangenberg and Physicus Müller, and the larger themes they evoke, converge: it is the key to evaluating expectations about practitioners; to divining how people came to their medical decisions; to comprehending economic priorities; and to acquiring a "feel" for how politics worked at the level of the village and community. Admittedly, *quackery* is a loaded term. Thousands of publications devoted to improving general health standards and propagating medical enlightenment evoked the same vile image of the quack: quacks were parasites who sapped the vitality of a people more rapidly than either war or famine; quacks were secret agents of ignorance, who negated all laudatory efforts to better the provision of medical care; quacks were "murderers of mankind." According to Samuel Tissot, a Swiss physician and prolific publicist for medical enlightenment, quacks were creatures "born without talent, raised without education, often illiterate." They knew less about medicine than "about the customs of wild Asiatic peoples." Besotted with gin, they plied their trade, having "become doctors only because they are incapable of doing anything else!"[26]

If modern medical historians have grown far more tolerant of "quacks," and have come to see the term as one physicians used to denigrate competitors, they have often missed the fact that "quackery" in the context of early modern society bore multiple connotations; it was not merely the slur a professionalizing medical elite employed to discredit their rivals. The language denoting "quackery"—the most frequently used German term was *Pfuscherey*, the artisans' term for interloping—indicates that something more elemental was at issue here.[27] The linguistic battles between interlopers and guilds were fought in terms of territoriality. And this language was not the peculiar, anachronistic speech of guildsmen mired in economic stagnation.[28] Midwives, surgeons, physicians, the Collegium medicum, and the ducal privy council all spoke of quacks in ways that underscored their temerity in "disturbing" or "undercutting" the livelihood of others.[29] Quacks were poachers; they violated the domains of licit practitioners, they ate away at others' livelihoods, and offended economic proprieties. Thus, respectable society condemned them in economic, social, and moral terms. In the realm of medicine, such charges were, admittedly, never totally innocent of the allegation that quacks harmed people in very real ways. But charges of physical injury always appeared within the framework of the proper division of a market, and market demand was perceived as basically inelastic. Both the language of such accusations and that found in the process of mediating disputes echo more fundamental debates over livelihood, market, and traditional rights and privileges, all overlaid by a persistent corporatist mentality. This language shows how people circumscribed and discerned their economic, social, and political milieux, and how they situated themselves within these worlds.

These questions, which lie at the heart of this book, reach beyond the world of physicians, patients, and quacks to major issues in German and European history, yet they are also embedded in the social history of medicine. While the history of medicine has outgrown its Whiggish past and shed its preoccupation with the triumphs of great doctors and the march of scientific progress, it has only recently begun to enter the mainstream as a central thread of historical inquiry rather than a limited subspecialty of the historian's craft.[30] Several agendas have merged to make the social history of medicine what one observer regarded as a sleek analytical locomotive.[31] In 1985, Roy Porter complained that we have "histories of diseases but not of health, biographies of doctors but not of the sick."[32] Numerous scholars have taken up that gauntlet in striving to compose medical histories "from below." Their investigations have begotten works on "the therapeutic experience" and have done much to correct the deficiencies Porter remarked. But the larger objective Porter sketched out—of "prob[ing] the personal and collective meanings of sickness, of suffering and recovery, probing how 'illness experiences' were integrated within the larger meanings of life from the cradle to the grave"—remains largely unaccomplished, despite several recent studies that more or less successfully deal with part of the question.[33] Most of these, how-

ever, rely all too heavily on what Dorothy and Roy Porter have described
as the "ample documentary remains . . . [of] the urban middle classes and
the 'Quality' ";[34] on transmitted folk-wisdom, such as proverbs;[35] or on
the recorded evidence of physicians.[36] The whole range of the "ordinary
person's response to illness," with all its tricky problems of definition, still
needs to be explored on the basis of extensive archival research. This, too,
is something my book hopes to accomplish.

Perhaps even the ambitious "new" medical historians pose their central
questions too modestly. The greater value of studying the history of
medicine and the history of health does not lie in the elucidation of issues
in medical history. More important, such work leads us to reevaluate what
we know about the history of society, and, in this book, to reassessing and
reinterpreting some standard interpretations of early modern German
history. Investigations should neither stop at "prob[ing] the personal and
collective meanings of sickness, of suffering and recovery" nor be content
with illustrating "how 'illness experiences' were integrated within the
larger meanings of life from the cradle to the grave"; they must consider
what these "larger meanings of life" were.[37] Perceptions of health, of
healing, of doctors, of doctoring, and of the body, have legitimately
attracted the gaze of historians. More enticing, however, should be the
broader structures in which these existed and the mentalities that nurtured them. This book directly engages the larger frameworks of early
modern "politics" and Politics; moral categories and economic initiatives;
familial, communal, and neighborly relations; and gender.

But how? What documentation allows the historian to peer into the
dark corners of the human mind and to unravel mentalities without
psychologizing blindly? How do we know what people thought about
illness, or how they made their medical decisions? How do we filter out
distortions created by prejudice and concerns of party? How do we move
from the particular and the peculiar to the general and typical? And what
will this eventually teach us about the bigger questions of early modern
history?

The evidence adduced to address these questions has been collected
almost exclusively from government archives—principally from the State
Archive of Lower Saxony in Wolfenbüttel and from municipal archives in
Braunschweig, Helmstedt, Königslutter am Elm, and Hornburg. Many
historians, especially those drawn to questions of mentality, to Alltagsgeschichte, and to the new cultural history, raise serious questions about
how useful such materials are in exploring mentalities and popular cul-

tures. They charge that these sources reflect "a privileged discourse"—that is, the prejudices of elites, the views of "professionalizing" physicians, and of those who sought to master men and shape society. Critics regard these documents as indicative *only* of policies and programs, and as incapable of reflecting wider mentalities. These objections are cogent. There is little denying that one must tread gingerly in such archival minefields, especially if one seeks to extrapolate delicate strands of mentality from such coarse materials.

Yet these criticisms also go too far; if we pursue them to their logical endpoint, exaggerated caution would soon incapacitate us. These "old-fashioned" sources, with all their undoubted flaws and biases, are indispensable and prove less dangerous and misleading than their detractors often maintain. For my purposes, their "flaws" become positive virtues. Criticisms of administrative documents as inherently distorted, and as reflecting only the mentality of an elite, rest on a limited comprehension of what these archives have preserved and, what is perhaps more significant, on a faulty understanding of how states functioned in the late seventeenth and eighteenth centuries. The methods of information gathering were complex, the execution of directives entangled, and the process of policy making multilayered and ambiguous. The very imperfections of the entire system created precisely the kinds of documentation that are invaluable, indeed, essential, to my investigation. The tentacles of central bureaucracy—what there was of it—barely stretched into local areas. Information provided in response to government directives was colorful, confused, even idiosyncratic, often containing so much contradictory or "extraneous" material that even the proto-bureaucrats of the eighteenth century often judged it worthless. Yet it dishes up to the historian a slice of life that is almost too rich. These archives do not supply the precisely uniform paper trails and the neatly bundled files late nineteenth- and twentieth-century bureaucracies have left behind; instead, they reflect the world of nuance, flux, and innuendo that was early modern society. Moreover, as Spangenberg's letter reveals, biased documentation is especially revealing and rewarding, for in arguing a point of view, its very "lies" and its "fictional elements," its dissemblances and distortions, display the terms of debate, and thus, to an extent, the mentality of those who composed the documents and of the bigger world in which they moved. Their purpose was, after all, communication.

For these reasons, it is vital to let the documents themselves guide the research process. No one, of course, enters an archive a tabula rasa, yet crossing the threshold laden with too many preconceived notions and theories to be proved or discredited—such as that of professionalization for the subject at hand—destroys much of our ability to learn from the documents, to perceive which historical issues were important, and to work out our own agendas. Everyone, of course, approaches the documents with thoughts about how "things worked." So did I. Immersion in the sources over time led me to pursue some lines of inquiry rather than others, persuading me that the stories often told of the medical worlds of the seventeenth and eighteenth centuries—those crystallized around professionalization and medicalization, about state control and issues of policy implementation—were less relevant to that world than many historians would have us believe.[38]

I have also attempted to avoid dichotomies such as those between "popular" and "elite" practitioners, "sedentary" and "peripatetic" healers, "popular" and "elite" cultures. These are hard to do without, but they are misleading. The boundary between "licit" and "illicit" practice was extremely permeable, for example, and even a heuristic isolation of "popular" and "elite" medicines proves unsatisfactory. Local studies are inherently atypical, but the amount of research to be done, and the need to control its sprawl, dictated some fairly narrow geographical boundaries, if more generous chronological ones. I have drawn extensively on the archives of the Collegium medicum and of the various other agencies—the ducal privy council, municipal governments, and the like—concerned with the business of public health administration. For certain localities, I have cast my net more widely in an attempt to reconstruct a milieu and to suggest the broader sociopolitical, socioeconomic, and sociocultural structures involved. These vignettes form the necessary basis for my discussion of mentality. Reports on population and vital statistics; extensive "village descriptions" (the *Dorf-Beschreibungen* composed from 1746 to 1784); and guild proceedings all proved pertinent and instructive. In addition, I turned to a massive antiquarian literature (written over four centuries), which falls in between the nominal categories of primary materials and secondary literature.[39] In Braunschweig-Wolfenbüttel, however, nothing compares to the marriage and postmortem inventories that David Sabean and Sabine Sander exploited so effectively for Württemberg.[40] Tax registers are fragmentary and wills are preserved only for the period 1808–13. But archival lacunae always exist and much can be done with what is available.

My first goal, therefore, is to describe the medical worlds we have lost:

the landscape of medical practice in late seventeenth- and eighteenth-century Germany. We still know woefully little about the day-to-day activities of even those practitioners—physicians and surgeons chief among them—who have long formed the primary foci of medical historical investigation.

A second major objective is to use the workings of the medical worlds of seventeenth- and eighteenth-century Braunschweig-Wolfenbüttel to illuminate larger issues in German and European history. Throughout the book, I follow the twisted skeins tying medical topics to larger issues of mentality, politics, and social and economic structures. Several arguments will become clearer as we move deeper into the daily world of medical practice. The socioeconomic credo of the age was a complex one, which in many ways still reflected a corporatist mind-set, but also provided the fertile cognitive subsoil for a growing commercialization of life. A rising tide of consumerism flowed from the new possibilities opened by a wider market, as even small territories like Braunschweig-Wolfenbüttel forged links with a precocious, often unstable, but increasingly potent, world economy. Politics, too, responded to these changes in the character and the complexity of life with new initiatives in information collection, record keeping, and local administration, even though governments continued to be more concerned with everyday matters of governing than with the formulation and implementation of future-oriented policies and programs.[41] The book also breaks with common and misleading appositions such as "insider/outsider," "urban/rural," and "popular/elite." These are only crude means of catching sophisticated historical realities. I argue—if somewhat cautiously—that the "peculiarity" and the purported backwardness of German social, economic, and political life have been overstated. The tendency to view the German states as caught in a Sisyphean task of catching up with Britain and France has imposed a tyranny of western models on German historiography and generated an array of false questions about German society, as to, for example, its relative "modernity."[42]

One should also wonder whether Braunschweig-Wolfenbüttel can be taken to stand for Germany. In short, how typical was it? In terms of political structures, little differentiated Braunschweig-Wolfenbüttel from most other small to medium-sized secular German states. Most were governed by a council of ministers (*Geheimer Rat*) with the generally desultory participation of the estates. This state of affairs basically pertained—if perhaps in a more elaborate form—to the larger entities of Austria, Prussia, and Bavaria. It may be, however, that governments in smaller states "worked better" and could be more flexible than in larger ones, although the "matchbox" kingdoms of the highly fragmented areas (such as in the southwest) were also sometimes those where flagrant abuses abounded and rulers' follies played havoc.[43] More important for our purposes here, the general flow and rhythm of governing in Braunschweig-Wolfenbüttel seems to have diverged little from that in Württemburg, Saxony, Hesse, and other similarly sized states.[44] This is not, of course, to argue that Braunschweig-Wolfenbüttel had no peculiarities, or that it differed in no respect from these other territories. Still, significant underlying congruities, not the least of which were the importance of cameralism and, later, enlightened principles, marked the governments of almost all these places. The transmission and publication of decrees, the drive to assemble more accurate information, the use of the system of Amtmänner to administer districts, and the continued reliance on village self-government were characteristic aspects of eighteenth-century governing. All play a major role in my story here. The dissimilarities in the realm of health and health policies seem fairly inconsequential, to judge, for example, from my own brief forays into Prussian archives and from the secondary literature on Prussia.[45] More research will perhaps revise this position.

As to religion, Braunschweig-Wolfenbüttel, like many of its contemporary north German states, was overwhelmingly Protestant, in its case, Lutheran. Can this predominantly Protestant composition account for a relative dearth of superstitious cures? Were Catholic regions more riven by superstition, more given to religious interpretations of disease, and more prone to attribute illness to hexing and supernatural intervention? This has often been argued, along with the concomitant assertion that higher levels of literacy and the more thorough suppression of popular religiosity had, by the eighteenth century, gone far to wipe out magic and superstitious practices in Protestant areas. It *may* well be true that magical healing persisted in Catholic regions longer than in Protestant ones, but it is perhaps wise to reserve judgment until meticulous investigations are completed for the Catholic parts of Germany in the late seventeenth and eighteenth centuries.[46]

This book is divided into five longish chapters. The first chapter sets the historical stage and opens with a discussion of the interplay of state and society in Braunschweig-Wolfenbüttel. It then takes up the story of how medical policy was "made" at all levels. Chapter 2 concerns the people responsible for the on-the-ground administration of health, and it focuses mainly on the physici, but also, if more fleetingly, on Amtmänner, pastors, schoolteachers, landowners, tithe-holders, and village notables.

Chapter 3 highlights the panoply of healers active in eighteenth-century society: physicians appear again in these pages, but so, too, do all those consulted in medical situations, including friends, neighbors, executioners, and old wives, surgeons, barber-surgeons, bathmasters, midwives, feldshers, operateurs, and apothecaries. Here, I am far less interested in determining a ratio of practitioners to patients than in ascertaining what practitioners saw as their role in society and how they related to their patients.

Chapter 4 begins with a survey of the statistical information available (mostly in the form of vital statistics), then turns to more impressionistic narrative accounts, such as demographic reports and medical topographies, which are (for Braunschweig-Wolfenbüttel) mostly available only in manuscript form. Here, I try to reconstruct patterns of diseases, as well as how such patterns were perceived and interpreted.

Chapter 5 moves the manner of defining and responding to illness to center stage, addressing questions such as when people saw themselves as too ill to work, as sick enough to stay in bed, to turn to a home remedy, or to consult another person for advice.[47] In short, this chapter scrutinizes the process of becoming a patient. It analyzes the effects of the social, economic, political, and cultural milieux on how medicine was practiced and on how medical decisions were made in the everyday world of the village, the neighborhood, the town. In so doing, it ties together, not only the multiple perceptions I have sought to introduce in this book, but the common history of people, medical practitioners, and bureaucrats in early modern Germany that is the purpose of this study.

Medicine, State, and Society

The state's role in the formation of modern society remains enigmatic. While almost everyone agrees that something critical occurred in the development of the modern state and of modern society in the late seventeenth and the eighteenth centuries, the character and timing of the changes, their impetus and direction, their success and pervasiveness linger as contested points of historical debate. The historian can choose among several well-developed models of state building: enlightened absolutism,[1] the Weberian bureaucratic state,[2] the social disciplining analyses of Gerhard Oestreich and Michel Foucault,[3] and Marc Raeff's "well-ordered police state."[4]

Enlightened absolutism has over several decades generated thousands of pages, but, as Charles Ingrao has observed, "few controversies have endured so long and resolved so little."[5] Recent West German historiography has generally (if not unanimously) responded favorably to enlightened absolutism, valuing its ability to adapt enlightened and humanitarian precepts to practical governing, as well as lauding reform initiatives that purportedly improved many aspects of social and economic life. Other historians have pointed out that the reform programs actually implemented were few in number, essentially cosmetic in nature, counterproductive (economic policies have been denigrated as stifling or as scatterbrained),[6] crassly self-serving (especially as regards military policy), or at best what Hans-Ulrich Wehler has termed "defensive modernization."[7] While these questions in their entirety are too big to tackle here, the role of the state looms large in my investigation. Braunschweig-Wolfenbüttel (more properly, Braunschweig-Lüneburg, Wolfenbüttel division) was one of those smaller polities where, Ingrao has argued, "enlightened government functioned best." Here, enlightened rulers and their ministers supposedly effected more immediate responses and acted more directly on the population than in other territories, as they were less burdened by the interference of estates, entrenched administrative units, local notables, or powerful nobles.[8] While this is certainly true on one level for Braunschweig-Wolfenbüttel, it is unwise to assume that a governmental consensus existed or that resistance was absent.

In his study of the "well-ordered police state" (which draws much of its evidence from the duchy of Braunschweig-Wolfenbüttel), Marc Raeff has bestowed upon the seventeenth- and eighteenth-century state a major role in the making of modern society. Raeff rates the state's ability to effect significant sociocultural and economic changes as high. "It is no accident," he maintains, "that the foundation and rise of the so-called modern state and the very process of its formation gave the political establishment a role of leadership in the development of society and the evolution of culture."[9] For scholars who see the seventeenth-century police state and the enlightened absolutism of the eighteenth century as major protagonists in the unfolding drama of modernity,[10] and even for those who admit that the ability of the early modern state to flex its muscles was finite, Raeff's contentions have been canons of faith.

Raeff and others have argued that the authority this state wielded was never to be equated with mere brute force: what made these states remarkable and effective was their ability to inculcate new behaviors and reshape mind-sets, achieving these metamorphoses through social disciplining. Such ideas of disciplining ultimately derived from Max Weber's concept of *Disziplin* as the defining characteristic of modern societies.[11] For the early modern period, first Norbert Elias in analyzing the "civilizing process," then Gerhard Oestreich and Michel Foucault, in their depictions of social disciplining, portrayed similar processes as ultimately having spawned modern society and begotten modern individualism. Pierre Bourdieu's arguments about the application of *violence symbolique* expressed basically the same principles in a somewhat different form.[12] All evoked a dynamic affecting every level of social, cultural, and psychological life: a process that was subtle and unseen, yet encompassing and prophylactic, and that, at least for Weber, Foucault, and Bourdieu, did not emanate solely from the political authorities. The result was, in Foucault's

words, both the "trained" body and the "trained" mind, whose internalized standards and norms of behavior further patterned ways of thinking, perceiving, and ordering the sociocultural environment.[13] For Weber
(as also, for example, for E. P. Thompson), these internalized standards
linked up closely to economic, and particularly capitalist, modes of surplus extraction. For others, like Foucault and Elias, the connection is less
materially determined, although they did not deny the consequences of
production and distribution systems.

The process of social disciplining seems an inevitable part of any study
of mentalities, even if the exact relationship is difficult to pin down.
Both notions have, however, a discomfiting slipperiness about them. One
problem arises when we try to set boundaries and specify what is *not* part
of a history of mentality or *not* part of a process of social disciplining.[14]
The seductive all-inclusiveness of both concepts partly explains their at-
traction as explanatory models, yet presents major problems for historical
research. Where do we look for the mainsprings of social disciplining? At
what point does mentality become plain? The solutions are neither easy
nor uncontested.[15] I aim at a middle level: what a study of medicine and of
health and healing in late seventeenth- and eighteenth-century Germany
can tell us about the larger mental frameworks people worked with, how
they perceived or conceived of their social, political, economic, and cultural environments, and to what extent they formed these milieux or
were molded by them. This inevitably returns us to the question of the
state: Did the state assume a decisive role in the creation or modification
of early modern mentalities? To answer this, one must consider the intentions of governments and the actuality of state power in the early modern
centuries.

It is in no way original to insist that older historiography grossly overstated the progress of the seventeenth- and eighteenth-century state toward a monopoly of power. Likewise, the intention of the state deserves
closer attention and more skeptical analysis. Scholars have often adduced
its actions, and the motives behind them, from the activities and gestures
of a small circle of dukes and princes, advisors, ministers, legalists, favor-
ites, and creatures, who were, however, by no means unanimous in their
views. Something subtler is called for. The purposes of those who formu-
lated state policies were rarely as clear-cut or as single-minded as Raeff,
for example, has suggested.[16] Many historians recognize that government
in the late seventeenth and eighteenth centuries was unable to consolidate
its power and had not yet unfolded as Weber's "bureaucratic state," al-

though many accept that the future lay with the bureaucratic state.[17] This may be true, but there is really not much evidence to support a claim that the state drew up and pursued timetables of rationalization in the seventeenth and eighteenth centuries, despite the undeniable proliferation of personnel and offices of state bureaucracy. James Vann, for one, has emphasized the significance of a bargaining process, rather than a linear evolution, in the construction of the state (in his case, Württemberg). "State builders," according to Vann, had "no 'five-year plans,' and they never spoke of the future as differing fundamentally from the present."[18] The cardinal aim of "governors" was to govern on a daily basis. That does not mean, of course, that they harbored no schemes or launched no long-term projects. Still the vast majority of decisions that seem "conclusive" or "pioneering" or appear to mark "turning points" were merely single actions in a lengthy series of daily decisions, whose primary purposes were the preservation of domestic order, the maintenance of internal integrity, and—especially—the resolution of individual, quotidian dilemmas.

It is also likely that the bureaucratic state of the nineteenth and twentieth centuries may well have been the accidental outcome of "autonomous forces" rather than the end product of plans and strategies.[19] Certainly, both Wehler and Raeff credit the power of "autonomous forces," yet when they speak of the state (in, as Wehler nicely puts it, "all its imaginable hybrid forms"),[20] it is usually as the protagonist of the drama. The state acts, others react. At times, of course, the state also reacts to external pressures: a sense of falling behind other states, in response to population growth, or in self-defense.[21]

Thus, the actions and intentions of the state need to be set against a backdrop of autonomous forces, socioeconomic structures, and individuals acting. The bulk of the ordinances and laws promulgated in the period have repeatedly been interpreted as interlocking cogs in the well-oiled engine of modernization, but they should not be viewed in that light at all. Collation and codification, whether by eighteenth- and nineteenth-century legalists, or by later historians, have fashioned a congruity of purpose that is comforting, but largely illusory. Grouping documents by topic—for example, gathering together all regulations pertaining to the butchering of cattle—endows them with a smooth but misleading developmental symmetry. If one returns these documents to their original chronological order, however, one is struck more by the welter of instances and the dissimilarities of intent than by the constancy of purpose.[22]

In one day, the same minister might countersign several orders with widely differing contents and even contrary aims. Thus, the word *pastiche* characterizes the reality of early modern governing better than the term *design*. This does not, of course, mean that particular plans could not be conceived of and set in motion.[23] It does, however, undercut any idea of a premeditated, clearly articulated scheme driven by sweeping demands for modernization. The exigencies of day-to-day administration and the need to work with existing laws and legal structures (such as the Amt and the village commune) frequently short-circuited innovative sparks, often preserving status quos quite intentionally. Decisions continued to be made overwhelmingly in response to individual cases: instances that might later, of course, become precedents, but that were seldom originally devised as general precepts.

Concentrating on the exercise of power at the apexes of government casts only reflected light on an equally fundamental topic: how the state worked in a many-tiered administration.[24] Resistance at local levels to state interference from above (for example, from entrenched local notables, known in Braunschweig-Wolfenbüttel as the *Honorationes*)[25] was never chimerical, but a reality habitually linked to a spirited defense of traditional rights and customs. Yet not even small villages closed ranks so tightly that no signs of internal discord escaped. Groups and individuals in seemingly homogeneous communities could envision and relate to the state in widely disparate and inconsonant ways: some feared and fought outside assaults, clinging doggedly to what they defined as traditions, dreading any loss or diminution of the rights they enjoyed under the status quo, while others saw the state as a shield against nearby enemies. In these internal combats, some willingly called in the state or appealed to outsiders in waging parochial battles. Such inclinations, and the frequency with which they turned into action, confound simple analyses that pit insiders against outsiders in representing the relationship between the early modern state and its subjects. There is no denying, of course, that the insider/outsider mechanism functioned and offers a plausible interpretation of some patterns of resistance to state authority. But the insider/outsider interpretation quickly exceeds its elucidative limits: it is too clumsy and unidimensional to explain the great variety of ways the state interacted with its people, or they with it.[26] Moreover, governors and subjects alike reconceived and re-formed the idea of the state as they joined in internecine battles or reached out to pluck patronage plums.

One constant point of interaction between the state and its subjects was law. Legal statutes—in particular the scores of ordinances (*Polizey-Ordnun-gen*) regulating aspects of civil life and ordering social relationships—are ostensibly obvious indicators of the role the state played, or sought to play, in the seventeenth and eighteenth centuries. While we cannot overlook these laws as a historical source, content analysis uncovers less than might be expected about the purposes behind the legal instrument: it provides almost no information about the effect such ordinances had or the reactions they aroused.[27] Ordinances are therefore *faux amis,* whose overt clarity often eclipses social realities.

These apparently substantial and unambiguous sources generate problems that go beyond the dissonance between rhetoric and reality. Edicts and ordinances formed the judicial and prescriptive superstructures within which administrators operated. They functioned as guidelines, yet these guidelines were constantly being renegotiated. And only at the level of the daily application of these laws can we recover some part of the actual workings of the early modern state. To grasp the actions of the state, it is essential to peer beyond the written instrument. The actual provisions of a law or ordinance become less meaningful than the question of how they found their way into customary usage. No ordinance existed as a pure entity: it was used and reused, sometimes repeated verbatim, sometimes subtly altered or significantly modified over the years. This observation suggests only one level of complexity, one that does not begin to address the more conspicuous questions of whether the state enjoyed an ability to implement its will, and of how that will could be recast or subverted in practice.

This reshaping perhaps evidenced itself nowhere more forcefully than in laws that touched everyday life most intimately. The formulation and execution of health policies in Braunschweig-Wolfenbüttel was the duty of the ducal privy council (*Geheimer Rat*) before 1747, and thereafter jointly of the privy council and the Collegium medicum.[28] In order to evaluate the impact and scope of health policies, one must observe the actions of the privy council and the Collegium and also examine the entire corpus of laws that pertained to public health and medical practice in the duchy. In the process of codification, medical laws were ripped out of their historical context and chronological order.[29] Valuable though they are to the historian, such collections frequently fail to take into account other legislation equally germane to an understanding of how medicine worked, yet that had, strictly speaking, no *medical* content. Thus laws are one source of knowledge about the relationship between state

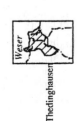

Braunschweig–Wolfenbüttel in the Eighteenth-Century

and society, but they are only instructive when looked at within the larger contexts that enfolded them.

Braunschweig-Wolfenbüttel, 1648–1820

The geographical focus here is the territorial state of Braunschweig-Wolfenbüttel, which today lies mostly in Lower Saxony, a modern German state whose borders stretch from the Elbe River in the north (where Lower Saxony abuts Schleswig-Holstein) along an uneven line in the south, running roughly on a downward slant from the Dutch-Belgian border in the west through Göttingen to the edge of what used to be the German Democratic Republic in the southeast. Like "Germany" itself, Lower Saxony was, until recently, a geographic, not a political, designation. In the seventeenth and eighteenth centuries, several states made up the region: most powerful was electoral Hannover, but the duchy of Braunschweig-Wolfenbüttel was an important political entity in its own right.

Like their cousins, the mightier rulers of Celle, Lüneburg, and Hannover, the dukes of Braunschweig-Wolfenbüttel were Guelphs. Throughout the later Middle Ages and into the early modern period, the lands of the older duchy of Wolfenbüttel were repeatedly divided to create ministates for all ducal offspring.[30] Fortunately for the state (and also for the historian forced to grapple with the minutiae of territorial divisions), the last major distribution occurred in 1635. From 1635 through 1807, boundaries changed little. In 1634, when the reigning Duke Friedrich Ulrich died, Braunschweig's "Middle House" became extinct. The Guelph heirs then settled on a final partition of their lands, which created the duchy of Braunschweig-Wolfenbüttel. The duchy fell to a collateral branch of the family headed by an extraordinary scholar–prince and bibliophile, Duke August the Younger of Dannenburg, who thus founded the "New House" of Braunschweig. Some minor land adjustments took place during August's long reign, the most significant of which led to incorporation of three-quarters of the communal Harz in 1642, of the county of Blankenburg in 1651, and of the county of Warburg in 1654 into Braunschweig-Wolfenbüttel. August retained the important district of Lutter am Barenberge, which was enfeoffed to the cloister Hildesheim. Duke August's two sons, Rudolph August and Anton Ulrich, subdued the fortified free city of Braunschweig in 1671 and, in the same year, took over the cloister Walkenried. In 1703, the house of Braunschweig-

Wolfenbüttel added the rich Amt of Thedinghausen to its domains. In 1735, the court moved from Wolfenbüttel to Braunschweig. Finally, in 1803, the *Reichsdeputationshauptschluß* ceded the abbey of Gandersheim and the cloister of St. Ludgeri in Helmstedt to the duchy.[31]

Throughout the eighteenth century, the territory of Braunschweig-Wolfenbüttel was divided into eight administrative regions and its land mass into a total of nine pieces, each encased in either Prussia or Hannover.[32] While this fragmentation was not extreme when compared to the miniature states in the German southwest, it meant that almost every area in the duchy was a frontier. Still, too much weight should not be attached to this apparent profusion of administrative units. For the most part (although less rigorously so for Blankenburg and Walkenried), the same ordinances and laws pertained throughout the duchy, except, of course, where peculiar circumstances dictated distinctive measures.

Largest in area and population was the Wolfenbüttel district, where about 46 percent of the total population lived in 1793. The duchy's two major cities and its administrative centers, Braunschweig (with about 22,500 inhabitants in 1768 and 27,301 in 1793) and Wolfenbüttel (7,201 in 1768 and 6,388 in 1793) were located there. The only other city, or rather town, of any size was Schöppenstedt (with 1,588 people in 1768 and 1,642 in 1793). This district demonstrated the greatest urbanization; in 1793 about 43.3 percent of its population lived in cities and about 56.7 percent in villages or isolated settlements. In the other districts (with the exception of Amt Thedinghausen), countryfolk outnumbered urbanites by a ratio of almost four to one. Because of the proximity of Braunschweig and Wolfenbüttel, there were none of the market towns (*Flecken* or *Markt-Flecken*) in the Wolfenbüttel district that assumed local prominence elsewhere.[33]

A quick survey of the other districts highlights the pronounced rural character of Braunschweig-Wolfenbüttel. Only in Amt Thedinghausen, where there were no cities, did a substantial number of inhabitants (42.2% in 1793) reside in market towns. In the Schöningen, Harz, and Weser districts, 70 to 80 percent of the population lived in villages or scattered across the land. Overall, in 1793, 50,424 people (28.4%) lived in 12 cities, 7,800 (4.4%) in 8 market towns, and 119,155 (67.2%) in 439 villages.[34] The population had increased steadily, if not dramatically, since the end of the Thirty Years' War. In 1765, the population was 157,696; by 1788 it had grown to 184,708; and by 1793 to 191,713. And, despite the economic decline of some cities, this population was distinctly more urbanized than earlier. Some parts of the duchy had, however, expanded more rapidly than others: the Wolfenbüttel and Schöningen districts increased their populations only slowly; slightly greater population gains were recorded for the Harz and Weser districts; while the population of Thedinghausen and Blankenburg (including Walkenried) rose strikingly (by 68% between 1765 and 1788, and by 74% between 1788 and 1793). Of this population, 84.3 percent lived under immediate ducal rule. Only 15.8 percent fell under the jurisdiction of the nobility, the cloisters, and religious foundations. Yet even this small percentage rarely escaped ducal regulation, especially in domestic affairs.[35]

Structures of Government

If economic configurations molded lives and social structures, so, too, did politics and political forms. Several levels must be drawn into the discussion here: territorial councils, "mediating branches" of government, and the personnel involved, from local and village notables to the governed.[36] The last are in many ways a largely unexplored topic. The quest for the "political peasant" in Germany has centered on the sixteenth century and on the Peasants' War. Historians have often sought traces of peasant political awareness and political culture in the protests that erupted into violence against landowners or tax agents, and, if less frequently, against central government. Yet the active participation of peasants and ordinary people in the construction of political culture in normal times has been consistently undervalued. And it remains a neglected issue.[37]

By the late 1620s, government in Braunschweig-Wolfenbüttel had assumed the form it would retain almost unaltered until 1806.[38] At least theoretically, the territorial estates checked the supremacy of the duke. The estates flourished in the sixteenth century when their decisions (the *Landtagsabschiede*) served as the law of the land. In the seventeenth and eighteenth centuries, however, the estates gradually forfeited much of their power. The duke, for example, no longer consulted with the full estates but met only with a standing deputation (the *Schatzkollegium*). After 1702, ducal resolutions replaced the Landtagsabschiede. Tellingly, from 1682 to 1768, the estates did not convene. Only the financial catastrophe of the late 1760s beckoned the estates back onto the political stage and occasioned reforms in government. The most important of these was the restoration of the estates' (admittedly limited) right to participate in the formation of law. Yet the duke and his privy councilors managed to retain substantial control over legislative decisions because conflicts among the estates frustrated the coalescence of any effective counter-weight to ducal authority.[39]

Throughout the eighteenth century, real political power therefore rested with a privy council composed of the duke flanked (usually) by four privy councilors. The duties of the privy council encompassed all govern-mental matters, including drafting laws; appointing officials and judges; distributing privileges and concessions; and auditing the accounts of Ämter and estates.[40] The execution of police ordinances was farmed out to several civil and ecclesiastical authorities, often causing a serious mud-dle of competencies. Special police bureaus existed only in the cities of Braunschweig, Wolfenbüttel, and Helmstedt.

In addition, the privy council created several permanent commissions. The most important of these regulated the grain trade, attended to the improvement of roads and waterways, oversaw pawnshops and pension funds, and carried out an extensive land survey between 1746 and 1784.[41] Another one of these special boards was the Collegium medicum, which reported directly to the privy council. Before 1747, the privy council executed many of the functions the Collegium later assumed.[42]

The structure of central government often had little direct impact on the lives of the vast majority of ducal subjects, however, and the laws promulgated and instructions dispatched from the hub were never real-ized (or probably even communicated) in a pure form. A host of mediat-ing authorities transmitted and implemented, but also reinterpreted, al-tered, or subverted, directives emanating from the higher councils of government. It was at the lower rungs of ducal administration that the complexity of relationships tying governors to the governed operated most decisively and most effectively coupled state and society. As subse-quent chapters will show, it was here that the political culture of the governed evidenced itself best in the quotidian exchanges and negotia-tions between subjects and sundry administrative agencies. For example, reactions to state initiatives, or, more intriguingly, the expectations people had of the state, their grasp of politics and political realities, their ability to articulate political concepts, political philosophies, and practical desires, all crowded within this more intimate political environment.

An analysis of political culture must thus begin at the level of local government and center on the Amt or *Gericht* (district or jurisdiction). Originally, the Amt was a form of seigniorial jurisdiction designed to manage the ducal demesne. By the late seventeenth century, however, it had taken on a collateral role as an extension of the central government.[43]

Each of the individual Ämter was entrusted to an Amtmann, with whom the privy council dealt directly. The original criteria for the selection of an Amtmann were his talents as a ducal husbandman, although he was also expected to possess some abilities in judicial and policing matters. Later, when the office became a unit of the central government's apparatus, the range of tasks entrusted to him and the number of officials directly under him expanded. By the seventeenth century, many Amtmänner had acquired two special aides—a *Justiarius* for matters of justice and an *Actuarius* for finances—and one or more secretaries to assist them in executing their various duties. These were chosen and paid by the Amtmann himself, thus allowing him considerable discretionary control over inferior Amt posts. The division of authority and allotment of competencies was never especially clear: an ambiguity remained, which inevitably spawned jurisdictional disputes, allowed delaying tactics to work, and created opportunities for graft and corruption. When the central government began to select and salary officials directly, it generated a bureaucratic network that reached into local affairs at the Amt, although not usually at the village, level. The Amt's offices were usually found in the largest town or market center in the area, where the Amtmann himself normally resided. The Amtmänner of some of the larger Ämter (or of Ämter of special importance) tended to enjoy more respect, more influence, and better pay than others, and Amtmänner jockeyed among themselves for such promotions. Amt government perpetuated a typical early modern piling up of inequalities, and there was little attempt to standardize Ämter or the emoluments of Amtmänner. Perhaps this was to preserve diversity, perhaps it indicated an inability to eliminate vested interests, or perhaps it was simply a result of not questioning established practices.[44]

The loosely defined structure of the Amt allowed Amtmänner to exercise a limited degree of patronage power, and they often cultivated an out-and-out patron-client relationship with their subordinate officials (physicians, too, could be caught up in this business), while at the same time, of course, being themselves locked into a larger web of favors and preferments.[45] Moreover, the Amtmann had many jobs: he was caretaker of ducal lands, administrator of justice, chief fiscal official, police magistrate, and more.[46] This multiplicity of roles engendered conflicts of intention and action. Jurisdictional hassles arose often and were aggravated by lower officials, who jostled one another for power and advantage. The garbled procedural instructions and the jumble of overlapping jurisdictions meant that central agencies such as the Collegium medicum, which had to rely on the local authorities for their facts, to carry through investigations, to enact decisions, and punish offenders, could never count on the unquestioning or sincere cooperation of local officials. The crispness of control, the veracity of information, and the degree of coordination differed enormously from Amt to Amt. The death, retirement, or transfer of one Amtmann, and his replacement by another, redrew the lines of coalition and of conflict within the Amt, easing or exacerbating the tensions of governing. In a milieu of competition and deference, the decrees of the ducal government often lost momentum, to be batted about endlessly in the layers and instances of Amt and village authority.

Village government, which was only incompletely integrated into the ducal bureaucratic network, presented another stratum of jurisdictional complexity. Village society worked on many levels and involved many variables—among them economics, religion, and custom. Later, I shall show that understanding how Amt government and village society functioned provides essential insights into medical decision making and, conversely, that comprehending the process of medical decision making helps identify the configuration of village politics and explain the terms of the political negotiations that went on. Only at the level of day-to-day interactions can these workings be extricated and scrutinized. What remains at this point is to look more closely at the social and economic structures of villages and towns, and to suggest how these might shape power relationships. Finally, it is necessary to consider the associations between town and countryside, and the degree to which similarities submerged differences.

Agriculture and Manufacturing

Considering the overwhelming preponderance of rural over urban environments, it is hardly surprising that agriculture was the principal form of economic activity and set the pulse of life. While other economic activities, such as forestry, mining, and manufacturing, could play major economic roles in particular places, farming predominated.[47]

Throughout the eighteenth century, grain was the principal agricultural product. All sorts thrived on the fertile loams around Wolfenbüttel, Helmstedt, Schöningen, and Eschershausen, which were then, as now, among the foremost grain-growing regions in Germany. Grain surpluses from these areas offset low yields in other districts and allowed the duchy to export grain throughout the century. The rich flatlands supported extensive cultivation, stock-breeding, and valuable cash crops such as tobacco, chicory, and dye plants, but hillier districts and less productive soil could also be fruitful in other ways. Where little terrain suited grain, fruit trees could be cultivated, gardens tended, and flax planted. Exported flax was the raw material for large-scale manufacture of linen thread and cloth outside the duchy. A wide assortment of vegetables were grown, among them legumes, turnips, cabbages, and hops. Potatoes were introduced in 1747, first into poorer areas like the Harz and Blankenburg, to stimulate their economies, where they were originally used to brew spirits and fatten animals. Later they were planted everywhere: "English" and "Dutch" potatoes for people, "pig" potatoes for the livestock.[48] Animal husbandry was important in several areas: Amt Thedinghausen gained a reputation for its good milk cows and fine horses. Throughout the duchy, sheep were raised for mutton and wool, and swine flourished everywhere, as did geese, chickens, and pigeons. In the Harz mountains, songbirds were bred for sale, and beekeepers were found there, too, as well as on the edges of the Lüneburg moor. Contemporaries regarded the entire duchy as fertile and domesticated; it was a landscape where "fecund fields . . . ennoble nature herself." "Nowhere does one find those uninhabited sandy steppes, those mile-wide wastelands, where man and beast have [both] gone wild."[49]

All in all, at least in the second half of the eighteenth century, the cultivation of an array of crops created a diversified agricultural economy that usually resisted the hardships monoculture could wreak on farming communities.[50] It was, moreover, an economy that fed its own and even exported grain. There were, of course, significant individual, regional, and temporal variations in the distribution of these agricultural riches. Hard times—the devastating cattle plagues of the 1770s, the subsistence crises of 1771–72, war and occupation (especially during the Seven Years' War)—could diminish or even reverse general trends of sufficiency and prosperity.[51]

The agricultural landscape of the duchy had been much bleaker in the seventeenth century, when potatoes were as yet unknown, as were good cash crops like chicory and tobacco, and the legumes useful for soil revitalization. Peasants owned few large animals, rarely overwintering those they had, and thus rarely accumulated sufficient manure for fertilizing crop-weary soils; transportation was poor, and pockets of want and even famine could rarely be relieved by speedy assistance. Some areas of the duchy took considerable time to recover from the devastation of the Thirty Years' War, returning to prewar production levels only near the very end of the seventeenth century.

In sum, cycles of sowing and harvesting governed the daily routines of most people in the duchy. Even in the Harz and in Blankenburg, where hills covered with thin, stony soils were poorly suited to farming, and where forestry and mining were the major sources of employment and income, people never completely turned their backs on agriculture. Likewise, cities never totally shed a bucolic aura and odor: the cultivation of modest kitchen plots and the keeping of small farm animals like pigs and chickens were common features of urban life.

Mining and refining, particularly in the Harz and in Blankenburg, grew to be major industries. State-run ironworks in Seesen, Delligsen, and Holzminden turned out iron bars, nails, and wire. Five glassworks manufactured clear and green plate glass, mirrors, and blown glass, as well as scientific instruments. Other state-supported manufactories included a stone-grinding works in Holzminden, a marble mill in Blankenburg, and several saltworks. Of all the state-fostered projects, however, the Fürstenberg porcelain factory, founded in 1744, achieved the greatest reputation and longevity: it continues to turn out fine porcelain today. None of these establishments were large, and few busied more than 50 workers each.[52] Despite the modest profits of some government-sponsored initiatives, few factories demonstrated much economic vitality. The most prosperous private enterprise was a chemical works run by the Gravenhorst brothers. Only a few industrial branches—the processing of chicory and tobacco, dyeing with madder, and the manufacturing of lacquers—assumed modest prominence in the general economy. The ducal government did not pursue a strong protectionist policy: the successes of glass and porcelain manufacturing were anomalies. Other attempts at economic nurturing fell flat. Several endeavors to introduce silk manufacturing, for instance, failed dismally.[53]

Such manufactories fitted well into the early modern model of *Manufakturen* or *Fabriken*. That is, each was "a workplace where articles [were] turned out in quantity by non-guilded workers." In terms of product and technology, the difference between guild work and manufacturing was slight, although the methods of organizing work and of marketing reveal some striking differences. The government occasionally distributed concessions to *Fabricanten*, allowing them, among other things, freedom from guild restrictions, tax reductions, some market protection, and, occasionally, monetary incentives. Not surprisingly, bitter conflicts between guilds and manufacturers sprang up, especially over the right to fabricate new items.[54]

Artisans and manufacturing workers were not evenly scattered over the duchy, of course. Whereas artisans made up a numerically significant and visible portion (50% or more) of the population in cities and market towns, their numbers were less noticeable in villages—about 16 percent. Goods manufactured or processed in Braunschweig included textiles and yarns, tanned leathers, tobacco, chicory, vinegar, liquors, and metals. Still, despite the not inconsiderable numbers involved in manufacturing and the range of goods, its contribution to the total economy of Braunschweig-Wolfenbüttel has been appraised as "meager" by its best historian.[55]

Industry often coexisted with agriculture in the form of domestic manufacturing (a conjunction some have analyzed under the rubric of proto-industrialization). Spinning, especially flax spinning, spread widely. Many people throughout the duchy—in cities as well as in the countryside—spun yarn for domestic use and export. Linen weaving began to flourish in the eighteenth century. Concessioned linen weavers controlled domestic production in Wolfenbüttel, Schöningen, and especially in Blankenburg. In the Harz and Weser districts and in Amt Thedinghausen, locals supervised all phases of the industry—from the planting and harvesting of flax through the spinning, bleaching, and weaving of cloth—and marketed their merchandise at home and abroad. Increasingly in the eighteenth century, some villages specialized in particular products, which, on the one hand, drew locally manufactured goods out into a regional or even an international marketplace, and, on the other, brought long-distance trade right into the village. For example, in the Amt Wickensen (Weser district) and in the eleven villages in Amt Gandersheim, the weaving of a special linen fabric called *Löwendleinen* occupied peasants in whole or in part throughout the year. They shipped the finished cloth down the Weser to Bremen and from there on to Portuguese, Spanish, or Dutch ports. To take another example, the processing of madder—the plant's cultivation and harvesting, the distillation of the dye—dominated the daily existence of many around Königslutter.[56] These are excellent examples of the variety of structures in manufacturing that could exist in one small duchy. Thus, although agriculture remained important everywhere, agriculture alone did not govern the lives of countryfolk. "Peasants" wore many hats: they were farmers, domestic workers, lumberjacks, agricultural workers, artisans, land brokers, petty merchants, and so on. Such multifaceted activities engendered a broad range of actions and attitudes, structures and mind-sets that are not adequately explained by the simple phrase *peasant mentality*. It is also rather difficult to deduce ideas and attitudes from patterns of land distribution and farming practices. Other factors played a significant role as well in shaping mentalities: among them, the size and demographic structure of a household, and its "moral reputation."[57]

The organization of village society threaded itself into this economic system. This is not to argue, however, that mentalities or social structures were epiphenomena tossed to the surface by "seismic shifts" in the economic crust.[58] But there can be no doubt of an economic component to the way people perceived their environment or cast their realities. Knowing how people earned their daily bread, how they came to calculate their economic chances, whether they thrived or suffered, adds to the mosaic that, when completed, fixes and reflects their mental states. Because agriculture remained the principal occupation, the size of fields, how they were cultivated, the communal rights and privileges enjoyed, the influence of landowners and tithe-holders, and the dues and taxes owed determined the specific social structure of the village and contoured the way villagers thought.[59]

The few large estates in the duchy were primarily held by the cloisters and nobles, and were either farmed by their owners or leased to managers. The duke let his domains, too, and usually in lifelong contracts. Still in 1800, in the district of Wolfenbüttel (the largest and most fertile part of the duchy), 67.4 percent of land was farmed directly by peasants, who, while they rarely owned the ground they tilled, very often held it in hereditary tenure on favorable terms. If, on average, the land *not* held by peasants tended to be the more productive, peasant land was not marginal.[60] Moreover, recent research suggests that peasants, often in the face of stiff opposition from more conservative owners and overseers, frequently pioneered agricultural innovations. For instance, the residents of Amt Warburg recognized the agricultural problems they faced and were equally aware of the solutions. Their poor soil required much fertilizer to yield an adequate crop return. Producing more dung meant keeping more cattle, which proved exceedingly difficult as long as the pasturage available was inadequate. Yet when the village of Raebcke requested permission to lease forest land from the government to turn into meadows for their animals, it was denied. Here peasant initiative clashed with the government's desire to preserve forests as economic assets.[61]

Small farms, worked by a peasant, his family, and servants, were the norm. There were no serfs in Braunschweig-Wolfenbüttel. All duties and services attached to property. *Meierrecht* ruled northern Germany: that is, most peasants held land in hereditary tenure and could not be alienated from it except for gross negligence, and then only after a legal process. They paid a modest, set fee, the *Meierzins*, which had, moreover, been reduced by about one-third after the Thirty Years' War. In times of catastrophe—crop failures, hailstorms, fire—the *Meier* had a right to "remission," that is, reduction or deferral of tithes and taxes. *Meierland* was generally impartible and passed to the selected heir on the Meier's death.[62] Despite being personally free since the fifteenth century, however, the peasant still served many masters: the *Grundherr*, the *Zehntherr*, and the duke (or, alternatively, nobles, monasteries, and foundations). The Grundherr, or landlord, received from each holding annual payments in grain and other fruits of the soil in addition to a small cash amount. Commonly, a single holding had two or more landlords. The Zehntherr collected tithes, and a single village could owe tithes to several persons. The third master for most peasants was the duke, to whom peasants owed corvée, either with a team and plow (*Spanndienst*) or as manual labor (*Handdienst*); in the eighteenth century, this amounted to no more than one or two days a week.[63] Most peasants enjoyed the use of common lands and participated in rights to woods, streams, and meadows according to the size of their holdings. Almost all paid ground rents, taxes, and tithes, and also owed cash or produce to village or district officials, for example, oats for their horses. In addition, the village assumed other duties to the church, the pastor, the teacher, the sexton, and even the village shepherd or swineherd, and, sometimes, the midwife, all of whom might receive firewood, manure, and free pasturage for an animal or two. General repairs, such as the upkeep of the church and communal buildings, were formal parts of peasants' burdens.[64]

At the top of village officialdom, and at the head of communal self-government, stood the *Bauermeister*, or village headman. He determined who had to render ordinary and extraordinary services, thus giving him a splendid opportunity to vent his ire on individuals by allotting the more distasteful or time-consuming tasks to those in his bad graces, although, of course, his power was in no way absolute, and he had to seek consensus if village peace were to be preserved.[65] The *Dorfgericht*, or village council, took responsibility for minor policing and was mostly involved in making agricultural decisions and settling boundary disputes. Members of the council were chosen from the full members (the *Erben*) of each commune. Through the council, the village decided how taxes and duties were to be allocated. Other people filled out the lower rungs of village officialdom. These included the men responsible for setting boundary stones, collecting customs duties and tithes, and even shepherds, swineherds, gooseherds, and midwives.[66] More loosely affiliated with the commune were minor ducal officials, pastors, schoolmasters, sextons, and foresters. Most enjoyed some land use and some (albeit limited) communal rights. In terms of intangibles, such as rank and deference, pastors rated with the full members of the commune, and teachers and sextons with the less privileged, such as the more recent settlers.[67]

Social and legal distinctions based on communal rights, property holdings, services due, and the number of horses or oxen owned divided peasants into several groups, for which it is difficult to come up with exact English equivalents: *Ackerleute* (or *Vollmeier*), *Halbspänner* (or *Halbmeier*, or *Kärner*), *Großkotsassen*, *Kleinkotsassen*, and *Brinksitzer* or *Anbauer*. Those at the top usually either owned their houses and lands or held them in hereditary tenure: they possessed full rights in the commune and formed a peasant elite.[68] Cottagers and settlers while also holding land and often owning houses, did not benefit from the same range of communal entitlements.[69] The lines separating the lower groups of peasants from each other were not very distinct, and various terms were often used interchangeably. The *unterbäuerliche* class, that is, those with no plowland, first emerged after the middle of the seventeenth century. The peasant elites probably earned their living exclusively (or almost so) from agriculture. Some of the cottagers also survived from agriculture alone, but a significant percentage of them, as well as almost all of the settlers (and the many landless persons) engaged in manufacturing in one way or another. On the basis of village descriptions composed mostly in the 1760s and 1770s, Walther Achilles calculated that in the unterbäuerliche classes, at least one of every twenty-two persons listed was some sort of artisan. Of these, fully one-third were linen weavers. The boundaries dividing those who wove full-time and those employed part-time are difficult to distinguish, especially for the linen weavers. In areas where linen weaving was widespread, for example, in the Harz and Weser districts, almost all members of the unterbäuerliche groups (and probably some of those above them as well) drew some part of their income from weaving.[70]

Each village generally had some craftsmen, often a smith, wheel-wright, carpenter, cobbler, and butcher, and perhaps a grocer or stall-keeper. Keeping a tavern was a special right, for which one had to pay a fee to the communal treasury. This was also true of mills and the homes/workplaces of millers, executioners, and knackers.[71]

Experts on the subject generally agree that during the eighteenth cen-tury, the economic position of peasants in Braunschweig-Wolfenbüttel gradually improved. Their enrichment derived largely from population growth and a concomitant rise in grain prices, especially pronounced after 1770.[72] A fortuitous conjunction of circumstances generated greater incomes from agriculture, while the prices of other commodities and wages stagnated. Thus, the real income of peasants climbed. Agricultural improvements, in particular, the introduction of more intensive methods of cultivation and new crops, began long before 1770. As early as the first decades of the eighteenth century, farmers had begun planting their fal-low with peas, beans, and rape, returning nitrogen to the soil and forestall-ing weed infestations, as well as adding to nutritional stores for both animals and humans. All this accrued to the peasant's advantage by allow-ing him to boost yields of winter wheat and feed more livestock. An improved three-field system (rotation of summer and winter crops with legumes) spread rather quickly and typified planting routines almost ev-erywhere in the duchy.[73]

We should be careful, however, not to equate improvements in agri-culture and a rising standard of living with prosperity. Walther Achilles's study of a peasant holding in Lutter am Barenberge (admittedly one of the poorer parts of Braunschweig-Wolfenbüttel) in 1756 shows that the aver-age harvest yielded only about four times the seed sown. This peasant sold much of his grain—rye, wheat, and barley—to raise cash for taxes, and another portion went for ground rent. The small amount of grain left over for family consumption meant that rye and barley had to be mixed in equal measures to produce sufficient bread. The peasant kept three cows and could only afford to slaughter one every two years. Very little beef appeared on his table. Milk, likewise, was in short supply: the peasant household consumed less than two pounds of butter a week in addition to the curds. Swine were more plentiful, although even in a good year, the family could only hope to kill and dress three pigs. At that rate, for a short time, all members of the household ate an extravagant (and rather over-whelming!) ten pounds or more of pork a week. But this was unusual.[74]

The overall agricultural picture, then, looks something like this. Peasants farmed the major portion of all land in Braunschweig-Wolfenbüttel, holding under very favorable conditions of tenure at least two-thirds of the best land in the duchy. Taxes were high, and peasants were overtaxed. Tax burdens were unequally distributed among peasant groups, and that disparity bred resentment. Still, rising grain values, growing population, and the steadiness in prices of other goods gradually reduced the pressure of all taxes by the closing decades of the eighteenth century.[75] Yet sharp differences divided villagers. Most striking were the inequalities of power, privilege, and wealth separating full peasants and the members of a growing agricultural proletariat. Finally, patterns of affluence and hardship differed markedly throughout the duchy. While myriad ingredients merged to determine the structure and dynamics of village life, many were indisputably tied to economics. Political power and social position derived ultimately from the rank of one's holding in the commune. This decided whether a peasant possessed a full vote in selecting a headman, participated in decisions as to how the fields should be cultivated, ruled on who had rights to communal lands, and determined who was responsible for special services to the village or Amt. Social decisions, such as who invited whom to weddings, who chose whom as godparents, or who sat where in church, were just as clearly linked to the prestige of one's farm.[76] The position of an "outsider" in the village often rested on the extent to which he achieved the communal rights the village council controlled. Property usually circulated within a community, and outsiders often had difficulty acquiring it. Villagers tended to be cash-poor, and a network of debts and credits constituted an important social, as well as a material, reality.[77]

Guilds

Not everyone lived on and from the land, of course. The economic, social, and political configurations of cities and market towns evolved differently from those in villages. While urban centers tended to be more closely linked to broader European affairs of the purse and the mind than were more agricultural areas, it is unwise to overemphasize either the magnitude of the split separating urban and rural worlds or the disharmony between urban and rural mentalities.

The duchy had only three cities of any consequence: Braunschweig, Wolfenbüttel, and Helmstedt. One characteristic defining urban environments in early modern Europe was the presence of guilds. In all three cities, artisans were plentiful and made a notable contribution to production. They outnumbered manufacturing workers and constituted a more significant social category. The commercial classes were perhaps socially and economically more important than artisans in both Braunschweig and Wolfenbüttel, but they never achieved the political influence or the wealth of the incalculably more powerful *commerçants* in mercantile centers like Hamburg and Frankfurt.[78] In Wolfenbüttel (and in Braunschweig after it became the official residence in 1735), the court and its entourage stamped the urban character more profoundly than trade and commerce did, although Braunschweig's trade fairs were major stops for commercial travelers in the eighteenth century. In Helmstedt, the university, its professors and students, imparted a (slightly musty) academic scent to the atmosphere.

In the smaller towns—Gandersheim, Holzminden, Königslutter, Schöningen, Schöppenstedt, Seesen, and Stadtoldendorf—artisans were sometimes numerous, although their impact was nothing like that of citizens who owned land in the surrounding countryside.[79] The further a market town or village lay from a city, the more craftsmen it would likely have. Such artisans generally found it impossible to live from their craft alone and also farmed.[80] Thus, although artisans and an artisan culture showed more visibly in the towns than in the villages, the ability of the guilds to dominate the social structure and determine the culture of small towns, as they did in Mack Walker's "home towns," remained limited, partly because ducal administrators governed these towns and cities directly.[81]

Guilds were originally urban prerogatives, and the wealthier the commune, the more leverage its guilds wielded throughout the territory. Guilds in smaller places usually formed as offshoots of the Braunschweig guilds. While many guildsmen in cities enjoyed a certain degree of comfort, rural artisans eked out a living. Their circumstances improved somewhat after 1749, when the government offered them more protection in order to entice skilled laborers. Country guildsmen possessed fewer rights than their urban colleagues: they were forbidden, for example, to take on apprentices.[82]

Knowing the numbers of artisans active in the cities, towns, and villages of the duchy, however, throws little light on more complex questions: What was the condition of the trades in the eighteenth century? How did that situation change over the course of time? And, finally, to what extent can we argue that the artisans' mental constructs pervaded and configured broader sets of attitudes? While there has been considerable scholarly work done on the first two questions, the third has attracted much less attention.[83]

The artisanal world in early modern Europe was polyfunctional; that is, despite the primary "occupational–economic function" of the guilds, it existed "alongside the social, political, legal, and religious dimensions, in a comprehensive, binding lifestyle that encompassed everything."[84] In the economic sphere, guilds attempted to divide the market equitably among all masters, to restrict competition, to offer fine workmanship at "fair" or "just" prices, and to establish a monopoly over production (in terms of both quality and quantity) and distribution. In short, they "typically aimed at securing continuity of work and income of their members, that is, 'a burgher's livelihood.' "[85] In addition (and not in truth clearly detached either in fact or in the minds of guildsmen from the economic sphere),[86] the guilds also sought to maintain standards of acceptable conduct for their members, to punish by fine or ostracism those who infringed these rules, to protect members from the taint of dishonor, and to supply a range of social services, such as burial and sick funds, help for widows, orphans, and injured journeymen and masters. Traditionally, then, guilds were not unions but the arbiters of a unique way of life in its entirety.[87]

This special position of guild artisans, moreover, "completely harmonized with the organizational principles of an estate-corporative society."[88] Yet in the eighteenth century, that world and the artisans' place in it were changing. Older craft traditions had come under attack from governments seeking a monopoly of legal power and, less obviously but perhaps more potently, from new methods of production and distribution. The political attack came to a head in Germany with the passing of the Imperial Trade Edict of 1731 that forbade the guilds to proscribe economic practices considered prejudicial to their own self-interests; banned their tactics of denunciation and ostracism; denied requests to close guilds; prohibited obstacles to the attainment of future mastership; and condemned guilds' refusal to accept members who came from society's "dishonorable" groups.[89] It also endeavored to place the guilds under the control of municipal authorities and to prevent empirewide organizations of guildsmen. In Prussia and Austria, both of which energetically enforced the edict, the guilds forfeited much of their autonomy and much of their judicial power. Concomitantly, the guilds lost a good deal of their control over the social and moral conduct of their members.[90]

The edict of 1731 did not, however, seek to crush the guilds. The

Prussians, for example, supported a modified requirement for guild membership, agreed to tighten boundaries around production territories, and permitted each guild a certain monopoly of production. Still, in Prussia, the guilds no longer represented "a universal social model" in the government's eyes. They were on their way to becoming something like an occupational group or union, which would retain the right to regulate its internal affairs, but would no longer exercise legal prerogatives or possess the ability to coerce or punish.[91]

What happened in Prussia was not the norm, however, and in the imperial free cities and the home towns "[w]here the authorities were in political fact hometown governments in which the guilds themselves participated, . . . the edict served *their* purposes or was not observed at all." In these home towns, "the period of guild decline was precisely that at which guilds were best able to defy state or public policy broadly conceived." Just when the guilds were losing these rights in other places, guild control of all aspects of life in such towns intensified as "a system of mutual defense by guildsmen-citizens" aimed at protecting the home town's "soundness and autonomy."[92]

Braunschweig-Wolfenbüttel's experience approximated the model of Prussia more than that of the home towns. The privy council's struggle to gain control over the guilds reached back into the seventeenth century. An ordinance of 1692 had sought to break the autonomy of the guilds and "integrate them completely into the ducal administrative system."[93] The triumph of the government over the guilds was never complete, and was not intended to be. The guilds in Braunschweig-Wolfenbüttel retained a limited right to fine their members, for example.[94] Still, when taken together, the guild ordinances passed in 1692, 1731, and 1765 did indeed seek to strip the guilds of much of their legal power and their independence.[95]

The crucial question here is, to what extent was the mentality of the guilds transformed, or to what extent did they maintain their exclusivity in a less sympathetic environment, where they had, at least on paper, surrendered a great deal of the lawful power they had once wielded and the right of self-government they had once exercised? The reform movement, which intensified in the middle of the eighteenth century, did not, of course, abolish the guilds. While the privy council sought to master the guilds, it had not in fact worked out alternative economic, legal, or social structures to replace them. The privy council therefore continued to protect guilds and even sustained some of their privileges, often taking with one hand and giving with the other. For instance, in 1790, the privy council refused to allow the closing of guilds—that is, it rejected the demand of the guilds to be allowed to set a fixed number of masters. At the same time, however, the privy council permitted guilds to lengthen the apprenticeship period and to restrict each master to only one apprentice, thus helping guilds buffer themselves against economic changes. Throughout the eighteenth century, the government tried to promote the settlement of guildsmen in places that lacked them.[96] Although the initiative was not successful, it spoke volumes about how the privy council itself had not shed a guildlike mentality. The attempts of the privy council to found new guilds took up the same refrain. New guilds were most frequently established in towns far from major urban centers, and by the end of the century more guilds, as well as more country-masters, plied their trades in Braunschweig-Wolfenbüttel than in 1692.[97]

Laws and government initiatives do not, however, accurately reflect daily life. Even if in Braunschweig-Wolfenbüttel, as in Prussia, the government fairly effectively bridled the guilds, the guild mentality as well as the guilds' fight to assert themselves did not disappear. The guilds resisted the erosion of their position, and complaints about infringements on what they viewed as their rights and privileges multiplied: they disputed issues of livelihood and public role, and they complained vehemently about the many who undermined their livelihoods. Denied the right to close their memberships, the guilds intensified their campaign against encroachers— against nonguild artisans, against the despised *Pfuscher*. The government prohibited any unrestricted harassment of nonguild artisans, but such persecutions continued unofficially well into the nineteenth century, and when they occurred, the government often turned a blind eye. At the same time, the government tried to sustain guildsmen's rights by passing regulations against encroachment and by pursuing cases brought to its attention.[98]

It is within the context of these battles and within the framework of shifting economic, social, and mental structures that the world of medical practitioners must be set. Apothecaries, surgeons, barber-surgeons, and bathmasters were themselves organized in guilds and were, like other guildsmen, feeling the pressures of government initiatives and novel social and economic circumstances. Some practitioners, like the midwives, who were not gathered in guilds, tended nonetheless to work on guildlike principles, as an examination of their disputes and their language, as well as how civil authorities treated them, shows. More important, we must consider the extent to which the guild mentality defined a way of life even for those who were not organized in guilds. Certainly, in Walker's home towns the guild presence colored the urban environment. What about in other places where guildsmen did not predominate, and where their legal prerogatives were fast fading? Did others participate and accept the guild's idea of livelihood and rights and privileges? To what extent did such acceptance help condition people's way of making economic—and medical—choices?

E. P. Thompson's idea of the "moral economy" suggests that there was considerable overlap between the worlds of the artisan and his client, and between the agricultural/rural world and the artisan/urban one. Notions of just price and fair marketing procedures defined both. The craftsmen's mentality was thus one of the pillars supporting the "mental structure of the corporate world of old Europe." Yet alongside the nobles' "catalog of virtues" and the artisans' code must be placed the peasant's "sense of right with his ideas of the equilibrium of duties and rights," and, increasingly late in the eighteenth century, the ideas of enlightenment.

Town and Country

Equally consequential, then, was the mental world of peasants, whose environment was likewise being transformed, often by the very same forces that rocked the artisans' world.[99] When Walker, for example, spoke of the "citizen's livelihood," he placed it within the framework of the German home towns, but the concept of the "citizen's livelihood" as "the economic security and stability of the solid citizen" was just as relevant to guilds in larger cities and to the village community.[100] In villages, in home towns, and in cities, the concept of a "citizen's livelihood" combined with an old (and in the eighteenth century almost vestigial) sense of Hausnotdurft, or usage, as a definition of property. Each household was entitled to its "appropriate needs." This concept by no means dictated equality of rights and privileges; rather, it institutionalized disparities. It accepted that households differed in their "proper wants." This notion was giving way in the eighteenth century to the more modern idea of property as a personally disposable thing, but it had enough life in it to sustain the idea that each member of a village or community possessed rights to an appropriate measure of goods and services, and to support the expectation that these prerogatives would be safeguarded.[101]

The forces that threatened to subvert the polyfunctional world of the artisan were likewise recasting the rural world. There, too, population growth was at the root of the problem. Peasant underclasses and nonpeasant groups expanded, producing new social tensions in villages. Only a minority of prosperous peasants could fully exploit the agricultural upswing of the second half of the century. This resulted in a growing gap between rich and poor in the villages, and the increase of population and the rise in agricultural prices only widened the rift. Village fat cats grasped the principles of agricultural reform and introduced innovations (in the shape of new crops, new methods, and new marketing strategies) for their own benefit,[102] which threatened to disrupt time-honored methods of planting and sowing that were intimately linked to village political structures.

Stubborn resistance of peasants to innovations from outside was not, however, the real source of rural conflict. In Braunschweig-Wolfenbüttel, as in many other places in the Germanies, the real battles were staged within villages and within families.[103] In his exhaustive study of Neckarhausen in Württemberg, David Sabean has pointed out that a 70 percent increase in village population corroded socioeconomic structures and allowed "a tripartite structure composed of relatively wealthy landowners, local resident craftsmen . . . and a mobile group of workers" to supplant the duopoly of agriculture and petty commodity production.[104] Tensions seethed within villages between "haves" and "have-nots," and between those who participated fully in communal decisions and those who did not, as well as between the more- and less-advantaged members of families.[105] All this should weaken any belief in the theory that confrontations in the countryside arose between closed, homogeneous villages that mulishly resisted modernization and fought the unwelcome, innovative forces of central government and enlightened reform. As we shall see, villagers often called on the help of external powers or imported ideas and ways of acting and speaking that profoundly challenged "good old usages."

Moreover, every German town, and even the cities, still lived close to the countryside. Towns and market towns, as well as Wolfenbüttel, with its unique court life, and Helmstedt, with its university, retained "burgherpeasant" traits, with many town dwellers owning and tilling fields in the vicinity. Even when Braunschweig's population neared 30,000, many of its inhabitants, especially those living near the urban fringes, possessed or farmed land themselves. Despite apparently dissimilar social structures, nothing really cut cities and towns off from rural areas. The urban maw did not merely gulp up the products streaming in from the countryside. Rather, the urban and rural economies flowed together. Urban merchants could, for example, become integral parts of rural economies. One need only reflect on the structure of many domestic industries to appreciate how this interpenetration occurred. During the late seventeenth century and throughout most of the eighteenth, the division between city and countryside was neither abrupt nor well-defined. We should also not uncritically accept a picture of municipal affluence and rural poverty. Toward the end of the eighteenth century, rural inhabitants tended to enjoy greater prosperity than their urban cousins (with the obvious exceptions of the wealthiest merchants and court personages).[106]

In sum, it appears impossible and undesirable to firm up the boundaries sundering rural from urban life. Likewise fruitless is the quest to isolate specific traits defining rural and urban cultures: they shared too much. Undeniably, there were contrasts. The cities could accommodate more sophisticated guild structures and a larger number of artisans, and cultivate more intense and regular contacts with the wider worlds of commerce, ideas, and politics. The court in Braunschweig and Wolfenbüttel, like the presence of the university and its clientele in Helmstedt, added unique flavors to their urban cultures. Yet the rural world hardly languished in isolation, untouched by urban influences. Braunschweig-Wolfenbüttel was a small territory, and few rural areas were so remote that people there imagined city streets were paved with gold. Rural dwellers knew the cities and towns quite well through frequent contact while conducting business, seeing the sights, pursuing legal claims, or visiting friends and relatives. And one should not forget that towns in Braunschweig-Wolfenbüttel, as elsewhere in the seventeenth and eighteenth centuries, grew because of migration from the countryside.[107] Those who came did not shed their attitudes and mentalities like an unneeded skin as they passed through the gates. Traffic flowed in the other direction as well. Ducal officials, pastors, schoolteachers, and the state-salaried physici usually (if not invariably) moved from the center to the periphery, from the urban to the rural environment, or shifted from place to place, stirring up settled patterns. Lines of communication and contact stretched both ways. No distinctive mentality imprinted either urban or rural milieu.

Policy Making

These settings—the territory of Braunschweig-Wolfenbüttel, the Amt and the village, town and country, economic and social structures—provide the essential backdrop for an examination of the ambiguities of policy making in early modern society. It often remains unacknowledged that policy making proceeded on many levels, and that the agencies and individuals involved held many perspectives and cherished sundry objectives. Variables of advantage and purpose, personality and program, combined. Moreover, no one "policy-making body" existed. Policies sprang up in the course of concrete interactions and represented a process of bargaining, mediation, and compromise, rather than the exercise of arbitrary authority in the pursuit of well-coordinated programs.[108] In this context, any attempt to ascertain what policy "was" and then examine how "it" was implemented is misconceived. Policy was fluid, and consequently is slippery to analyze historically. For example, health policies in Braunschweig-Wolfenbüttel unfolded in an environment of diversity: involved were the ducal government in the form of the privy council, the Collegium medicum, the physici, local officials, pastors, landowners, philanthropists, and last, but not least, the people. People acting within a specific historical environment—here, in late seventeenth- and eighteenth-century Germany—are the main focal points of this book, but it is almost impossible to penetrate the interactive dynamics involved without first separating out the protagonists and viewing them in isolation. The last section of this chapter deals specifically with the privy council, the Collegium medicum, and the finely textured fabric of medical legislation; the following chapter concentrates more narrowly on the physici, the Amtmänner, the Honorationes, municipal and village officials, and pastors. This division is entirely artificial, even arbitrary. Unfortunately, it implies precisely what I wish to argue against: that policy making occurred in the palaces of dukes and kings and in the cabinets of councilors and secretaries, totally independent of influences bubbling up from below. Yet, apart from convenience, other reasons determine this form of presentation. We remain lamentably ill-informed on how organs like the Collegium medicum did business. For too long we have fixed on programmatic statements, disregarding the demands of practical governing and the force of personal drive and ambition. Scholars have written a great deal about the broad outlines of organizational history,[109] and far too little about how individuals conducted their affairs as they sat round the council table.[110] Finally, if past historiography has consistently overestimated the efforts of central government in its intent and ability to act, one way to illustrate the relative lack of consistent or future-oriented policies is to examine how such bodies as the privy council and Collegium medicum defined their missions and functioned on an everyday basis.

Members of the privy council and of the Collegium medicum often voiced distinctly different positions, and no uniformity of opinion drew the two councils, or their members, together. In addition, the matters that pushed or galvanized these groups into action usually called for ad hoc solutions to impending problems. Almost all of the countless molding forces at work illustrate the basically reflexive nature of policy making at the level of the privy council and the Collegium medicum.

The duchy passed two comprehensive medical regulations in the eighteenth century: the medical ordinances of 1721 and 1747.[111] These ordinances cannot claim historical pride of place and were in no way extraordinary. The Prussian government, for example, had established a collegium medicum as early as 1685. The provisions of the two ordinances, moreover, approximate those of a whole series of similar statutes promulgated in the late seventeenth and eighteenth centuries.[112] Despite their conventional form and content, despite their undoubted character as programmatic statements, they cannot be ignored. First, they form the legal tissue enveloping the administration of public health and medical practice. Second, they offer a picture (admittedly incomplete) of what their authors felt government should be doing in the field of public health. Finally, they serve as useful indicators of general trends in medical policies and policy making. They do *not*, it should be emphasized, define policies; at best they only mark a stage in more extended processes of policy making and policy implementing. Intriguingly, neither ordinance merely expresses the goals and intentions of a well-defined and distinct elite medicine. Both imply the plurality of sanctioned medical practices.[113] They cannot, therefore, be seen simply in the light in which they are so often placed: as the manipulative tools of an academic or elite medicine, and of state-sanctioned medicine vigorously engaged in fixing standards and in promoting a medical monopoly for physicians.[114] An undeniable aura of norm-setting and ordering clings to these ordinances, but it was not their only, and perhaps not even their most salient, feature. These are texts to be read as the admittedly distorted reflections of a complex medical reality.

The medical ordinances of 1721 and 1747 complemented each other. The earlier piece of legislation laid out an ethical code for practitioners and published fee tables. The ordinance of 1747 elaborated on an extant, if decentralized and flimsy, medical bureaucracy, placing a Collegium medicum at the summit. The same incentive drove both ordinances: the rectification of abuses. The ordinance of 1721 remarked that "for numerous years abuses have spread in the practice of medicine; [and they have involved] physicians, apothecaries, surgeons, midwives, as well as patients, and also 'petite' apothecaries, oculists, lithotomists, herniotomists, and all sorts of corrupt and seedy strangers, old wives, and [those] others who, driven by greed and impudence, are found here as false physicians and interlopers." The 1721 medical ordinance endeavored to control such misconduct, as well as to "instruct [medical personnel] in their proper duties [and to set] fees, not only for physicians, but for all who are licensed to help and advise the sick, as well as [to inform] patients about their obligations."[115] The subsequent paragraphs established guidelines for the conduct of medical activities, defined the right to practice, outlined ethics, and set rates for medical services, yet created no mediating or executive structures and only scantily sketched out procedural conventions. For example, there was no mention of any body empowered to administer or formulate health policy. The method for licensing physicians was rudimentary: each physician who wished to practice was required to prove that he had attended "a respected academy," passed his exams, and was able to produce appropriate certifications of his degrees.[116] Curiously, the ordinance offered no clue as to what constituted a respected academy or as to who would review credentials.

The medical ordinance of 1747 likewise spoke of the correction of "rampant abuses and prevailing disorders," but now administrative mechanisms—the Collegium medicum and, more informally, the medical societies—were established to handle them. The desire for such an administrative and executive body had appeared several years before. In June 1744 a plan submitted to the privy council referred to "the great . . . value of properly established collegia medica for promoting the happiness and the prosperity of the state's inhabitants." After praising the Prussian medical ordinance as the best example of its kind, the author pointed out that nowhere "is the medical status quo . . . more properly ordered than in those places where public collegia medica have been set up, [are] properly maintained, and [endowed with] appropriate powers." This proposal was not unique, its author noted: in his father's and grandfather's time, similar suggestions had been advanced, but had always foundered on the "great problem" of securing adequate salaries for the men involved.[117]

The medical ordinance of 1747 at least on paper resolved some of these problems. For example, it defined rights more stringently. Physicians had to submit to an examination by the Collegium medicum before they opened a practice, and had to swear to fulfill their duties faithfully and attend their local medical society regularly. Likewise, the Collegium medicum would henceforth conduct the mandatory examinations of apothecaries, surgeons, barber-surgeons, military as well as civilian, throughout the duchy, and of all midwives in Braunschweig (outside the city of Braunschweig, the local physicus continued to examine midwives).[118]

The mandate given the Collegium medicum exceeded that of licensing; the privy council also held the Collegium accountable for everything touching on public health in the duchy. Thus the members of the Collegium were also involved in collecting and evaluating vital statistics and morbidity lists; in censoring medical publications; in rendering expert medical opinion; in responding to inquiries from the privy council on matters requiring special medical knowledge; and in drafting new regulations (such as the new pharmacopoeia of 1777 and the midwifery ordinances of 1757 and of 1803).[119] Their brief encompassed an incredibly broad range of obligations in theory; in reality the individual paragraphs of the ordinance echoed the overwhelming concern of government for the control of epidemic disease.[120] The Collegium directed the attention of all physici primarily to "all *casus notabiliores*, especially epidemics [and] epizootics."[121] The medical societies, too, were admonished to assemble their observations on epidemics. Possibly the government intended the medical societies to function as informational clearinghouses, or to perform as ad hoc local boards of health in times of disease emergencies.[122]

What is most striking about these medical ordinances is, however, their murkiness on matters of jurisdiction, competency, and personnel selection. The ordinance of 1721, for example, while interdicting an array of illicit activities and fixing minimum criteria for the practice of medicine, did not explain how standards were to be upheld—how, for instance, doctors were to be examined or licensed. Little spoke of the physici and their functions, and there was nothing on the manner of their appointment, specific duties, or salary. (Physici had, of course, long existed in towns and cities, where municipal or ecclesiastical authorities selected them.)[123] In fact, there was almost no hint of a centralized medical bureaucracy; the administration and supervision of medical matters in the broadest sense remained in the hands of the privy council and with the municipal and local governments.[124]

Here the medical ordinance of 1747 offered improvement at least superficially: it created a Collegium medicum and entrusted it with the "supervision of all medical affairs."[125] However, the prerogatives of the Collegium fell within narrow bounds. Although it technically answered only to the privy council, it actually enjoyed no substantive executive power and depended on the cooperation of civil, military, and ecclesiastical jurisdictions at all levels. The medical ordinance specified that "each and every magistracy" was to "uphold [the Collegium medicum] without question" in all cases pertaining to public health, but the Collegium possessed little ability to compel that cooperation and, in fact, more often than not, failed to obtain it.[126] Before the creation of the Collegium, the privy council had tussled with comparable problems of obstructionism, recalcitrance, and the assertion of local privilege without much success. In 1744, for example, the privy council complained that "in several places the medical ordinance is not adhered to as it should be, nor pursued with requisite vigor . . . [and] in some places, the local magistrates . . . entirely overlook matters of medicine and public health." These authorities used all sorts of "judicial flimflammery" to bamboozle the hapless whistleblower, while burdening him (often a physicus like Spangenberg) "with [filing] written protests and [producing] proper evidence . . . and treating [such persons] as if they were litigating on behalf of their own selfish interests" rather than acting for the public good.[127]

Even after 1747, these problems persisted, although the Collegium medicum's decisions and pronouncements de jure carried with them "the force of an immediate ducal authorization."[128] In a way, the creation of the Collegium actually impeded the execution of medical decrees by furnishing another way to entangle appeals in jurisdictional overlaps and bureaucratic red tape. Many circumvented the Collegium entirely by going over its head directly to the privy council. This happened so frequently that the privy council was forced to reiterate that the proper venue of medical instances was the Collegium.[129] To no avail, of course. Thus at crucial points the Collegium was really never more than an advisory council: its decisions filtered slowly through a series of often hostile, or perhaps only diffident, intermediate organs. And, in fact, the privy council never intended to disencumber local and ducal authorities from their obligations in the sphere of medicine, recognizing that public health involved too many particularities to be detached neatly from the wider affairs of governing.[130] The privy council itself added to the dilemma; at an important moment, the privy council defined the Collegium as "in most cases only an *advisory* organ," whose decisions were to be implemented "in conjunction and cooperation with [those] other agencies possessing executive powers."[131] The Collegium was bereft of executive powers of its own and at the mercy of other authorities, whose cooperation proved tricky to obtain. The 1770–71 reorganization of the ducal administration,[132] prompted by the insolvency of the government, allowed the "faithful estates" to object to how the Collegium conducted its affairs. The estates demanded that the Collegium no longer be permitted to issue "direct citations, summonses, decrees," but must instead only "request" the co-operation of local authorities in all executory instances. The estates and the government compromised, granting the Collegium the right to make *medical* decisions, but left their enforcement to the Amt and magistrates. Of course, the Collegium had never been able to exert its will unequivo-cally, but under its dean, Dr. Johann von Meibom,[133] had ruffled the feathers of numerous local notables.[134] And others had complained about the highhandedness of the Collegium. The surgeons and bathmasters, for example, protested that the Collegium failed to address them with proper respect and meddled in guild business.[135]

The discussions in 1770–71 also commented on the effectiveness of the Collegium medicum since 1747.[136] Privy Councilor von Flögen dis-paraged the existing Collegium as "not what I understand a collegium medicum to be." Von Flögen deplored "the currently wretched state of this body, the general antipathy and disdain in which, unfortunately, the entire public holds it" and spoke of "disgruntled physicians." He stressed the need to foster more cordial relations between the Collegium and medical personnel, as well as for more courteous cooperation between the Collegium and other authorities, and bemoaned the lack of both. The fault lay not only with intransigent and uncooperative authorities. He blamed the Collegium, too, for not proceeding with the tact and diplo-macy the situation required. Von Flögen regarded the proper function of the Collegium as "to animate, to encourage, to test, to know, to maintain in good order, and—if possible—to engage the attention [of physicians]; never, however, to act in a domineering manner." Apparently relations between the Collegium and medical personnel were just as contentious as its relations with local authorities. Von Flögen suggested that a new dean—Johann Martini was his candidate—might reduce the friction, al-though Martini, too, had in the past been embroiled in several nasty conflicts (and would again be in the future).[137] Even within the Col-legium, disputes—personal and intellectual—often boiled up and led to bitter exchanges of words and insults, and, while no duels were fought, on at least one occasion blows were narrowly averted.[138]

Circumventions and obstructionism characterized the relationship be-tween local magistrates and the Collegium medicum as well. The tone of

communications as they passed back and forth was often rude and some- ·
times downright insulting.[139] Conflicts with local authorities were legion.
In many places, including the capital, quarrels ran on for years. The
magistrates complained that the Collegium intervened in matters exceeding its authority, while the Collegium commented acidly about the lack
of good will and the obstructionism the magistrates showed.[140] Thus,
even legally, policy making never rested solely with the Collegium, but
was mediated in confrontations between it and other agencies, whose
interests rarely overlapped neatly and who often acknowledged very different priorities.

There were, moreover, the related problems of how best to promulgate
orders and preserve documents. In 1749, the government mandated the
publication of all laws within four days of receipt. Each official was to keep
a ledger, noting the date the document was received, when and how it
was publicized, and a short digest of its contents. As far as was feasible, the
actual order, or a good copy, was to be appended. The ledger was to be
passed on to his successor in office. This was a seldom-attained ideal, and
most jurisdictions kept poor records. For instance, in 1768 the new Amtmann in Seesen reported that he was unable to locate most of the original
documents. The previous Bürgermeister, a man named Tiemann, ran a
store and had used the fine paper of ducal ordinances to wrap up his
customers' purchases of butter and cheese. Wider publication was also
neglected. Village headmen were supposed to read newly promulgated
orders before the church doors each Sunday after service. Still, in the
1790s the complaint that "scarcely one person in a thousand" knew anything about the provisions of the various medical ordinances was at best
only a modest exaggeration.[141]

Yet even the Collegium medicum did not pursue a monolithic set
of well-defined goals; nor did the aspirations of individual members
smoothly coincide. A look at how the Collegium dealt with individual
cases will make these contradictions more apparent. The makeup of the
Collegium itself engendered competition between members for patronage and favors, allowing pecuniary interests and individual ambitions to
exacerbate personal dislikes. Members included honorary fellows who
were not necessarily physicians; the chief of these was a privy councilor
who functioned as president. The men who held this post, especially the
privy councilors Heister, Hantelmann, and von Flögen, represented the
wishes of higher authority and kept uppermost in their minds the broader

objectives of governing. Presidents were often quick to criticize the accomplishments and the individual members of the Collegium.[142]

The chief medical member was the dean (*Decan*), a position briefly held by Rudolf August Behrens, and then, after his death in late 1747, assumed by the hot-tempered and assertive von Meibom. Later, in 1772, the smooth and polished, although equally forceful, Johann Martini became dean. He was succeeded in turn by Johann Pott, the onetime garrison physician in Wolfenbüttel and Braunschweig. Meibom in particular tried to imprint his personality on the council and tended to rub his colleagues the wrong way. He often gleefully provoked steamy battles with other officials and individual medical practitioners, gaining a reputation for arbitrary and arrogant behavior. The other medical members consisted of three assessors and a secretary. A financial officer kept the books, and after 1770, a clerk and a copyist handled the mounting volume of paperwork.[143]

Salaries and preferments could drive wedges between individual members. The first dean, Dr. Behrens, and his successor, Dr. von Meibom, both enjoyed a stately salary of 500 thaler. The secretary, besides receiving free writing materials, drew the still substantial amount of 200 thaler.[144] If the salaries of ordinary members, the assessors, were roughly equal, about 100 thaler a year for their services (about the same salary that was paid to the physicus in Braunschweig, Dr. von Hagen), their *incomes* were not. In 1761, besides his 100 thaler, Dr. Höfer gleaned an additional 120 thaler from his position as physician to the garrison in Braunschweig, and another 60 from the hospital. Thus his annual income (not counting private practice) was 280 thaler. Dr. Martini earned a little more. His salary as assessor of 130 thaler was supplemented by 50 thaler he received in his capacity as physicus, by another 60 thaler for his services to two local cloisters, by 50 thaler from the poor relief, and by 20 thaler from the Braunschweig workhouse—a total of 310 thaler. Dr. Seebode had 100 thaler as a member of the Collegium medicum and another 20 from the orphanage. In addition, the three assessors split a percentage of the fees paid by examinees.[145] This pay scale demonstrates how the government regarded its servants. They were expected to acquire multiple posts through patronage, connections, professional skill, and personality. Together these constituted their livelihoods. Most perforce assumed several jobs and identities. Sitting on the Collegium medicum also, of course, raised opportunities for further advancement. The right of members to pocket a part of fees and fines led not infrequently to the charge (unsubstantiated) that members were trying to feather their nests by pursuing pointless cases and demanding unnecessary examinations.[146]

The members of the Collegium medicum were perhaps proto-bureaucrats, yet they remained in significant ways creatures of the duke. Nominally appointed for life, they in fact served at ducal pleasure. None was ever dismissed for incompetence or misuse of office, although some charges were leveled. They relied on patronage networks to secure their own incomes, and were themselves able to pull strings by sponsoring candidates for appointments. The privy council retained control over placements and actually conferred the office, but neither members of the Collegium nor privy councilors were deaf to the petitions of locals and individuals, and they did not inevitably opt for their protégés.

The lower echelons of public health administration replicated to a degree the pattern of preferments and patronage at the top. The physici, for example, were allotted a salary set higher or lower depending on several factors: what other positions they held; the relative wealth or poverty of their districts; how much private practice they could expect. Even in the 1770s, after methods to make salaries more uniform were introduced, discrepancies still existed. Pay ranged from a low of 35 thaler yearly for the prosperous town of Gandersheim, where the physicus enjoyed ex officio the lucrative post of "body-physician" to the noble abbess of the cloister and to the nuns, to the higher salaries distributed to physici in poor districts like Seesen (85 thaler) and Stadtoldendorf (84 thaler). Physici were at the mercy of the Collegium medicum for support and advancement, and they relied on it to back their authority against local officials. Over time, they acquired little sense of themselves as civil servants and continued to regard themselves as clients of the Collegium.[147]

The medical ordinance of 1747 delineated the duties of the physicus only sketchily—he was to observe epidemic diseases, supervise apothecaries, report on medical abuses and unusual medical events, instruct midwives—and left unspecified procedures for selecting, paying, and dealing with physici. Neither was there any firmer delineation of the powers of the physicus vis-à-vis other local and ducal officials. More extensive discussion of the physici, who long before 1747 were familiar faces in towns and, to a lesser extent, even in the countryside,[148] must be left to the next chapter, but the lack of specific regulations regarding them in the 1747 medical ordinance highlights three points: (1) the ordinance did not create an effective or extensive medical bureaucracy; (2) it did not establish policies that were then implemented; and (3) it did not specify how the human gears of the machinery were to function. The Collegium medicum was empowered to elaborate the fundamentals sketched in the ordinance but in fact the Collegium rarely drafted more detailed regulations, instead occupying itself with deciding individual cases and debating appropriate responses to immediate problems.

Medical societies were another aspect of the 1747 legislative initiative that either never came to fruition or wilted rapidly. Apparently, these were stillborn almost everywhere. Despite desultory attempts of the Collegium medicum over the years to animate the local branches, there is no evidence of success. In 1758, when the president of the medical society in Wolfenbüttel called the society to order to discuss the epidemic situation in the city, only one person (of five) attended. In 1770, for example, Privy Councilor von Flögen pointed out that only in Helmstedt did a "shadow" medical society still meet.[149]

Rules and Reality

The most effective way, then, to read the medical ordinances of 1721 and 1747 is as a series of sketches that briefly and incompletely delineated jurisdictions, laid down codes of ethics, published fee tables, and outlined duties. These ordinances expressed dissatisfaction with existing circumstances and a desire to improve medical care, or to eliminate what the ordinances called abuses. The definition of abuse, however, was a variegated one, which did not merely refer to what twentieth-century observers would regard as intolerable conditions, fraud, or *mal*practice. Moreover, the language of "correcting abuses" was a common legalistic formula and every reformer's platitudinous justification for action. Another way to read the medical ordinances is to ignore their fitful prescriptive content and try to pry out of them something about the actual conditions of medical practice.[150] It is striking how broadly the legitimate practice of medicine was depicted, and how feeble attempts to define any type of practitioner or specific group out of existence were.

Typically for the genre, both medical ordinances permitted a wide range of legitimate medical practitioners: physicians, of course, but also apothecaries, surgeons, barber-surgeons, military surgeons, bathmasters, midwives, *and* a colorful assortment of healers that fell outside these categories, including "half-surgeons" and operators such as "oculists, medicastris, bullatis, those who cut for the stone, repair hernias and harelips, dentists, mountebanks, and snake-charmers," whose practice was authorized in certain circumstances. "[T]here are certain surgical operations," the ordinance of 1721 specified, "[such as] the couching of cataracts, cutting for the stone, the repair of hernias and harelips, that are done so infrequently that ordinary surgeons lose their touch." The ordinance stipulated that these persons were to be "tolerated and protected in their practice as useful members of the human community."[151] While the medical ordinance of 1747 drew tighter restrictions on legitimate practice, it, too, countenanced such practitioners under special circumstances.[152] Although both ordinances explicitly prohibited "all illicit, fraudulent, superstitious, [and] forbidden treatments," neither specified what these were.[153]

Although the logic justifying a right to practice changed between 1648 and 1820, the metamorphosis was never completed. One can document a shift from a justification based on corporatism to a practice legitimized on a test of competency. Yet the corporate mentality never died out entirely, nor did the Collegium medicum distance itself completely from a corporate language and mind-set.[154] According to the ordinance of 1721, in "well-policed republics, the accepted rule is that no art or craft may be exercised by anyone who cannot show adequate proof that he was taught his trade by skilled and reputable persons."[155] The ordinance of 1721 demanded nothing more than "proper testimony" to capability, and accepted proof of guild membership and a masterpiece as sufficient validation.[156]

After 1747, the government mandated that each medical practitioner undergo an examination subsequent to his training or to his admission to a guild.[157] Still the guild standards, its language, and the corporatist mindset that accompanied them did not vanish totally, to be supplanted by a more streamlined idea of administrative competency. Corporatism lived on in the discourse on medical practice, and it influenced the practice of medicine and the administration of public health at least through the early nineteenth century.[158] A clear illustration can be drawn from the situation of surgeons and bathmasters. The whole educative process and examination system intricately entwined state and guild regulations. For example, those who wished to practice surgery outside the city of Braunschweig had to present evidence of their skill and propriety (i.e., their apprenticeship contract, their masterpiece, and proof of legitimate birth). In addition, they needed the testimony of local officials that they had inherited or purchased a bathhouse. If no such facility existed in the community, then the authorities had to justify the feasibility of establishing one. This last dictated that calculations be made on several levels: size of population, possible market, position of surgeon, ability to meet contractual obligations and pay property taxes.[159]

At this point, the issue of defining "quackery" in historical context comes into play. The terms *Quacksalberey* and *Pfuscherey* appear almost interchangeably in the contemporary medical discourse, although the second is commoner. And while the former applied only to medicine, the latter referred to illegal practices in all crafts. The medical ordinance of 1747 acknowledged the continued, cooperative authority of guilds in regulating and legalizing a whole range of medical practitioners. The medical ordinances reproduced most of the traditional, corporatist logic embodied in the guilds' endeavors to shelter their members from competitors and interlopers; it was a line of reasoning congenial to a world still perceived as having limited resources and a basically inelastic market system. After 1747, all "grievances about [medical] *Pfuscher*" went before the Collegium medicum, and these complaints constituted the vast majority of the cases the Collegium heard on quackery.[160] The concept of *Nahrung*, or livelihood, assumed a central position in the mind-set of the Collegium, conditioning its responses to a large number of issues. Nahrung, for example, largely determined how duties and privileges were allotted to civilian and military surgeons. Military surgeons were expressly forbidden to seek clients among the civilian population, in order not to disadvantage "those who practice a citizen's livelihood."[161] The concept of livelihood, and the essentiality of preserving that livelihood, was far more than merely a convenient way of marking off the territories of civilian and military medical personnel: it supplied the reasoning for categories of licit and illicit practices in medicine as well as in a wide variety of economic pursuits. Nahrung underlay the thinking both of the Collegium and of a government that above all sought to preserve the economic integrity and social stability of entire communities and groups of people.[162] It was a conservative, although by no means a reactionary, orientation.

But this mentality no longer snugly fitted the world that surrounded it. New forces, new methods, and new ideas challenged its premises, and questioned its logic.[163] As E. P. Thompson has illustrated, tensions heightened and conflict broke out when a mentality rooted in one moral economy clashed with the newer acquisitive ethos of a different marketing world.[164] While many continued to circumscribe their world within the perimeter of corporatism and, more vaguely, within traditional boundaries, these were no longer (and, for that matter, probably never had been) the only moral, social, and economic abstractions available. As population grew, as the market economy expanded and penetrated more deeply into local economic affairs, as new products and new manufacturing techniques developed that could no longer labor comfortably within older guild structures, as the balance of supply and demand shifted, and as a new valuation of individual over common property arose, the hostility between an older corporatist mentality and new mental paradigms heated up. This is not, however, to suggest that guilds were hardened and implacable foes of progress, as they are often portrayed to be.[165] The guilds often adapted to these changes, demonstrating more flexibility than typically assumed. Guildsmen themselves could pioneer ways of doing things. I am not positing here a fierce and implacable enmity between two opponents—for example, between "guildsmen" and "capitalists"—squared off against each other. I am suggesting a proliferation of models and a changed awareness of the socioeconomic world that affected everyone and required modifications in how all groups and individuals thought and acted.

In the realm of medicine, while many remained wedded to the idea of a just price and to an equitable division of the marketplace, economic necessity and economic opportunity fashioned other reactions. In choosing medical care, people often clung steadfastly to older notions of neighborliness and livelihood, but they could also vigorously assert their right to choose freely among the abundance of offerings displayed in the medical marketplace. Roy Porter has interpreted this behavior in eighteenth-century England as typifying a pubescent consumer society.[166] Perhaps for central Europe the situation can be less clearly linked to growing consumerism, although it is hard to judge, as almost no work on the subject has been done for Germany, in comparison to the lively interest in the topic displayed by historians of France and England.[167] Certainly, however, the tensions between an old lifestyle and a newer one account for some of the complexities involved in medical decision making, for the proliferation of medical possibilities, and, thus, for the changing relationships between medical practitioners in the seventeenth and eighteenth centuries.

These topics cannot be explored on the evidence of the medical ordinances alone. In order to understand the structure of medical legislation in the late seventeenth and eighteenth centuries, we must move beyond medical ordinances per se and survey the legislation that supplemented and completed them. Throughout the period 1648–1820, medical legislation was overwhelmingly reactive, not proactive. Characteristically, the privy council and the Collegium medicum responded to situations as they cropped up and based new legislation on the decision of individual cases that could became precedents for the future. To a significant extent, emergencies, such as epidemics, produced conditions demanding speedy attention, and these spurred the Collegium medicum into action. It may also be surprising how much governmental business was stimulated "from below" in answering petitions and complaints. Motivations "from below" could come from physici or others acting in their official capacities. Yet, as the Spangenberg report cited above graphically illustrates, the borders between official business and personal suit were easily crossed.

One way to analyze medical legislation is to group laws and regulations as they pertained to discrete clusters of practitioners, to apothecaries, physicians, midwives, surgeons, or to specific instances, such as plague. I prefer to attempt something slightly different here. The normal frameworks in which the discussion of medical legislation is so often cast tend to obscure the forces at work and blur lines of continuity and change. Instead, I have selected several motifs as best illustrating issues of causation and mentality: epidemics; popular medical enlightenment; corporatism; quackery; the rise of consumerism in medicine; and populationism and statistics. Obviously, this chapter can only discuss part of what subsequent pages will flesh out.

The most constant concern of public health legislation was epidemic disease. In the late seventeenth century, legislation regarding epidemics, especially plague, formed the principal initiative of the ducal government, assuming a salience and urgency equaling that of impending invasion by hostile forces.[168] In Braunschweig-Wolfenbüttel, as elsewhere, plague's imminence or presence exerted a formative influence on the early history of public health legislation, while assuming a central place in the consciousness of magistracy and people alike. Yet over the eighteenth century, the memory of plague and the heritage of plague institutions were probably more determinant than the actual experience of the disease itself. Plague had attacked Braunschweig, Helmstedt, and Schöningen repeatedly in the fourteenth and fifteenth centuries. Braunschweig in the sixteenth century reeled under several waves of the disease; in 1550, reportedly, 6,000 died; in 1566–67, 8,000. In the same century, plague also struck Wolfenbüttel (most severely in 1597), and the smaller settlements of Schöningen, Stadtoldendorf, Gandersheim, Holzminden, and Bockenum. Repeated, if less destructive, outbreaks marred the first half of the seventeenth century, but only once did plague menace Braunschweig-Wolfenbüttel after the Thirty Years' War: in 1657 both Braunschweig and Stadtoldendorf suffered serious loss of life. This pretty much marked the end of plague's career in the duchy, although there were some subsequent alarms. Plague appeared briefly, but ultimately mildly, in Königslutter and near Blankenburg in 1680–81. The last documented epidemic ran its rather clement course in Stadtoldendorf in 1721.[169] Thus, for most of the period 1648–1820, plague was a peril to be held at bay, not a personal tragedy that shattered lives. That fact did not make plague any less crucial in shaping public health legislation through the middle of the eighteenth century.

Plague determined at least two major aspects of health legislation that persisted long after the disease had virtually disappeared. First, there were the cordon sanitaire measures that constituted a state's main defense against an encroaching biological enemy. Second, plague initiated a genre of pamphlet literature written to instruct the population on prevention and cure. Cordon sanitaire measures—that is, the interdiction of trade and communication with suspicious areas by setting up blockades and requiring health passes, the quarantine of patients, and the fumigation of clothes, homes, and merchants' wares—were hardly new; they had been standard public health tactics in the sixteenth century. Governments again took this approach when plague raged in northern Europe in 1710–14 and when it struck to the east and south in the 1730s and 1740s, but as the threat diminished, the cordon sanitaire ceased to be a primary public health measure. After the 1721 outbreaks, plague vanished from the landscape. Although it continued to affect language and actions, it was no longer a proximate menace. Other epidemics, and also nonepidemic diseases, posed more immediate threats to the health of the population.

One legacy of plague continued. During the epidemics of the sixteenth century, the first plague edicts appeared in Braunschweig-Wolfenbüttel. During the 1657 epidemic, a nine-page printed pamphlet instructed inhabitants on how to identify, prevent, and treat plague.[170] Such printed instructions became routine in the later seventeenth and early eighteenth centuries.[171] Born under the sign of plague, they soon began to discuss other diseases, especially dysentery. Later, as the memory of plague receded further, broader concerns of public health emerged in a literature that began to concentrate on the health of children and the prevention of childhood scourges like smallpox; the provision of better care for expectant mothers, lying-in women, and infants; and the avoidance of accidents that turned laborers into cripples.

Dysentery provoked a series of pamphlets designed for distribution to peasants and to local notables such as pastors and Amtmänner. Dysentery could be fearful. Sufferers perished miserably from massive dehydration and fatal debilitation, although the young and strong often recovered. Yet it was less lethal than plague and thought more predictable. Weather, lifestyle, personal habits, and food consumption patterns were all held responsible. Dysentery struck with seasonal regularity, tending to reappear in the late summer and fall, seemingly related to the harvest. It appeared to be a disease of surfeit, not scarcity. Gorging oneself on certain fruits, especially unripe plums, was popularly regarded as near-lethal. If less amenable to cordon sanitaire measures than plague, personal adjustments in lifestyle and eating patterns seemed able to control dysentery's ravages. Plague moved from one place to another with a frightening, almost malevolent, inexorability; dysentery, while perhaps contagious, could pop up anywhere. Thus, control, prevention, and cure of dysentery followed other rules than plague prophylaxis. Still, pamphlets advising peasants about dysentery were published simultaneously with those on plague (often combined in the same brochure) and continued throughout the eighteenth century as one of the commonest forms of hygienic literature.[172] As these were supplemented and expanded, they were eventually allied with an extensive, if controversial, program of popular medical enlightenment.

Popular Medical Enlightenment

No issue provoked greater controversy among the eighteenth-century philosophes and reformers than that of the definition of enlightenment. Although most conceded the desirability of a limited degree of enlightenment, almost no consensus existed on where to draw its boundaries and declare "this far but no further." Both the desirability and extent of popular enlightenment were hotly disputed. Despite this, only a conservative minority distrusted the objectives of a popular enlightenment predicated on utilitarianism and whose goals "for the lower classes" were "to root out indolence and the poverty, mendicancy, and vice that grow from it and to replace [those faults] with industry, diligence, and every social virtue."[173]

How this type of popular enlightenment might best be spread sparked lively debate in the numerous learned journals of the day,[174] and various answers eventually appeared as a literature written especially for peasants. The most famous of these were Rudolf Becker's *Noth- und Hülfsbüchlein* (Handbook for emergencies), Friedrich Eberhard von Rochow's *Der Kinderfreund* (The children's friend), and the didactic novels of Johann Pestalozzi and Christian Salzmann, all of which had some (sometimes quite expansive) health content.[175] Other books explicitly preached popular medical enlightenment. Samuel Tissot's *Advice to the People on Their Health* and Johann Zimmermann's work on dysentery, *Von der Ruhr unter dem Volke*, counted as pioneering achievements in the popularization of health and hygiene.[176] Others quickly followed these exemplars and churned out a plethora of straightforward instructional manuals and schoolbooks, as well as tables, catechisms, didactic poems, and articles in calendars, journals, and newspapers. Of the literature published in Braunschweig-Wolfenbüttel, Friedrich Schlüter's *Immerwährende Gesundheits-Kalender* (Perpetual calendar of health),[177] whose 826 pages did not belie its title, was particularly well-known. Its length and elevated language probably did not serve the purpose of popular medical enlightenment very well.

A brief examination of the activities of the government in framing popular medical instructions reveals the various forces and initiatives involved. The discussion turned on three points: the need for such popular enlightenment in view of the actual health conditions in the duchy; the level of medical knowledge considered suitable for popular consumption; and the method to be employed. Three parties entered the debate: the privy council (usually assuming the role of initiator), the Collegium medicum, and a group of physicians and pastors.

The government eschewed any attempt to make each man his own physician. In 1761, when the privy council asked the Collegium medicum to draft a health *règlement*, it emphasized that "the instructions are to be directed merely to preservative means and the observation of a proper diet."[178] This general point of agreement between the privy council and the Collegium left considerable latitude for dissenting opinions on content, tone, form, and the overall advisability of such directives. More than once,[179] the privy council requested the opinion of the Collegium on whether standard works such as Tissot's book and Johann Krügelstein's *Noth- und Hülfsbüchlein in der Ruhr und epidemischen Krankheiten* (Handbook for dysentery and epidemic diseases) could perhaps be introduced in the schools, as Bernhard Faust's *Gesundheits-Katechismus* (Catechism of health) had been in Hesse.[180] The Collegium repeatedly raised the objection that such books "did more harm than good" and pointed out that while they were anything but inherently bad, the intended audience was too raw and unlettered to interpret their message accurately. In 1803 the Collegium opined "that the intended purpose of properly instructing the peasants about their health cannot be achieved because of the continued faulty and mechanical character of the school curricula . . . and because of the great ignorance of schoolmasters in the countryside, who are totally incapable of explaining the content of this catechism."[181]

For its own part, the Collegium medicum much preferred editing reliable popular works, like Tissot's, or composing its own short instructions for publication in the widely read calendars and almanacs, thereby targeting an existing readership. Calendars traditionally published advice on health and illness. Until 1751, every issue of the *Verbesserter Schreib-Calender* (Improved almanac) carried an astrological "prognosticon" of health, listing "propitious days" for bloodletting, shearing hair, bathing, and cupping.[182] In the mid eighteenth century, many governments sought to purge calendars of just this sort of superstitious content and to refurbish them into organs of enlightenment.[183] In the course of such laundering, the zodiac men and the prognosticons disappeared entirely from the *Verbesserter Schreib-Calender* by 1752. Between 1769 and 1790, each calender then offered instead a further installment of the "health instruction for the people," composed by two members of the Collegium medicum. This semiofficial health manual emphasized a group of dietary prescriptives and hygienic practices reckoned to fit the requirements of the common man, and above all directed to the health problems of the peasant. Its first rule admonished the peasant to seek competent advice in illness, preferably that of a physician, but if none were available, that of a pastor or other "knowledgeable person." Instructions on care for the sick lauded the healing virtues of fresh air, cleanliness, and good diet. Lengthy sections devoted to childrearing and the treatment of childhood diseases like convulsions, smallpox, measles, scarlet fever, whooping cough, and worms reflected a strong populationist impulse. Other installments handled those complaints and injuries—rheumatism, pleurisy, asthma, hernias, sprains, and fractures—thought to be the hazards a life of toil occasioned. A special section advised pregnant and lying-in women and nursing mothers on their proper regimen and repeated all the cardinal rules of eighteenth-century pediatrics.[184] The "health instruction" was prosaically and clearly written, the instructions simple but thorough, fully describing the remedies recommended, advising how to procure medicines, and explaining their effects. It stressed prompt action as the most effective way to combat oncoming illness. The usual warnings about the insidious damage done by quacks rounded off a rather conventional presentation of the elements of health care.

The last segment of the "health instruction" appeared in 1790. Despite having produced this piece of popular medical instruction itself, the Collegium medicum doubted that much good had been done. In 1784, after reporting to the privy council that "almost all the vital instances, [those] having the greatest effect on the public welfare" had been covered, the Collegium cautioned against more adventurous excursions into the field of "medical knowledge," because "apathetic and shiftless peasants would not understand much more . . . and the [unfortunate result would be] that of further encouraging medical quackery."[185] Ten years later, the Collegium expressed even less optimism and classed this endeavor among "so many unhappy efforts at enlightenment." The "health instruction" proved unpopular with its intended audience as well. The editor of the *Vebesserter Schreib-Calender* complained "that ever since the health rules have been appearing in the calendar, peasants have bought few of them."[186] (The actual reason for this flagging circulation might better be sought in the changing taste of the reading public, as well as in the availability of a wider selection of cheap literature.) The Collegium had become increasingly convinced that the single hope for improving the health of the people lay, not in increased distribution of popular instructions, no matter how excellent, but in an improved public health administration that relied on integrating physici, village authorities, pastors, and schoolmasters into a comprehensive system. This plan, the Collegium argued, posed less danger to the public as a whole than an education whose products had only "a smattering of knowledge."[187]

Not only the government experimented with contrived forms of popular literature. Private groups and individuals, minor government officials, philanthropists, pedagogues, physicians, and pastors among them, contributed mightily to the campaign. Their endeavors often collided with those of the Collegium medicum, and, to some extent can be classified as part of a contest for authority and influence between the ecclesiastical and the political powers in many arenas.[188] Several newspapers and periodicals of this genre circulated in Braunschweig-Wolfenbüttel.

By far the most popular, the most journalistic in tone, and the most widely read of these was the *Gnädigst Privilegierte Braunschweigische Zeitung für Städte, Flecken und Dörfer* (Privileged Braunschweig newspaper for cities, towns, and villages), dubbed the *Rote Zeitung* (Red newspaper) because its title was inked in scarlet.[189] Until his death in 1797, Hermann Braess, pastor to the community of Dettum, edited the *Rote Zeitung* and wrote most of the articles. Although his collaborators cannot all be identified, many were pastors, like Johann Helmuth (who also composed a popular natural history).[190] A network of clerical colleagues facilitated the distribution of a semiweekly paper that found subscribers in Berlin, Hamburg, Leipzig, Rostock, and Stade.[191] The *Rote Zeitung* by no means rivaled the literary merits of its more illustrious contemporaries, such as Matthias Claudius's *Wandsbecker Bote* (Wandsbek messenger) or Johann Hebel's *Rheinischer Hausfreund* (Rhenish house companion), for Braess set a more modest goal: the common man need not become a scholar, but "he must know what a person must know, must recognize his duties [in life], and must judge what he himself does, and be able to improve his imperfections."[192] Besides reporting on current political and diplomatic events, the *Rote Zeitung* carried articles of geographic and historical interest and inserted agronomic information and advice on domestic economy in series like "The Industrious Farmer in the Month of. . . ." Encased within short, simply written stories for children to copy out, in polemics against superstition, and in prosy tales about fictional peasants (Braess invented "My Neighbor Heinrich," a less famous version of the Austrian philosopher-peasant Kleinjogg) could be found a goodly portion of the paper's medical teachings.[193]

The *Rote Zeitung* was not, of course, the sole example of such literature in eighteenth-century Braunschweig. The first popular journal with a predominantly economic slant published in the region, the *Wochenblatt, der Wirth und die Wirthin* (Weekly for the husbandman and his wife), predated it by three decades. The latter paper taught few specifics of health and hygiene, but its sweeping messages about prudential husbandry and austerity in household management linked up easily with sound precepts of personal and community health. For example, an article on the marketplace exposed sharp practice and deceits, while cautioning against the medical swindler as well.[194] The *Holzmindisches Wochenblatt* (Holzminden weekly), which appeared from 1785 to 1796, was more belletristic, but it, too, made room for a measured dose of medical enlightenment. Two erstwhile theology students, August Raabe (the postmaster in Holzminden) and Heinrich Widemann, edited the paper.[195]

The instructional content of these popular periodicals paralleled that presented in the "health instruction" sponsored by the Collegium medicum or, for that matter, that found in the denser works of Tissot and Becker.[196] All campaigned against quackery and medical superstitions, all admonished peasants to place their full trust in Aesculapian competence, all worked to discredit home-grown therapies, and all endeavored to convince the laity of the efficacy of treatments, such as clysters, emetics, and laxatives, they supposedly abhorred and avoided.[197]

Thus, several agents labored within the context of what might be termed "popular medical enlightenment" in Braunschweig-Wolfenbüttel, often pursuing different goals and preferring different methods. The Collegium medicum sought an improvement of the health of the people through the progressive extension of a still rudimentary public health apparatus and continually foundered on its structural weaknesses. Although the Collegium did not deny the desirability of stimulating public awareness of health, it worried about striking out too energetically on a path that might dead-end in medical dilettantism. The Collegium foresaw a role for pastors, particularly in collecting vital statistics and informing the physici of outbreaks of disease and even specific illnesses in their areas. Many pastors, however, balked at being so used and embarked on a more active involvement in health, partly through the writing of their own popular papers. Pastors were quick to pillory in print physicians who failed to fulfill ethical standards of compassion and service. Churchmen also argued that the real stumbling blocks in the way of improving health in the countryside were the exorbitant price of medicines and the excessive fees of physicians, as well as a shortage of physicians in the countryside, because they selfishly sought lucrative practices in the cities. Many complaints from licensed medical practitioners about pastoral quackery also suggest how often the ambitions of pastors and medical practitioners collided. Many pastors shirked the duties they were allotted in matters of public health. The collection of vital statistics proved fraught with difficulties. Delays, inaccuracies, and real intransigence on the part of sextons and pastors were common and cannot only be attributed to indolence on their part. It appears that a power struggle was in progress.[198]

The various instances sketched here do not, of course, exhaust the possibilities and realities of medical legislation and popularization, especially as the vast majority of government actions focused on the resolution of individual cases. Nor do they fully reveal the multiplicity of agents involved in what is so often loosely known as "medical policy making." Yet these collected instances, and the general themes I seek to draw from them, are meaningful. First, they define how the major moments of medical legislation entwined with broader social, moral, and economic forces. They show how medical matters are only explicable when considered within these greater fields of influence. In doing so, they allow us to peer into the workings of a society while revealing to us much more than information about medicine and health. Indeed, one might seriously argue that there was no such thing as a "medical decision" at all; "medicine" was (and probably still is) so thoroughly plaited into the larger worlds of morals, economics, and politics that no separate or specific logic sustained medical choices. Second, these instances of medical legislation, in particular those that resolved or mediated individual cases, generated most of the documentation upon which this book is built. It is a history that testifies to the richness of the medical worlds we have lost and reveals the contours and deeper makeup of the mental motifs seventeenth- and eighteenth-century Europeans employed. And while it seems foolish to maintain that only an examination of medicine or health or healing can reveal substrata of attitudes and mind-sets, the complex interactions of individuals, state, and society in early modern Europe are illuminated with surprising subtlety by the immediacy and intimacy of these records of health and illness.

The Physici

Health policy became real only away from the cabinets of ducal government. Thus, in order to capture this reality, we, too, must push ourselves back from the council table and journey out into the world of the Amt, the town, and the village. Here the role of the privy council and the Collegium medicum diminished, and the significance of this handful of men faded rapidly. What happened every day often bore only a very imperfect resemblance to the resolutions of higher authorities. The routines of public health and medical administration fell to the physici, the Amtmänner, local notables, magistrates, pastors, landowners, and, in some places, nobles and religious foundations.

If all these people were at times intimately and intensely drawn into the business and politics of medicine and public health, only one—the physicus—drew his very raison d'être from health and medicine.

The Office of Physicus

Despite the central importance of the physici, surprisingly little research has been devoted to their lives. Most scholars have been satisfied with portraying them as the underpaid and overworked pioneers of science and enlightenment in a benighted countryside. And many physici, like Christian Gruner, saw themselves as the "miserably compensated or unpaid servants of the state, drudges without thanks or reward, slaves called upon [to help] the poor, whom the state otherwise scorns, diligent researchers of [the qualities] of mineral waters for the benefit of the state's purse, and overworked examiners of herbs for [both] man and beast."[1] By the middle of the eighteenth century, the physici in most German territories were becoming common features of a developing state apparatus. Historians have thus linked the expansion of a network of physici to the spread of the enlightenment in northern Germany and characterized them as extensions of an increasingly intrusive absolutist state. Surely any investigation of the physici must consider their position in the governmental bureaucracy and their relationship to the Enlightenment. But other aspects of their existence should not be ignored: physici were also, we tend to forget, members of a community and the creatures of an extended patronage-clientage system. Their self-image mirrored all these facets.[2]

Attempts to locate the physici (and, more generally, all physicians) in more inclusive medical and historical frameworks have often imposed ahistorical dichotomies. In looking back on the medical past, historians have almost always perceived—or constructed—two separate medical worlds. At first the boundaries between the two seemed ludicrously apparent: there were quacks and then there were "real" doctors. As social historians began to enter the field of medical history, these easy distinctions dissolved under a barrage of new questions and perspectives, both historical and sociological in nature. It soon became routine to speak of a conflict between "popular" and "elite" medicines. Gradually, however, this dichotomy also came under fire, and what had once seemed clear-cut lines dividing the two tended to smudge. The days of writing "autonomous histories" of each and of distinguishing between "saints and sinners" are now pretty much over, and scholars "of all stripes agree nowadays . . . that the frontiers between orthodox and unorthodox medicine have been flexible."[3]

Purportedly to correct old misconceptions, historians then employed other divisions, which, however, are themselves theoretically leaky and offer only imprecise resemblances to reality, as their architects sometimes readily admit. Some have accepted the new categories as heuristic and analytic conveniences, while remaining skeptical of their ability to represent reality. As a result, the scholar can now choose among a variety of bifurcating models. Matthew Ramsey, for example, has recently devoted a long volume to analyzing medicine in France between 1770 and 1830 in terms of the professional/popular pairing, "join[ing] two major lines of inquiry that have attracted growing attention in recent years but have generally been pursued separately: the history of popular culture and of the professions."[4] Other combinations have their proponents. We now see in the literature a proliferation of describers: on the one side are adjectives such as *professional, academic, orthodox, regular, proper, learned, official, commercial, licit,* and *enlightened,* while on the other we find *popular, lay, irregular, unorthodox, improper, customary, traditional, vernacular, home, fringe, illicit,* and *unenlightened.*[5] All have their uses, all their snags.

Complicating the situation are other sets of dichotomies, which have proven as fallible as the more familiar ones based essentially on the "popular/elite" distinction. Among these, the use of the dyads *sedentary/peripatetic* and *rural/urban* to describe practitioners has been the most common. Historians now can chose among a large number of nouns and adjectives to characterize medical practices in the past, yet all of these have been severely criticized. We cannot, it seems, do without them, but did the entities they supposedly depict ever exist? Interminable arguments as to which are perhaps more valid, and even more honest historically, have often wound up in sterile debates about semantics. Consequently, even those historians most cognizant of the dangers of razoring historical realities into bits labeled *popular* or *elite* (or whatever the preferred terms are) have found it impossible to eliminate such jargon from their vocabularies. Attempts to supplant it have often produced a welter of awkward, uglier, and equally imprecise words.

We can, of course, jettison the idea of a dichotomy and turn to other approaches: front-runners here have been the concepts of a spectrum, layer, level, and field. This obviously does not solve the problem of how to construct an inclusive medical and historical framework either. More important, I believe, is to embrace plain speaking, while taking pains to accept the confusions and difficulties as they arise, and indeed to make them integral parts of the argument. The most we can hope for is that such a laborious unraveling will eventually lead us closer to an understanding of a historical situation that we can perhaps never fully recreate. The danger always exists, of course, that thereby a richly textured description of the activities of the physici will emerge, marvelous perhaps in its intricacy, but with little analytical power.

These theoretical musings relate intimately to any discussion of healers in the early modern world and are especially germane to any treatment of physicians and physici. Where do *they* fit in the medical worlds of the late seventeenth and eighteenth centuries? If an older historiography could easily portray physici as the workhorses of medical reform and the mouthpieces of enlightenment, as path-blazers slashing away at thickets of superstition and ignorance, such comforting simplicity has now been denied us. Today, few historians will argue that seventeenth- and eighteenth-century physici (and physicians) were knights of hygiene and science who sallied forth under the banners of enlightenment and medical science to battle ignorance and confound superstition. Now we are far more likely to encounter analyses that pin the physici in the jaws of a vise composed of local interests on the one hand and the aspirations of central government on the other; or to view them as the protégés and creatures of territorial governments that ran on patronage and clientage relationships. Yet the experiences of the physici as a group, in particular the lives of those who never scaled the ladder to become body-physicians or to sit on a territorial collegium medicum, who never attained a professorship or authored a significant piece of medical literature, have not been examined in detail.[6]

The physici have a history all their own, and one that has rarely been told from the perspective of the personal, the immediate, and the human. While numerous works exist on the professionalization of medicine and on the multitude of legislative ordinances that elaborated the duties and obligations of the physicus in town or countryside, few have addressed the quotidian realities of his existence, or compiled collective biographies that reveal the actualities of life at the level of the everyday.[7] The physici are important to this book for other reasons as well. With some regularity, they composed detailed assessments of conditions in the countryside and in small towns throughout the duchy. The very subjectivity of these narrative descriptions and analyses is a great boon: the reports document the power relationships, the conflicts, and the tensions that characterized the daily workings of health policy. Moreover, the physicus served as a lightning rod: he experienced local opposition to health policies intimately and immediately; he drew down upon his head the animosity of those who contravened policies; he felt the consequences of not fitting into an elaborately structured village or neighborhood environment. And, as representative of the ducal government, he was the one who often came into conflict with other practitioners, with ducal officials, with local notables and nobility, pastors, and with ordinary people on matters not only of health but of politics, economics, propriety, property, customs, and usage. By focusing on his position, on his triumphs and tribulations, on his place and function in a community, we learn a great deal about the men perched on the bottom rung of the health bureaucracy, and an equally great amount about the workings of late seventeenth- and eighteenth-century society.

Furthermore, an examination of the physici allows us to peer into a particularly dim corner of medical practice in early modern Europe: that where the physician is found. Contrary to what many believe, it is often easier to learn about apothecaries, midwives, surgeons, and even quacks, than it is to open up the lives of ordinary doctors to historical scrutiny. The archives tend to be far more loquacious (if simultaneously more misleading and mendacious) about the careers and lives of the "other" medical practitioners. For many physicians, however, we tend to know considerably less. Case books and ledgers rarely exist; I have not turned one up in Braunschweig-Wolfenbüttel. The published case books that we have for many famous physicians are just not there for the ordinary doctor, and I suspect that the paucity of materials is not merely a matter of preservation. It seems that few physicians took case notes; the minority who did intended to publish them. At best, perhaps, physicians kept account books, but I have not found these either. Even the case books—manuscript and published—of celebrated physicians have only just recently begun to be exploited for the purposes of social history.[8] How ordinary practitioners lived, what they earned, how they viewed themselves and their surroundings, how they constructed their identities, have remained hidden.[9]

A meticulous examination of the physici answers many of these questions, and this chapter examines the physici in their multifarious roles. Still, although the physici are the protagonists of this chapter, they do not appear alone on the stage, for they were not the only ones caught up in the "on-the-ground" functioning of medicine and public health policy. The Amtmänner, who oversaw the general well-being of the district entrusted to them, and who exercised police and judicial powers, were equally central figures. Without their cooperation, no law could be implemented, no case decided, no quack pursued, no fine collected. An Amtmann could expedite or block the execution of all directives and ordinances, including those affecting health. Other persons participated in the local affairs of government, and village notables wielded enough power to thwart or delay the wishes of Amtmänner, physici, and the central government alike. Far from being the "mere tools of enlightened government," pastors often pursued their own agendas, dabbling in medicine, shaping programs of popular medical enlightenment, promoting smallpox inoculation and, later, vaccination.[10] And one must also not forget that although the physici made up a large portion of all licensed physicians, they were by no means the only physicians engaged in medical practice. Even in relatively isolated and remote areas, the physicus often had to compete with another *physician*—that is, with a licensed, approved, and university-educated practitioner—for clients and fees. The discussion must have room for all of these, too. Yet despite their undeniable importance, it is not my intention to focus on this supporting cast directly; they come to share the limelight with the physicus as they entered the orbit of his life.

The origins of the office of physicus lie shrouded in historical darkness, and need not, in fact, concern us here very much. Numerous medieval and early modern cities appointed "plague-doctors," who may have been the forerunners of the eighteenth-century physicus.[11] By the early sixteenth century, German cities were hiring physici with some regularity. The first proper contracts between magistrates and physici appeared in the sixteenth century. These documents became more common in the seventeenth and eighteenth centuries, when their forms also became more standardized.

The duties and definition of the physicus changed over time. In the late seventeenth and early eighteenth centuries, the tasks assigned to the physicus were still primarily forensic: "The physicus is a physician appointed by the authorities [and] who in the special medical instances that come to court must render his opinion [on them]." Indeed, another common name for the physicus was *Medicus forensis*.[12] By the end of the century, the description of the physicus's task had expanded: he was to see that all "the rules of medical police were properly observed."[13] When Johann Schwabe published a two-volume handbook delineating the duties of a physicus, he listed healthy air, potable water, safe beer, wine, whiskey, bread, meat, and all other food products as falling within his normal purview. The physicus was to provide care for all, but especially for the needy, during epidemics. He was to instruct nurses, to investigate epidemics, epizootics, and occupational diseases, and "to care for the health of the common man in general." In addition, he was responsible for lifesaving measures, oversight of midwives, care for the sick poor, and the supervision of surgeons and apothecaries. Moreover, he was to do everything possible to "extirpate quackery."[14] The compendium published for Braunschweig-Wolfenbüttel in 1793 by August Hinze, physicus in Calvörde, listed all these chores and more.[15]

Stolpertus,

ein

junger Arzt am Krankenbette,

Von einem patriotischen Pfälzer.

Vita brevis, ars longa, occasio præceps, expe-
rimentum periculosum; judicium difficile.

Hipp. Aphor. I.

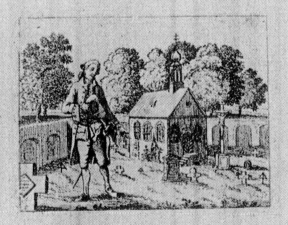

Neue Auflage.

Mannheim,
bei Schwan und Götz,
1800.

Title page, *Stolpertus, ein junger Arzt am Krankenbette,* by Franz Anton May (Mannheim: Schwan und Götz, 1800). Reproduced with the permission of the Wellcome Institute Library, London.

After the Thirty Years' War, numerous territories began to rebuild and reorganize their war-torn lands. This initiative led to some basic codification of medical legislation, as well as spurring efforts to appoint physici responsible for nonurban areas.[16] The distinction between *Stadt* (city) physici and *Land* (country) physici is not, however, of much importance. Physici in capitals, or in university towns, often found themselves in a particularly profitable situation, being at one and the same time professors (of physic, botany, anatomy) and civic officials as well as physici. In territorial capitals, the range of options was wider, allowing one man to accumulate a number of offices. A city physicus could be a member of the Collegium medicum, as was Dr. Martini in Braunschweig.[17] Less illustrious or less aspiring men could likewise acquire several posts, often adding the position of garrison physician to an already bulging occupational portfolio. Johann du Roi, secretary of the Collegium from 1765 until his death in 1785, was physicus in Braunschweig from 1776 to 1785, as well as physician to the garrison there.[18] Johann Pott, secretary of the Collegium from 1785 to 1800, served as professor of botany at the Anatomical Institute in Braunschweig in 1776 and *Garnison medicus* in 1786; he became dean of the Collegium in 1800.[19] Johann Martini, the forceful head of the Collegium from 1772 to 1800, united in his person several positions. In 1761, while still an ordinary member of the Collegium, he was also physician for the poor relief and to the workhouse, as well as for the cloisters of Crucis and Riddagshausen. His total income was 310 thaler.[20] While combining such positions always created some problems, and quickly elicited complaints from those passed over, it was neither illegal nor unusual. In fact, it was more or less expected that a man needed to fill several posts synchronously to make a decent living.

The habit of stringing together offices was not, of course, limited to the upper echelons of official medicine. Everybody did it. Those on the lower rungs of the ladder battled perhaps more frantically to secure further appointments: as physicians to ducal mining companies, to factories (for example, to the porcelain works in Fürstenburg), as spa physicians, and as body-physicians to the many ruling and nonruling members of the ducal family. These were all plums, and no one hesitated to thrust his thumb into the patronage pie.

Patronage might, of course, play an invaluable role in winning a situation. Many eighteenth- and nineteenth-century medical authors stressed the decisive influence of family ties, "pull," and even outright bribes in attaining a post in the early modern world.[21] Pulling strings was so integral to the functioning of early modern government and society that it seems willful to deny the strength and importance of the bonds of patronage and clientage, of favors and honors, that honeycombed early modern society and government. Contemporaries were sure that those who lacked benefactors had little hope of success. Friedrich von Hoven was a student-comrade of Friedrich von Schiller's and among the first class at the famous Karl's School in Ludwigsburg. He later became a professor at the University of Würzburg and headed the Julius Hospital there. His memoirs relate how he maneuvered for the position of first physicus in Ludwigsburg. In 1785, at the age of twenty-six, and with remarkably little fuss, he had become second physicus. Then his luck ran out. His official post did not help him surmount the obstacles impeding the establishment of a practice in the town. According to von Hoven, it was next to impossible for a physician without powerful friends and alliances to make his way.[22] While von Hoven readily admitted that to some extent his youth made him appear unsuitable for quick promotion, he also attributed his failure to his maladroitness at flattery, and especially to his inability to "cultivate the favor of the fair sex." More telling was his lack of a patron (only later did he find such a powerful friend among the nobility) and the venality of others. His next application for the position of first physicus likewise went awry. The successful candidate was employed as physicus in the small town of Vaihingen, and was, von Hoven conceded, "a talented physician and honest man." Yet "these reasons [alone] would have hardly been enough to elevate him to the position of first physicus in Ludwigsburg, if he had not . . . paid the duke 200 louis d'or."[23] Only by personally interceding with an obliging privy councilor (and with a bit of luck) did von Hoven finally obtain his objective some years later.[24]

Friends and patrons formed the necessary accoutrements gracing a successful man in a world that still worked to a large degree through a network of personal acquaintances and face-to-face relationships. Support ran horizontally as well as vertically. Useful patrons might be older, influential mentors perched near the top of the patronage ladder, but friends and schoolmates were often equally valuable in locating and securing positions, serving as an extended web of eyes and ears ready to put in a good word for a comrade. Ernst Heim, famous, as were few other doctors in the eighteenth century, for his practice rather than his writing, was helped to his first post by the timely intercession of a friend. In 1777, when Heim was already thirty, and still unable to earn an independent income, a school chum of his, then physicus in Spandau, asked Heim to substitute for him during an illness. When the friend died of tuberculosis soon after, Heim was well placed for advancement.[25] Friendships struck while studying medicine, or even earlier, often paid off. Such relatively tight networks of friends and acquaintances secured that all-so-vital first post for many a young and struggling physician.[26] And connections remained crucial. For example, Physicus Rörhand in Schöppenstedt felt the competition of Dr. Carl Spohr acutely. Spohr's father was the ecclesiastical superintendent and, according to Rörhand, had circulated a personal note to all the pastors in the area "asking them to recommend his son to the schoolmasters, and [the latter to do likewise] to their pupils and their families," as physician and man-midwife. Father Spohr's status made it easier, Rörhand not implausibly insisted, for his son to connect with the members of the community than Rörhand could do.[27]

All this is undeniable, yet the question that remains unanswered is to what extent such relationships—ties to higher authorities, family connections, and the patronage of friends and school companions—dictated the choice of physici? Were *all* positions decided on such calculations? Mary Wessling presents an excellent case study of a physicus in Württemberg who was caught up in competing webs of patronage that spun up to the highest circles of government and vibrated to the motions of larger political animals. And here, too, the influence of local notables—the *Honorationes*, as they were known in Braunschweig-Wolfenbüttel—played an undeniably critical role.[28] While my story has its share of these kinds of ties, it turns more on the relationship of the physicus with his neighbors, whose connections with the greater seats of power were tenuous and equivocal.

Districts and Duties

The history of the *physicate* in Braunschweig-Wolfenbüttel parallels the history of similar institutions in other territorial states. The general outlines are well known. As in most places, physici first appeared in cities. In these early years, the existence of the office of physicus tended to correlate with the threat or reality of epidemics. The plague years of the late sixteenth and early seventeenth centuries, especially the epidemic years of 1577, 1597, and 1609–11 in Braunschweig, occasioned a plethora of new ordinances. After the Thirty Years' War, renewed threats of plague and dysentery buffeted the duchy, initiating new endeavors in the realm of medical policing. These efforts aimed at reforming and upgrading the state's medical apparatus and culminated in the passage of a medical ordinance in 1721.

About the same time, and particularly in the larger cities, it became less common for the office of physicus to go unfilled for years on end. Throughout the seventeenth century, and well into the eighteenth, the appointment of physici remained a prerogative of local authority, exercised in most cases by city councils and magistrates. These localities hired and paid their own physici and defined their responsibilities.[29] In 1750, for example, the city of Braunschweig specified that its physicus would examine and supervise all other physicians, surgeons, and midwives, and decide whether to grant or withhold concessions to "mountebanks, dentists, and oil-peddlers" during trade fairs, as well as treat criminals and those held under investigative arrest. For performing these tasks, he earned 200 thaler yearly and received a fee for each examination performed. His replacement, however, fared less well. The city justified its decision to reduce the physicus's salary in terms of "the current [poor] state of our finances, and [the fact] that often years go by when the physicus is not required to render his *judicium* on either wounds or corpses."[30] The earliest contracts thus pertained to specific individuals and were written for specific terms of office. Antonius Macholdus, the first recorded physicus in Braunschweig's history, was selected by the magistrates in 1591, and was paid 150 thaler. His contract ran for six years.[31] The city likewise engaged his immediate successors on its own authority and under very similar terms, although their wages and the duration of their contracts varied. Friedrich Spiess was appointed in 1610 for a term of only three years, receiving 80 thaler yearly in addition to "suitable lodgings, or lacking these, 20 thaler in coin." The city council renewed his contract under identical conditions in 1613. His successor, Peter Fincci, earned 130 thaler plus housing. When the position was again filled in 1640, it was apparently a probationary appointment: Viktor Gregor's initial contract ran for only a single year, and he was paid a mere 50 thaler. When the city renewed his contract in 1642, this time for a three-year term, the magistrates raised his salary by 70 thaler. The last physicus selected directly by the magistrates was Laurentius Giseler, who contracted for a term of five years. He earned 100 thaler, collected another 20 thaler for housing, and exercised the right to "draw [each year] a *Wispel* [about 24 bushels] of rye free" from the municipal granary.[32]

Unfortunately, other than their names, and with the significant exception of Gieseler, we know very little about these men. We do not know why the city council selected them over their competitors, whether they fulfilled the expectations of their employers well or badly, or even, in some cases, exactly how long they remained, or the circumstances under which they left.

We know less about the physici of Wolfenbüttel, the city that served as the duke's residence until 1735. It is possible that the duke's body-physicians filled this post until the late 1730s. Significant documentation first exists on physici in Wolfenbüttel from around the middle of the eighteenth century, when the ducal government began appointing all physici—in cities and in the countryside.[33]

For the city of Helmstedt, the home of the ducal university since 1576, we have a more complete record. The position of physicus had existed in Helmstedt at least since 1652. From 1652 through 1808, nine men filled the post; four of the first six (through 1752) held only the licentiate of medicine, one, Voß, was a "candidate" (who, however, took his doctorate immediately before swearing his oath of office), and the status of another, Christian Richter, physicus from 1673 to 1676, is uncertain. The last three were all physicians with the academic degree of doctor. Despite the presence of a medical faculty at the university and several professors of medicine in the city, not one of these academics assumed the position of physicus. In fact, there was a clear distinction between *civic* physicians— that is, those who were members of the commune—and university professors, who were not.[34]

Helmstedt's city council chose all physici between 1652 and 1735. With the selection of Johann Voß in 1735, however, the city's right to choose its own physicus abruptly ended. By then, the reigning duke had regained most of the rights of sovereignty his predecessors had once bargained away. He, or rather his privy council, now exercised the exclusive right to appoint the physicus. In fact, Voß's appointment stirred up quite a conflict between city and territorial governments, with the magistrates in Helmstedt flatly refusing to pay Voß's salary. Although eventually a compromise was reached (the ducal government agreed to pay half of Voß's salary), Voß was a just a marker in the larger struggle between the duke and one of the cities he was seeking to pull more tightly under his sway. The privy council had come to regard the physici as servants of the duke, to be chosen by the privy council (later with the consultation and approval of the Collegium medicum), and to be sworn in as *ducal*, not municipal, officials.

The privy council and Collegium medicum exercised these prerogatives cautiously, however, and not only initially. Voß was, one thinks, a good choice for the city's first new-style physicus. His father, a surgeon and bathmaster in Helmstedt, had married the daughter of a prominent brewer in the city and acquired property there. Voß had studied medicine in Helmstedt. He was thus the son of a citizen and a property owner, boasting a background very similar to that of the men the city council had previously favored for the post. For instance, the father of the earliest physicus mentioned for Helmstedt, Johann Bosse, had sat on the city council. Dr. Bosse himself had studied medicine in Helmstedt. Physicus Just Kreyenberg had a similar history. Born in Helmstedt as the son of a wealthy merchant, he had also studied locally. In his application for the position of physicus, Kreyenberg stressed his civic affiliations and his status as "a local," to which the city council responded positively: it held *patria* to be the best guarantor of diligence and probity in office. Not all physici were homegrown, although many had studied in Helmstedt. Local ties, while not the sine qua non of office, helped a lot.

The Collegium medicum also kept such affiliations in mind when faced with numerous candidates for one job. While one might expect that a central bureaucracy would wish to avoid those with strong local affiliations, preferring men with no previous connections to the area as less biased civil servants, the Collegium knew better. Although the members of the Collegium and the privy council appreciated the advantages of impartiality, they were even more aware of the precariousness of the physicus's position in a community. The privy councilors and the members of the Collegium recognized that a man who was hated and resented had little chance of achieving any of the goals they cherished, and, as we shall see, they were generally circumspect in their choices, listening and at times yielding to suggestions and objections locals raised.

This does not mean, of course, that conflicts such as the one that brewed up between the magistrates in Helmstedt and the privy council over Voß did not occur: they were ubiquitous. The reasons for quarrels were legion, and pay was only the commonest note of discord. It is enough here to stress that the central government acknowledged its limitations. Caught up in the daily necessities of governing, privy councilors often felt the wisest and, in the long run, the most expedient route was that of least resistance. In a world of power relations and individual circumstances that dictated malleability and compromise rather than rigidity and fiat, negotiation was the byword of the day.

If the office of physicus had long existed in towns and cities, in the form of a contract between a doctor or licentiate of medicine and the city's magistracy, the buildup of a network of physici throughout the duchy first commenced in the 1690s. In 1696, the estates proposed creating the office of *medicus provincialus*, and including in his jurisdiction the Braunschweig and Wolfenbüttel districts.[35] The *medicus provincialus* was to work "for the preservation of the general health and prosperity of the subjects in the countryside." His duties—the estates had in mind appointing *one* man to cover this very large area—would extend to the supervision of the entire apparatus of rural medical care. He would be required to test the abilities of all those who practiced medicine in any form before they would be permitted to continue their practice in the area. He would visit and supervise all the apothecaries and draft appropriate pharmacopoeias for them. He was to investigate all "contagious diseases, such as intermittent and petechial fevers, throat distempers, bloody fluxes, and similar sicknesses," as well as all "dangerous wounds and murders." In his forensic capacity, he also would perform the *cadaveris dissectio* criminal law mandated. In order to combat sudden outbreaks of serious diseases more expeditiously, the *medicus provincialis* should carry along with him a "traveling apothecary chest," and he was to be granted a special right to dispense medicines from it. If necessary, he was permitted to send a "skilled medicus" as his substitute. He was enjoined to treat "high and low, rich and poor" alike and to conduct himself so as to offend "neither God nor conscience."[36]

On 26 March 1696, the ducal government drafted instructions for a physicus that adhered closely to the recommendations of the estates. "Especially in times of dangerous and infectious diseases," he was "to [aid] our loyal subjects . . . in the countryside, [who] out of poverty, simplicity and negligence fail to employ expedient means [and thus needlessly] sacrifice their health and their lives."[37] These precepts eventually formed the general guidelines for all physici appointed in the duchy throughout the eighteenth century, although, of course, the physicus's duties became more numerous and encompassing as time passed and as the network expanded.

Besides sketching out general principles, the ducal government took the more practical step of arranging a salary for its provincial physicus, allotting him 90 thaler.[38] By early 1696, the government had hammered out a scheme providing for the appointment and salarying of at least one physicus. But the plan misfired, and not until 1714—and almost certainly as a result of the last great plague epidemic to shake northern Germany—

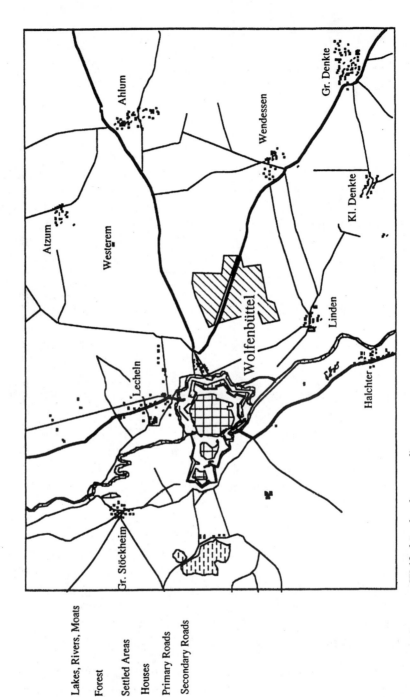

Wolfenbüttel and surroundings

Legend

Lakes, Rivers, Moats

Forest

Settled Areas

Houses

Primary Roads

Secondary Roads

did the privy council actually select Rudolf Held to fill the post. His "district" stretched over the whole of the Wolfenbüttel and Schöningen regions, including three towns (Königslutter, Schöningen, Schöppen-stedt) and all the areas surrounding them. One expected Held to carry out a "health visitation" much on the model of the religious visitations introduced in the sixteenth century. The government assessed a certain amount on each locality to cover Held's salary, which totaled 250 thaler, plus 50 thaler expenses.[39]

Over the next few months, protests rolled in; each community objected at having to contribute to Held's salary. Amt Bettmar, for instance, reminded the ducal government of "the anxious and truly miserable, worrisome times [we live in]." "Our situation is such," the Amt continued, "that most of us hardly have our daily bread in our homes; much land has remained unplanted for lack of seed; we can no longer pay the ordinary taxes, let alone this new impost. Moreover, we do not use this doctor, but rely on home remedies [to cure] our ills, as did our fathers before us."[40] The government's response to these supplications, and to the reality that the localities simply did not pay up, was to fire Held, effectively abolishing the post. Nothing indicates that Held had not performed up to the expectations of the privy council. The document releasing him cited the obstacles encountered in raising his salary as the sole reason for terminating his contract.[41] In fact, when Held complained in 1715 that, despite having served as physicus for almost a full year, he had received only less than a quarter of what was due him, the privy council pushed the localities for payment. By September 1715, Held had received (almost) all his back pay.[42]

The initial attempt to create a system for dispensing medical care and providing medical supervision in the countryside thus skidded to an ignominious halt. Thwarted by the intransigence of local authorities, which the central government either could not or did not want to break, the provincial physicus disappeared almost as soon as he came into being. That no effective means of paying him could be worked out was fatal, but the whole idea was ill-conceived. If—and this was doubtful—one person might indeed be able to cover the duchy, perhaps at a bare minimum regularly visiting apothecaries and examining medical personnel, it was totally unrealistic to expect him to monitor outbreaks of disease and function as a doctor to rural communities. Such a roving official offered perhaps the worst of all possible worlds. He could not fulfill the tasks the privy council envisioned for him, and, because he was constantly on the move, never had the chance of becoming part of a community, of winning the trust of locals, or of settling down as property owner and taxpayer; he remained the worst kind of outsider.

When the privy council tried again in the 1740s, it modified the old plan in some striking ways. Most important, it decided to appoint several physici and to settle them permanently in their districts. This second attempt was an integral part of efforts to revive the medical ordinance of 1721.[43] Yet it would be mistaken to assume that physici did not exist between 1715 and the 1740s. Cities continued to select their own physici. As the ducal government reacquired its sovereign rights over various cities (Braunschweig in 1671; Helmstedt by 1735), however, those cities forfeited their *jus nominendi* in regard to a number of offices, including that of physicus. Thus long before the medical ordinance of 1747 went into effect, the ducal government was regularly designating physici. There were physici even in the smaller towns and in the countryside, although the extent of their duties and the method of their appointment remain unclear.

Dr. Georg Hieronymi, for example, assumed the office of physicus for Wolfenbüttel and its environs in 1739.[44] Similarly, there was a physicus in the Weser district from at least 1723 on. A Dr. Bismarck was appointed physicus in 1738, and when he died the following year, Amtmann Hantelmann in Holzminden (the governmental seat for the Weser district) passed on suggestions for possible replacements to the ducal privy council. Hantelmann's top choice, and the eventual appointee, was Dr. Johann Wachsmuth, a Halle-educated physician who had published several articles on panaceas.[45]

Apparently only in the Weser and in the Harz districts were physici regular features of the administrative landscape before 1743. In that year, the treasury proposed creating similar physici for the other two administrative districts, Wolfenbüttel and Schöningen. These districts eventually proved far too cumbersome for one man to manage,[46] and over the next thirty years, they were split up and reorganized, significantly multiplying the number of physici. The Wolfenbüttel district had existed in one form or another before 1743, but in 1743 it was rearranged. The Schöningen district was first created in 1744. The duties specified for the new physicus in Schöningen, Dr. Johann Centner, paralleled those incumbent on Held some thirty years earlier. Centner was promised a salary of 40 thaler, "which includes [compensation for] the performance of the *inspectiones* and *sectiones* that need be done in these Ämter, for which he will receive nothing [extra] except transportation to be provided through the corvée."[47] The general regulations that pertained to the other districts of the Weser, Harz, and, now, Schöningen, were likewise extended to the Wolfenbüttel district.[48]

The duties of all these physici, as well as their relationships with local authorities and with the central government, can perhaps best be understood by examining the instructions local authorities received about these newfangled officials.[49] Such guidelines, while they mirror reality only imperfectly, delineated the general space in which the physici moved. They also highlight the points where conflicts and controversies would arise. For example, the circular the privy council sent to all the authorities in the Harz district in 1743 specified the Amt's responsibilities vis-à-vis the new physicus, as well as reminding them of their more general obligations in the administration of public health.[50] In 1749, the government repeated these instructions, and extended them to all physicates and Ämter in the duchy.[51] At the same time, perhaps unwittingly, the privy council initiated a conflict over privileges, prerogatives, finances, and bookkeeping that would nag at the physici and the Collegium medicum throughout the century.

Dr. Conrad Blum was the first physicus appointed to the Harz district under this new regime, and in spelling out his assignments and the duties of the authorities in the realm of medical police, the privy council began to elaborate a rudimentary public health network for the duchy. These principles would remain intact throughout the eighteenth century and into the opening decades of the next century. "When dangerous or very contagious diseases appear in your districts," the local authorities were ordered to send a "detailed report" to Dr. Blum, and to inquire of him whether and when he wished to inspect the place where the outbreak occurred. The locality had to supply him with transportation, usually a horse, which the commune should pay for if the patient(s) could not. Sending a horse meant that a peasant had to place an animal at the doctor's disposal as part of his corveé. Peasants resented this as a novel, and therefore improper, demand, and local authorities realized that peasant manpower used in this way was unavailable for other tasks. Nobody much liked the idea. Similarly, the Amt was to pay for the medicines the physicus ordered. If patients could reimburse the local treasury, that was fine, but for paupers, the locality was accountable. Here was where the difficulties began, spawning bitter and often absurdly protracted arguments over who should pay for what, how much, and when. *Every* physicus got

bogged down in these almost unending struggles over the disbursement of
his salary or, just as commonly, for the cost of the medicines and care he
dispensed, and for the transportation costs he incurred. Physici rarely
found the assistance they wanted or needed, often waiting in vain for
peasants to show up with horses and carts. Physici waited even longer to
be reimbursed for costs they incurred when they hired transport on their
own. Likewise, the room and board that localities were supposed to offer
was rarely forthcoming.[52]

The government never regulated the whole business adequately. When
the mechanism concocted in the 1740s quickly proved very unsatisfactory, the privy council tried a new one. It was far too easy for the community to dodge the responsibility of providing transport. Authorities could
complain about peasant recalcitrance; peasants could protest that such
duties exceeded their obligations; and the whole conflict could bounce
around for months, even years, defying any resolution. The new rules set
up a per diem of two thaler intended to cover all costs, which was to be
paid by the community.[53] This was supposed to streamline the whole
procedure, but it merely created new quandaries. The physici experienced exactly the same problems collecting their per diem as they had
when they had submitted detailed bills, and communities—which now
bore all of the costs incurred—became even more reluctant to inform a
physicus of a medical emergency or to request his services. Authorities
had to justify such expenditures to their communities and often chose not
to raise such bones of contention, especially when the physicus did not
reside in the village or town. Thus, both the physicus and the central
government could very easily be kept in the dark about outbreaks of
disease. And although the responsible men were often (although not
invariably) ducal officials, that link in no way secured their eager cooperation and good will. Amtmänner were appointed by the ducal government
and were as such, technically, its creatures, yet they exercised a certain
independence of action, partly made possible by their distance from the
center, but also surely in fact necessitated by their need to work with a
community, as well as by the various economic, social, and familial ties
they forged over time.

Concealing suspicious outbreaks of disease could be motivated by fear
of financial losses should news leak out that a deadly disease gripped a
community. The situation was, however, far more embroiled. The poor
were not necessarily most opposed to the "interference" of a physicus, for
the commune was responsible for their care. Wealthier peasants, those

who paid higher taxes, less willingly countenanced the presence of someone who cost them money. Internal divisions within a community could result in someone informing the physicus or privy council directly that procedures were being flouted. Sometimes pastors were informants. Less altruistic reasons also played a role; a charge of negligence was the perfect weapon for would-be troublemakers. Such problems persisted and perhaps even worsened after the privy council began to extend the network of physicates in the 1750s.

In 1743, then, city physici were to be found in Braunschweig, Wolfenbüttel, Helmstedt, and Königslutter, and country physici in the four large districts: Schöningen, Wolfenbüttel, Harz, and Weser. While the life of the physici in cities was by no means without adversity, the position of these four district physici was wholly unworkable. By placing the physici "on call," the central government essentially made them dependent on the cooperation of local authorities, which seldom materialized. Furthermore, the districts sprawled so widely that a physicus often encountered obstacles in traveling where he was needed; he could easily be caught in one place when his help was required elsewhere. Moreover, it proved virtually impossible for him to carry out the broader supervisory tasks the government foresaw for him. Consequently, the privy council soon began to create new physicates, or to split up the older ones, eventually quadrupling the number of physici and their districts from four in 1743 to sixteen by 1808.[54] It also became an occasional practice to appoint adjuncts or subphysici to assist men grown old in office, or whose districts presented special challenges.[55]

The story of how the Weser district was split in twain began in 1754 when the ageing physicus Johann Wachsmuth requested that young Dr. Carl Struve be appointed his adjunct and designated his successor. Although still quite inexperienced (he had received his doctorate from Jena just two years before), Struve appeared a desirable candidate in many ways. A member of the scientific society in Mainz, he had already contributed to a learned journal in Erfurt. While Wachsmuth admitted that two physicians would be hard put to support themselves in Holzminden, he nonetheless pushed the young man's case zealously. Struve, Wachsmuth pointed out, could spend his time writing and tutoring pupils in mathematics and philosophy at the newly established cloister school in Holzminden. Having a second physician in Holzminden promised other advantages: a medical society could be constituted; more work would be generated for the apothecary; he could substitute for Wachsmuth; and last but not least, Struve would make an excellent husband for Wachsmuth's only daughter. Struve's appointment went through. As adjunct, he earned a minimal salary of 30 thaler, with which he had to make do, despite much grumbling, until Wachsmuth died in 1757. But then things did not proceed as Struve and Wachsmuth had desired. The promise of a smooth transition was frustrated by the recommendation of Amtmann Wilcke in Stadtoldendorf, who wished to divide the Weser district. Wilcke argued, plausibly, that the size of the district exceeded the ability of one man to handle, and he proposed that the region be rearranged into two smaller physicates, with seats in Holzminden and Stadtoldendorf. Dismayed at the prospect of his future income fading by half, Struve quickly protested, charging Wilcke with favoritism: "Under a contrived motive he seeks his own interests in trying to split the district and to play part of it off into the hands of Dr. Kahle in Stadtoldendorf. Dr. Kahle, however, is neither a *litteratus* nor a member of a scientific academy, but rather wastes his time making porcelain and writing poetry, lives a disreputable life, and is in no way capable . . . of running a physicate." All this availed Struve little. The privy council divided the district in 1759. Struve received the new Holzminden physicate, while a Dr. Hoffmann became physicus for Stadtoldendorf.[56]

The creation of new physicates presented equally great problems in those parts of the duchy that retained special rights and privileges; rights and privileges that the Collegium medicum and the privy council were reluctant or perhaps unable to dispute. In 1782, for example, the recently licensed Dr. Maximilian, then resident in Blankenburg, sought the post of physicus in Hasselfelde, requesting a hefty salary of 200 thaler and the right to dispense medicines. The privy council apparently felt Maximilian's petition possessed enough merit to follow it up with the local authorities. In particular, the council wondered if giving Maximilian the right to deal in medicines would contravene any existing privileges, and whether the government in Hasselfelde would be able to provide him with an adequate salary.[57] Officials in Hasselfelde quickly said yes to the first query and no to the second. Granting Maximilian the right to dispense medicines would interfere with the privileged apothecary in Hasselfelde, whose concession prohibited the intrusion of any rival. The authorities quoted chapter and verse of teritorial law to the privy council, a law that forbade physicians from dispensing in order to avoid undercutting the business of the apothecaries.[58]

Local officialdom in Hasselfelde admitted that, while a physicus in every Amt was theoretically desirable, it was not *faisable*. Hasselfelde could not finance a physicus; moreover, "the common man [here] seldom consults a physician, and when he is forced to do so, can pay him only very little." The report referred back to the experience of a Dr. Kratzenstein, who had functioned as physicus in Hasselfelde from 1751 to 1761, and who, despite a 30-thaler salary, was unable to sustain himself. The prospects for a physician in Hasselfelde had dimmed since then, "for there are enough physicians in the surrounding area, who have won [people's] trust . . . and who are consulted in illness."[59]

Clearly preferring to husband its resources and spend its money in other ways, the Amt sketched out plans for repairs to public buildings, for poor relief, for stone chimneys to be constructed, for fire fighting, and for the diversion of a mountain stream to fountains and reservoirs in the town—all projects to which it attached a higher priority than to the appointment of a physicus. Faced with such obduracy, the privy council backed down and decided not to appoint a physicus in Hasselfelde just then.[60]

The debate on establishing a physicate in Hasselfelde was first raised by an individual's desire for such a post. It is indicative of the workings of the central government that even this late in the century, such petitions formed the basis for action. And if the attempt to establish a physicus in Hasselfelde failed in 1782, it would succeed in 1797–98, when an individual once again set the machinery grinding into motion.

In 1797, Johann Vibrans had been physicus in Königslutter for about a year when he requested a transfer to Hasselfelde. He complained that "the concession granted Dr. Samuel Hahnemann [the founder of homeopathic medicine] to dispense his patent remedies," had rendered him "breadless."[61] This reanimated the idea of appointing a physicus in Hasselfelde, and the Collegium medicum once more set to work. What did the local authorities in Hasselfelde think now? Although still not thrilled with the idea, and still pleading poverty—the fire of 1794 had played the very devil with local finances—they responded in a more conciliatory fashion: if the size of the physicate were expanded to include surrounding areas, a physicus's private practice *might* serve to support him—but the Amt could contribute only 30 thaler to his salary.[62] After further deliberation, the privy council appointed Vibrans, mandating a salary of 100 thaler, plus seventeen cords of hardwood for fuel and nine shocks of wheat.[63] Vibrans decided to stay in Königslutter after all, however. Dr. Hahnemann had just put his house up for sale, and Vibrans awaited his imminent departure.

With something of an exasperated sigh, one imagines, the privy council selected another man for Hasselfelde.[64]

A pattern thus emerges. Individual cases spurred the central government into action, but the government's ability to create physicates or appoint physici was always limited. Local people sometimes raised objections that the privy council and the Collegium medicum felt powerless, or at least reluctant, to override. Some of this hesitation arose from an inability to propose suitable alternatives. Although the central government always provided some part of the physicus's salary, it was unwilling—and after the financial debacles of the late 1760s unable—to pay it all. Local treasuries were the only other feasible sources of money for a physicus's salary. Yet the arguments of impecuniousness swayed the privy council, partly because they were true (especially after the Seven Years' War), but also because the privy council thought in terms of the general financial stability of a locality, a financial stability and an economic equilibrium that often forced specific programs to be modified, eviscerated, or simply abandoned altogether in name of the greater good.

This pattern at best roughly and partially corresponded to a more complex reality. For instance, it would be wrong to believe that the impetus for action always lay with the central government, which was then forced into bargaining with intransigent locals over technicalities such as salary. Sometimes the wish for a physicus developed within a community, and the Amt or local authorities pushed most vigorously for his appointment, although this was far more likely to happen toward the end of the century rather than at mid century. At least some localities had internalized the notion that the state was responsible for the welfare of its subjects and understood, indeed even fostered, the need for state intervention.

In 1794, for example, Superintendent Eggers laid out to the Collegium medicum the pressing need for a physicus in Harzburg. Eggers complained about the prevalence of quacks in his area, singling out Joseph Schmidt in the nearby village of Neustadt as a notorious example. Even the presence of a physician, Eggers admitted, would probably do little to stop Schmidt. In time of illness, locals either resorted to home remedies, visited Schmidt, or traipsed over to Goslar (outside Braunschweig-Wolfenbüttel) to consult physicians there. Eggers believed that a physicus might take business away from the quacks, could supervise the apothecary, and would prevent money from flowing out of the state. A doctor named Schrott resided in Harzburg, but Eggers deemed him unsuitable because he was "stubborn, arrogant . . . and not in the least able to please local inhabitants." The Collegium medicum agreed with Eggers's estimation, recognizing that the poor roads in the area, the distance the physicus in Seesen would have to travel to visit patients, and the need to attack "rampant quackery" all dictated the appointment of a physicus. Again the complication was payment, and that hurdle more than anything else contributed to the tardiness with which the appointment proceeded. Perhaps the Collegium medicum was waiting for Schrott to die or move away. When the Collegium finally dispatched Johann Welge as physicus to Harzburg in 1799, he received a pitiful salary of only 30 thaler.[65]

Certainly, there is enough evidence to suggest that by the end of the century, some districts, or rather some people in many districts, had begun to assert a right to a physicus—especially, one gathers, if they did not have to pay him, or pay him much. For instance, in June 1794, Pastor J. F. Altenburg in the town of Bisperode near Stadtoldendorf wrote to jog the memory of the Collegium medicum; the man who had been appointed physicus some months earlier, Wilhelm Borges, remained on maneuvers with the Prussian army. Dysentery had broken out in Bisperode, and Altenburg knew of no one to whom patients could turn, other than the local apothecary, Laurentius, "or those without expertise." In December, he repeated his plea, which was this time signed by the magistrates and local notables (a total of fifteen persons), all of whom pointed out that Borges obviously had no real interest in the post: he had been appointed in March 1794 and had yet to be seen in Stadtoldendorf. They reminded the Collegium that they lacked all medical assistance, and that Dr. Eicke in Eschershausen, who had been delegated interim physicus for Stadtoldendorf, had proven of little use during the current epidemic of putrid fever. They complained that "he [took] no pains about them" and visited them "only very seldom." Not only did the citizens of Stadtoldendorf wish to see the position filled, they also put forward their own candidate, a certain Dr. Härtel in Alfeld.[66] Their demands demonstrated that they had a definite sense of state obligation to localities. Their comments about both Borges and Eicke likewise articulated strong feelings about the proper conduct of physicians.

Qualifications and Appointments

By the middle of the eighteenth century, the power to appoint a physicus lay exclusively with the privy council. The Collegium medicum suggested candidates, evaluated their abilities, and then forwarded its recommendations to the council. The council generally heeded the advice of the Collegium, but not always. When the Collegium selected 29-year-old Dr. Stolze as the new physicus in Stadtoldendorf, for example, the council objected and required the Collegium to subject Stolze to a "more rigorous examination" (it seems possible that the Collegium had appointed Stolze without seeing or examining him). During this second examination, held in August 1755, Stolze responded poorly. He was unable to answer questions posed in Latin, and his knowledge was judged by the Collegium to be "mediocre" at best. On the basis of this miserable report, the privy council concluded, "[T]his physicus is not of the quality that one can trust him . . . with [the] health of so many people. You [the Collegium] are to inform him that he must seek another post and leave his present position."[67]

While the Collegium medicum exercised the official consultative role, the privy council solicited local authorities as well both for names of candidates and for their reactions to the candidates submitted by the Collegium. The process of selection thus involved negotiations among the three groups, with the occasional "interference" of others, such as pastors, abbesses, widows of high-ranking officers, and nobles.

A vacancy (most often caused by death) set the machinery in motion. Almost immediately after the death or departure of a physicus (and sometimes before!), applicants besieged the Collegium medicum and the privy council with their petitions. The list of candidates typically included a range of fresh-baked doctors, physici from other places who hoped to better themselves, and doctors from outside the territory. There were always several candidates for each post, even for the least inviting and least lucrative ones. As early as 1745, Dr. Behrens, found that in Braunschweig, one could not speak of a dearth of physicians; rather, there was "such an overwhelming number of them as never before."[68] An examination of their applications reveals quite a bit about the qualifications supposed desirable, and about the self-understanding and self-representation of the candidates. The letters often contained personal and individualized information, but they tended to emphasize a series of attributes and present a certain picture of the candidate. A guiding ideal of what qualified a man for the office and, fully as important, what justified his claim to the position shaped the petitions. A case from 1766 illustrates some of these points, while documenting the life story and early career of a man who served as physicus in Helmstedt for over forty years.

In 1766, Friedrich Meyer, a 37-year-old native of Osnabrück, requested the right to practice medicine in the duchy. He had studied in Gießen and received his doctor's degree from Göttingen.[69] His petition recounted his skills as well as his personal history:

After having worked as *medicus* in several lazarettes, I settled in the town of Lauterberg am Harz in Schartzfeld and have been practicing there since 1759. Before Schartzfeld was fully destroyed [during the war], I managed to find my living in this area although only just barely. Since then, however, as the last war greatly impoverished the place and its inhabitants, . . . it became so that no physician could survive there: so I turned to the government of the Kingdom of Hannover to seek some improvement.

There were, however, at that time no vacancies in Hannover and as it is no longer possible for me to maintain myself in this miserable place, where I have been forced to sell many of my possessions, so I have determined to seek my living elsewhere. Now I aspire to set myself up [in practice] in Your Excellency's lands, especially because my nearest relatives live in the city of Braunschweig. [However], I have learned from Drs. Brückmann and Seebode that there is no shortage of physicians in Braunschweig. [I] also understand that [only] an old, no longer active medicus is to be found in Schöningen, and that the inhabitants wish to see another physician move there. . . . I request that I be allowed to go to Schöningen, settle there, and practice medicine.[70]

Little happened for many months, but in September Meyer retracted his petition after learning that the physicus in Schöningen was still alive, and that, as he discovered, his earnings would probably be insufficient to support him.[71]

By October 1766, things had changed to benefit Meyer. In July 1766, Johann Lange, physicus in Helmstedt since 1757, left the city to assume the better post of physicus in Lüneburg. A position was now vacant, and applications quickly flowed in, from Meyer and other physici. In November, the privy council named Meyer to the post, allotting him a salary of 85 thaler.[72]

There is nothing particular unusual about either Meyer's petition or the privy council's decision. Meyer possessed all the general qualifications: a respectable degree, considerable experience, a good reputation. Meyer's petition reveals as well the way in which so many applicants shaped their pleas. Meyer stressed his academic and medical qualifications, but also, and just as prominently, his need. He could, he insisted, no longer maintain himself and his family without a more remunerative position, and he clearly expected this logic to work favorably on the privy council. He was equally careful to avoid the impression that his motives were solely monetary. Yes, he needed money to survive, especially as he had just started a family, but he also underscored (repeating it twice) that he was not greedy; he had been satisfied with a "scanty" income in Schartzfeld and had only considered leaving when "scanty" shrank to "nonexistent." Likewise, his mention of kin in Braunschweig was calculated: the information that his relatives lived there suggested that reputable members of the community (one assumes they were) would vouch for him, and also that he could draw upon their assistance in terms of money and connections. In addition, he pointed out that the wish for another physicus in Schöningen had already been independently registered by the inhabitants, and that he would thus be welcomed and not viewed as an intruder. These themes are endlessly repeated in almost all the petitions received by the privy council or Collegium medicum from physicians seeking government-controlled posts. The physicians had not reasoned wrongly: as two further examples from Blankenburg illustrate, the deliberations of the Collegium and council turned, if not exclusively, on like considerations when they weighed candidates' qualifications.[73]

The physicate in Blankenburg was a "splendid post."[74] An independent principality that had often served as a mini-fiefdom for younger sons, or as a residence for dowager duchesses, Blankenburg was also the preferred summer home of the court. It was a fairly populous place, with over 11,000 inhabitants in 1793, and had suffered little in the Seven Years' War, thanks to a useful marital connection between the Habsburgs and one of the duke's daughters.[75] Compared to his occupational peers, the physicus in Blankenburg enjoyed an excellent salary.[76] The possibility of treating members of the court, the faintly cosmopolitan atmosphere, and the admitted enticement of a princely salary dictated that competition for the Blankenburg post would be fierce.

In 1767, Dr. Johann Schulze, physicus in Blankenburg since 1761, left to take up a post at Clausthal in Hannover.[77] Schulze must have been offered a very nice position indeed to turn his back on what he already had in Blankenburg. From ducal funds, he received, besides fuel, 164 thaler. Other sources added to this an additional 200 thaler, raising his total income (without counting his private practice) to 364 thaler. One supplicant was Dr. Georgi, who had been subphysicus in Blankenburg since 1762. Georgi felt he had served his probationary period and was owed the post.[78] When the privy council consulted the magistrates in Blankenburg, however, their conclusions were not promising: "[A]lthough we do not doubt his medical knowledge, we submit that he has not the requisite experience, and the discernment that comes with it, to carry out [such] important duties."[79] The council hardly lacked other candidates. Besides Georgi's application and that of the ultimately successful candidate, Dr. Philip Sandart, two physici in Braunschweig-Wolfenbüttel, two doctors in Braunschweig, one in Wolfenbüttel, and two physicians from outside the duchy's borders had applied.[80] The council decided to offer the post to Johann Pott, then secretary of the Collegium medicum, at a salary of 224 thaler. Politely yet firmly, Pott refused, insisting that while 224 thaler represented a fine salary for a young physician with little practice, in his circumstances not less than 300 thaler yearly could induce him to leave Braunschweig. He knew Blankenburg was not "so promising as it seems to be on the surface." So while Pott remained in Braunschweig, Sandart went to Blankenburg, where he remained until his death in 1785.[81]

The play repeated itself when Sandart's successor in office, Dr. Friedrich Krebs, died of a "nervous fever" in 1793, leaving a very pregnant widow and five young children in "not the most advantageous economic circumstances."[82] Georgi was still around, but his reputation had not improved over the years. The magistrates now regarded him as a "weak and dull man," who had, moreover, pretty much abandoned medicine. This made the appointment of a "suitable physicus" all the more imperative, as did the onset of spring, with its myriad diseases.[83] Throughout May 1793, applications rolled in from physicians both within the duchy and from outside. J. Schiller, physician in Quedlinburg, stressed that he was "a born Blankenburger" and had studied medicine in Helmstedt. He had been practicing for seven years in Quedlinburg, where "my conduct and indefatigable diligence [have] won me popular acclaim." He asked the privy council to allow him to return to his birthplace, to "bring with me the money that has come to me from my wife, and serve the public."[84] Dr. Christian Loeber, then physicus in Vorsfelde, focused on his poverty. He longed to leave Vorsfelde, and move, preferably to Blankenburg, although he would consider other appointments: "In the three years I have been here in Vorsfelde, even though I live as simply as possible, I have eaten up all my substance, except for 300 thaler; and [my practice] among the locals is severely restricted by the prevalent quackery of the apothecary Röhle."[85] Other candidates included Dr. Reese, at that time physicus in Königslutter; Dr. J. C. Fahner, physicus to the county of Hohestein in Prussian territory; Dr. Friedrich May in Goslar; and Dr. Heinrich Apfel, then physicus in Stadtoldendorf. The deliberations of the Collegium medicum on these several candidates illustrate some of the principles that it followed in selecting physici.

Obviously, competence topped every list, but many men possessed an adequate degree of that. Almost equally valuable was a good reputation, and reputation meant far more than acclaim as a physician. Reputation included lifestyle; one had to be Christian and God-fearing, to be sure, but one also needed an adaptable personality, bespeaking an ability to fit into a community and win local respect. This could be, and was, judged from a man's previous record. For example, in the deliberations on replacing the physicus in Calvörde in 1803, the Collegium medicum considered two candidates unsuitable: Dr. Christian Ziegler for his "suspicious lifestyle" and Dr. Reinbeck because of "the notorious connection he [maintains] with that incorrigible medical quack the charcoal-burner Schmidt in Harzburg."[86] Similarly, in 1789, the Collegium was forced to choose between several candidates to replace the physicus in Holzminden. In many respects, Dr. Johann Dedekind (whose life story will concern us at greater length later in this chapter), then physicus in Königslutter, outstripped the rest of the field, "because he is one of the most senior physici . . . and there is no cause to doubt his medical knowledge." Yet he had "a bad reputation, he is stubborn, and at times unfair, but perhaps his great poverty has led him to make such mistakes, and if his position were improved, he might shed these faults." Dr. Rudelstaedter, a physician in Gandersheim, likewise possessed good practical experience and theoretical knowledge, although the Collegium was reluctant to recommend him because of his "coarse manner."[87] And physici were careful to protect their reputations from the slightest taint of impropriety, even that spread by petty gossip. Dr. Blum in Lutter am Barenberge prepared to take the wife of Pastor Baumgarten to court for spreading rumors about him, in particular, that Blum had accepted a bribe from the schoolmaster to conceal his syphilis.[88]

Diligence in executing the affairs of office was another desideratum, although other factors weighed in to tip the scales. For the Blankenburg post, the Collegium medicum noted that "native and foreign physicians have applied in great numbers," and the Collegium specified its preference for the former. It was, the Collegium insisted, often hard to judge the capabilities of men with whom its members were not personally acquainted. Relying on written testimony had its problems. In addition, the Collegium argued that it was "not expedient to prefer foreign over local physicians, for in this case we would soon lack diligent physici in the smaller towns if they no longer had any expectation of a future improvement [in their positions]."[89] The privy council often explicitly promised a physicus, as it pledged to Dr. Küster (the newly appointed physicus to the poor district of Calvörde) in 1788, that if there were another vacancy, it would "take him especially into account."[90] And the possibility of losing a man who despaired of promotion was quite real. When the position of physicus in Holzminden opened up in 1789, one of the unsuccessful candidates was Dr. Johann Schroll, who had been physicus in Vorsfelde since 1787. He now asked to be freed from his duties: "I can no longer deceive myself with baseless hopes, and, as I cannot exist here, am forced . . . to plead for my release from office." The privy council granted his request, and Schroll (like many others) set off for St. Petersburg to seek his fortune.[91]

All these factors came into play during the debate over candidates for the Blankenburg post. Dr. Martini, dean of the Collegium medicum, clarified his priorities. His first choice was Dr. Reese, because of his record of service with the Prussian army, and because he had a "good name" in Königslutter as physicus. "This man," Martini concluded, "not only commands the necessary skills . . . but also the praiseworthy qualities of diligence, zeal, and humanitarianism." As to Dr. Schiller, Martini felt he "could not be considered" because the magistrates in Blankenburg raised objections. Furthermore, "I know nothing about his qualifications [as a physician]." Dr. May was, Martini felt, a "skillful physician, but it is doubtful whether he would be satisfied with the proposal . . . that he share the physicate with another man at a salary of only 224 thaler." Neither Reese nor May agreed to these terms. May had an ample income. Reese, who earned no more than 75 thaler in Königslutter, apparently did not think the move worth the minor improvement in salary.[92]

And so back to square one. If May was uninterested, then the Collegium medicum suggested appointing Dr. Apfel, who had been physicus in Stadtoldendorf for over twelve years and had managed to make a living there despite the "well-known difficulties in the life of a practicing physician." Apfel desired the post in Blankenburg not least "so that I might better be able to educate my children." He stipulated a salary of 350 thaler, without which

I believe it is more advisable for me to remain in Stadtoldendorf and to withdraw my application. . . . My reasons are . . . the following: First, it is well known that each change of residence for a physician is a risky step . . . especially when he moves to a place that does not lack for physicians. Second, I am convinced that in Blankenburg, a place with about 350 households and hardly more than 2,300 inhabitants, and where several physicians live nearby . . . I would not find myself in as good circumstances as I enjoy here in Stadtoldendorf. . . . Third, I have many reasons to be satisfied with my life here and in seven years have bought my own house and other pieces of property, [and] . . . by selling or trying to rent my property, as well as in all other ways, I must fear great [financial and personal] damage.[93]

Apparently Apfel's remarks were not mere posturing; his first refusal served him well in the long run, and when he was finally appointed physicus in Blankenburg on New Year's Eve 1793, he got a salary of over 300 thaler.[94]

These examples illustrate the criteria that determined the choice of a physicus. First, the privy council and the Collegium medicum were unable or unwilling to impose their will either on physici or on local governments. The selection of a physicus followed a meandering course and involved prolonged bargaining. The privy council always took the complaints and preferences of the locality seriously, and even if the locals did not always get what they wanted, their wishes were never waved aside as immaterial or unimportant. Physici, too, exerted leverage: they called on friends, relatives, and patrons to assist them; they presented testimony in their behalf from places they had been or where they wished to go; and they haggled about salary. They could exercise a range of other options, and could, for example, move out of a patronage relationship with the duchy and into the service of another (they hoped) kinder and more generous lord. Several went to Russia in search of just these benefits. Second, the content and rhetoric of the negotiations took place within a larger governmental framework and governing mentality. Both the Collegium medicum and the privy council, and the latter in particular, always considered the viability of a community as a whole and were unwilling to disturb an existing (and often frail) balance by inserting a disturbing influence in the person of an unwanted and contentious physicus. Thus, the privy council was especially concerned about how well physici would fit—financially and socially, as well as medically—into the community. Third, the association between physici and the privy council was built on patronage and clientage networks, and, as in all such relationships, patrons were limited in their ability to grant or withhold favors, and clients were rarely impotent. Yet the physici regarded and represented themselves as clients of the government, and turned to the government first for assistance in a wide variety of instances. The reliance on patronage and the competition that the Collegium medicum fostered in physici, as well as the physicus's often precarious position in a locality, worked effectively against the formation of any strong sense of corporate or professional identity.

Objections

If questions of salary constituted the most frequent stumbling block to the appointment of a physicus in any locality, more than monetary concerns drove locals to resist the appointment of physici. Communities also protested against individuals, and based these objections overwhelmingly on the personalities and personal conduct of the men in question.

In May 1789, for example, the magistrates in Holzminden registered the death of "our only physician," Dr. Sievers, who had succumbed to a putrid fever. His loss weighed "heavily" on a town gripped by dual outbreaks of putrid fever and smallpox. The nearest physician lived "a good three hours away" in Stadtoldendorf. The magistrates wanted a quick replacement for Sievers and trusted that the privy council would "take proper care in replacing our loss with a skilled [man] and one of great experience, because Holzminden is the largest of the market towns in the duchy, and the physicate [is] rather profitable. [Because] no other physician lives anywhere in the vicinity, the person placed here will not suffer any competition for practice or for his [rightful] fees."[95]

By the end of May, several men had put forth their names for the post. Among these was Dr. Hellwig, a physician then practicing in Fürstenberg. He pointed out that, "because of the large number of poor people [here], medical practice . . . is not profitable and [it is] bound up with great financial disadvantages. I can prove that I have never received the least payment for most of the medicines I have distributed; my wage from the porcelain factory does not cover my expenses."[96] Apparently, the news of Hellwig's application spread rapidly to Holzminden, causing a public "sensation." Twenty-five prominent citizens protested. While these people raised no questions about Hellwig's "honesty and devotion," they suspected that Hellwig was too inexperienced to assume the role of "only physician for 9–10,000 people." Moreover, "everyone here knows that Dr. Hellwig after he abandoned the vocation for which he was trained, that of apothecary, and studied for a short time to receive his doctorate, was never able to earn his living by practicing medicine. About ten years ago, therefore, he took the post of controller at the ducal porcelain factory in Fürstenberg. . . . [which he received] principally so that he could serve in emergencies as physician and apothecary to the few factory workers in that secluded spot." He practiced little medicine there. The two notables residing in Fürstenberg never consulted him and preferred to call on a physician in Höxter or on Dr. Sievers in Holzminden.[97] In view of such vigorous opposition from the community, the privy council decided that Hellwig was not a suitable candidate for the position in Holzminden and continued the search.[98]

Likewise, earlier, when Dr. Johann Centner, physicus in Schöningen, died in 1769, he left behind a legacy of twenty-six years of generally harmonious relationships with the local authorities. In its request for a replacement, the Amt stressed how very popular Centner had been. He had died literally with his boots on. Despite his age and his infirmities, he had undertaken a strenuous trip to visit a patient in Salzdahlum, collapsing with a fatal stroke on his return. As much as the Amt had liked Centner, it disliked his adjunct, Dr. Johann Bühring, whose three-year stay in Schöningen had won him few friends and many enemies. "In his medical practice, as well as in social intercourse, he acts without discretion and has caused great misgivings to well up in everyone [here]." The magistrates in Schöningen presented similar objections, pointing out that Bühring had few patients "either among locals or foreigners"; nor had they seen "any evidence attesting his skill and experience." In short, neither the Amt nor the city's magistrates wanted Bühring as physicus. They preferred another Centner, but if that proved impossible at the moment, then they suggested that perhaps the apothecary Graf, "because of his long experience in *arte medica*," might be licensed to practice in the interim. This would also increase the apothecary's business.[99]

The recommendation of the Collegium medicum to the privy council reflected these concerns. The Collegium concluded that Bühring should probably not be appointed physicus in Schöningen, both because of the dissatisfaction of the local authorities, who wanted a more seasoned man, better versed in medicine, and because of the "lack of trust" the public showed. Consequently, Bühring did not get the post in Schöningen, but was sent to Vorsfelde, where he served as physicus until 1783.[100]

Similar objections stymied the appointment of Dr. Carl Spohr as physicus in Schöppenstedt in 1791. The village administrators and "the public" in Schöppenstedt were wary of the man, having heard "disturbing rumors" about Spohr's lack of practical experience, and, more alarming, "about his [suspect] character and morals." Amt Schöppenstedt expressed much satisfaction with its previous physicus, Dr. May. It praised May for his skill as a physician, his congeniality, and—tellingly—for his ability to draw business into the city, arguing that "the reputation . . . [of a physician like May has] a not inconsiderable impact on a city's economy" by attracting people and generating trade for the apothecary. One should not underestimate the force of such material motivations. Whereas the apothecary in a town could be the physicus's natural enemy, their relationship was basically symbiotic. The apothecary Hohmann in Stadtoldendorf added his plea to many others for the speedy replacement of the physicus in 1794. By April of that year, the post had gone unfilled for months, and Hohmann complained that "with no physician in the nearby area, my business is so bad that I earn absolutely nothing."[101] In its report to the privy council, the Collegium medicum insisted that no evidence supported the rumors about Spohr. The members of the Collegium uniformly regarded Spohr as a good and skillful physician. In the five years he had been in Seesen, they had received no complaints about him. And yet the privy council still passed over Spohr and appointed another man to Schöppenstedt.[102]

Local protests could also *promote* a candidate. An unusual incident in Schöningen in the mid 1770s illustrates how persistently locals maintained their own ideas as to who suited their needs and who did not. One can read out of their objections a sense of the qualities they desired in a physician as well. In March 1776, Dr. Georg Scheibner died, after being physicus in Schöningen for seven years. In the Amt's request for a replacement—"for the satisfaction of the local public, [to serve] . . . the [surrounding] countryside and the neighboring Prussian territories, for often patients from nearby places consult our physician"—the town administrator could not resist emphasizing the community's dissatisfaction with Scheibner, especially in his declining years. "We will not mention the justified complaints that . . . could be raised against him. [They do] not concern his medical skills . . . but touch on his religiously and morally reprehensible conduct. We did not [object before] because, on the one hand, we remonstrated with him, and, on the other, we could expect that his *curriculum vitae*, considering his delicate constitution, would soon run to an end."[103] This was an obvious and not so gentle slap at both the Collegium medicum and the privy council for appointing Schreibner in the first place.

Applications for Schreibner's position flowed in. One came from Dr. Johann Holdefreund, physicus in Königslutter from 1767 to 1769. Holdefreund then lived in Oschersleben (near Schöningen), and his petition remarked that it is "well known [that I have enjoyed] the trust of the entire

city of Schöningen and its surrounding area for the past twenty years."
The president of the Collegium medicum quickly quashed his application, noting that because Holdefreund had fled an investigation into
charges of adultery and incest, he certainly could not be considered for a
governmental position until the courts resolved the case. The Collegium
then appointed the 29-year-old Dr. Friedrich May.[104]

What here seems the end of the matter was in fact just the opening
salvo. Holdefreund would not let the matter drop and renewed his application with letters to the body-physician Wageler and the president of
the Collegium medicum, Privy Councilor von Flögen, arguing that he
had a "right" to some physicate, citing a promise made him when he first
went to Königslutter in 1767. He repeated his claim that he had won the
"love and trust" of those in the Schöningen district, and moreover, could
boast of drawing "annual honoraria" from numerous "distinguished persons" in the area.[105] And the town of Schöningen arrayed itself on Holdefreund's side. In November, the magistrates complained that May had not
yet arrived to take up his post and repeated their plea that Holdefreund—
"this talented and hard-working physician"—be appointed physicus instead, "as all the citizenry and entire region devoutly wish."[106] May excused his dillydallying, protesting that he had found it impossible to locate
suitable housing in Schöningen despite having made several trips there.[107]

The Collegium medicum found this dearth of housing "suspicious"
and very quickly cut to the heart of the predicament: the owners of empty
properties did not wish to rent or sell to Dr. May, "thus obliquely supporting the application of Dr. Holdefreund for the position of physicus in
Schöningen." Caught between a rock and a hard spot (the Collegium
could not after all force someone to deal with May), the Collegium
temporized, then compromised, eventually appointing neither May nor
Holdefreund to Schöningen, but Dr. Johann Dehne. May went to Schöppenstedt, and Holdefreund to court.[108]

In some areas, negotiations between center and periphery were especially thorny. The presence of the abbey in Gandersheim, for example,
added another dimension to patron-client relationships, since the abbess
belonged to the ducal family. When Physicus Conrad Blum died there in
1761, the Collegium medicum proposed moving Dr. Jacob Müller, then
in Seesen, to the more lucrative and attractive post of Gandersheim, thus
rewarding a physicus who had served several years in a small, poor post
with promotion to a better one, a procedure it was slowly developing in
these years as a precedent. To replace Müller in Seesen, the Collegium

suggested a young man, Friedrich Eicke, who had been practicing in
Gandersheim. There was a catch: what did the abbess think of these new
arrangements? Elisabeth Ernestine Antoinette was not amused.

I hope that Doctor Eicke can remain here so that I can [continue] to draw on his
wisdom and his medicines in the future. For the last two years he was Blum's
right-hand man, prepared Blum's prescriptions in [his mother's] apothecary, and
adhered faithfully to [Blum's] methods. Since Blum's death, [Eicke] has achieved
notable cures and won over almost all of Blum's clients and is already very
experienced in his practice. . . . [I would like, therefore, to see] that Dr. Eicke be
given the physicate here, as he was born here, raised here, has his property here,
and lives with his mother in the apothecary. As he previously learned the apothecary trade, he can continue to maintain the apothecary . . . which is already
one of the best in the land. Even foreigners prefer the medicines compounded
there . . . and His Royal Highness [her nephew], heir to the throne, has ordered
entire boxes of these medicines for the allied army and for his own troops. All this
will deteriorate and fall into disorder if Dr. Eicke leaves.[109]

Consequently, Eicke stayed in Gandersheim, becoming physicus with the
very modest salary of 65 thaler. The Collegium medicum reasoned that
because "so many people of means live[d] in or near Gandersheim," he did
not require as much as did physici in less remunerative spots such as Seesen.
And Dr. Müller, left in Seesen, also benefited: he received a new title, that
of first physicus in the Weser district, and, perhaps more useful, a higher
salary of 95 thaler.[110] Here, too, the Collegium was not pursuing firm
guidelines, but working out ad hoc solutions to everyday problems.[111]

Finding a Place

Achieving an appointment was, of course, only the initial step in a physicus's official life. Now he must assume his assigned responsibilities, while
simultaneously building a practice and finding a niche in the community.
This succession of events moves us into the *Alltag* of the physicus's life:
what happened once he was inserted into a community. His duties were
numerous, often onerous, sometimes impossible: he was to gather and
interpret information, monitor public health, track diseases, prepare a
number of reports at regular intervals, supervise surgeons, midwives, and
apothecaries, and function as forensic expert. The execution of each
of these tasks required the cooperation of various local authorities to a
greater or lesser extent.[112]

The position of the physicus was therefore a nodal point in early modern public health, although one situated in something of a geographical and cultural limbo. A physicus was in metaphoric terms the bureaucracy's sensitive fingertip placed on the pulse of public health. By casting the physicus exclusively in the role of bureaucrat, however, we set him too firmly in a bureaucratic hierarchy and risk losing track of the richer and more complex milieux that enveloped—and sometimes threatened to suffocate—him. It is also thereby too easy to overlook the fact that he fulfilled multiple roles in a community, roles that had little—often nothing—to do with medicine directly. These extraofficial and extramedical aspects of his life—his position as property owner and paterfamilias, as debtor and creditor, his propriety, his piety, his bearing, even his dress and mannerisms—largely determined whether his neighbors accepted him. The behavior of a medical officer in these, his several roles, conveyed potent social and cultural messages. Because medical practice lay deeply embedded in everyday routines and was poorly distinguished from other aspects of life, the relationship between patients and practitioners was as sharply contoured by perceptions of probity, common sense, and piety as by any objective weighing and measuring of the ability to cure or by careful calculation of costs.

In this world, lifestyle was never a matter safely left to individual volition. Personal traits were immediately and irrevocably situated in social, cultural, and moral frameworks and carried broader implications for the community and communal life. Villages and neighborhoods ran on face-to-face politicking, and a community judged its members in a multiplicity of roles, rarely filtering the doctor out from the father, from the property owner, from the churchgoer, from the debtor or creditor. Moreover, most communities were becoming increasingly locked into and dependent on regional and even global trade networks, and thus were no longer (if they had ever been) tight, homogeneous, and distrustful little knots of resistance to external pressures or innovations. This gradual "opening," a growing suppleness in what remained a somewhat stiff communal system, makes the eighteenth century pivotal.[113] Still, in this world, medical decision making continued to rest chiefly on broader judgments about the personal characteristics of healers, inclinations that seldom turned—and perhaps even today, rarely turn—solely or principally on medical variables. This comes perilously close to asserting that "medicine didn't matter" in the early modern world, or that it was not terribly important. That is not quite the intent. Instead, it must be stressed that *medical* practice in the eighteenth century was one element of many, was locked into complex series of relationships, and cannot be comprehended in more limited and exclusionist terms of "good" or "bad" or "enlightened" and "unenlightened" medicines.

The available documentation strikingly demonstrates how poorly many physici seem to have adapted to their communities. Clearly, there were exceptions: men who had won the trust and good will of their clients and fellow villagers, if perhaps only after years of struggle. This inability to adjust has often been blamed on insiders responding harshly to outsiders and strangers, or as unenlightened resistance to enlightening initiatives. Both interpretations need to be applied with great care and tact. Little, for example, tied the explicit rejection of enlightened medical programs to any prevailing sense of disapproval or dissatisfaction with a particular physicus by a community or group. And, despite the frequent, bitter complaints of physicians about the benightedness of peasants in respect to all aspects of health and medicine, there seems in fact to have been remarkably little concentrated resistance to the introduction of a whole series of what scholars have traditionally considered enlightened innovations. There was, for example, no frenzied reaction to the introduction of smallpox inoculation. Paradoxically, many physicians remained skeptical. Village councils cautiously calculated the costs of projects to improve water supplies, drain swamps, and clean up middens, to be sure, but seldom rejected them out of hand as either undesirable or pointless. Nor were they all fruitless.

The insider/outsider confrontation, which historians have frequently invoked to interpret the defiance of villagers in the face of innovations, or to explain the preference for local healers (variously quacks, wisewomen, and executioners) rather than "more qualified" outsiders, also has its limitations. Appeals to outside authority were common, and even habitual. Villagers called upon more distant mediators and sympathetic advocates to help them assert their rights or defend their positions against internal rivals. And finally, villagers and the common folk as a whole never avoided physicians with the rabid fear and intense distrust that medical pamphleteers and medical publicists fondly described, although admittedly patterns of serial or simultaneous consultation, which often sandwiched visits to a physician between trips to the cowherd and the apothecary, did not exactly correspond to the physician's ideal. By and large, however, annoyance with the resident physicus grew out of personal experiences and from a perception of his inability to adjust to the rules, social structures, and idiosyncracies of a specific community. Complaints clustered overwhelmingly around lifestyle and behavior. Dissatisfaction with cures may have been common, but it was not often remarked, and malpractice charges were so rare as to be almost nonexistent.

When a newly minted physicus arrived in his district, he often entered a terra incognita. Although some men went to places where they were already well known, or where they had friends and relatives, or held property, most were encountering a new community and one in which they had few friends or protectors, and whose rules and privileges were alien to them. Their welcome must have varied enormously. The most important ties for these men in the first weeks and months remained those to the Collegium medicum and privy council as their employers and patrons. These bonds were, however, tenuous and not all-important, and could either tighten or loosen with time. A physicus who banked solely on the "authority" granted him by his office was in for a rough ride. Although in one sense employees or creatures of the central government, the physici relied on the community for part of their salaries and for the natural products that constituted a goodly portion of almost every physicus's wage. They equally depended on the acquiescence of the local bureaucracy in calling upon them for forensic investigations for which they were allowed to collect extra fees, to pay for their transportation, and to reimburse them for their services to the poor. The entitlements accorded the physicus, whether in the form of fuel, fodder, or the right to fatten a pig, also demonstrated his rank among the privileged of the community. By withholding or cheating on these, village officials (even very base ones, such as goose- and cowherds) could signal their acceptance or rejection of a man. Thus the physicus rapidly found himself on his own and in a sometimes difficult (although not completely untenable) position as the servant of two or more masters, whose interests diverged as often as they converged.[114] Some physici steered skillfully between Scylla and Charybdis, while others quickly foundered on the rocks of provincial intransigence or disappeared altogether in a whirlpool of drink, dissipation, and despair. One could, and all did, appeal to the Collegium medicum for help or for redress of injuries, but that help was often too little, too late, too remote, or too feeble to circumvent local obstructionism. Yet physici and locals could get along famously. Physici, like physicians and Amtmänner, could forge bonds of friendship or marriage and reach positions of trust and communal responsibility, often to the extent that the village would block interference from outside, even from the physicus's putative employer, the Collegium medicum, as Schöningen did for Dr. Holdefreund.

Physici seem frequently to have been poorly informed about their duties. Three years after sending Dr. Fahrenholtz to Königslutter, the Collegium medicum sharply admonished him for his dilàtory perfor- mance in reporting mortality and morbidity statistics. He protested that although he knew he was supposed to collect such statistics, he was com- pletely unaware of any further responsibilities. "It is true," he continued, "that from time to time in the past two years I have received such lists from some of the sextons and schoolmasters." But he had no notion what to do with them. When he questioned the Amt's clerk, the latter responded that "he, too, had no idea." Dr. Ernst Pini, who went to Schöppenstedt as physicus in 1758, found that the Amt had only preserved copies of the medical ordinances of 1721 and of 1747: everything else was missing.[115]

Most physici entering their new realms tended to see unfavorable conditions, or ones that were harsh or bluntly hostile. To some extent, such grim reports were platitudinous and self-serving: it was obviously to the physicus's advantage to exaggerate the obstacles that confronted him. Not surprisingly, men sent to the less desirable regions were quickest to stress the impossibility of living on what they were able to earn, as well as to detail the problems bound up with executing their duties graphically. In 1753, the newly appointed physicus to Calvörde, Dr. Johann Hoff- mann, was soon murmuring about the meanness of the place and the poverty of the citizens, "who when they do consult a physician, can only pay him very little, and would prefer to have him perform *gratis*." More- over, Calvörde was overrun with quacks.[116] Dr. Küster, who coveted and got the Calvörde physicate in 1788, later complained about this hardship posting: "The Calvörde physicate is insignificant. There are a great num- ber of common and indigent inhabitants here, and almost no Honora- tiones. Thus, a physician can only expect a very meager income. [Under such conditions] my courage and diligence must fail me if I cannot hope for improvement in the future and must waste myself here."[117] Sometimes physici did not even reach their districts before protesting about lack of business and insufficient salaries. Georg Beltz, who was awarded the post of physicus in Hasselfelde in 1740, quickly expressed dismay at the prob- lems he knew would face him, and that would, in his words, make his survival there a very close-run thing.

[The people] living in and around Hasselfelde are mostly impoverished and cannot pay even half of the legally set medical fees. [They are], in addition, accustomed to taking homemade remedies and will not turn to a medicus except in [times of] the most desperate need. . . . [I]n search of cheaper prices, they swiftly run to foreign empirics and [scorn] real physicians, and thus one does not have enough to do. Without a more generous salary, it will be impossible [for me] to find a reasonable income there. Fearing that I shall have to leave again after suffering great [financial] harm, I have lost almost all my desire to go to Hasselfelde, while I know from my previous experience just how much a physician can lose in reputation and property by moving about too often.[118]

Dr. Johann Vibrans, who was transferred from Calvörde to Walkenried in 1794, had an equally dismal introduction to his new domain. In fact, he insisted, the move had damaged rather than improved his financial state. Walkenried was a "small, unimportant place" with no notability except for a few ducal officials, foresters, and churchmen. The rest of the inhabitants, according to Vibrans, "are not even farmers, among whom one occasionally finds prosperity, but are [merely] laborers and artisans—all equally penurious." With a population of 320, Walkenried was "for a physician, a place with practically no earnings." Almost paradoxically, however, Walkenried proved expensive, inasmuch as "all necessities, such as lodgings and food, when one does not have one's own house and property, cost more than is usual in [large] cities." In addition, Vibrans felt harassed by the competition of physicians in neighboring areas, from the apothecary in nearby Grünenplan and from the surgeon Cramer, "who combines the practice of internal medicine with his surgical practice, his grocery, and tavernkeeping, and who hawks internal and external medications."[119]

If the smaller, poorer, and less desirable physicates inspired the most pitiful pleas for more salary, even the best postings, such as Blankenburg, also left physici plenty of room for disenchantment. Dr. Friedrich Krebs, who went to Blankenburg in 1785, quickly asked for more money. Part of his duties included caring for the nearby miners, a task for which he received an extra 60 thaler. He felt this to be insufficient recompense and requested 40 more, arguing that he was responsible for over five hundred miners, "whose daily work greatly predisposes them to accidents." Help came from what may be thought an unexpected quarter; from the magistrates in Blankenburg, who conceded that Krebs's position was "not particularly lucrative," involving as it did expensive and time-consuming trips into mountainous regions. The local Honoratiores expressed their satisfaction with Krebs overall, for "[unlike] his predecessors in office, he does not order expensive medicines when cheaper ones can be substituted," and his bills to the city's treasury were modest. The magistrates concluded that because Krebs endeavored not to overcharge the Amt, the treasury could well afford to advance 40 thaler.[120]

To understand the situations in which physici found themselves, to comprehend how public health policies functioned, indeed, took shape, within communities, it is worthwhile to follow the careers of several men. Local battle lines appear here, but also bands of solidarity.

Johann Siegesbeck was physicus in Helmstedt from 1731 until 1735, when he left for St. Petersburg.[121] Before going to Helmstedt, Siegesbeck had practiced medicine for twenty years in nearby Magdeburg. Persistent, caustic controversies with the city council in Helmstedt hallmarked his stay there.[122] "Although ever since [I became] physicus [here in Helmstedt], I have carried out each and every duty incumbent on me with all diligence, and with no complaints, still the city council here, and especially its head [Bürgermeister Cellarius], nurse a *jalousie* toward me." The only reason Siegesbeck could find for this animosity originated in his appointment. After receiving his post, he had failed "to give someone or other a *presente*," that is, a bribe or token of his appreciation. The city council refused to issue him a written contract, "despite my patience," and withheld all his fees, including "my piddling little salary," even though "my predecessors received these punctually."

Particularly galling were the tricks pulled on him when he tried to obtain his firewood or fatten his pigs.[123] One quickly sees how newcomers such as Siegesbeck might be easily duped. Siegesbeck referred to the failure of the city to extend to him what it had freely given the previous physicus, Just Kreyenberg. But Kreyenberg had been born in Helmstedt, the son of a respected merchant, had studied at the university there, and served for over thirty years as physicus. Such a man was not easy to deceive, and almost certainly his strong Helmstedt connections made his life run more smoothly.[124]

When Siegesbeck arrived in Helmstedt, he was promised wood for fuel. As he wanted to spare himself the "wasted time and expense" of felling and carting the wood to his lodging, he and the city council agreed on a 4-thaler supplement to his salary instead; "and as a newcomer I believed this [was a good deal]." He soon discovered that he had been hoodwinked. Kreyenburg had gotten "six to eight cords of beech wood and some oak," which had been "felled, split, and hauled to his door free, for only a tip to the driver." The previous physici had also enjoyed the right to fatten two pigs. That privilege had never been mentioned to Siegesbeck, and he only heard about it by word of mouth. Locals regularly shortchanged and insulted him. His predecessor had been paid 4 thaler for each autopsy; he was told they were to be done ex officio. Kreyenburg had always been asked to attend the annual festive meeting of the city council; Siegesbeck was never invited. He protested that "although I have never held much with such ceremonies, still, [the city council] thereby openly snubs me."[125] Public demonstrations of rank and deference weighed heavily in such communities, and one member of the city council specifically insisted that "as city physicus, he [Siegesbeck] shall yield place to members of the city council."[126]

Points of contention arose not merely over intangibles such as respect, or irritations such as the skulduggery over the wood; Siegesbeck also clashed with the city council on medical matters. In 1731 "a foreign vagabond," who went "by the fabulous title of court dentist to the elector of Mainz," popped up in Helmstedt. Siegesbeck, referring to the medical ordinance of 1721, which did not permit such practitioners except after they had been examined by the resident physicus, and then only during fairs or annual markets, wanted to prohibit the court dentist's activities. Despite this, the city council allowed the man a "free passport" to peddle his skills and wares house to house. Similarly, according to Siegesbeck, the council permitted, even encouraged, mountebanks to erect their booths with no further formalities. When he protested, Siegesbeck was told that while it lay within his province to alert the city council, it was the council's decision alone whether or not to act on his advice. And when he cited the relevant section of the law, the council insisted that "it knew about no such medical ordinance." Moreover, the city council was not about to yield to Siegesbeck, or, for that matter, to the privy council on this point. In a short, curt, rely to the privy council, Bürgermeister Cellarius— Siegesbeck's bête noire—refused to respond to the physicus's charges, merely noting that Siegesbeck was exempted from property taxes in the city until he bought a "taxable house" and still paid no personal taxes. The implication was that Siegesbeck should be satisfied.[127] The problem lay not only with Siegesbeck. His successor in office, Dr. Voß, ran up against similar obstacles.[128] Clearly, in both cases (and although the city council itself had chosen Siegesbeck), the municipal government was waging a rearguard action. That the duke would eventually reassert his sovereignty over the city was an inescapable and distasteful fact, but the city council played the game to the end, obstructing where it might and asserting its independence where it could.

Even in places where ducal sovereignty was less hotly contested, physici clashed with magistrates. In 1756, friction began to develop between the physicus in Gandersheim, Conrad Blum, and an imperious Amtmann, Ludolf Granzien.[129] Granzien was a strong personality and a can-tankerous soul, apparently very used to having his way in Gandersheim and piping the tune to which the physicus danced. Granzien had had what he regarded as a very fruitful and cooperative arrangement with the previous physicus, Dr. Wachsmuth (a man he had recommended for the job), principally because Wachsmuth deferred to his authority. The appearance of what Blum called a "raging epidemic disease and petechial fever" in Gandersheim occasioned a major confrontation between the physicus and the Amtmann. Granzien dutifully reported the incident to the privy council and quickly took steps to contain the epidemic. He downplayed the gravity of the incident, arguing that what Blum had alarmingly, and inaccurately, termed an "epidemic and petechial fever" was in fact only a severe outbreak of "the purples." Of the twelve deaths in the city, most were of "old and lived-out persons . . . who thereby paid nature's debt."[130] Granzien believed he had taken the appropriate steps by fumigating infected houses, ordering the apothecary to dispense free medicines, distributing money to the sick poor, providing nurses, and so on. And the Collegium medicum agreed that he had acted quickly and appropriately; they expressed less satisfaction with Blum's conduct, ad-monishing him to furnish more information.[131]

Granzien was careful not to let the reins of power slip from his hands. He refused to allow the physicus to take control of the situation even in an obviously medical matter. He relied on his own judgment, insisting that

physicians tend to blow up such illnesses all out of proportion in order to puff their cures. . . . Such [tricks] are well known to me. . . . While [I was] in Holzminden, the physicus once demanded of me that I shut up a citizen's home because a servant there suffered from a contagious disease, and that I immediately inform the ducal government. I went to the specified house myself, took a close look round, had the body buried forthwith, arranged to have the house well ventilated, and thus ended the danger once and for all. Had I followed the suggestions of the physicus, the city would have acquired a bad reputation, and all commerce on the [river] Weser would have come to a halt, closing off the city for a long time and doing extreme damage.[132]

Granzien knew his priorities, and he would listen to the physicus with one ear only. This conflict over authority lay at the bottom of the prob-lems between Granzien and Blum during the course of the 1756 epi-demic. Blum blamed the large number of deaths in the city on bad beer. Granzien castigated Blum for his unwillingness to visit and treat the poor, and for shifting that burden onto the surgeon, Blumenberg.[133] The battle, which dragged on for two more years, had just been joined. Granzien accused Blum of not carrying out his duties correctly and of exceeding his authority. According to Granzien, Blum was never to be found at home, especially, curiously, in the afternoons, and moreover, he was "not someone with whom you can have a reasonable conversation." In addition, Blum had taken up gemstone grinding and made an infernal racket with his grinders, which disturbed all his neighbors. He also stuck his nose into things that, according to Granzien, "in no way belong to his métier." Blum went around testing wells, and "arrogantly" barked out orders, for example, to the apothecary Seitz that he was not to unpack the wares he had purchased in Braunschweig except in Blum's presence, so that he might inspect them.[134]

The privy council took a far milder view of Blum's "transgressions." They tended to excuse Blum's late reports as resulting from overwork. They reminded Granzien that analyzing well water was part of a physicus's business and observed that Granzien's judgment of Blum, who had only been in Holzminden for a few months, was "premature" and smacked of bigotry. The council regarded Blum's hobby as a completely harmless, if eccentric, pastime. In regard to the apothecary, the council admitted that while Blum had not acted quite properly and had been impolite to the magistrates, his behavior was rooted "not in ill-will but in ignorance or maladroitness." Granzien's conduct, however, they found more objectionable. Granzien should not have overridden Blum's orders to the apothecary; he had every right to give them. Furthermore, the privy council warned Granzien that it was "in the interests of the common good to maintain a good relationship with the physicus" and reminded him that "when you have some complaint, you are to phrase it in a seemly and dispassionate manner.[135]

Not surprisingly, this did not subdue Granzien; in fact, it probably inflamed him. He obviously found Blum's initiatives presumptuous. Granzien referred to his years of harmonious cooperation with the physicus Wachsmuth in Holzminden, where the physicus "was not permitted to do anything about the apothecary without my knowledge. Thus much controversy was avoided." At this point the privy council again reminded Granzien of his duty and enjoined him, in a somewhat exasperated tone, to live "in peace" with Blum.[136] One suspects that such was not the case.[137]

Not only Amtmänner like Granzien and important municipal authorities, such as the members of the city council in Helmstedt, could render a physicus's life miserable. The physicus in Holzminden, Dr. Carl Struve, found himself embroiled in a conflict neither with a city council, nor with a ducal Amtmann, nor even with an ecclesiastical dignitary, but with a simple forester named Grotian. Struve had the right to fatten two pigs and pasture a cow at village expense, and had done so since his arrival in Holzminden in 1759. Then suddenly in 1764 Grotian informed him that in the future he would have to compensate the communal treasury for what he had once enjoyed free. Until Struve paid what he owed in arrears, Grotian would hold his swine hostage. Struve complained that he saw no reason why he should suffer this outrage, since "all other ducal and city officials here, even the midwife, enjoy this right with no fuss [being raised]."[138]

Far more usual (if less amusing) than such chicanery was the withholding of compensation for services rendered. Physici submitted bill after bill and often waited months in vain to be satisfied, while those in control of local purse strings disputed their claims. Frequently, for instance, the Amt or magistrates did not call upon the physicus for a forensic opinion, preferring to delegate the job to another physician, surgeon, or bathmaster. Partly the authorities did this to favor friends or relatives, or to spite a physicus with whom they were feuding by denying him his legitimate fees. Sometimes, the authorities were merely being tightfisted; surgeons received considerably less than the fee set for the physicus, and complaints from physici about this sort of fraud were common. Dr. Carl Rörhand, physicus in Schöppenstedt, protested such "infringements." A fight in nearby Amt Sambleben had left one person seriously wounded. Rörhand went to Sambleben, but was thwarted by the authorities, "who not only authorized Doctor Seiffart to do the investigation of this judicial case, but also accepted his certificate as valid, although he is not sworn in as physicus" and was not permitted such work.[139] This undermined Rörhand's authority as much as his income. In 1783, for example, Physicus Apfel in Stadtoldendorf turned to the Collegium medicum for assistance in collecting fees owed him by Amt Wickensen for his treatment of several poor patients some months earlier. He had sent his bill—"which I calculated according to a very modest scale of fees"—to Amtmann von Rosenstern, but the latter replied that poor relief funds in Wickensen only allowed reimbursement to the apothecary for medicines, not payment to a physician.[140]

The medical treatment of the poor often occasioned disputes. Was the physicus responsible for treating the poor ex officio, or was he to be paid additionally for extra duties? The legal position was indefinite. Some agreements detailed that the physicus was to care for *all* the poor free of charge and submit no bills for this work. Other contracts read differently, allowing a special supplement for the treatment of the poor. Many were maddeningly vague on the subject. Apparently, the amounts set aside for such charity cases seemed (at least in the physici's eyes) to lag considerably behind the costs incurred. This perceived gap formed the meat of a major confrontation in Helmstedt soon after Meyer's appointment as physicus in 1766. In 1767, Meyer complained about the large number of paupers—he specified 172—the city expected him to treat for a meager 25 thaler. The magistrates rebutted his charges with the counterclaim that Meyer ordered too many expensive medicines from the apothecary. In 1768, Meyer protested that the magistrates refused to call on him for autopsies in legal cases, denying him his legitimate fees. Nor would they pay him for the medicines he used to treat prisoners, those wounded in brawls, or those involved in accidents. Increasingly acrimonious allegations flew back and forth throughout 1768 and 1769.[141] The city council in Helmstedt argued that Meyer exaggerated his troubles vis-à-vis the poor. The director of the poor relief related how Meyer had contractually agreed to handle the sick poor free of charge; that was why he enjoyed a salary "ex publico." When Meyer was appointed physicus, the director of poor relief had given him a list of all the registered poor, "so that no one could pester him unnecessarily and without right." The director now accused Meyer of misusing this list. Meyer intimated that all those found on the list required medical assistance, which was by no means the case. The director estimated that Meyer probably treated no more than thirty-two charity cases a year. The Collegium medicum and privy council, hoping to patch over the dispute, proposed allowing Meyer a supplement from poor relief funds. The magistrates in Helmstedt never accepted that suggestion, and eventually the privy council itself paid Meyer the additional sum.[142]

In rural areas, conflicts also turned on questions of medical care for the sick poor. More frequent, however, were the disputes over who should bear the financial burden for dispatching the physicus on official business. In 1798, Amt Stauffenberg sent Dr. Carl Spohr, the physicus stationed in Seesen, to visit the village of Münchehof when smallpox appeared there. The authorities armed Spohr with a mandate addressed to the village officials ordering them to show him "all those lying ill." While in most cases the parents of children infected with smallpox refused his help, Spohr nevertheless asked to be paid the two thaler owed him. The Amt argued: "[I]t is so often the case that we are required by the Collegium medicum to send the physicus out to these villages. Generally, however, the ill do not want to accept his assistance. The peasant cannot be persuaded to submit himself [or his family] to a cure that might last several weeks; rather, he turns to potions from amateurs, which shake his body to its very foundations, so that either a quick improvement or an equally quick end results." In light of these obstacles, the Amt felt that the central government should compensate Spohr. The privy council refused and ordered the Amt to reimburse Spohr not only this time but in all future instances, "because the entire area must be concerned about containing outbreaks of disease wherever they occur," as the spread of epidemics could best be prevented "through the purposeful treatment of patients already ill."[143]

The physicus was not always the minnow caught in the waves whipped up by a melee of leviathans. Local authorities and physici fought over issues that had little or nothing to do with resistance to interference from above. It is often hard to disentangle the two arenas of conflict, however, because they overlapped. Physici could always argue that complaints about their actions in office, or about personal misconduct, merely masked struggles over medical authority and power. Separating the political from the personal, and the medical from the sociopolitical, is an almost hopeless task. Both physici and local authorities willingly cast their cases at the feet of privy councilors for decisions, and this modus operandi looks suspiciously like ill-concealed obstructionism rather than any sincere effort at mediation. In addition, we must add to this already murky brew the competition physici experienced from other practitioners, including physicians, which will be treated at greater length in Chapter 3. Enemies usually knew each other's names and had all-too-familiar faces, and specific cases vividly illustrate how alliances shifted and motives changed.

Altercations and Alliances

The career of Dr. Jacob Müller, physicus in Seesen from 1755 until his death in 1786, was one filled with controversy, although not in other ways unfortunate. Despite some early disputes with the magistracy in Seesen, and some serious conflicts with the Collegium medicum and privy council, when he died in 1786, he was still physicus, and also Bürgermeister.[144] When Müller first applied for the post of physicus in 1755, he was twenty-eight, had studied medicine in Jena for three years, and had practiced in Eltze for another three. He had not yet taken his doctorate. The Collegium medicum, initially unimpressed with his credentials and displeased with his examination, finally agreed to appoint him physicus if he acquired his degree from the University of Helmstedt without delay. Two years later, he was sworn in as physicus. Once in Seesen, Müller related tales of the same problems that plagued other physici. The Amt held back his fees in *casibus medico-forensibus*. He suffered "intolerable" incursions into his private medical practice, but also into his duties as physicus, "and the authorities, who are supposed to prevent such abuses, abet them instead."[145]

Like so many other physici, Müller literally bombarded the Collegium medicum with endless requests for more money and special favors: in 1767, he wanted a larger salary; in 1768, he requested an appointment as physician to the miners at the iron works.[146] Müller's performance as physicus did not much please the Collegium either. In 1766, the Collegium complained that "for some time now," Müller had failed to supply regular reports. Müller responded that if one expected a physicus to amass such data, he must have accurate information. To secure that information, he needed the cooperation of the local authorities. Pastors, schoolmasters, and sextons all failed to inform him of outbreaks of disease: "From the entire Amt of Harzburg, and also from Amt Lutter am Barenberg, I have never received a single communication. From the village of Engelade, the schoolmaster occasionally forwards a report, and, in Amt Langelsheim, from the schoolmaster Henser in the village of Wolfshagen, and from the cantor Kriebel in Langelsheim, [I receive information] rather regularly. From all the other places, I have never heard a word."[147] The local authorities, according to Müller, failed to notify him "until some evil disease is so widespread that everyone becomes alarmed." Likewise, they "feared the expense" involved in bringing him to their area.[148] For example, in September 1766, the ducal forester Schmidt informed Müller of an outbreak of dysentery in the market town of Langelsheim. The local authorities refused point-blank to authorize transportation to Langelsheim until the Collegium medicum ordered them to do so. As Müller felt the situation warranted his immediate attention, he walked the few miles to Langelsheim. When he got there, the village headman named three or four patients, adding "there are perhaps more, but when people are not bedridden, they keep their illnesses secret." Dysentery had, in fact, been present in the town for about three to four weeks, and ten persons had died. The fragmentary account Müller obtained from the surgeon Stube in Langelsheim did not, however, permit him to compose the *historiam epidemia* the Collegium medicum demanded. When Müller requested payment from the forester, silence was the only reply.[149]

The resistance of the local authorities was, however, only one of the reasons Müller listed as to why he was unable to execute his duties as physicus properly. Equally deterrent were the distances between villages, "the cool and unrestrained, totally impermissible, but up to now uncontrollable quackery" that persisted in his district, and the widespread reluctance to consult a physician. The end result was that he had "a medical practice hardly worth the name."[150]

The dissatisfaction of the Collegium medicum with Müller matched Muller's disenchantment with his district. By 1770, the Collegium was hounding Müller for his increasingly slipshod performance. Despite sharp reminders to attend to his duty more painstakingly, he acted "as if he wishes to withdraw himself wholly from the subordination he owes the Collegium medicum." Weary of nagging, the Collegium fined Müller 10 thaler, ordered him to complete missing reports, and threatened him with severer penalties if he dared ignore these warnings. Müller promised to mend his ways in the future, but in fact did nothing to satisfy the Collegium. As a last resort, the privy council ordered the Amt to garnish his wages.[151]

Not only the Collegium medicum was displeased with Müller. In 1781, an anonymous denunciation related how Müller slighted his duties as physicus and detailed his bothersome eccentricities.[152] The letter referred to Müller's "giddy whims": He exhibited a "clever mechanism" and assembled "peep-shows, like those the Italians carry around, . . . in which one is allowed to look for a few pennies." In addition, he constructed a "solar microscope" and turned his home into a workshop "more like a smithy" than one fitting for "a man who holds the health of our district in his hands." He frittered away his time cutting glass. If, the letter continued, anyone approached Müller for medical help, "he reacts very unpleasantly at having been disturbed at his hobby." He refused to visit patients unless they were very ill, and his whole demeanor drove people away. For these reasons, he probably wrote no more than thirty prescriptions annually in the local apothecary. "He excuses his time spent with cutting glass and other extraneous things as essential because no one or only very few people consult him, and he cannot live from [his medical practice] alone." Preoccupied with his projects, "he only fulfills half of his duties as Bürgermeister and not the tenth part of his tasks as physicus." Not surprisingly, the Collegium medicum did not act on an anonymous

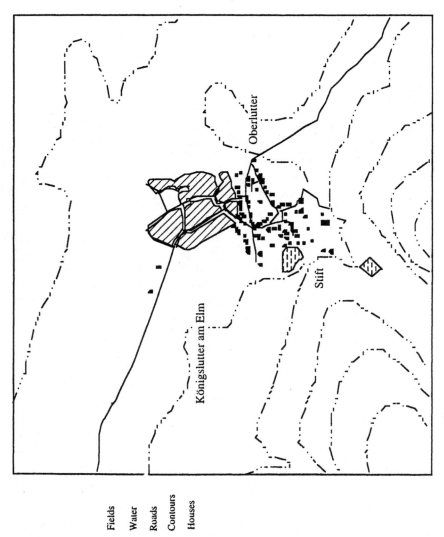

Königslutter am Elm

Legend

Fields

Water

Roads

Contours

Houses

Oberlutter

Königslutter am Elm

Stift

denunciation, and perhaps we should not make too much of it here either, although other witnesses confirmed his odd behavior. One wonders if the identity of the penman is not so obscure: was it perhaps the apothecary who felt his own business hampered by the dying trade of the one doctor in town?[153]

If the story of Dr. Müller has its unique little twists and turns, its general outline is familiar. These conflicts and confrontations cannot be written off as epiphenomena of the sources. "Contentious" or "eccentric" physici are not necessarily overrepresented in the archive. Of the 110–120 physici who served in Braunschweig-Wolfenbüttel between approximately 1730 and 1808, all but a handful—and these were usually men whose tenure in office was so brief as to be inconsequential—were involved in some kind of scrappy encounter (often resembling a Hobbesian war of each against all) with local and central authorities, peasants, petty officials, and innumerable others. This was so because it was that sort of world, a world of infinite compromises and clashes, where individuals, individual decisions, and tiny events made history, and, for that matter, shaped—one might say, personalized—the health policy of the regions. A few additional illustrations only bolster this perception, as well as fleshing out the *Alltag* of medical practice, health policy, and life.

Dr. Johann Dedekind, physicus in Königslutter from 1769 to 1789 (and later physicus in Holzminden from 1789 to 1799), was one of the relatively few physici in Braunschweig-Wolfenbüttel whose accomplishments merited an entry in August Hirsch's biographical dictionary of "famous physicians of all times and places." Dedekind had studied medicine at Helmstedt and received his doctorate there in 1777. He is often credited with developing an early (perhaps the first) plan to extract sugar from beets.[154] Typically, nothing in Hirsch hints at the strife that dogged the man, both in Königslutter and in Holzminden.

In December 1768, the Collegium medicum granted Dr. Johann Holdefreund's request to be relieved of his position as physicus in Königslutter (Holdefreund, as we have already seen, was in his own sort of trouble).[155] In his stead, the privy council appointed Dedekind, whose medical practice in Schöppenstedt was ailing.[156] A few years later, and throughout 1773 and 1774, Dedekind repeatedly petitioned the Collegium for an increase of salary, claiming that he donated medical care to inhabitants of the local cloister lands. It appears that Dedekind was not quite representing the matter accurately. When the Collegium investigated, it came to light that the cloister already paid Dedekind 20 thaler annually to medicate the poor. The privy council denied Dedekind's supplication, reminding him that he was ex officio obliged to treat the poor of his district.[157]

Apparently all was not well between Dedekind and the community of Königslutter. For example, in 1775, in the midst of deciding on a replacement for the physicus in Schöppenstedt (a post Dedekind was seeking), Dean Martini remarked that "Dedekind has spoiled his nest in Königslutter and wants a transfer."[158] Dedekind was not transfered, and the relationship between him and his district deteriorated. By 1779, the Collegium medicum verbalized its extreme exasperation with Dedekind, complaining to the privy council about his "inappropriate conduct." He bickered with all and sundry, but fought most vehemently with the notables in town, constantly badgered the Collegium for more money, improperly asked the Collegium to take his part in all manner of disputes, and so on. The Collegium specifically pointed out that Dedekind's "reprehensible conduct toward the apothecary and toward several of his patients has made him a laughingstock." Particularly offensive were his "biased and egotistical opinions." By 1789, when a position opened up in Holzminden, the Collegium shuffled appointments to accommodate Dedekind, as well as several other men who had problems with their communities, trusting thereby to heal several festering sores. Dedekind's medical abilities were unquestioned; his deportment was not. The Collegium hoped that moving him to a somewhat better position in Holzminden would improve his financial circumstances and sweeten his disposition.[159]

Life ran no more smoothly for Dedekind in Holzminden than it had in Königslutter. One resident complained to the privy council, for example, that "Dr. Dedekind habitually leaves the city without informing anyone where he is to be found." The Collegium medicum warned Dedekind that this was highly inappropriate behavior and would not be countenanced.[160] And Dedekind was soon voicing his own disappointments. In 1794, he bitterly protested the encroachment of young Dr. Eicke from Gandersheim (the son of the onetime physicus there). In no uncertain terms, Dedekind accused the Collegium of favoring Eicke. Such partisanship was grossly unfair, Dedekind charged, because the Collegium "cannot produce one document to show that the public is disaffected with me and that I deserve such shabby treatment." Dedekind felt it unconscionable that "in my gray age" the Collegium would allow a rival to pilfer part of his income, especially after his many years of faithful service in both Königslutter and Holzminden. Holzminden, Dedekind insisted, had too little work for two physicians, and both would starve. He asked the Collegium to tell Eicke to establish his practice elsewhere, for everyone's sake. Dedekind insisted that no evidence called either his ability or his dedication into question, and "those occasional accusations against me are based totally on prejudices, on hypotheses, and on suspicions, none of which have a factual basis. . . . But if the Collegium medicum wishes to destroy me . . . [it] should at least wish to avert a similarly tragic fate for Dr. Eicke, and should counsel such a talented and honest man not to seek his fortune here, [in order to] . . . prevent his total ruin."[161]

Disingenuousness got Dedekind nowhere. The Collegium medicum labeled his protest "inadmissible," pointing out that no licensed physician could be denied the right to settle wherever he pleased. Moreover,

> Dr. Dedekind . . . falsely maintains that he enjoys the confidence of the entire public [in Holzminden]. We are forced to remark that this is unfortunately not in the least true. His peculiar, often brusque, and insolent manner . . . has caused him to forfeit affection and respect as well as public trust. Everyone in Holzminden is witness to this. But it is also sufficient testimony that the previous physicus in Stadtoldendorf, Dr. Apfel, now in Blankenburg, visits patients almost daily in Holzminden, or sends his advice in writing. Moreover, we believe that size of the population in Holzminden, as well as its location bordering the abbey of Corvey, where good physicians are lacking, warrants the presence of a second physician [in Holzminden]. This appears all the more necessary in that the physicate in Stadtoldendorf is currently vacant. [In addition], as Dr. Dedekind can no longer ride because of the delicacy [of his health] and the frailty of his frame, he must make all his journeys in a wagon, which, however, the peasant is seldom able to furnish [him]. . . . We have for a long while now wished that a younger, more active man would establish himself in Holzminden. . . . If Dr. Dedekind indeed enjoys the trust he says he does, he will do immeasurably better than Eicke.[162]

Here, as elsewhere, the Collegium medicum did nothing to hinder competition between physicians. It never granted physici an exclusive right to medical practice, as much as they might desire one, and as much as they protested the incursions on their practice by other *licensed* physicians living nearby (or by others *legally* practicing some branch of medicine). The only rights the Collegium and privy council consistently defended were those connected with official duties. A physician's private practice was his own affair; it was not sacred, and no physicus received a monopoly on medical practice in his district.[163]

Dedekind's problems rested on the personal animosity he evoked and on his inability to fit into a community. He failed to fulfill the expectations of the populace in Holzminden. It was not so much his medical practice as his human relations that stuck in the throats of his neighbors.

One might wonder why the Collegium medicum bothered trying to favor or placate ornery fellows like Dedekind by shifting them from place to place. And Dedekind was hardly the only physician moved for such reasons, nor was a single relocation, or a single second chance, anywhere near the rule. The Collegium shifted some men, such as Dr. Vibrans, several times and for similar reasons: from 1793 to 1796, Vibrans held four different posts as physicus.[164] One might postulate that sheer lack of talented candidates forced the Collegium to make do with the admittedly less than ideal material that presented itself. This may well have been true early in the century, when physicians were scarce, but that the Collegium did not really lack for candidates by mid century is indicated by the volume of applications, the number of complaints about competition from other physicians raised by physici, and the (admittedly fragmentary) evidence we possess on the density of physicians in several areas.[165] Why then did it hang on to troublemakers like Dedekind? Clearly, part of the reason was the persistence of a sense of noblesse oblige and of a patron-client mentality. The Collegium acted as patron, trying, often with great patience and admirable restraint, to locate suitable positions for its clients, the physici—and even for ones who seemed undeserving of sustained sponsorship. The case of Dr. Pini, the only physicus I have found who was actually dismissed from office (although not in fact forced from his position) indicates the lengths to which the Collegium would go before abandoning a man.

In 1758, Pini, then a practicing physician in Wolfenbüttel, became physicus in Schöppenstedt, a market town of about 1,500 inhabitants.[166] Apparently the first ten years of his stay in Schöppenstedt went well enough. No major problems surfaced, or at least none reached the ears of the Collegium medicum, but in 1768, a decade-long feud began between the local authorities and the Collegium medicum, in which the former repeatedly requested Pini's dismissal on grounds of incorrigible drunkenness. There is little reason to doubt the basic truth of the magistrates' claims about Pini's impudence and inebriety. The privy council was worried enough to ask the magistrates to submit a detailed report on Pini's behavior and "to check with the local apothecary . . . to find out if and how much Dr. Pini owes him for liquors, to give you a detailed bill, including the dates of consumption."[167] The magistrates confirmed the worst rumors and suggested that the distressing metamorphosis in Pini's until then generally satisfactory behavior had come as a result of bad investments Pini had made in Berlin, which had practically bankrupted him.[168] When first attempts to sober him up failed, the privy council tried to induce Pini to move. Amtmann von Juncker in Schöppenstedt tried to persuade Pini to resettle in Goslar. Pini and his wife considered the suggestion, and Pini, in fact, communicated his own frustrations about losing the trust of the community. He was not that enamored of his situation in Schöppenstedt either, "since one person by the name of Siemens had caused an uproar against him in the Küblingen manufactory and said he should go to Goslar." Pini complained that the (unspecified) promises that Dean Meibom had made him when he was appointed physicus in Schöppenstedt had never been honored. In addition, he hoped to attract more patients in Goslar. But he did not move, and there was a brief improvement in his conduct after the privy council warned him that if he did not shape up, he would not only be "immediately dismissed," but also punished.[169] Certainly, Pini's report to the magistrates in Schöppenstedt on the conditions in the area in 1770 is lucid enough, and in fact is quite perceptive in its comments on the underlying economic causes of poor health.[170] Yet these were only moments of industry in what was a long, slow slide into alcoholic oblivion. In 1770, Pini griped that despite his renewed diligence, his patients and the public still treated him with "ingratitude."[171]

If things turned for the better for Pini in the early 1770s, this recovery did not last. By 1775, he had begun his final decline, which was not halted until his death in 1777. The last years of his life are a litany of bizarre incidents, "final" warnings, drunken stupors, threats of dismissal, and repeated pleas for "just one more" chance. When the privy council dismissed him in January 1776, he did not go, and he was not replaced until after his death in late February or early March 1777.[172] Why had the Collegium medicum not removed Pini earlier? There were plenty of other candidates available. Why did it allow him repeated second chances even though he flubbed every one of them? In January 1776, Amtmann Schüler wrote that Pini had been found several times "in deserted buildings dead drunk." One winter afternoon, they stumbled across him on the floor of the local customshouse "having drunk himself into a stupor . . . lying there with his mouth open wide, his saliva frozen into a long icicle."[173] In June 1776, he went on a binge (*paroxismus*) that lasted eleven days, in which he raged like a madman, threatening and abusing his wife (at least verbally) and giving all the signs of having fallen into a deep melancholy.[174] Despite this, the Collegium retained some sympathy for the man, and its deliberations perhaps give some sense that the authorities in Schöppenstedt may have been exaggerating their accusations, although no one doubted that Pini drank. Pini admitted his failings, but proposed that people had often mistaken his "vexation" over an unhappy domestic life and debts for intoxication.[175]

Dr. Martini, who "wished for the sake of Pini's wife and children that one could retain him," did not really expect that anything would change as long as he remained in Schöppenstedt. He could never regain the trust of its inhabitants. The best solution might be to send Pini to another place, with the very strict warning that if he did not behave himself there, he would not only be dismissed immediately, but also thrown into the workhouse. Perhaps "this transfer will remove him from his [evil] associations, which it may be hoped will raise his spirits. He will also see that we mean business."[176]

Pini had his advocates. In 1775, four members of the community wrote in support of Schöppenstedt's beleaguered physicus. The picture they drew of the man was by no means as sinister as Schüler's. Pini was a skillful, "very diligent and commendable" physician who had served the community for seventeen years, they argued. The letter listed several "nobles, pastors, and officials" in the area who stood behind Pini and desired to retain his services. "Almost the entire city and region," the message went on, "takes his part." "Only a very few prejudiced [people]" had painted "that very dark portrait of Dr. Pini." He had been "unjustifiably maligned, suppressed, and pilloried." The widow of Lieutenant Colonel Bötticher took up his case. She admitted that he drank, but said that he had good reason and hinted at an affair between his wife and "a certain lodger." The widow and these others hoped to keep Pini in the city as physician if he could not continue as physicus.[177]

What at first seemed a clear-cut case of dereliction of duty thus soon reveals itself to be a bubbling cauldron of factional disputes. Those who supported Pini found him to be a good physician, who had some problems, but whose failings the authorities had unnecessarily embellished. On the other hand, the authorities regarded Pini's drunkenness (and their own impotence in dealing with it) as sufficient reason for his immediate dismissal. One thing is clear; in the increasingly shrill accusations against Pini, he is rarely portrayed as a bumbler. Although the authorities speak of his "neglect" of patients, they seem more offended by his "dissipations" and "orgies of drunkenness" than by any malpractice. Curiously, they do not mention any specific case where his inebriation resulted in a total inability to function or caused harm to a patient. One wonders if the magistrates felt that a man who supposedly represented authority and a certain social position should also adhere to a standard of decorum that he parodied. Some of Pini's patients might have been less offended by his drinking, which they excused as a quite understandable consequence of his "misery." The position of the Collegium medicum, too, reflected some of these contradictions. It was extremely patient with Pini, restoring his post when his wife pleaded for him after he was first dismissed. And when Pini was finally and irrevocably relieved of his office in late 1776, he was not driven from Schöppenstedt.[178]

Pini, like Dedekind and Müller, was unacceptable to a good number of the best citizens in his district because of his lifestyle. More shocking, however, was the behavior of Dr. Christian Loeber.[179] As in the case of Dedekind, none of the five short lines in Hirsch's authoritative biographical dictionary breathes of scandal. Loeber's life seems unremarkable. Born in 1743, he studied in Erfurt and died while physicus in Vorsfelde. Over the years, he wandered restlessly from Hornburg to Heßen to Schöppenstedt to Vorsfelde, seeking but never quite finding his niche. He published a little, adding his moiety to the mountain of literature the physician-authors and physician-scribblers of the eighteenth-century ground out.[180] But if we probe the life of Dr. Loeber more deeply, we retrieve a story highlighting how medical practice, even in the closing decade of the eighteenth century, remained so implanted in everyday routines of life that it cannot be detached from them historically. While Loeber's case is in no way typical, it demonstrates (if in an exaggerated manner) how a certain lifestyle could generate tensions and initiate actions against a physicus.

Hair-raising rumors swirled around Dr. Loeber. His behavior was, if reports were to be credited, eccentric, macabre, perhaps even criminal. He had, it was whispered about, dug up his own child and "painted him blue," displaying the resultant "mummy" on his mantelpiece; he had set up an "outlandish self-styled 'Philanthropie'" from which his students fled, driven away by hunger, and also, it was intimated, by the unwanted sexual advances of its director; he had erected in his garden a number of "gravestones painted with large crosses, as memorials to the deceased poet [Christian Fürchtegott] Gellert and to an old man by the name of Hubrig who supposedly attained the age of 108"; he denied the "miracle works" of Christ; he had constructed a summerhouse, installing in it three windows and a ventilator, although it was "nothing more than open leafwork from top to bottom." Moreover, he led a "wild and disorderly" life, and his neighbors held against him that "he parades up and down the streets with a burning pipe [in his mouth] and even goes into the barns with it." He quickly forfeited "all the trust, esteem, and credit" he might otherwise have enjoyed. In Heßen, where he first served as physicus, the magistrates admitted that "initially [he] was well-liked" and probably could have earned a decent living "if he had pursued an upright and prudent life and if he had not drawn upon himself the distrust and scorn of almost everyone because of his immoral lifestyle and his uncouth manner." Thus, despite a good start, and despite the important support of friends and relatives there, he was soon in deep trouble, personally and occupationally. It is not, of course, terribly relevant whether such stories were true or false, vastly exaggerated or basically accurate, or whether his enemies wove a web of lies around him. The charges cannot be dislodged from their historical and cultural habitat, from a conceptual world that rendered particular actions culpable or repellent and that mandated the exclusion or at least avoidance of those who perpetrated them.

When Loeber went to the graveyard in Schöppenstedt and had his child exhumed, he violated one of the oldest communal taboos—that separating the living from the dead. If early modern people still cavorted in cemeteries, they nevertheless avoided the recently dead. Touching a corpse or dissecting it constituted moments of tension and liminality in early modern societies, even if some of these taboos were dissipating at the end of the eighteenth century. Only slowly did people conquer their horror of dismemberment after death. Fear of dissection remained vivid and was connected with a prevalent popular religiosity.[181] Thus Loeber's deeds seemed all the more grotesque: to dig up his own child's body, anatomize it, and, in the words of one person, turn it into a "mummy" deeply disgusted the average observer. What Loeber had done, of course, was to perform an autopsy: he examined the child's esophagus, tongue, and cerebrum to determine the cause of death. Then he dissected out these parts and turned them into anatomical *praeparate*.[182] If his neighbors and the magistrates in Schöppenstedt, as well as churchmen (he was fined for desecrating a grave), found Loeber's behavior monstrous and sacrilegious, Loeber's own perception and representation of his activities, as well as the opinion of the ducal Collegium medicum, the privy council, the medical faculty at the University of Helmstedt, and what may be called an "enlightened" public, was quite different. These people could, and did, interpret Loeber's acts as the laudable, if perhaps somewhat clumsy, efforts of an enlightened man to discover why his child had died and to pursue legitimate research, unfettered by superstitions and religious prejudice.

Similar misapprehensions dogged other aspects of Loeber's life. He was not only a ghoul, he was a fool. One cannot miss the biting sarcasm the magistrates in Heßen lavished on Loeber's many projects. They labeled his "Philanthropie," his monuments to Gellert and the "old man of 108," and his garden house *cum* hermitage "laughable." Other circles might view all these more sympathetically and even admire them, but that was not the reaction in the small towns and villages of Braunschweig-Wolfenbüttel.

For instance, one of Loeber's pet projects was the establishment of a "Philanthropie," a school for teaching poor boys the respectable trade of surgery. Faith in the ability of education to improve the human race and the pedagogical reforms that accompanied it were, of course, cherished goals of most of those who congregated under the banner of enlightenment, although the types and extension of education were hotly debated. But by any measure, Loeber's attempt was miserable. Conditions at this "starvation school," if reports are to be believed, were Dickensian. It was not merely Loeber's inefficiency that his neighbors scorned; it was the entire enterprise, both in concept and execution. He took in the 11-year-old son of an impoverished locksmith as his servant and "dressed him in an outlandish garb just like his own"—a long, loose robe decorated with stars. He persuaded a young vagrant, who made his living by harp-playing and begging, to lodge with him, "for what purposes we can only surmise and dread." To these "pupils" he added a day laborer's boy and a village lad from nearby Veltheim. His choice of pupils enhanced the general impression that his was more a school of crime and mendicancy than of surgery. Little could come of this sort of training, locals insisted, except to breed a burdensome band of "lazybones and scamps," who "now plague our citizens with their incessant pleas for alms." And one apprentice "showed the results of *his* godly education" by filching money from his teacher.

Equally anathematizing was his blasphemy. He had converted to Catholicism to please his first wife, and his subsequent return to the Protestantism of his youth left good citizens suspicious of the firmness and orthodoxy of his beliefs. His naturalistic interpretation of a miracle of Christ's—he imprudently broadcast the idea that Christ had used a salve made from soapstone shavings to cure a blind man—only reinforced existing doubts about his godliness, leading observers to comment that it was "indeed a good thing for his young pupils' souls that their 'instruction' only lasted a few days!"

Like many other enthusiasts of this pre-Romantic age, Loeber tended to choke up in the presence of unspoiled nature. Many planted gardens, constructed mazes, and enjoyed communing with nature in the open air. All this aroused the vast amusement and undisguised contempt of "less enlightened" but perhaps more practical souls, who dismissed such efforts as a waste of good land and a misuse of valuable time and money. Those who still conceived of nature as an enemy to be conquered rather than a goddess to be worshipped saw little point in paying homage to an environment that thwarted their comfort rather than enriched their lives.[183] Yet this was not merely another clash of the forces of light and knowledge against the marshaled troops of darkness and superstition, as many eighteenth-century writers and historians since then would have us believe. What we see here is the resistance thrown up by an older style of life founded in prudent husbandry and calculating parsimony, and reinforced for that matter by the cameralist and agronomic reforms of the century, against the wasteful artifice of show and sentimentality. Likewise, Loeber's monument to the poet Gellert, whose fanciful tales stirred the imagination and jerked the tear glands of hundreds of eighteenth-century readers, could only appear ludicrous to the residents of a tiny town in northern Germany. And one is left, I fear, with a certain sympathy for peasant materialism and hardheadedness in the face of a "Grub Street" enlightenment that quickly descended into gimcrackery and looniness.

Most of all it is necessary to see how one group might perceive behaviors as sane and praiseworthy, or, at the worst, as character quirks that presented no serious dangers to society, while others regarded them as preposterous or malevolent. Loeber's veneration of the old man who lived to be 108 is a perfect example. Most of his neighbors in Schöppenstedt were more than faintly amused, while some expressed severe doubts about the sanity of an individual who frittered away his assets apotheosizing such an absurd object. A world of restricted resources, particularly one marked by a shortage of arable and inheritable land, did not value the aged. While Loeber's exaggerated esteem for this modern Methuselah caused his neighbors to shake their heads, and forces us to smile somewhat condescendingly, many other contemporaries shared his enthusiasm for macrobiotics and the science of prolongevity. As we know, macrobiotics flowed easily out of the mainstream of medical theory in the eighteenth century, attracting the attention of major figures like the Berlin physician and medical writer Christoph Hufeland.[184]

Thus, while Loeber's neighbors and the local notability regarded his actions with a skepticism bordering on odium, others judged his sins as less besetting and his flaws as nothing more than minor defects of personality. The Collegium medicum, for example, while its members worried about Loeber's propensity for mounting up debts, deemed mere foibles the very behaviors that deeply distressed his neighbors and that formed the basis for their overwhelmingly negative judgments on his suitability as a fellow citizen *and as a physician*. Locals worried about defaulters and bankrupts in their midst, and communities tended to praise physici for their economic restraint. Dr. Schulze, although he enjoyed only a small salary and had a practice hardly worth the name in Calvörde, won the respect of the community because he "avoided debts and maintained himself through his prudence and frugality."[185] In the written comments of the members of the Collegium medicum as they deliberated back and forth on the question of Loeber's appointment, it is evident that while they all agreed that Loeber was perhaps not the most desirable candidate imaginable, little could be held against him as a physician. They all judged him "knowledgeable." One member pointed out that the man who penned the damning report from Heßen was "indeed no friend of Dr. Loeber's." Moreover, the document contained in his opinion, only "simple calumnies," and proof rested "merely on gossip." The real question in his mind was, "Can Dr. Loeber be faulted as a physician?" And to that query the answer was an unequivocal no. Another member concluded that what the magistrates in Heßen reported "only concerns his *moral* behavior of eight years ago, and it was then not well substantiated."[186]

Yet the findings of the Collegium medicum and the opinion of Loeber's occupational peers miss the critical point here: for the vast majority of people, medical decisions and medical decision making never depended solely on medical issues and medical judgments. As Loeber's case illustrates, we need to observe the medical world of the eighteenth-century physician against a broader historical backdrop. The tensions between a physicus and his public were not merely skirmishes in the war between the Enlightenment and its enemies. Enlightenment was just one variable here, and by no means the deciding one at that.

Nor can Loeber's extravagances be seen as a typical manifestation of the Enlightenment among physici. While we know less than is desirable about the private lives of the physici, what their families were like, how they amused themselves with hobbies, what their other intellectual aspirations were, some must have lived like Carl Spohr. Physicus Spohr was the father of Louis Spohr, whom contemporaries regarded as the greatest living composer after Beethoven died in 1827.[187] The fame of the son sheds light on the father. The Spohr family had resided in the vicinity of the Harz mountains since the middle of the sixteenth century. The family tree branched into limbs bearing pastors and medical men. Christoph Spohr (1605–79) was a surgeon in Alfeld; his descendants were property owners, pastors, and physicians. Louis's grandfather was a pastor, and his father was a physician, of course. Carl Spohr spent an unsettled youth, fleeing the family home for Hamburg at age fifteen, supporting himself there by translations and language lessons. His medical studies reflect his innate restlessness. He moved more than was customary (even in a century of chronically peripatetic students) from one university to another, attending the universities in Leipzig, Göttingen, Straßburg, and finally Altdorf, where he took his doctorate in 1780.[188] Later in life, he formed a friendship with the father of homeopathy, Samuel Hahnemann, who once practiced in Königslutter. After marrying in 1782, he established himself as a physician in Braunschweig, where he did not prosper. Louis, the couple's first son, was born in 1784. In 1787, Spohr was appointed physicus in Seesen, where he sired five more children. His life as physicus in Seesen— he remained there until his transfer to Gandersheim in 1812—seems to have been relatively uneventful. It was marked, of course, by a certain number of the same conflicts with authorities, difficulties with quacks, problems with payment, and the like that characterized every physicate, but no major flare-ups occurred, and certainly nothing matched the experiences of Loeber or Pini. Indeed, in 1791, when locals in Schöppenstedt objected to the possible transfer of Spohr there, the Collegium medicum defended him as a good physician about whom it had received no complaints (although the Collegium did not move him to Schöppenstedt).[189] In 1829, he received the title of medical councilor in recognition of his services. He filled the post of physicus for fifty-four years until his retirement in 1841.

In many ways, Spohr's lifestyle deserves the adjective "enlightened." Perhaps even more clearly, it represents a certain kind of *Bürgerlichkeit*— that is, the middle-classness typical of the late eighteenth century. Spohr *père* translated numerous texts from English, Spanish, French, and Italian into German. He and his wife were enthusiastic amateur musicians; she enjoyed the piano and had a trained voice, while he played the flute.

Musical evenings were frequent in the Spohr household. Thus, if perhaps Loeber can be seen as the lunatic fringe of the Enlightenment as lived in late eighteenth-century Germany, Spohr was a more mainstream figure, whose apparently very respectable personal life (once he matured) and descent from a family of landowners and citizens long resident in the area made him more acceptable to his community.

And where do the other physici fit—into the model of Loeber or Pini, or that of Spohr? Were they part of the party of enlightenment or of what Peter Gay once termed the party of humanity? And how did they fashion themselves?

A good number sought to maintain or achieve the type of Bürgerlichkeit Spohr exemplified. Many of their petitions, despite their platitudinous tone and special pleading, articulate the aspirations of an emerging middle class.[190] They speak of their desire for a "suitable income" (perhaps unconsciously reworking and updating an older terminology derived from *Hausnotdurft*) and a modicum of comfort, and, almost as frequently, of the need to educate their children properly. Securing good schooling for their children, of course, tied in closely to both enlightenment and middle-class ideals of the value of education in attaining generational social mobility. Physici often asked for transfers to places where their children might be better educated, or for their admission to special schools as part of their perquisites of office. For instance, in 1803 when Dr. Spohr unsuccessfully applied for the position of physicus in Holzminden, the Collegium medicum sugarcoated the rejection by promising "free school in Holzminden for his children [this included Louis Spohr] when they come of that age."[191] Later, Louis Spohr also relied on the special assistance of middle-class, noble, and ducal patrons.[192] Earlier, education for their children rarely seems to have been one of the favors granted physici; rather, they were more likely to receive at their funerals "free ringing of the bells and free interment in the church," as did Dr. Giseler and his predecessor, Dr. Jordan, in Braunschweig. And during the general land survey in the 1750s and 1760s, the commission in charge set aside garden land (valued at 70 thaler) for the physicus in Vorsfelde, specifying that it could be left to his heirs.[193]

The physici themselves often embodied the results of education linked to social mobility. Dr. Müller in Seesen had, for instance, first trained as an apothecary, as had several others, including, much earlier in the century, Dr. Conrad Blum, who had learned his trade at the court apothecary in Eisenach.[194] Generational mobility could be striking; Dr. Krätzer's father and grandfather were horseleeches and executioners.[195] While the eighteenth century tended to regard the flocks of poor students entering fields such as theology and medicine as a growing social and intellectual problem, the very fact reflected a strong faith in the ability of education to elevate, even if that hope was painfully dashed for the many who eventually eked out miserable existences as tutors (the stock literary character of the penniless, frustrated *Hofmeister*) or struggling and impoverished physicians, but who also—let us not forget—formed an underground of enlightenment.[196]

Many physici (although certainly not all) belonged in one sense or another to the party of enlightenment. Many deliberately shaped their lives according to its principles as they understood them, and if that shaping deformed some of these men—as it perhaps twisted Dr. Loeber—it exercised a more benign influence on others, forming their lives as much as did their often tenuous connections to medicine. If we take at face value (which, of course, we should not) the complaints of physici and physicians that their practices were small and provided insufficient employment and income for them, what *did* they do with their time?

Some, like Loeber, drafted plan after plan for the "betterment of humanity," and especially for educational ventures that would also profit them. Loeber's "Philanthropie" had both objectives. Earlier in the century, Urban Beltz had approached the privy council with a scheme for "improving the livelihood and prosperity of the city of Hasselfelde" that was predicated on cameralist and mercantilist principles. He proposed elevating Hasselfelde to a minor commercial and manufacturing center that would contribute to the wealth of the duchy and, indirectly but significantly, improve his own lot. He directly asked the government for employment: "[A]lthough it is not a *medicus*'s principal task to concern himself with matters of *Oeconomica* and *Cameralibus*, it is also not alien to him. Such fields have their basis in nature and the experimental and observational knowledge [gained from nature] by physics and chemistry." He pointed out that in all times, rulers had employed physicians in such realms.[197]

Agronomy, or rather agronomical projects, concerned a few physici in Braunschweig-Wolfenbüttel, most notably Dedekind, with his plan for extracting sugar from beets.[198] Dr. Johann Bühring, after serving as physicus in several places, abandoned medicine in 1783 to take over his father's estate in Kochstedt.[199] Others, like Johann Hoffmann, botanized, as did the secretary of the Collegium medicum and physicus in Braunschweig,

Johann Philipp du Roi, who published botanical articles and supervised the Veltheim tree nursery in Harbke near Helmstedt. Dr. Johann Siegesbeck acquired quite a reputation in plant morphology and after leaving Helmstedt in 1735 went to St. Petersburg, where he directed the botanical garden for almost twenty years.[200] Some, often in their later years, devoted themselves to the natural sciences, as did Urban Brückmann (a member of the Collegium medicum and body-physician) who assembled a notable mineral collection, or Wilhelm Gesenius, physicus in Walkenried from 1795 to 1805, who published a well-respected encyclopedia of butterflies.[201] And Dr. Holdefreund wrote extensively on German antiquities.[202]

More common than these pursuits was medical publication. The vast majority of the medical writing done by the physici (and physicians) in Braunschweig-Wolfenbüttel was ephemeral and brought them little fame, although there were some exceptions, especially among the members of the Collegium medicum and among those who taught at the Anatomical-Surgical Insitute in Braunschweig. Carl Wageler, a student of Roederer's in Göttingen, had come to Braunschweig as professor and body-physician in 1763 and become a member of the Collegium medicum. He taught obstetrics and later in life built up a sparkling reputation for his work on typhosoid illnesses. Johann Sommer, another student of Roederer's, replaced Wageler as teacher of midwifery and director of the lying-in house. He devoted his writing almost exclusively to obstetrics. Theodor Roose, another member of the Collegium medicum and its onetime secretary, in Hirsch's opinion "was one of the most respected physiologists and forensic experts of his day." Another professor at the institute, Karl Himly, wrote extensively on ophthalmology, winning himself a prominent place in its history. The publications of Georg Hildebrandt, the professor of anatomy in Braunschweig, included an important four-volume text on human anatomy, as well as his observations on the small-pox epidemic of 1787 in Braunschweig and a popular medical calendar.[203]

The writings of the other physicians and physici in Braunschweig-Wolfenbüttel won most of their authors only a more fleeting celebrity, but their publications reflected a similar fascination with statistics, medical geography, and topography, as well as popular medical enlightenment and more strictly medical topics. One important contribution was Johann Lange's work on home remedies in Braunschweig.[204] A few other titles must suffice as illustrations. Unlike Lange's volume, almost all of these were composed in German. Several men published works on specific illnesses; Brawe on fevers and on ergot, Bücking on quartan fevers, Dehne and Spohr on rabies, Gesenius (when not off after his butterflies) on putrid fever, Harcke on measles, Holdefreund on croup, Krebs on tuberculosis, Lange on petechial fever, Mümler on scarlet fever, du Roi and Brückmann on scabies, and Zimmer on yellow fever.[205] This list is hardly exhaustive and surely differs little from one that could probably be produced for any similar group. Likewise, the physici and physicians in Braunschweig-Wolfenbüttel contributed articles on spas and waters, on child health, on prevention of illness, on treatments, on lifesaving measures, on statistics, on forensic medicine, on quacks and superstitions; in short on all the myriad topics that crowded the medical journals of the eighteenth century.[206] Perhaps most frequent among the medical articles that filled the pages of the Braunschweig newspapers and journals were those devoted to smallpox inoculation and, later, vaccination.[207] Advocacy of smallpox inoculation and vaccination was a touchstone of enlightenment beliefs, as much as was an article attacking superstition, or quackery, or, for that matter, discussing resuscitation, the better care of the sick in hospitals, and plans for providing more medical care in the countryside. Authorship of such articles linked a man to the network of enlightenment, and, in Braunschweig-Wolfenbüttel, tied him as well to those with the ear of the duke and his privy council. Georg Mühlenbein clawed his way up to power and authority in the duchy and to membership in the Collegium medicum mostly through his efforts in introducing vaccination, both in his first physicate (Schöningen) and through his publications. Not until he converted to homeopathy in the early 1820s did his star, and his influence, fade.[208]

One can thus reconstrue the Enlightenment; it was a way of moving into a new kind of patronage relationship, this time with its partisans. One spoke the same language, promoted the same causes, and lived the life of the enlightened: one wrote, publicized, deplored ignorance. Whereas the language of patronage and clientage was perhaps once almost exclusively that of favors given and services done, it now became one of enlightenment, which attracted those who listened for its tones. Petitions, not only from physicians, but from an array of others as well, continued to be framed in terms of livelihood and need, but increasingly also in cameralist terms of the "common good," and in the even newer language of humanitarianism. This does not, of course, mean that those who penned such articles were sycophants: rather enlightenment, identified through the use of certain key words and phrases, became a part of their consciousness and a part of their identity. That refashioning could take place within the older structures of patronage and clientage. The clique of the enlightened, despite the rhetoric of meritocracy, and despite the growing supply and expanding market of goods and services, was still a clique that sought disciples and rewarded those who followed well.

Assessments

Loeber's case, Spohr's life, and, for that matter, many of the other physici in this book can thus be scrutinized under the lens of the Enlightenment. But the lens of the Enlightenment is fish-eyed, and while it sharpens certain features, it blurs others. The historian must keep switching lenses to avoid being blinded by the seductive and apparently clear image cast by any one—whether it is that of the Enlightenment, professionalization, or medicalization—to the extent of obscuring the others. This chapter has looked at the role of the physici through several lenses, sometimes panoramically, sometimes microscopically. One major theme emphasizes the role of the state at the level of the everyday. We can never comprehend the actions of the "state" unless we first appreciate that the terms *state* and *state policy* represent little more than an imprecise shorthand for an extraordinarily complex mélange of the ideas, the ambitions, and the self-promotion of individuals and groups—here, of physici, Amtmänner, members of the privy council and Collegium medicum, local communities (who themselves were not, of course, monolithic in their wants and desires), with the occasional strong influence of miscellaneous others. The often volatile alliance of agents who made up the "public health apparatus" was rarely directed or fused together by general and inflexible principles. Neither did the central authorities (represented by the privy council and the Collegium medicum) "relentlessly [push] for a uniform way of life to be shared by all members of society" as Marc Raeff has claimed. If there was any ideology here, it was the rough-and-ready one of mediators long used to steering in the murky waters of competing interests, where the coldly rational principles of men who "no longer had any understanding of rural 'primitive' culture" would have soon gone under. These mediators were by no means so eager to destroy the "ancient social ties, communal groupings, and loyalties" as some scholars have depicted them; nor, apparently, did they reject older, admittedly convoluted, administrative pathways out of hand.[209] I seek to show here (and even more in the following chapters) that in health policy—sometimes seen as an arena where the rationalizing tendencies of the "state" nicely meshed with the professionalizing tendencies of academic medicine to suppress alternative healing and to construct a cadre of medical and public health professionals—a far less proactive agenda prevailed.[210]

This state governed overwhelmingly in the decision of individual cases and relied on personal, if invariably ever less immediate, knowledge and observation. The Collegium medicum, like the other mediating agencies in government, stood between the privy council and the duke's subjects. It was defined as a supervisory and information-gathering body, and its mandate included the regulation of all matters touching medicine and public health. Yet the ordinances creating and empowering it were ambiguous and generated, rather than abolished, thorny jurisdictional problems. Indeed, the *executive* powers of the Collegium remained weak.

Most policy rulings were articulated in connection with judgments on individual cases, which then *might* serve as precedents. Consequently, the formulation of health policies in the duchy remained throughout the period ad hoc, involving a process of give-and-take to satisfy numerous individuals and groups, which often cherished conflicting goals and harbored disparate motives. Furthermore, if we insist on viewing the Collegium medicum as a rationalizing agency, we run the danger of ignoring the prominence the privy council and the Collegium gave to preserving existing socioeconomic structures. They often pursued quite different, or contradictory, policies and demonstrated a pronounced degree of flexibility in dealing with unusual or unique local circumstances. This can be seen in many ways. One can find it in the Collegium's own waverings in the realm of medical theory, one can see it in an otherwise inexplicable toleration of illicit practice, and one can observe it as well, as I have chosen to do here, in how the ducal government recruited and dealt with its physici.

The physici were the men on the spot, those who enforced health policies on a day-to-day basis in areas removed from the controlling oversight of the Collegium medicum and the privy council. Because of this distance, because of the world they inhabited, and because policy decisions overwhelming derived from the resolution of single cases, they were in a certain sense equally the *formulators*, or at the very least, the *arbiters* of health policies in their districts. Most became permanent clients of the ducal government, which moved them from one district to other, more lucrative districts as better positions opened up. Undeniably, the physici functioned as critical mechanisms in the public health machinery. But it would be naive to assume that they were the only purveyors of medical information and medical care in their districts. Nor were they the only negotiators of public health policies. Working together with them, or often thwarting their efforts, were a host of others: local officials, school-teachers, pastors, landowners, noblemen, and their wives, to mention only some. Thus, at this level, a multiplicity of agents competed for authority in the field of medicine as elsewhere.

In respect to the physici, the Collegium medicum and the privy coun-cil pursued a strange policy for a purportedly "rationalizing" organiza-tion. Instead of trying to create an independent, salaried bureaucracy of experts, the Collegium nurtured a patronage relationship with its physici. Education and merit counted in their selection, but loyalty and longevity in office, not special skill or talent, went further to explaining a man's ability to retain a position or advance.

In addition, the archival evidence demonstrates that the Collegium medicum and the privy council were by no means out of touch with the desires and concerns of the local notability. Both kept abreast of problems in local communities and often sympathized with the positions repre-sented. For instance, the Collegium suggested moving physici from one district to another when friction developed between a physicus and his community. The Collegium sought to respect and respond to the wishes of those within the community and rarely advanced nominations without testing the waters. It frequently solicited in advance some indication of the possible reactions of the village or town to various candidates. If we turn to the actual appointment of physici, this pattern of conciliation becomes more striking, as is the consideration the Collegium and the privy council gave to preserving socioeconomic integrity and communal peace within local areas. And this also reflects, it seems to me, some realization of a need to husband materials in a world perceived as limited in its ability to mobilize resources or expand production.

The strong inclination to conserve assets and to divvy up a meager economic pie as equitably as possible, rendered the payment of physici a difficult matter. A positively Byzantine salary schedule existed. Each time a new physicus was selected, complex negotiations took place to devise a respectable living for him. Despite several feeble endeavors to upgrade physici's wages, no regularization or general augmentation of salary was achieved. For its part, the ducal government held to the maxim that while entitled to some support from the ducal treasury, physici were to receive only supplements. The localities were to pay most of their wages.[211]

The usual manner of designating physici also does not fit well into the

Procustean mold of a government unswervingly set upon rationalization. The ducal government and the Collegium medicum almost always *negotiated* with communities when appointing new physici. Those eventually named were sometimes well known (if not always in a positive sense) to the communities. Communities themselves frequently raised significant exceptions to the physicians proposed and often recommended others. The Collegium and the privy council went to some lengths to assure that the candidate would be acceptable to the community affected.

It was by no means uncommon for objections raised by local notables to override the Collegium medicum's choice of physicus and promote the appointment of another. Sometimes these petitions smacked clearly of attempts to push for a candidate connected to the notability in some way or other (for example, through marriage), but frequently the Honorationes protested that a physician was inexperienced, or incompetent (thus almost reversing roles with the Collegium medicum), or, just as telling, lacked the requisite familiarity with local circumstances.

Transfers were also gauged to local circumstances. When the Collegium medicum resolved to move Dedekind from Königslutter to Holzminden, it was following one of its few well-established principles: to move faithful officers from less lucrative or less honorific positions to more desirable ones. The physici themselves, as well as notables in the various places, clearly perceived the selection of a physicus as a minor political prize that could fit well into local frameworks of clientage and patronage. Of course, the two (or more) lines of patronage and clientage often clashed. The privy council and the Collegium always hoped to supply physici with opportunities to rake in perquisites in addition to their often meager salaries. This system of perks and favors held sway throughout the eighteenth century and well into the next. Simply put, physici continued to live, for the most part, off the good will of the local notability and the ducal government. Little was done to modify their own understanding of this clientele relationship.

The physici quickly internalized this position, viewed themselves as clients, and acted as such in their recurrent petitioning to the Collegium medicum. And for many of them, their status must have been reinforced, at least at the time of their postings, by their relative youth and inexperience. Most appear to have been in their late twenties when appointed.[212] They often asked the Collegium for higher wages, but just as frequently requested that they be allowed to expand their occupational portfolios by acquiring other posts. They also tried to invoke the authority of the Collegium in coercing local authorities to fulfill pledges of housing, schooling, and grants of food, clothing, and fuel. Physici assumed that the Collegium and the privy council were their vehicles for obtaining favors and justice. These sorts of negotiations were constants and made up a major part of the work done by the Collegium, as did mediating disputes between medical personnel. Even those with attractive postings, such as that of physicus in Holzminden or Blankenburg, used the Collegium as the venue to plead their cases for other advantages. But when physici applied for additional posts, they were often denied on the grounds that they would then monopolize several incomes, robbing others of their proper livelihoods. This was exactly the sort of economic reasoning that continued to drive the actions of bodies like the Collegium and the privy council, which concentrated less on rationalizing and streamlining administrative procedures and more on sustaining the viability of a community as a whole.

Quacks, Bread-Thieves, and Interlopers; Friends, Neighbors, and Kin

Perhaps no myth in early modern medical history has held on as tenaciously as that of the paucity of practitioners. Despite noteworthy studies demonstrating the existence of a plethora of healers, the image of a "medical badlands" simply will not go away.[1] Likewise persistent, if equally false, is the view that for most people the physician was a figure almost as strange and fabulous as the crocodiles and hippopotami that were the featured attractions of eighteenth-century menageries and traveling freak shows. A physicus was present in numerous communities, and the frequent disputes between physici and others testify to the familiarity (and often contempt) that repeated encounters bred. Yet mapping the medical landscape of the eighteenth century is a Sisyphean task. It is impossible, for example, to chart the ebb and flow of practitioners (except for some areas), or to trace out neat statistical trends. What can be reconstructed, however, is equally valuable: a snapshot of a medical landscape peopled with myriad practitioners entangled in a web of wider social, cultural, and economic forces.

The Varieties of Medical Practice

In 1773, Johann Pott, secretary of the Collegium medicum, inventoried as best he could the medical practitioners in the duchy. In Braunschweig, he noted thirteen *medici practici*, four apothecaries, and fourteen surgeons; he did not list the eight midwives practicing there. In Wolfenbüttel, he found five physicians, five surgeons, and one apothecary. Helmstedt had, "besides the members of the medical faculty," one other physician; a physician also lived in Harzburg. Interestingly enough, the secretary did not include the thirteen physici. As to surgeons who practiced outside cities, Pott commented, "I am not in a position to know about them, or to tell if any of them has died or moved."[2] In 1799, Braunschweig had twenty-six physicians, a number that included the members of the Collegium medicum. In addition, sixteen surgeons resided in the city. None were involved in obstetrical work. Ten midwives delivered children. A court apothecary and three others provided medicines. There were, of course, a host of other practitioners, including both those who enjoyed concessions and those who practiced without them.[3] Several university-trained physicians lived outside Braunschweig. The city of Helmstedt had the largest concentration of academically trained physicians in the duchy—five professors and two other physicians—which was hardly surprising considering the presence of the university there. The smaller towns of Goslar, Fürstenberg, Gandersheim, Heßen, Königslutter, Schöppenstedt, and Stadtoldendorf each had one physician in addition to a resident physicus. A Dr. Kraus could be found in the market town of Bodenburg. And this list was not complete. Smaller market towns and villages may well have boasted their own resident physician even much earlier in the century, or their inhabitants may have regularly consulted a physician living in an adjoining territory. Besides the physicians, each city in the duchy had its own apothecary, and there were, moreover, a host of smaller apothecaries scattered about. Likewise fifty surgeons and "a proportionate number" of licensed midwives lived in the countryside.[4]

Conditions in Helmstedt were somewhat different. The university founded there in 1576 was home to several professors of medicine and a whole flock of medical students, almost all of whom engaged in medical practice. Their presence imparted an Aesculapian odor to traditional town/gown rivalries.[5] The physicus there was yet another academically trained physician. But this catalog by no means tallied up the number of "licensed and concessioned" practitioners in the city. For example, at mid century, in addition to Physicus Voß, the census reveals two surgeons, two bathmasters, an apothecary, and three medicine peddlers. Two or three midwives held licenses for the city and its suburbs. A whole series of others—grocers and druggists chief among them—compounded and sold medicines. The odd regimental surgeon, or feldsher, was also, if illicitly, involved in providing medical care to the civilian population.[6] In 1805,

August Jurgens was granted the right to practice veterinary medicine.[7] In addition, a number of traveling specialists, such as oculists and corn doctors, periodically visited Helmstedt.

This picture reproduces itself in miniature for almost every other place in the duchy. The kinds of practitioners found in cities, in market towns, and in the countryside varied in number, but hardly at all in type, aside from the fact that physicians were seldom resident in villages (although they could be found in nearby towns), and few villages had their own apothecary.

For example, in Amt Blankenburg in 1747, there were four physicians, including the 80-year-old holder of the medical licentiate, Blume, who was "no longer able to leave his house"; the "Medicus" Spangenberg; the body-physician Keck, who, however, lived on his sinecure and apparently did not practice medicine; and Dr. "Medicus Practicus" Hummel, who managed to get by on his 60-thaler salary as librarian to Duchess Christine Louise.[8] In the Weser district in 1747, there was only one physician, the physicus, Dr. Wachsmuth. Yet only about an hour's journey away, in Bevern, there was a *medicus practicus* named Goesche (in truth, an apothecary). Wachsmuth categorized him as "no *litteratus*," saying, moreover, "[He] earns but little from his practice, and prefers instead to deal in beer and textiles, and travels about . . . buying flax and selling barrels of his brew." There was only one licensed apothecary in the region, in Holzminden; debts had closed down the apothecary in Stadtoldendorf.

In the Weser district, there were three surgeons and thirteen bathmasters, of varying quality. Just two of them, one surgeon and one bathmaster, belonged to a guild. Four of these men lived and worked in Holzminden. Premier among them was the surgeon Ernst Schmidt. Forty-eight years old in 1747, he had served in several Prussian regiments in Poland as company surgeon and had lived in Holzminden since 1740. He was a member of the surgeons' guild in Nordhausen. Another was Ernestus Happe, aged forty-five. After serving in the army for six years, he had settled in Holzminden twenty years earlier. He had, however, lost his guild papers and had not rejoined the surgeons' guild. He asked to be allowed to practice as a free master (that is, unaffiliated to any guild) "because he is poor and both his eyesight and hearing are bad, and thereby his livelihood suffers . . . and he can take on no apprentices." There were two bathmasters, the identically named brothers Johann Berger, senior and junior. Both had been born in Holzminden, where their father had once run the bathhouse. The elder brother was thirty-three and could not produce his articles of apprenticeship, because "his deceased father had refused to give them to him, so that he would not go off to foreign places [on his *Wanderjahr*] and leave him." The younger brother told the same story. He had no interest in enrolling in a guild, pleading that he was "very weak, infirm, and seriously ill with tuberculosis and does not expect to live much longer."

Although one found no surgeons in the smaller town of Stadtolden-dorf, there were three bathmasters. The oldest, Ernst Scheibe was eighty-one. The next, August Knopp, was somewhat younger—only sixty-four—and had lived in Stadtoldendorf for many years, having come there in 1703. The 27-year-old Georg Riedt, who had arrived in the city just two years before, probably did the lion's share of bathhouse business there. He was not a guild member either.[9]

Gandersheim, which had a population of 1,354, boasted one apothe-cary, three surgeons, and eleven bathmasters in 1769—a not insignificant percentage (8%) of the 172 artisans in the city.[10] Only two groups of artisans in Gandersheim—the tailors and the cobblers—were larger (there were, by contrast, nine merchants, eight linen weavers, seven smiths, six cabinetmakers, and eight butchers). And in the first decades of the nine-teenth century, the number of medical personnel was about the same. Two physicians lived in the city in 1814. One was the physicus, Carl Spohr, who had been there since 1786; the other was a younger man, Dr. Johann Liebrecht, who had settled in 1806. Of the three surgeons in the town, two, Ludwig Martini and Otto Thilo, had practiced there for al-most a quarter century; the other, Ludwig Martini's son, had become city surgeon in 1795. None received a salary. The apothecary, Josua Höfer, was a newcomer, having arrived in 1812. Of the two midwives, Marie Kön-necke had "reputedly" been examined and appointed by the Collegium medicum twelve years earlier. The other, Johanna Misch, had been ap-pointed by the magistrates in 1806. Neither received a salary. By 1818, little had changed in the district. Two physicians resided in Gandersheim proper, and there were twelve surgeons (four in Gandersheim, and the rest in other places), thirty-one midwives (two each in Gandersheim, Greene, and Delligsen, and one each in twenty-five smaller places), and two ani-mal doctors (in Gandersheim and Greene).[11]

It was thus a tiny, remote, and indigent settlement indeed that neither figured on the itineraries of traveling oculists, oil salesmen, and peddlers nor had a resident surgeon, bathmaster, or retired or furloughed feld-sher.[12] This sufficiency, or even surfeit, of practitioners became the rule only after about 1730, however. Lutter am Barenberge, which in the mid and late eighteenth century was no more poorly endowed with practitioners than other similarly sized places, had only one bathmaster in the late 1600s, and he lived as a small cottager and had "but little to do."[13] For more immediate types of medical attention—self-help or the assistance of neighbors, friends, root-wives, and others—there was probably little to choose between the rural and urban settings.

Of course, such surveys and descriptions are quantitatively and qualitatively deceptive, perhaps even fanciful. Obviously, the size of practice varied, often enormously. Johann Barthold, for example, who held a privilege as "Operateur & Medicinae Doctor" in Braunschweig, treated about 330 people over an eighteen-month period in 1712–14. His large practice, which spanned the entire city and virtually the whole social spectrum, encompassed both medical and surgical cases. He treated men and women, children and adults, officers and gentlemen, artisans and laborers, among them a large number of cobblers, whose guild had contracted with him for medical care. He did far more internal medicine than surgery; only seventeen cases were exclusively surgical in nature, such as repairing hernias, treating kidney and bladder stones, soothing eye injuries, and couching cataracts. To judge from these selected records, he bound no wounds and treated no accidents. Rather, he attended numerous cases of fever (ardent, quartan, and tertian), consumption, influenza, and dropsy, as well as worm fever and convulsions (especially in children), panic attacks and cardiac arrhythmia (mostly among his female patients). He did no midwifery at all.[14]

While practical physicians like Barthold would have been found on Pott's list, it excluded the myriad other practitioners who did not slide neatly into the categories of physician, surgeon, apothecary, or midwife. Most damning, however, is the fact that such registers say little about the aspects of medical practice that make up the meat of this chapter: how practitioners got along with others, how they thought of themselves, related to their patients, conceived and verbalized their right to practice. To ferret out these imponderables, one must examine the full range of medical practice, while bearing in mind the larger environment in which medical practitioners moved. Particularly important here will be an analysis of how practitioners described themselves and their actions. By looking at the language they employed to make sense of their activities and their position in this world, it is possible to enter a bit into their mental universe. Especially critical here are *changes* in their discourse as they grappled with the transformations of their environment and tried to adapt their self-images, their ways of representing themselves to others, and the language they used to deal with local authorities, the central government, other practitioners, neighbors, clients, and friends. Simply put, what were the elements of their consciousness and identity? Did these change over time and, if so, how?

To answer these questions, we need to look at many practitioners and how each fitted into extant medical hierarchies. Perhaps more important, we must come to see how these hierarchies corresponded to the larger social structures of city, town, or village, and how the men involved adapted to informal, yet nevertheless densely structured, networks of friends, neighbors, and kin. Here we must avoid facilely dividing practitioners into tidy groups of midwives, bathmasters, surgeons, druggists, and apothecaries, if by doing so we mean to erect impenetrable barriers around them. Throughout this chapter, we shall repeatedly observe how practitioners fought to defend their own rights and privileges, and to secure their livelihood (Nahrung), and how this continual bickering over territory formed the core of their consciousness. While medical ordinances tried to distinguish among the sundry forms of medical practice, and while practitioners of all kinds were perfectly capable of using these legal statutes to argue their cases, the overlap of practice everywhere and the constant violations of the territory of one practitioner by another were so common as to be normal parts of the medical world of the eighteenth century. Patients, as we shall see in Chapter 5, tended to be fairly oblivious to the legal niceties, either because they did not know them or because they did not care.[15]

While the 1721 medical ordinance explained the proper conduct for all medical personnel and laid down criteria for determining the boundaries between "licit" and "illicit" actions, the time-honored ducal prerogative of granting privileges and concessions to petitioners, including dentists, oculists, and peddlers of wonder cures, deposited obscuring strata of medical practice onto already equivocal distinctions between licit and illicit practices.[16] When the Collegium medicum was established in 1747, it held the exclusive mandate to examine medical practitioners, grant or refuse them the right to practice, or limit that right medically, geographically, or temporally. In addition, the 1747 measure charged the Collegium medicum with investigating and punishing "all unauthorized, fraudulent and superstitious treatments, [and] prohibited operations, whether or not they involve dispensing medicines."[17] Herein, the "terrible race of quacks" (*Quacksalber* or *Pfuscher*), "those man-eaters" (*Menschenfresser*) were blamed for the "wanton slaughter" of thousands of the duke's subjects, "who could have been useful to the state [had they lived], for no pestilence, no natural catastrophe, no war can rip people away from their loved ones and from mankind" as quickly as the quacks supposedly did. In the rhetoric about quacks, no word, no description was too brutal. Animalistic metaphors tended to prevail. Georg Mühlenbein, physicus in Schöningen, compared quackery to "a many-headed monster . . . when one head is lopped off, ten appear in its place."[18]

Yet years of interleaving the "permitted" with the "forbidden" created large gray areas of medical practice and made it almost impossible for anyone to discern easily who was and who was not a quack. A bewildering array of "ordinary guild surgeons, privileged bathmasters, veterinary empirics, among them executioners and shepherds, manufacturers of medicines and their agents, dealers in patent remedies, 'emergency' apothecaries, sellers of cosmetics and arcana, sedentary and peripatetic *operateurs*, including oculists, lithotomists, dentists, and corn doctors; laymen, who inoculate the cowpox, or promise to restore hunchbacks, twisted limbs and clubfeet to straightness; 'experimentalists' who apply electricity, galvanic fluids, and magnetism . . . and those who claim to possess the touch or to heal by sympathy" populated the countryside.[19] As almost all of these purported to have, and many could actually prove, a *legal* right to practice, we need to look much more closely at what a quack was in this context, or was supposed to be.

In legal terms, the medical regulations of 1721 and 1747 limited internal medicine to physicians; compounding and dispensing medicaments to apothecaries; major surgery to first-class surgeons; minor surgical techniques, such as bloodletting, bandaging, and fitting trusses, to lower-level surgeons; barbering and cupping to barber-surgeons or bathmasters, and so on. The fault of such a minutely structured hierarchy was that it never corresponded to reality. Exceptions had to be made, and the Collegium medicum made them by the hundreds, muddling its own distinctions between legitimate and illegitimate practices of medicine.[20] Furthermore, and just as important, the law permitted no practitioner to poach or encroach on the protected terrain of others: physicians were not to dispense medicines; surgeons were not to barber; bathmasters were not to bleed.[21] Poaching or encroachment was called *Pfuscherey* in Germany, and *empiétement* in France.[22]

And it is clear that in the literature and legislation of the times, if not necessarily in the minds of practitioners and their clients, the definition of a quack hardened during the course of the eighteenth century. The medical ordinance of 1721 accepted a broad range of persons as legal, or at least tolerated, practitioners of the healer's craft. Internal medicine was most rigidly circumscribed, being declared off-limits to everyone except physicians. All others—surgeons, for example—were expressly denied the right to prescribe "innerliche Medicamenten." The Collegium medicum warned them to restrain their "presumptuous natures," as their "Ignorantz der Fundamental Theorie" rendered them unable to ascertain the "true causes" of diseases, so that their therapeutics could only rest on a "dangerous empiricism." Surgeons and army surgeons were also admonished to admit their limitations and "well consider that you who lack all knowledge of the *fundamentis mediciniae* might easily cure someone into his grave."[23] Still, both ordinances condoned the medical activities of a variegated crew of "half-surgeons, operators, and snake-charmers."[24] Even root-wives were not totally banned from practice, although they were forbidden to distribute "powerful, blood-stimulating herbs." The Collegium medicum conceded that several types of operations—the couching of cataracts, lithotomies, the surgical correction of cleft palates—were so infrequently performed that "regular surgeons [could] lose their touch," and it therefore granted special licenses to "skilled operators" who offered these "needed services." At the same time, they were ordered to eschew "viewing the urine and prognosticating from it . . . [as pursuits] which bamboozle the common man and inveigle him into unnecessary treatments."[25] The others in this category, the roving dentists, mountebanks, and drug-dealers, were required to obtain special dispensations if they wished to ply their trades. Each year they had to petition the authorities for renewal of their concessions, be examined by a physicus, and pay a 1-thaler fee. These privileges retained their validity only for the duration of a fair or market, and "immediately upon its close, [they are to] pack up and depart."[26]

The medical ordinance of 1747 and laws passed subsequently further constricted the boundaries of allowed medical practice, although by no means eliminating the niches certain operators inhabited. Traveling medicine men, dealers in patent remedies, carnivalists, and the like, however, found it increasingly difficult, and after 1791 theoretically impossible, to obtain permission to erect their booths and peddle their wares unmo-

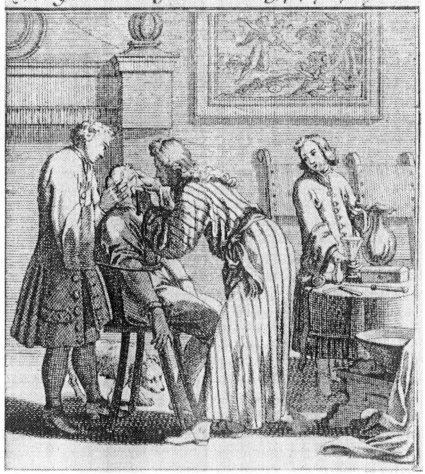

"Der Oculist," from Christoph Weigel, *Abbildung der gemein-nützlichen Haupt-Stände,* . . . (Regensburg: n.p., 1698). Reproduced with the permission of the Wellcome Institute Library, London.

lested.[27] Mobility itself had become suspect to the medical elite, although some of the most dexterous operators continued to move from place to place.

Oculists are an excellent example of the peripatetic operators for whom transience was an inescapable fact of life.[28] Early modern oculists demonstrated surprising successes with operable cataracts. Still, even highly respected and superbly talented men, like Georg Bartisch (who composed the first ophthalmic text in German) in the sixteenth century, and the Prussian Dr. Hilmer in the eighteenth, never found it economically feasible to settle down permanently.[29] Master Jochimb Schmidt, who had successfully treated the 74-year-old reigning duke, August the Younger, for cataracts in 1653, himself lamented how "the innumerable mountebanks and quacks about in this land . . . have taken the food out of my mouth and have destroyed my livelihood" and that even in his declining years, he was forced "by cruel necessity to cast about for my living in strange and inhospitable places."[30] Thus, unquestionably, the word *quack* was by no means the sole property of physicians as a weapon against their rivals.

The traveling oculists, as well as the other peripatetics (although the separation of roving and sedentary healers is misleading and probably misconceived),[31] differed vastly in their abilities and honesty. Some proved outright crooks, seeking only to fleece their victims; some believed in their cures. Many offered panaceas in every imaginable guise, praising rose water as a "universal balsam," simple glycerine as anodyne for the pains of strangury, or exalted tonics guaranteed to lift melancholy, thicken (or thin) the blood, and restore one's lost manhood. Breathing out promises of eternal (or almost eternal) health and beauty, they hawked distillates and tinctures of lead or mercury and caustic substances like lye as cosmetics, or mixed them into their "wonder cures." They often accompanied their sales pitches with magic tricks and illusions, troupes of jugglers, contortionists, tightrope walkers, animal acts, and curiosity shows. Many surrounded their healing with the hoopla of show business, such as the oculist Seiffert in Braunschweig, who himself told the magistrates that he intended to entice customers with the spectacle of his small daughter dancing on a tightrope.[32] Some, like "Councilor von Köring" from Berlin, paved their way in advance, flooding the next stops on their tours with ornately printed advertisements. Köring proclaimed his ability to restore vision to those sightless since birth and "to many others who are stone-blind, all within the time it takes to utter an Our Father." He also pledged

Duke August's handwriting before his cataract operation. HAB, Cod. Guelf. 236.8 Extrav. Blatt 52. Reproduced with the permission of the Herzog August Bibliothek, Wolfenbüttel.

Duke August's handwriting after his cataract operation. HAB, Cod. Guelf. 236.9 Extrav. Blatt 50. Reproduced with the permission of the Herzog August Bibliothek, Wolfenbüttel.

sure cures for deafness, cosmetic surgery for harelips that would make the sufferer "as beautiful as one of the Muses," palliatives for cancerous growths, relief for those writhing in the "hellish tortures of the stone," and more. He arrived in Braunschweig accompanied by a retinue of six men clad in blue livery with yellow trim. After examining him and his instruments (the optical needles "neatly displayed in a red morocco case"), the Collegium medicum felt confident of his ability to couch cataracts, but refused to allow him to treat other ailments and insisted that he distribute no more "booklets of lies." While the Collegium quite amenably licensed oculists, lithotomists, and dentists, albeit for only short periods of time, it demanded that they refrain from all "inappropriate display and histrionics." Others hoped the puffery of titles—*court* dentist, *ducal* surgeon, *royal* oculist—and the grandeur of their documentation would impress the Collegium and their prospective clients. Thadaeus Meyer, "operator and oculist," proudly presented his credentials—eleven folio sheets written on fine parchment and graced with an imposing seal—to the council in Gandersheim, but not to good effect.[33]

Oculists, corn doctors, and lithotomists were frequent sights in towns and villages. The government tolerated and encouraged them throughout the eighteenth century, as their special talents were valued. In the wake of the first territorial medical ordinance of 1721, the government seemed to crack down on the "dissipated hordes" of "mountebanks, hoaxers, con men, tricksters, tumblers, and ropedancers," who "swindle money from Our faithful subjects" at fairs and markets. An order from 1723, for example, sternly warned that "these will no longer be tolerated." But they were. The rest of the paragraph, which allowed those who had "special concessions" from either the duke himself or the privy council to practice openly, considerably attenuated the harshness of the ban.[34] As late as the end of the century, some of these operators, oculists, and cutters for bladder and kidney stones enjoyed the right to practice.[35] Both the ducal privy council and, after 1747, the Collegium medicum, continued to receive and consider requests for concessions, which ran the gamut from men such as one Girault, who billed himself as dentist to the duke of the Palatinate and Cologne, carried documents from the Academy in Paris, and sold an amulet guaranteed to help children with teething,[36] and oculists like the Italian "eye-doctor" Cassamata and the well-known and widely traveled Dr. Hilmer, to less famous purveyors of universal balsams and other remedies, such as Ferdinand Knupf, who petitioned for the right to sell his medicines, as well as to exhibit, among other curiosities, "a great crocodile from Egypt," the Asian Jokus fish with two legs, a long tail, and a head "round as a ball," and an "ingenious mechanism" that in the space of two minutes could accurately reproduce any portrait in miniature.[37]

There was substantial opposition to the granting of such concessions. Resistance came from the Collegium medicum, of course, but also in large measure from magistrates in big cities and, perhaps even more vehemently, from those in smaller towns. The last were almost viscerally suspicious of vagrants.[38] And the public was not always easily duped. Protests about such practitioners, while not exactly common, were hardly unknown. For example, in 1686, the draper Christian Schindler complained about a mountebank who had sold his son medicines during the Braunschweig fair. Schindler protested that his son, "who contributed to my livelihood and fortune in no little degree," after swallowing the pills, purged so strongly that he swooned, then fell into a fever. Schindler had had to consult a physician and "several clever surgeons," who prescribed "the use of very dangerous mineral doses" but could not guarantee his son's recovery. He asked for restitution of the costs of the cure now under way, as well as for the loss of livelihood his son's incapacity occasioned.[39]

Government itself sometimes scrupled little. Fees paid for concessions (and they cost between 5 and 6 thaler toward the end of the century) were, after all, revenue.[40] Still, as we shall see, the granting of concessions most threatened those who *already* held other concessions and privileges, and the members of various medical guilds, such as bathmasters, barber-surgeons, and surgeons. Over the course of the eighteenth century, the ducal government gradually closed the aperture, allowing fewer concessions. The surgeons, apothecaries, and bathmasters of the duchy supported such measures as long as they were not directed against them individually.

It was—typically—a single incident that provoked the passing of the final ban in 1791, as the case of Gottlieb Schamler, an erstwhile actor, illustrates. Schamler's printed advertisement promised, among other things: "To soothe the most awful toothache in a quarter hour; to set artificial teeth [so skillfully] that one cannot distinguish them from natural ones." In addition, he offered tooth powders for sale, as well as an "English water . . . which is not a kind of lacquer or paint, but rather a secret and a masterpiece of beauty" and "a balsamlike pomade, which restores lost hair and makes thinning hair once again fresh and alive." He promised as well to remove birthmarks, goiters, pimples, unwanted hairs, corns, and bunions, besides curing frostbite and chilblains.[41] In 1785, he appeared in Braunschweig, petitioning to be permitted the practice of dentistry at the fair. He had enjoyed a similar concession in 1784 and brought with him a testimonial from the police director, Fredersdorf, to the effect "that he and his wife during their stay here caused no complaint to be lodged against them."[42] He received a three-week concession allowing him to vend "his innocuous salves." When, however, he violated its terms, "in that he tried to force an internal powder on a person to treat [his] deafness," the dean of the Collegium medicum refused to extend his concession. Here the city authorities rendered their opinion, noting that while the Collegium indeed possessed the right to judge the capabilities of those who applied for concessions, "for our part we would not allow such mountebanks and dentists to hawk their wares" in public places. "Such is," they continued, "not of public benefit," as "like medicines can be obtained just as cheaply and of the same good quality in the local apothecary."[43] While the 1791 edict forbade such practices, not until 1798 did the Collegium finally stop distributing concessions to "roving druggists, oculists, lithotomists, dentists, and their like" entirely.[44]

It would, however, be a grave mistake to think that opposition to wandering practitioners came solely from the Collegium medicum, the privy council, and local governments. Their hostility did not arise solely from principles of good medicine, and they were not attempting to suppress irregular healers to the benefit of physicians: the reality was more labyrinthine, as several examples show. The type of person who applied for concessions varied hardly at all from the beginning of our period until the end. What did change was the way they hawked their wares: with the passage of time, extravagantly worded, if cheaply printed, flyers appeared in greater numbers; they were more elaborate; the language was more engaging, more "salesmanlike"; and, perhaps most striking, the range and number of products greatly expanded.[45] Whereas in the seventeenth and early eighteenth centuries, the traveling dentist might have sold tooth powders and brushes, by the 1740s and 1750s, his items of merchandise numbered in the tens and twenties. An advertisement Johann Lucas circulated in 1766 listed twenty-eight different products and services. This growth of inventory and its diversification marks the times and goes far to verify Roy Porter's thesis about the convergent evolution of quackery and consumerism in the eighteenth century. More attention will be paid to the dynamics of this interaction later in this chapter.[46]

The idea of licensing was less obviously connected to an early form of "quality control" than to a desire, on the one hand, to augment state revenues, and, on the other, to protect and promote industry and commerce by granting special, sometimes almost monopolistic, rights. In the seventeenth century, the privy council and the duke himself distributed "consent and privilege letters" in various trades. It was equally necessary for academically trained physicians as for surgeons and operators to obtain such patents. Most who applied spoke of their "art" (*Kunst*); in fact, the majority practiced some sort of surgery. Martin Petzold in 1647 received a concession to present his "skills, medicines, and treatments" to the public, and to sell his preparations "freely [and] unhindered."[47] In 1660, Hermann Meyer received permission to practice and "otherwise to be tolerated in Our duchy and lands, be allowed to exercise his *Profession* without prejudice . . . and to reside permanently with his family and household here as is right and proper for a *Medicus* and *Chymicus*."[48] In 1662, Dr. Johannes Fabricius, described as "especially skilled in cutting for ruptures and the stone," likewise secured the right to practice "without impediment" everywhere in the duchy.[49] In 1697, the regimental feldsher, Johann Kaspar Witte, who had served with the colors for twenty-eight years, wished to be allowed to "establish my household" and open his practice in the districts of Lichtenberg and Gerbhardtshagen. The privy council granted Witte's request, and it extended his privilege to his widow when he died in 1701.[50]

The decision to bestow or deny the right to practice turned on several variables, of which competence was only one, and perhaps not the most important. Equally central to the negotiations were questions of territory, of livelihood, of settlement, of civil status, and of the taxpaying capabilities of the petitioner. The central government, the guilds, and local authorities shared these concerns and the language that expressed them. The privy council followed the path it had set down in dealing with the guilds. That is, while trying to loosen the guilds' stranglehold on production to some extent and to break their legal authority, it remained committed to analogous goals of providing suitable and sufficient livelihoods; and it expressed its decisions in a language that embodied these objectives. As the government tried to exert more control over economic life in the duchy, it repeatedly mixed into disputes among claimants, including those who asserted the right to some particular branch of medicine. Local authorities, however, worried about the economic viability of new residents. Settling in a village meant that the recent arrival had to find his own niche, politically and socially as well as economically. Local authorities based their decisions to a large extent on their estimation of where the newcomer might fit in the village hierarchy and not merely on the basis of his or her *medical* competence. Ability was never a matter of indifference, but it alone was not paramount. Or perhaps it is better to say that competence had many components: economic and political as well as occupational.

For example, in 1745, the "tooth and mouth doctor" Christoph Siegreich petitioned the Collegium medicum for a concession. He described his abilities, accenting his skill in extracting rotten teeth and in replacing them with artificial ones, and in cleaning teeth "with comfortable and subtle instruments." Dr. Behrens reported approvingly on Siegreich's competence, stressing the proficiency he had gained through long experience. While Behrens felt that Siegreich's capabilities would "certainly prove valuable to the public," he nonetheless raised doubts. Would Siegreich be able to wrest an adequate living from dentistry, even if he proposed "traveling occasionally to nearby places and [visiting] the annual markets and fairs"? Or would he be forced to resort to illicit practices? If Siegreich settled in Braunschweig, what impact would his trade have on the local surgeons and bathmasters? When Siegreich finally obtained a concession, it went with the title of privileged dentist and entitled him to the exclusive practice of dentistry in the city. That was unusual, although the other conditions of his appointment were not—for example, it was "in no way permitted him to allow his wife or any other person to substitute for him in his absence or in any other circumstance." There is no sure way of determining the extent of Siegreich's business. He performed dentistry in Braunschweig until his death in 1781 or 1782, when his son, Johann, asked to "inherit" his father's privilege. After determining that as a dentist Siegreich *fils* was "not totally without talent," the Collegium medicum granted him, like his father, a *privilegium exclusium*, for which he paid 5 thaler 33 mariengulden.[51]

The possession of this entitlement hardly created an economically secure world for either Siegreich. In 1756, the Collegium medicum noticed how many dentists peddled their wares and their services at trade fairs, thus "much prejudicing" Siegreich and the city's surgeons.[52] A more serious threat appeared in the form of a "French actor" named Julien, who applied for a dentistry concession in 1764. The Collegium examined Julien and found him and his skills in no way exceptional. The report noted that he possessed only one dental tool, a pelican, used for dislodging teeth, "but lacks the other necessary ones, such as a dental elevator, clasp, and English key." The Collegium argued that as there was insufficient work for two dentists in Braunschweig, Siegreich deserved preference. Still, Julien secured a concession for half a year, which was then extended for at least one more six-month period. After that Julien became a regular sight at the Braunschweig fairs.[53] The Collegium was never quite happy with him; and Siegreich was vociferously unhappy. In 1770, Siegreich protested that "his small livelihood, from which only and alone he must survive, has been conspicuously reduced over the years." The Collegium took Siegreich's part, disapproving in equal measure Julien's "very ordinary skills" and his outrageous prices. Moreover, Julien "draws money out of the city." On the other hand, Siegreich was so modest in his demands "that no one complains about him." The Collegium found Siegreich's desire for protection fully justified, the more so because, unlike Julien, Siegreich paid *onera publica* from his earnings.[54] The outcome of the conflict between Siegreich and Julien is unknown, although Siegreich was still practicing dentistry in Braunschweig over a decade later. The terms of the Collegium's defense of Siegreich's privilege are most meaningful here; they form common threads in the definition of practice and in determining the "territory" of a practitioner. The Collegium and Siegreich both spoke of a livelihood—a Nahrung—that warranted, merited, and demanded protection.

Nahrung meant livelihood in a very broad way. The citizen's livelihood (*bürgerliche Nahrung*), as Mack Walker has aptly described it, was "not a static property qualification nor even a requirement of technical skill. These might contribute to it, but they were not its essence. It meant the economic security and stability of the solid citizen, a trustworthy man because he was committed to local society and totally reliant on it." Walker spoke of the citizen's livelihood within the framework of the German home towns, but the concept of livelihood as "the economic security and stability of the solid citizen" was just as relevant to guilds and village economies elsewhere.[55] Everywhere the ideal of livelihood was allied to that of the "appropriate need" (*Hausnotdurft*) that sustained inequalities by working to guarantee that each household and each citizen could demand that his rights of livelihood and his unique socioeconomic position be defended.[56] In this vein, when the Collegium medicum stressed the moderation of Siegreich's prices as well as his links to the city, it singled out no unimportant or trivial features, or qualities solely indicative of Siegreich's unimpeachable character. Siegreich was a taxpayer, Julien was not; Siegreich owned property, Julien could not; Siegreich spent his income in Braunschweig; Julien leeched money out of the duchy. We shall explore these topics in more depth later, as they are the essence of how the seventeenth and eighteenth centuries defined the limits and proprieties of medical practice, and such considerations did not, of course, apply only to medical practitioners.

Perhaps these concerns are mostly easily exemplified in the production and sale of things. Issues of money, commerce, and livelihood (alongside those of purity and safety) determined how the government dealt with a particularly numerous and varied group of medicine manufacturers and vendors. The medical ordinances of 1721 and 1747 allowed only approved and privileged apothecaries to prepare and sell medicines. Physicians were specially forbidden to compound and dispense medicines themselves, with the exception of specifics and arcana deemed their "secrets" and part of their personal property.[57] This conflict between physicians and apothecaries over the right to distribute medicines was already hoary with age, and had been repeatedly, if vainly, resolved in favor of the apothecaries. In 1696, for example, the municipal government in Braunschweig sought to uphold the rights and shield the livelihoods of apothecaries against the encroachment of physicians. To prevent the "ruination" of the apothecaries, the privy council admonished physicians to desist from self-dispensing and have their prescriptions filled at licensed apothecary shops.[58]

Competition for the apothecaries did not only come in the guise of the physician. In the eighteenth century, as colporteurs traveled the improved roads of the duchy more rapidly and distributed themselves more widely over the countryside, as the number of products proliferated, as the means of advertising increased, and, in fact, as economic life, especially after mid century, geared up, more and more dealers in medicines popped up to compromise the apothecaries' business. Increasingly, complaints from apothecaries focused, not on the competitive threat from physicians, but on "corner apothecaries" (that is, those not members of the guild), on wholesalers who sold "their elixirs and tinctures, and other fraudulent potions" directly to patients, and on surgeons, feldshers, "begging hags," and soldiers.[59] To fight these, municipalities cautioned all physicians and shopkeepers to refrain from the trade in medicines "whether *simplicien* or *compositorum*" and ordered that a vigorous watch be kept for all peddlers who dealt in "tonics and cordials."[60] Nothing suggests that such prohibitions worked, and the trade in medicines grew rather than diminished.

"Oil-peddlers" in Helmstedt around the middle of the century, for instance, handled a wide range of products. A list of what three stallkeepers could always supply suggests the breadth of their business: sieves "in wooden frames, and hair-sieves from Bohemia"; oils and medicines bought from traders at the Braunschweig fairs or in "German-Bohemia," which included theriacs, scorpion oils, sulphur balsam, oils of amber, caraway seed, juniper, almond, aniseed, and turpentine. From merchants at fairs they also purchased, and then vended, distilled substances, including essence of pomegranate, "mixtur simplex," stomach drops, tincture of bezoar, and Hungarian water. In addition, they could also furnish their customers with dry goods and notions, such as strings for shoes, belts, buttons, penknives, combs made of ivory and horn, snuffboxes, thimbles, needles, sealing wax, incense, scissors, and eyeglasses.[61]

In this battle between the apothecaries and their rivals for control over the sale of new items, we see the signs of a consumer society expanding within an economic framework that still, however, spoke in an older, corporatist idiom. Although the apothecaries' tough competitors—the wholesalers, retailers, grocers, and peddlers (especially the "oil-peddlers")—were hardly novel figures in the middle of the eighteenth century, there were simply more of them and many more of their wares.[62] And the economic world they inhabited was changing. It took time to adopt new ways of talking and new ways of dealing, and for the socioeconomic structures to adjust themselves. At first, procedures and practices mingled the old and the new in tolerably jury-rigged ways. Throughout the eighteenth century, therefore, battles were waged verbally in the corporatist discourse, even as that discourse was growing obsolete and less able to phrase current themes and tensions.

This dissonance would eventually become almost deafening at all levels of government and society, but those involved in the daily fray over livelihood and rights perceived it first and most painfully. One way governments had traditionally tried to cope with issues of encroachment within the guild system was simply to *list* the products each guild was entitled to fabricate and sell, thus delineating market boundaries.[63] Some broader logic always governed the distinctions made, even if it was often tenuous or, more frequently in the eighteenth century, extremely tangled. Still, as products proliferated, listing rapidly became outdated. Lists had to be revised at ever-shorter intervals or in an ad hoc manner. Listing now proved a crude discursive or linguistic way of dealing with a substantive problem. When lists no longer sufficed, when the older methods of dealing with production and distribution broke down, there was a period of flux, while new methods and new discourses evolved. One such moment occurred in the mid to late eighteenth century: old forms held on, people defended their rights and privileges with them, yet more and more adventurers, more and more fence-leapers, more and more encroachers pushed their claims. Those on the other side of the wall—the guildsmen and those who worked (and had long worked) with guild words and mind-sets (including governments)—no longer could fight either substantially or discursively merely on the territory of livelihood. Many of them no longer really wanted to. They, too, were being co-opted into, or were helping to shape, a new world of denser market relationships. Yet that transition was hardly complete by the end of the eighteenth century.

Several of these issues of encroachment, consumerism, and their languages in a medical context assume greater importance in the second half of this chapter, but before we consider them, it is necessary to enlarge further on a concept and word of special significance here: *quack*.

Quacks and Quackery

Two apparently—but only apparently—contradictory phrases have often been used to characterize the medical world of the eighteenth century: it was either "the golden age of the doctor" or "the golden age of the quack." Likewise, two themes have dominated the writing of the social history of medicine over the past twenty-five years: the rise of the medical profession and the subsequent medicalization of society.[64] Historians concerned with the development of professionalization have generally traced the beginnings of professional medicine to the late eighteenth and early nineteenth centuries. Simply (perhaps too simply) put, the play of market forces in a nascent capitalist system drove professionalization forward. Thus the push toward professionalization was intimately linked with the need to achieve cultural and social authority in order to fight the serious economic competition quacks posed.

A series of studies focusing on the rise of commercial capitalism and a consumer society from the late seventeenth century through the mid nineteenth has, however, significantly transformed the debate over the terms and dimensions of this rivalry. Roy Porter dissolved the "quack/ professional" conundrum by stressing the "parallels, not the antitheses" between quackery and orthodoxy. The "tenacity of quackery" and the successes of orthodoxy in eighteenth-century England were both due to the rise of "medical entrepreneurship in a consumer society," according to

Porter: "Far from disappearing, it [quackery] flourished, and it did so because of the specific orientation of a commercial capitalist, spectacle-loving, consumer-oriented society, in which the very goal of quacks—to persuade the public to consume medicine—was expedited by the same forces that explain why the society became more heavily medicine-consuming at large."[65] This sort of research has helped as well in the ongoing process of reversing the older stereotype that introduced this chapter: rather than a medical wasteland, we find a medical landscape pullulating with practitioners. Anyone who fell ill was faced, not with a dearth of possibilities, but (as Mary Fissell has phrased it) with "a profusion of health-care providers eager for his or her custom."[66] Such demonstrations of the superfluity, rather than the scarcity, of medical practitioners highlight interpretations that most medical historians now accept: that the lines between popular and elite medicines were very blurry; that there was little difference between what academically trained physicians and other healers thought and did; that people differentiated hardly at all among the claims of various healers, consulting practitioners of all types serially or simultaneously.

Perceptions of quackery, too, must thus be firmly situated in these contexts. To do so, we must first see how the representation of quackery depended on the sense of economic encroachment. And while this notion is critical in any understanding of the dynamics of quackery, it forces us at the same time to confront a bigger question. If a richly laden medical marketplace needed to feed on the fecundity of a pubescent consumer economy, should this not cause us to reevaluate the economic vigor and productive potential of an area—Germany—generally regarded as a commercial backwater? A closer look at the phenomenon of quackery therefore prompts a more general reassessment of larger economic issues. New products and new services, and their purveyors, strained existing perceptions of proper market behavior and required accommodations to be struck—substantively and discursively—among market forces, legal strictures, and older notions of the fair deal, the equitable distribution of the economic pie, and of the "appropriate livelihood" of a household. The introduction of new products and new services—proprietary medicines and treatments—disrupted this world. Later, I shall suggest the impact of economics on how people made their medical choices: to what extent, for example, did they come to regard medical advice as a commodity, something to be bought and sold rather than offered freely as the gift of a friend or as a neighborly kindness? Such investigations may help us find out if consumer mentalities had become rooted in everyday life by the end of the eighteenth century.

In a major work on the social world of medicine in eighteenth-century France, Matthew Ramsey has schematically related medical practitioners to the market: folk healers moved almost exclusively in the realm of the traditional economy; physicians were guided by corporatism; and empirics exploited the market economy. Ramsey argues that each of these groups was shaped by its own economic ethos—that is, by differing (and often contradictory) ideas of how the business of medicine should be conducted. For Ramsey, the charlatan or quack was the *chevalier d'industrie* most in tune with an emergent capitalist or entrepreneurial mentality.[67] While this tidy structure buckles under the weight of eighteenth-century economic and medical realities—it leaves out, for example, the thinking of those who selected practitioners; it portrays quacks and quackery too simply; it ignores the often aggressive marketing done by physicians; and it does not fully consider all the licensed medical personnel who were *not* physicians—it nonetheless offers a useful starting point from which to launch a broader survey of the relationships among business, economics, and medicine.

Pfuscherey, the guilds' term for proscribed activities, was the word used to describe medical quackery throughout the period.[68] Zedler's *Universal-Lexikon*, published before mid century, variously defines a *Pfuscher* as "a man unskilled in his craft" or, "among artisans," an interloper, or "ground rabbit" (*Bönhasen*). Under *Pfuscherey*, Zedler further directs us to the entry *Nahrungs-Störerey*, which means the disruption of a livelihood. Quackery in crafts and in many areas of medicine involved any infringement or encroachment that subverted another's livelihood. Zedler was clear that physicians, too, could be guilty of Pfuscherey by practicing surgery or dispensing medicines.[69] Such complaints about physicians were indeed lodged, and subsequently adjudicated, in the sense of encroachment. For example, the surgeons in Braunschweig complained about the "surgical Pfuscherey" of Dr. Othmer when he set a broken leg, reduced a hematoma, and lanced swollen glands in 1795, and the Collegium medicum forbade him such "surgical Pfuscherey" in the future, despite the fact that he had originally trained as a surgeon and had previously been city surgeon.[70]

In the documents, complaints, and petitions of the eighteenth century, the term *Pfuscher* generally meant infringement and encroachment, and appeared similarly in regard to craftsmen outside the field of medicine. For instance, in 1749, the privy council ordered that "no artisans should be tolerated in the villages, who properly belong only in the cities. All those Pfuscher and despoilers [*Nahrungs-Verderbern*] [and] all those not guild members are to refrain from such craft work."[71] The tailors' guild in Hehlen demonstrated how its members understood Pfuscherey: it undermined their livelihood and deleteriously affected the economic stability of the greater community. "We are . . . enclosing a list . . . of all tailors who reside in adjacent places in large numbers, who for the most part have not properly [*zunfftmeßig*] learned their *Profession* . . . [and] who sometimes work as schoolmasters." These, by their Pfuscherey, drew work away from the guildsmen in towns. Such troublemakers "rob us of our livelihood and the work from which we must feed ourselves, our wives, and children, as well as contribute to the guild's treasury, give to poor relief and the church, and meet our taxes and other public responsibilities."[72] Physicians, too, could cognitively and linguistically join medical Pfuscherey to the encroachment of other artisans. Benjamin Richter in defining the contrast between the "honest physician" and the despicable quack, reached for the artisan analogy to press his case home. If the authorities did not allow an unguilded shoemaker or cobbler—described as "deceivers"—to practice their trades, and in fact "drove them out of the republic," he wondered, why did they tolerate medical quacks?[73]

As economic rivalry increased in the eighteenth century, as the guilds felt the pressure of government initiatives introduced to stimulate commerce and the competition new products and new methods generated, this older language of corporatism often sounded shrill. Simultaneously, a new speech, set of terms, and meanings came into being, and if they first appeared merely to fortify and bolster the older language of corporatism, they would eventually come to replace it, although the process took considerable time.[74] For example, more and more frequently in the eighteenth century, the physici and the Collegium medicum, as well as Amtmänner and pastors, used the terms *Pfuscherey* and *Quacksalberey* to denote practitioners who menaced the health of the population and who lacked medical skills, as well as in the older sense of encroachment. This usage gained favor in several forums toward the end of the eighteenth century. Krünitz's *Encyklopädie*, the first volumes of which appeared in the 1770s, did not get to its *P*s and *Q*s until 1809 and 1811. And here, even in the opening decades of the nineteenth century, *Quacksalver* and *Pfuscher* retained much of the meaning found in Zedler, although they also gained more exclusively medical definitions, as well as being invested with a greater sense of incompetence and poor workmanship. Significantly, in discussing the pros and cons of tolerating or pursuing both medical and other Pfuscher, the editors embarked on an extended essay (taken from an earlier article by G. L. Woempner in the *Neues Hannöversches Magazin* in 1804) on the reasons for and against establishing freedom of work and abolishing the guilds. Opinion divided almost evenly: the harm done to competition by the guilds and the higher prices that resulted balanced nicely against the rights of guildmen, who had to pay taxes and fees where they lived.[75] Equally, as the century progressed, it became more common for those protesting the Pfuscherey of others to supplement this traditional vocabulary with neologisms or invest old words with new meanings. Quackery and the definition of the term *quack* in the early modern world, then, are loci where economics and medicine tightly entwined, linguistically and virtually. For the reasons suggested above, however, the historian needs to be exceedingly cautious with definitions. Whereas not very long ago one spoke unselfconsciously of quacks, quack medicines, and quack remedies, evoking unambiguous images of incompetence, superstition, gullibility, and willful deception, today this easy self-confidence has all but evaporated. Did not yesterday's quacks after all merely represent another, and not necessarily inferior, way of practicing medicine? Were they not in all their multifarious guises—as midwives, homeopaths, root-wives, Thomasonians, and the like—merely those who fell by the wayside or who were muscled aside in a struggle to monopolize the medical marketplace? Nowadays most social historians of medicine shy away from employing the term *quack* at all because of just these reservations. We substitute something less value-laden and less pejorative, preferring to speak perhaps of "fringe" or "popular" healers, while reserving the term *alternative medicine* for the more ornate theoretical constructs of the nineteenth century.[76]

Unfortunately, in our hurry to distance ourselves from the value judgments of the past (and present), we have perhaps succumbed to an equally distorting historical myopia. We have lost sight of the fact that the word *quack* as used in earlier centuries did not necessarily denote incompetence. Nor can we facilely equate the persons and practices thus labeled by contemporaries with "popular" or "fringe" healers and medicines. In fact, the definition of quackery pertained little to that often-postulated sharp rivalry between quacks and physicians (an interpretation that plays such a prominent role in the professionalization and medicalization literature) and hardly at all to perceptions of competence: instead, it reflected deviations from a set of accepted economic and ethical norms.

The answer to what constituted quackery in the seventeenth and eighteenth centuries therefore involves separating its individual elements from a complex amalgam of economic motives, social proprieties, and morals. A scrutiny of alleged instances of quackery exposes these as something considerably more than just a crusade on the part of the Collegium medicum, the government, or a coterie of physicians to eliminate the competition of other healers. Likewise, quackery cannot be fully subsumed under the category of malpractice, and neither can we group these practitioners with what the twentieth century usually terms quacks—that is, flimflam men and bunglers. Quack was not merely the sneer a professionalizing medical elite reserved for its rivals. The language denoting quackery alerts us that something more elemental was at issue here. Accusers usually attacked other *licensed* and *examined* medical personnel (including physicians) in terms of quackery. For example, in 1716, the Barber-Surgeons' and Surgeons' Guild in the city of Braunschweig renewed its complaints about an interloper who had settled in the city. Once a military surgeon, but neither a member of the guild nor a citizen, he openly went about the town "prescrib[ing] medicines *interna et externa*."[77] In the guild's eyes, this man was a quack.

Charges of quackery, or Pfuscherey, typically insisted that a particular individual had infringed on the complainant's rightful and traditionally sheltered source of income, and threatened properly behaving guildsmen and their families with inescapable ruin. As late as 1803, when the surgeons in Wolfenbüttel brought the Pfuscherey of the hospital administrator Oettinger to the attention of the Collegium medicum, they spoke in these terms. Oettinger, they claimed, "engages in every sort of minor surgical operation, sets blisters of Spanish fly, heals scabies, lances boils, extracts teeth, applies leeches, and leaves us nothing but barbering, from which alone we cannot survive." There is here *not one word* implying that Oettinger was either a trickster or a menace. The destruction Oettinger wreaked was principally economic and social, as well as moral, or, if the combination is not too jarring, econo-moral. Oettinger trespassed on the business of the surgeons and simultaneously violated their sense of economic and craft proprieties. He already enjoyed a salary from the hospital (in his capacity as administrator) and had thus "wrongfully" appropriated a second source of income with his "doctoring."[78] He had, metaphorically speaking, "stolen" the surgeons' "bread" and made it impossible for them "to preserve our integrity and respectability [any longer]." Oettinger was a mischief-maker and a knave. The surgeons did not merely appeal to the government to uphold the beleaguered and contested guild monopoly they enjoyed. Their petition voiced a widely accepted idea that the state somehow bore ultimate accountability for ensuring the livelihoods of all its inhabitants.[79]

Surgeons and barber-surgeons guarded their own rights in the same ways and in the same language that other guilds used to denounce interlopers who trespassed on *their* privileged and protected livelihoods. David Lehnert entwined arguments of livelihood and civil status in his petition to be allowed his trade in oils and medicines. He pointed out that he had been a citizen of Helmstedt for more than thirty years, and that "in this time I have always paid . . . [taxes] on my property and my livelihood promptly and correctly." If forced to sacrifice this part of his livelihood, then "I shall lose my bread, and I and my wife and children must leave the duchy."[80] As William Sewell has noted, such corporate language and the mentality behind it persisted well into the nineteenth century. Even in the middle of that century, there remained "something distinctly corporative about the working-class world . . . that fit with the continued usage of corporate terms in workers' language."[81] Physicians, especially those who did not sit on government councils, hold professorships, or attain the much-desired title, status, and salary of a body-physician, to a large extent also believed in corporatism, acting like anxious guildsmen in defense of their territory. They, too, were extremely wary of "improper" incursions on their practices; incursions they, too, most often articulated in corporatist ways.

Such deeper readings of the documents on quackery—readings that ignore the more "obvious" thread of professionalization—reveal some of the mental constructs eighteenth-century Europeans "thought with." The fact that the Collegium medicum eventually (in 1817) fined Oettinger for his "illicit practice" is in comparison to these other themes at best merely incidental.[82] "Illicit practice" here harbors different meanings than adherents of professionalization and medicalization arguments would have us believe. The documents establish a reality of quackery that a model postulated primarily on the efforts of a budding medical profession to assert control over its rivals can only inadequately accommodate.

The Oettinger case suggests that in the eighteenth century (and into the next as well), quackery was still overwhelmingly understood as *Pfuscherey*, a term borrowed from guild parlance, denoting an "unprivileged, nonguilded craftsman," an interloper, but not necessarily or even usually an incompetent.[83] In medical occupations with a guild, guildlike structure, or guild mentality, among surgeons, for example, the quack or Pfuscher was not culpable because he was a "human butcher" (*Menschenschlachter*), but because he disrupted their livelihoods. When two surgeons and a bathmaster in the market town of Voigtsdahlum complained bitterly about an assorted group of Pfuscher (three ex-soldiers, two army surgeons, a schoolmaster, a cobbler, and a linen weaver), it was because they "drive away our bread."[84] Repeated complaints to the Collegium medicum invariably stressed loss of livelihood as the prime, often sole, grievance, accusing the quack of a sort of theft, of stealing what was widely considered as property: a livelihood. In such and similar denunciations, the dangers quacks presented to the health of the people receded into the background as less egregious offenses. As the century wore on, however, denunciants themselves began to realize that including in almost talismanic fashion the phrase "the harm done thereby to the health of the population" augmented their chances of a sympathetic hearing from the Collegium medicum.[85]

A sense of economic propriety was, therefore, critical in ascertaining who deserved the epithet *quack*, and it underpinned as well the daily decisions patients made about whom to trust and consult. For most people in the seventeenth and eighteenth centuries, quackery continued to be cast principally in terms of a deviation from a more traditional division of labor and markets, as well as from an accepted moral and economic ethos. This perception is not peculiar, of course, to one German state. Medicine and medical practice for most people did not form discrete entities but existed in the interstices of a web of ties linking friends, neighbors, and kin, which governed a whole way of life. But at least by the middle of the eighteenth century, as more *chevaliers d'industrie* and more new products entered the economic lists, that way of life was facing stiff new challenges.

Medical Entrepreneurs

The flood of proprietary and specific medicines that washed over Europe demonstrated by its very existence the accelerated capacity of production and the greater absorptive qualities of eighteenth-century consumerism.[86] It eloquently testified to the extension of international marketing and distribution networks that crossed borders and penetrated villages and rural backwaters in the hinterlands of small German territories. Perhaps the most famous of these were the medicines the Halle "Medicamenten-Expedition" fabricated and shipped, literally throughout the world.[87] But the career of Jean Ailhaud's *remède universel* in Braunschweig-Wolfenbüttel at mid century illustrates as well the extended reach of such firms, and the process of negotiation and accommodation necessary to fit a new item into the somewhat creaky corporatist framework of production and distribution.

When Jean Ailhaud died in 1756 in Aix-en-Provence, he must have considered his life a smashing success. He had acquired three estates with seigniorial rights, amassed a vast fortune, received the title of *conseiller secretaire du Roi*, and enjoyed an almost Europewide fame, or rather notoriety. The source of this self-made millionaire's wealth lay in the *poudre purgative* he manufactured. Contemporaries knew it simply as *la poudre d'Ailhaud*.[88] In the 1740s, Jean *père* had obtained from the French crown an exclusive entitlement to vend the powder in France. He built, and his son impressively extended, a distribution network that included outlets for the *poudre purgative* in all the major cities of France, and that, under his son's guidance, opened marketing channels into central and eastern Europe as well. By the 1770s, Ailhaud *fils* was selling an average of 400,000 boxes (each containing ten doses) annually. Both father and son advertised widely, promoting their powders with brochures, which were quickly translated into most European languages.[89]

Despite (or perhaps because of) their stunning financial successes, the Ailhauds drew the opprobrium of academic medicine down upon their heads; the groundswell of disapprobation and criticism grew as the business prospered. In 1759 and 1760, the physicians Dupuy de la Porcherie and François Thiéry exposed the *effets funestes des poudres Ailhauds* in print. Tissot railed against Ailhaud and his system. Others at the beginning of the next century hyperbolically accused Ailhaud of destroying as many innocent people with his powder as Napoleon had on his campaigns. They classified this Ailhaud—"the inventor of a purgative that shat out a marquisate for him"—with the other great charlatans of that age of light: with Graham, "the inventor of the celestial bed," and with Mesmer, "that shady magnetist."[90]

What specifically was it that caused so many to rail against Ailhaud? First, he marketed his remedy as a *catholicum*—a panacea, or universal cure—and enlightened and academic eighteenth-century opinion tended to reject such claims as fraudulent and chimerical. The trade in proprietary medicines was not limited to men like Ailhaud, however, but was also exploited by medical luminaries such as Georg Stahl, Friedrich Hoffmann, and Johann August Unzer, as well as by several physici in Braunschweig-Wolfenbüttel. Johann Wachsmuth, physicus in Holzminden, for example, defended and sold several *catholica*.[91] Market demand for such remedies in the eighteenth century was prodigious; their sale produced a luxuriant crop of "toadstool millionaires."[92] Perhaps this was because the eighteenth-century pharmacopoeia held so few effective drugs (ipecac, digitalis, quinine, and opium among them). But perhaps Ailhaud and his like pulled off such stunning financial coups because they so adroitly played on popular resistance to increasing medical regulation in eighteenth-century Germany and France,[93] while skillfully meeting a burgeoning demand for "do-it-yourself" cures. More likely, they not only rode the crest of a consumer wave, but were themselves instrumental in stimulating and then satiating market requirements.[94]

For all these reasons, the makers of panaceas and specifics enjoyed a heyday, and not only in England, where the profusion of proprietary medicines has been most extensively investigated. The most important eighteenth-century writer on catholica, Bernhard Schreger, lists over 450 of them, including the ever-popular Halle medications, Hamburg fever drops, the "wonder drugs" of Count Cagliostro, the Ragolosche powder for epilepsy, numerous supposed cures for rabies (including one whose main ingredient was the common oil beetle), and, of course, the ubiquitous "sure cures" for venereal diseases.[95] Schreger condemned Ailhaud's powder for its ability to evoke "the most violent reactions, vomiting, colic, dysenterylike diarrheas, and bloody stools." Furthermore, he charged that it often brought on "sudden death with all the symptoms of poisoning." Chemical analysis yielded only indefinite clues as to its composition, both because the mixture varied over time and because of the unreliability of early analytical chemistry when confronted with organic (in eighteenth-century terms, vegetable) compounds. All agreed that a strong cathartic was present, and most analysts identified a mixture of scammony and jalap or ipecac, cut with sugar, licorice, or a decoction of tamarind to enhance palatability.[96] How such medicines were distributed, and what the demand for them was, reveals, at least in part, how marketing strategies developed and consumerism evolved in the late eighteenth century.[97]

Part of the Collegium medicum's job involved monitoring the sale of medicines. The medical ordinance of 1747 specifically forbade the advertisement or distribution of all medicines in the duchy before the Collegium had tested and approved them.[98] The Collegium examined a whole series of substances over the years. For example, in 1773, it found that "two very simply compounded unguents" indeed proved "unusually effective" in healing recent wounds and old injuries and permitted their sale. In the same year, however, they judged Dr. Lattmann's medicines, made of tobacco leaves and olive oil, to be "neither new nor useful." Likewise, the Collegium worried about the easy availability of poisons. When the medical student Ittershagen proposed a way to exterminate field mice, the Collegium judged it ipso facto a poison, and thus probably equally fatal to animals and humans, and opposed its sale. And, in the previous decade, the Collegium had waged a campaign to control all *drastionien*—that is, harsh laxatives and emetics, maintaining that "in fact no purgative whatsoever should be freely accessible to the common man to use as he pleases."[99] As in other instances, the Collegium did not necessarily get its way, however: the ducal privy council, which had to think in terms of the economy of the duchy as a whole, and was as much dedicated to stimulating commerce and industry as to protecting traditional rights and privileges, generally wanted a less strict interpretation of the law. While the privy council acknowledged the need to hinder the circulation of dangerous drugs, it was not always willing to restrict sales simply to uphold what it was coming to regard as outdated monopolies. And the Collegium also voiced concerns about the economic potential of new commodities. For instance, when Dr. Meibom tested a sample of locally produced "sal ammoniaco," he found it "as good as the Indian and Venetian varieties" and felt it would find a ready market with foreign wholesalers if properly handled. A few months later, however, he expressed far less enthusiasm for the commercial successes of a "sal seignette," as any apothecary could make it from Spanish soda and cream of tartar.[100]

The Collegium medicum also meticulously investigated the claims of the Braunschweig Gravenhorst brothers, who manufactured a "sal mirabile Glauber." The Gravenhorst factory in Braunschweig was a flourishing enterprise, perhaps the most prosperous in the duchy. It produced chemicals for industrial as well as medicinal use. The Gravenhorsts publicized the virtues of their Glauber salts as a purgative, for treating ague and dropsy, for alleviating stomach disorders and flatulence, and "for the common female complaints during pregnancy." Whereas the Collegium denied Ailhaud's claims and condemned his powder, it explicitly approved the Gravenhorsts' "miracle salt."[101] (But then again, the Gravenhorsts were leading members of the party of enlightenment in Braunschweig.)

In fact, these decisions paralleled the government's general attitude toward the regulation of commerce and manufacturing. Beginning roughly in mid century, manufactured goods and new methods of marketing began seriously to rival artisan forms of production and distribution. Although this change actually proceeded quite gradually, the competition seemed particularly onerous and offensive to artisans. While trying to promote commerce and manufacturing, the central government sought to prevent anyone being destroyed in the competition between old and new. And this produced a decidedly schizoid policy, both in the larger world of economic relations as a whole and in the smaller world of medicine, which was equally affected.[102] In rendering his opinion as to whether the young Dr. Pott should be excused his examination when he first wished to settle in Braunschweig, Dr. Behrens felt, for example, that this was not advisable. "I do not deny," he commented, "that it is a gain and a boon to the state when it attracts many talented subjects from other places," but he did worry about the unfair advantages that such newcomers would enjoy to the detriment of current residents, and this applied in his mind as much to physicians as to tailors.[103]

At the same time, the older standards of livelihood and moral economy were also slowly disintegrating, and the idea of the "best possible provision [Versorgung]" for the entire population began to push at, and push aside, the older principle of livelihood. As the government began to accept the idea of provision over livelihood, it also sought to prevent local producers from being driven out of the market entirely. This shift, however, signaled a new emphasis on the demands of the consumer over the rights of the producers.[104] New methods, new goods, and outside forces alone did not break up a more traditional economic world based on the mental abstraction of livelihood and the reality of craft production. Rather, many of those within that historic world themselves began to exploit the new potentials or create them; they helped subvert the world of Nahrung from within.[105] And, as we shall see, medical practitioners often employed the language of free competition and "good provision" to justify their practices, while eschewing or underplaying the older language of artisan life. Or, folding one into the other, they accented the benefits of competition for providing quality and quality control, which were among the time-honored functions of the guilds. Patients, too, mixed their language in justifying their own medical choices.

Ailhaud's poudre purgative was such a new offering.[106] Although undoubtedly a stimulant to competition, it also fell under the 1721 strictures on the sale and distribution of medicines. Just when the powder was first sold in the duchy, rather than purchased by mail order direct from Aix-en-Provence or from one of Ailhaud's distributors in France, is uncertain. It was well enough known by 1755 to provoke a condemnatory article in a Braunschweig learned journal.[107] It is, however, relatively clear how the powder crossed the Rhine: manufactured in Aix, it was shipped to Germany through Ailhaud's depot in Strasbourg. The agent in Strasbourg, a man named Lichtenberger, contracted with local distributors in northern and western Germany for the sale of Ailhaud's powder on commission. These factors merchandised the poudre purgative both retail and wholesale, softening up their markets by flooding them with Ailhaud's pamphlets, plying pastors with free samples, and widely broadcasting their intention to offer the medicine free to the destitute. Lichtenberger's man in Braunschweig was one Johann Aldefeldt, merchant and pastry chef, an immigrant from Strasbourg who had settled in Braunschweig in the late 1730s or early 1740s. He traded retail and wholesale in a wide array of commodities. He handled spices, sweets, and bulk chemicals. Many of the products he and others like him sold steered them onto collision courses with guildsmen who merchandised what they regarded as privileged wares. Frequent conflicts broke out with the apothecaries over the right to trade in certain medicines, particularly those medicines that were not compounded, or were not prescribed by doctors, but that, like Ailhaud's arcanum, represented consumer goods.

Although the confrontation over Ailhaud's powder is perhaps the best-documented one, it was hardly unique. Two wholesalers and the resident apothecary in Helmstedt disputed the right to vend certain wares, including particular pills and potions. The battle spread and eventually pitted the guild of merchants against that of the apothecaries. The list of goods offered by the dealer *en gros* Branden Meyer suggests the range of commodities handled by both merchants and apothecaries. In 1747, for example, Meyer's inventory ran to over five closely written pages. It included elixirs, essences, tonics, and distilled oils; sundry pills, powders, and salves; "fixed salts" including borax; miscellaneous spirits (vegetable and mineral); tinctures, snuff, and a broad palette of colors—carmine red, ultramarine, cerulean, Berlin blue, cinnabar, and several more.[108]

In 1750, the Collegium medicum adjudicated a dispute between the apothecaries on the one hand and the wholesalers and herbalists on the other by specifying—that is, by listing—what each might sell. Wholesalers were forbidden, among other things, to vend the following except in weights greater than one pound: Spanish fly, rhinoceros horn, Indian fever bark, snake wood, brown root, dried serpent, and "true" unicorn horn. They were likewise denied the retail trade (less than a half pound) in emetics, purgatives, soporifics, and sudorifics. Another list specified what they must not merchandise under any circumstances, except with special permission or outside the duchy. This catalog of forbidden items was lengthy, and included all sorts of tinctures, elixirs, medicinal salts, pills, syrups, electuaries, spirits, aqua vitae, emplasms, cataplasms, and unguents, as well as spices and herbs. The business of the wholesalers was restricted to bulk sales for the trades and manufactories: the government allowed them to sell, for example, only those salts that "artists and artisans need for their professions," like borax, crude nitrites, and "green, blue, and white" vitriols, as well as the common kitchen and sea varieties.[109]

Thus the apothecaries and medicine peddlers were enmeshed in a set of changes in marketing that reached deeply into community life, upsetting and eroding older bonds and conventions. Quarrels similar to those between wholesalers and apothecaries flared repeatedly between taverners or bathmasters and apothecaries. For example, the long-standing acrimony between the apothecary in Thedinghausen, Johann Pollitz, and the local taverners came to a head in 1759. The taverners claimed that Pollitz's sale of wine and brandy greatly diminished their trade. He insisted, however, that he only kept enough of each on hand as was usual for his business and "without which I could not find my living [*Subsistenz*] here." He also doubted that his little sideline in wine and brandy seriously harmed the taverners, whose main livelihood came from selling local beer.[110] Likewise, the bathmaster Pape in Seesen, who stocked large quantities of medicines, oils, and distilled waters in his bathhouse, provoked the triple ire of the local apothecary, the taverner, and Physicus Blum.[111]

As Ailhaud's agent, Aldefeldt was sucked into a similar controversy. In 1767, he petitioned the Collegium medicum for a right to distribute the poudre purgative "without restriction." He already handled the powder on commission and mailed out samples to pastors and other notables in the countryside. In addition, he had given numerous doses of the remedy away free to the poor. He placed before the Collegium a list of thirteen "men of account" who had used the powder, approved it, and would so swear. Yet the Collegium quickly found against Aldefeldt. It further argued that the sale of Ailhaud's poudre purgative be totally forbidden in Braunschweig-Wolfenbüttel, as it already had been in Hannover. This should have been the end of the matter, but, as was so often the case in these instances, it was only the beginning.

Soon after this ruling was made public, letters of support for Ailhaud's powder—and also, to some extent, for Aldefeldt's position—inundated the privy council and Collegium medicum. Some insisted that the powder was a true boon to "suffering humanity." Others felt that a prejudiced Collegium had not sufficiently explored the issue. Professor Just Friedrich Zachariä, editor of Braunschweig's most enlightened journal, cannily observed that if thirty years' opposition by the medical experts in France had failed to dam up demand for the powder, it was not to be expected that "sheer prohibitions will deter the public from [purchasing] this specific."[112]

Faced with this stream of protest, the privy council reopened the case. The closer investigation the Collegium medicum initiated in 1768 produced only inconclusive and contradictory evidence. The authorities in Braunschweig identified twenty-seven persons who praised Ailhaud's powder and reported no serious side effects. Some were wildly enthusiastic. A Lieutenant Delmer, who told of suffering for years from incessant "stabbing pains in the chest" that so affected him that he could "neither stand upright nor move about freely," experienced great relief after using Ailhaud's powder. Just three doses had caused the cramps to vanish without a trace, and since then he had felt "newborn." From almost everywhere in the duchy praise for the healing qualities of the poudre purgative poured in, outweighing the negative evidence the Collegium assembled. Significantly, the majority of support came from people prominent in their communities. Pastors tended to be the most outspoken of Ailhaud's allies. The pastor from Campen lauded Ailhaud's powder: of the many laxatives he had been forced to consume in his life, not one had "worked so well or so gently" as Ailhaud's, which produced not the "least discomfort." From Helmstedt, several *promenenti* (among them, a professor of medicine, a pastor, and a member of the city council) spoke unanimously of the good Ailhaud's doses had done them. All these had purchased their supply, or obtained samples, from Aldefeldt. And even the physicus felt there were many cases in which the arcanum had its uses.[113]

Pastors, ducal officials, magistrates, and other notables in more rural areas likewise detailed their experiences using the powder to treat everything from "hypochondriacal attacks" to cancerous growths, stomach cramps to gout, with results ranging from "beneficial" and "effective" to "astonishing" and "miraculous." Some pastors regularly purchased, or received free, packets of the powder from Aldefeldt, with which they dosed their flocks, brute animal and human alike. Several churchmen archly noted how favorably the generosity of Ailhaud and Aldefeldt contrasted with the notorious "tightfistedness" of the apothecaries with whom they regularly dealt. Pastor Hoerstal in Schöningen related that when he had ordered the drug from Aldefeldt to treat an impoverished schoolmaster in his parish, Aldefeldt sent a messenger with the doses and would accept no money. The position many pastors took in defending Ailhaud's remedy struck another blow in the (admittedly rather desultory) war they were waging with the government and the Collegium medicum over social and cultural authority. Although the pastors almost unanimously supported the idea of improving medical care in the countryside (and some did ally with health officers), most followed a path that diverged from the policy of strict medical regulation the Collegium preferred. The pastors advocated instead a widespread program of popular medical enlightenment and—as we have seen—many busily churned out popular medical advice for the common man. They were quick to pillory physicians, surgeons, and apothecaries for their unseemly "economic self-interest" and to scourge them verbally for dereliction of their duties. Thus, too, pastors positioned themselves against medical corporatism, and, if only for momentary strategic gains, on the side of medical consumerism.[114]

Among the physici, opinion diverged as well. Most were admittedly unenthusiastic, or hostile, but some had added Ailhaud's *remède* to their armamentarium and prescribed it regularly. Even crusty old Gottfried Beireis, professor of medicine at the University of Helmstedt, was by no means completely negative about the purported benefits of the medicine. He felt it useful in opening up "clogged visceral pathways" and expedient in the treatment of chronic problems caused by "obstructions." On the other hand, he objected to the high price of Ailhaud's powder and poohpoohed its claims to universal applicability. Of the physicians who did not regard it as totally worthless, most believed that its harsh cathartic action dictated caution: only a physician should administer it. They generally advocated restricting its sale, rather than proscribing it entirely. Most agreed that private persons, such as Aldefeldt, should not sell a medicine like Ailhaud's.

Eventually, begrudgingly, the Collegium medicum compromised. The members of the Collegium never wavered in their conviction that "this medicine does far more harm than good," but they bowed to the pressure exerted by the privy council for a milder interpretation of the law. The Collegium agreed that an uncompromising prohibition might actually be counterproductive, as "forbidden fruits are always sweetest, especially to the common folk." And so the Collegium retreated from its previous position, a retreat clearly effected by a combination of outcry from respectable people and by the privy council's refusal to stand stalwartly behind the Collegium's original decision. Thereafter, only the newly established government-run warehouse was permitted to stock Ailhaud's powder and supply it to apothecaries. The Collegium specifically excluded grocers, like Aldefeldt, from dealing in such materials. When Aldefeldt's widow and sons defied the ban and continued to merchandise Ailhaud's powder over the counter, their shop was raided and their valuable inventory impounded. But Aldefeldt's defeat was only a skirmish lost; the battle over the right to market such consumer goods continued and intensified. Eventually grocers like Aldefeldt, as well as druggists, wholesalers, and others, expanded their activities, successfully fighting off the efforts of some to preserve a more closely regulated system of monopoly and privilege.

No participant in this debate was unaware of the wider economic ramifications. Embedded in the rhetoric of "controlling the illicit sale of medicines" were good mercantilistic arguments for creating a government monopoly over the sale of all "the well-known foreign medicines," such as Scheer's Essence, Stoughton's Stomach Tonic, Unger's Digestive Powder—and Ailhaud's poudre purgative—because the "great consumption" of them drew "[enormous] sums of money out of the state, which could be retained if more common remedies were applied instead."[115] Yet not all arcana were imports. Local products entered the market in large amounts throughout the eighteenth century. Apothecaries compounded many of them. One of the most enterprising in this regard was Johann Praesun, who sold his special medicine throughout the duchy, trumpeting its value in cases of "chronic afflictions, such as epilepsy, [and] for arthritis, podagra, and kidney stones," until the Collegium medicum put an end to his trade.[116]

The saga of Ailhaud's panacea in Braunschweig-Wolfenbüttel in the third quarter of the century illuminates some of the central issues involved in the complex interplay between medicine as "science" and "profession" and medicine as "business." It should also suggest some of the tensions inherent in a society still ruled by the dictates of mercantilist protectionism and guild rights, unable to cast off these legal shackles, and yet also caught up in the rising swell of new items, new advertising possibilities, and new marketing methods.

Sometimes government and guild members wanted to eat their cake and have it too: they desired protection from competition, while asserting a right to exploit the market whenever the opportunity arose. Such contradictory goals were hard to mediate and created bizarre alliances and tense relationships, while proponents and opponents of protectionism jumped back and forth from one side of the economic fence to the other. This drama—or was it farce?—replayed each time a new product appeared. The government wavered, unable to silence its nagging paternalistic conscience definitively and unwilling to upset the social order that anchored such protectionism, but equally unable to close its ears to the siren song of a more open, more competitive market. Conscience and tradition counseled that it was necessary to protect one's subjects and shield those, like the apothecaries, whose survival seemed to depend on monopolistic concessions, as well as to cushion hothouse industries from more dynamic foreign competition. Possibilities of control diminished, however, as the number of commodities ballooned, and as many of those who had once sought protection enrolled in the ranks of their erstwhile rivals. Although the government of Braunschweig-Wolfenbüttel seldom granted special concessions (such as tax rebates) to help sustain infant industries, and rarely defended waning or outdated guild rights vigorously, it also mounted no major effort to destroy the guilds. Studied indifference on many economic issues characterized the government's attitude; old privileges were sometimes allowed to lapse, but were also fitfully supported. The range of government responses was wide and not always predictable.[117]

Among those committed to improving medical care, the debate continued as to whether the goal could best be achieved by regulation, by education, by allowing a free market to work, or by some combination of all three. We clearly also cannot ignore the fact that "the people" were not infinitely malleable. They, too, had a voice, which they often, and sometimes effectively, raised, and they, too, could stubbornly assert their own right to choose among the abundant offerings in the medical bazaar. This brings us to the question of what factors helped determine their medical choices. To what extent did a sense of proper economic behavior—or to employ E. P. Thompson's phrase, a "moral economy"[118]—drive people's decisions?

While a detailed discussion of the process of medical decision making must be left to a later chapter, a few remarks seem appropriate here in regard to communities and consumerism. The perception of economic propriety was itself in flux, as it almost had to be in an era replete with novel commercial possibilities for both buyer and seller. If people continued to embrace an older idea of moral economy—of a rather narrowly circumscribed proper realm of economic action—they also increasingly demanded their right to select from outside the realm of healers organized in guilds or prescribed by older laws. Thus while concepts of livelihood and suitable income were both declining, they had by no means disappeared in the eighteenth century. Both mentalities coexisted, as perhaps they always had, although the balance was shifting.[119]

For example, people bought and consumed proprietary medicines (even ruinously expensive ones) in enormous quantities and expended considerable sums in determined attempts to restore their own health or that of friends, relatives, and children. Entrepreneurs among the surgeons and apothecaries, too, were quick to seize on new market possibilities. Many manufacturers and consumers alike resented and ignored guild monopolies in asserting the right to free choice in the medical marketplace. And perhaps here, within the older system of corporatism itself, we find clues to the rise of market culture and of a new consumer orientation. The guild system had always allowed some room for guildsmen to innovate, to expand their markets, and to employ nonguild workers. There had always been conflicts among guilds as to the right to manufacture new products, and this was as true of medical products and services as it was of "populuxe" items such as fans and umbrellas.[120] Moreover, smoldering resentment against guild privileges was always ready to burst into flame when guildsmen themselves violated (or seemed to violate) the very standards that existed to protect them, and when they transgressed vague but still potent feelings about the "common good" and "public interest."

Surgeons, Bathmasters, Apothecaries

Despite the undeniably central importance of economic influences, the characteristic attributes of the eighteenth-century medical world can neither be subsumed under the rubric of marketing alone nor be explained simply by examining medicine as part of a growing array of commodities. There were other determinants. Issues of education and of local rights and privileges, for instance, need to be explored further, especially in the cases of those who provided a good deal of everyday medical care: the surgeons, bathmasters, and midwives, as well as the many others who cannot be neatly pigeonholed.

The surgeons and the bathmasters of Braunschweig-Wolfenbüttel

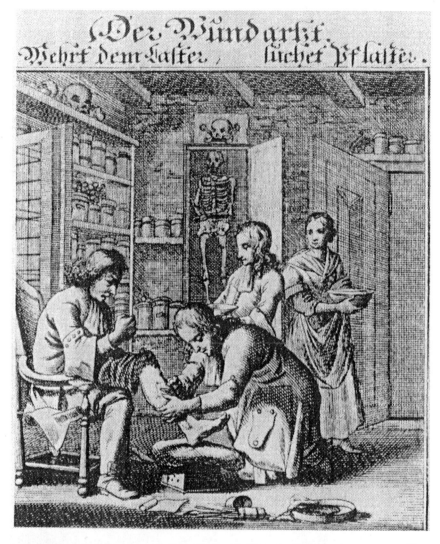

"Der Wundarzt" (The Surgeon), from Christoph Weigel, *Abbildung der gemein-nützlichen Haupt-Stände, . . .* (Regensburg: n.p., 1698). Reproduced with the permission of the Wellcome Institute Library, London.

waged a fierce and protracted battle over boundaries and encroachment, but this conflict was only a territorial skirmish in a much bigger struggle fought out at the level of the empire.[121] The dispute over duties, rights, territories, and titles continued until 1801, when the ducal government united the barber-surgeons and surgeons in a single guild.[122] Intermediate

"Der Bader" (The Bathmaster), from Christoph Weigel, *Abbildung der gemein-nützlichen Haupt-Stände*, . . . (Regensburg: n.p., 1698). Reproduced with the permission of the Wellcome Institute Library, London.

steps toward this eventual resolution included the specification that local authorities not appoint bathmasters or surgeons without first having them approved by the Collegium medicum (1765); that surgeons and bathmasters in places where no guild existed could not take on apprentices (1768); that barber-surgeons and bathmasters be viewed as identical (1769); and that the practices of surgeons, barber-surgeons, and bathmasters could no longer be inherited (1775).[123]

Disputed here were the rights to treat fresh wounds and to barber and shave, for as often as the bathmasters tried to practice surgery, the surgeons attempted to shave and cut hair. The tussle dated at least from the sixteenth century. In 1538, the Braunschweig city council forbade bathmasters to bind wounds, and then formalized these rules in the bathmasters' ordinance of 1580 and the surgeons' ordinance of 1618. The decision touched off a long dispute, with the bathmasters taking their case to the ducal and imperial courts in a legal snarl that lasted from 1635 to 1738 and makes Dickens's Jarndyce v. Jarndyce seem almost straightforward.[124] The drama in the courts, however, paralleled face-to-face confrontations among the bathmasters, surgeons, and barber-surgeons.

The bathmasters' rights were attached to particular pieces of property—the bathhouses—which cities, towns, and nobles regarded as valuable pecuniary assets. After thriving in the sixteenth century, bathhouses began to disappear in the next. In the seventeenth century, there were eleven of an original sixteen left in the city of Braunschweig. Bathmasters were allowed to shave, let blood, cup, and perform other minor surgical operations, but only within their bathhouses. The boundaries dividing surgeons from barber-surgeons and from bathmasters remained indistinct. The regulation of 1716 specified that bathmasters and barber-surgeons who lived in local bathhouses had to respect certain limitations; they were not allowed to barber or let blood except in their houses and were expressly forbidden to bind fresh wounds at all. This last prerogative fell to the surgeons alone. Surgeons who leased bathhouses assumed the right to do everything other surgeons did, but "grooming, shampooing, or shaving can only be permitted them in their homes and not elsewhere." The ordinance also prohibited military surgeons from engaging in private civilian practice and restricted barber-surgery and surgery to members of the guild.[125]

The surgical practice of barber-surgeons, who retained the right to shave and cut hair, was not linked to the possession of a bathhouse, but to membership in the barber-surgeons' guild and to the purchase of a surgical franchise, sold by the city for a fee of between 300 and 400 thaler. This franchise became the personal property of the purchaser, to be sold or willed to his heirs as he pleased.[126] In 1755, the Bathmasters' Guild had four masters, nine journeymen, and three apprentices; the Barber-Surgeons' had eleven masters, twenty-two journeymen, and five apprentices.[127]

In the middle of the eighteenth century, the government decided that those who wished to practice surgery must henceforth be tested by the Collegium medicum. This examination replaced the prior certification process, which the guild's masters had monitored and conducted.[128] After the founding of the Anatomical-Surgical Institute in 1750, those who intended to engage in surgery had to have passed its course.[129] In 1794, the Collegium medicum recognized the right of physicians to do major operations, while simultaneously warning them to leave minor surgery, such as bloodletting, blistering with Spanish fly, leeching, cupping, and pulling teeth, to the surgeons.[130] While these legal lines were hardly irrelevant to surgeons and barber-surgeons, particularly as they formed the basis for justifying daily complaints and sustaining more elaborate suits, they alone never defined the flow of a practitioner's life, his self-understanding, and his associations with his colleagues, the authorities, and his clients.

Relationships among bathmasters, surgeons, and apothecaries were often tense, or even combative, yet they could also be harmonious, mutually beneficial, and lucrative. Contests joined on medical turf cut into more general structures of village and town life and reflected larger communal concerns. Issues of livelihood and custom, for example, dominated the leasing of bathhouses, in the minds both of those who sought such posts and of those who controlled their distribution.

How the city of Helmstedt administered its bathhouse between 1749 and 1767 shows where medical care, privilege, communal responsibility, and poaching converged. In the 1740s, Heinrich Valentin Kraps held the lease, as he had done since 1722, and as his father had before him. A resolution of 18 November 1749 confirmed the status of the bathhouse as exempt from certain taxes, and also excused some older tax debts Kraps had incurred. In 1754, however, the city chose to lease the bathhouse to a man named Schramm, a decision that quickly drew a wail of protest from Kraps. Beginning his petition with old-fashioned politeness, Kraps portrayed himself as a 72-year-old "graybeard" who "with tear-swollen eyes, prostrate[d] himself humbly" to seek redress of grievances. Two weeks previously and without his knowledge, the city had transferred the bathhouse he had held in continuous lease for over thirty-two years to one of his former journeymen. He displayed complete surprise at this turn of events, saying, "I have paid my fees promptly each quarter." Previously, when the lease ran out, it had been renewed "without any negotiation." "My age, the destitution in which I live, and my inability to read and write, are the real reasons I, unsuspectingly and innocently, bypassed the deadline." Had he known, he would also have bid on the bathhouse. In fact, the sole other candidate was the journeymen, Schramm, who offered only two thaler more than Kraps normally paid. "The official Traut . . . said nothing to me about a new contract, let alone mentioned the deadline. Traut's own interests are involved in this affair. . . . [T]he new tenant admits that he did not wish to drive out his old teacher, but Traut egged him on, promising that he might marry Traut's maid, who some years previously had given birth to his [Schramm's] illegitimate child." Kraps painted a moving picture of the misery that awaited him and his aged wife, who was blind and lame. The ducal privy council found in favor of Kraps, "so that he will not fall burden on the poor relief." It allowed Kraps to retain the bathhouse and admonished Schramm to be patient and wait until the old man's demise.[131]

Over the generations, several members of the Kraps family were bathmasters in Helmstedt-Neumark. Johann Heinrich Kraps, a younger relative of Heinrich Valentin's, also settled in Helmstedt, but quickly trod on the toes of the man who then held the lease, the surgeon Anton Babenroth. Kraps had apparently been trained as a bathmaster, yet in 1767 also kept The Wild Man tavern. Two local officials complained to the Collegium medicum how Kraps "shamelessly" carried on his old trade and "marche[d] about openly with his surgeon's tools" under his arm, proffering his services to one and all. Kraps's conduct violated several customary rules of economic propriety, in that he already enjoyed three livelihoods (*3fache Nahrung*): he kept a tavern; he traded in rags; and he handled paper. The officials wanted to force Kraps to abandon his medical practice, not because he harmed anyone with his ministrations, but "because otherwise the Neumarkt treasury will lose money, as the bathmaster Babenroth cannot be released [from his contract] and he has already fallen behind in his payments."[132]

The associated issues of property, propriety, and practice are even more evident in procedures involving individual bathhouses. In 1726, when the town of Königslutter wanted to lease its bathhouse, it searched for "someone or the other who can offer more *locarium* than the current occupant" paid. In other words, despite the presence of a bathmaster in the property,

the town sought to augment its revenues. A good number—twenty-one—
of the town's citizens found it "in truth very commendable that one seeks
to contribute thereby to the *bonum publicum*," but they expressed dismay at
the thought of simply auctioning it off to the highest bidder. "In such a
manner, one might get a person not very experienced in his profession,"
and then, when a serious injury occurred, a "disaster" might result.[133]
Thus communities, or at least a number of their members, often looked
further than their pocketbooks, although the bathhouse remained an
important source of revenue, and a juicy bit of patronage, over which
neither nobles nor towns wished to sacrifice control. Altercations between the Collegium medicum and nobles over the right to name bathmasters to bathhouses owned by the nobility stoked the nobles' sense of
outrage at what it viewed as the highhandedness of the ducal government
and contributed to the fiscal revolt staged by the estates in the late 1760s
and early 1770s.[134]

The successful candidate in Königslutter did not, however, rest secure.
Writing to the Collegium medicum in 1762, the magistrate Hehn reminded it that the local treasury owned the bathhouse, which it was
permitted to lease to "any such bathmaster or surgeon . . . who has been
examined and found competent." Moreover, "no one besides this man is
permitted to shave and practice surgery." The city council was already
deep in negotiations with such a man, one Anton Uhlenhorst, and was
very anxious to obtain his services. Uhlenhorst had, however, been star-
tled by a rumor going round that the Collegium was considering giving a
concession to the person who had previously held the lease, a man named
Schneider.[135] Uhlenhorst refused to put his name to a binding document
until he was assured that the Collegium would deny Schneider the right
to practice in Königslutter. He asked further for protection from any
competition, except that of the other bathmaster resident in Königslutter.
The city council for its part worried that Uhlenhorst would be driven off
by these fears, and, if so, that they would never be able to lease the
bathhouse again except to Schönejahn, who was, however, an inappropriate candidate because he was neither a bathmaster nor a surgeon
and could not take on an apprentice.[136]

Schneider's loss was only temporary. In 1779, he took over the bathhouse for a yearly fee of 24 thaler. When Schneider died in 1784, the city
followed the ducal mandate of 4 May 1767 specifying that "instead of
frequently auctioning off [bathhouses]," cities should content themselves
"with an appropriately modest rent to avoid *inconveniengien* [*sic*]." The

Collegium medicum protested the "common habit" of magistrates in many smaller cities of leasing a bathhouse for a certain number of years and then offering it again on the open market. This effectively drove up the cost and put the lessee out of his post, often driving him to Pfuscherey or mendicancy in order to survive. In this case, the city council decided to lease the property to Johann Schönejahn (who was possibly a son of the bathmaster Schönejahn mentioned above), who had been examined by the Collegium, and who had already established himself in Königslutter.[137]

Schönejahn's tenure in Königslutter by no means ran smoothly. In 1791, a surgeon named Fischer from the nearby village of Supplingenburg, asked the city magistrates for the permission to move to Königslutter. He convinced the magistrates of his talents by pointing out that many patients in Königslutter had already expressed "great satisfaction" with him. Although conceding that there were already two surgeons in Königslutter, Schönejahn and another named Rüland, the magistrates spoke of "clear evidence" that "neither ha[d] been very successful in his practice" and opined that it was not wise to entrust the inhabitants to their ministrations alone.[138]

Schönejahn's problems went beyond lack of trust; he was also in financial hot water. Although he held the lease of the bathhouse "for an indefinite term," he was at least 100 thaler in debt to the treasury by 1791. Nothing was more certain to make the town begin to look elsewhere for a bathmaster, especially as Fischer volunteered to assume the lease in whole or part. And the magistrates in Königslutter supported Fischer, because they regarded him as "a skilled surgeon" and a good financial risk. There was seemingly little sympathy for Schönejahn. Pressure put on Schönejahn to repay his debts finally caused him to concede. Fischer did not at that moment appear worried that Schönejahn would stay on in the city as a surgeon. Two years later, however, Fischer tartly complained about Schönejahn's presence. Schönejahn continued to have an apprentice, thus cutting into Fischer's rights. And this battle continued through 1797.[139]

In 1796, Rüland, the other surgeon in Königslutter, died, and Schönejahn quickly petitioned the Collegium medicum for Rüland's concession. Schönejahn now had other competition for the post as well. Rüland's son, then serving as a company surgeon in the ducal army, also sought to acquire his father's post, "mainly in order . . . to stand by my mother and siblings," who lived in Königslutter. This time the magistracy decided in Schönejahn's favor, hoping that if Schönejahn received the post, the cause of his quarrel with Fischer would vanish. Moreover, they still felt that the "limited market" in Königslutter made it impossible for three surgeons to survive there. Yet they also argued that Schönejahn "is a resident here, whereas Rüland seeks residence only so that he might share the advantages of the parental home with his family." So although defeated in 1784, Schönejahn won in 1796.[140] Rüland's loss, too, was only temporary; after Schönejahn's death, he became city surgeon, and later he and Fischer's son were both involved in several protracted instances of Pfuscherey in Königslutter. These struggles continued unabated through the first decades of the nineteenth century, and the terms—livelihood, boundaries, poaching—changed not one whit.[141]

Surgeons, bathmasters, and apothecaries found rivals everywhere, within their own ranks, among other approved practitioners, and elsewhere as well. For example, the bathmaster Johann Futtermenger in Seesen gave the resident surgeons Pape and Fincke cause for complaint in 1758. They accused Futtermenger of letting blood, which he was not supposed to do. When called upon to testify, Futtermenger admitted that he had performed a venesection on the son of the local tavernkeeper, Wienhausen, but only after "the feldsher Fincke had struck the arm twice before and had been unable to draw blood." Futtermenger offered the fee to Fincke, who refused it. He also admitted that he had cupped the wife and sister of Wienhausen because Papen had refused to do so. Futtermenger argued "that he had had to take over his family home . . . and without [being able to exercise] his profession, he could not exist here."[142]

This was not an isolated incident, but rather just one of many clashes among the three men, which can best be understood as normal circumstances. Five years earlier, for instance, Fincke had accused Futtermenger of treating several people in the nearby village of Engelade. Two people related that Futtermenger had shaved them. A year later, the surgeon Pape charged that Futtermenger had cupped a corn hauler in Herrhausen and, in Engelade, had healed a child suffering from an ulcerated throat. Both claims were substantiated. The hauler knew of several people who had employed Futtermenger to cup them, and another man testified that Futtermenger had applied poultices to treat his stepdaughter's skin lesions, left by a bout with smallpox. The father related that "he was new in Engelade and knew not that Futtermenger was forbidden to practice his profession."[143]

Typically, the abiding rivalry between Futtermenger and Pape did not prevent the two from later uniting against a common foe. Futtermenger had in the interim received the right to practice in Seesen, and he now readily closed ranks with Pape and Fincke—his former rivals—against the Pfuscherey of another interloper. Pape once again took the offensive, raising complaints about his ex-journeyman, Hirsch. Despite having completed his training six months previously, Hirsch refused to move on and remained in Seesen, "earning his bread by Pfuscherey." Hirsch had allegedly compounded his crimes by stealing from Pape "a finely wrought writing-case" and several dentistry tools. Fincke and Futtermenger, equally worried, one assumes, by the specter of another competitor in the area, sprang to Pape's aid, arguing that "considering the unrelieved poverty of most people here, our earnings are very small, [and] yet the *onera publica* remain the same. [Thus] it cannot be permitted that one person to the disadvantage of his guild-brothers be allowed to tarry here and reduce their bread."[144]

Hirsch had violated several conventions: he had betrayed his old master; ignored guild custom, which required him to leave Seesen once his training was over; and arrogated an unwarranted share of the available livelihood. Moreover, he was a thief, and theft particularly dishonored an artisan, often leading to his ostracism from the guild and preventing him from ever becoming a master. As it was meant to do, the accusation stained his character.[145]

This almost open warfare between surgeons and bathmasters was customary, and was repeated in every Amt, in every town, and in every village as men fought to preserve and, in some cases, to extend their livelihoods.[146] If we look at the semi-independent duchy of Blankenburg, we see how the running battle surgeons and bathmasters fought over territory and income almost monopolized their daily existence. In 1768, there were only two guild surgeons, Schwancke and Schuster, in the entire area, and these two resided in the city of Blankenburg itself. Another surgeon lived in Hasselfelde, and one in Braunlage. The last was so impoverished that after paying his examination fees, he could no longer afford to join the guild.[147] According to the letter of the law, neither could accept apprentices. Even Schwancke and Schuster found it almost impossible to attract apprentices, "although they demand from them nothing more than a Christian upbringing, that they understand the rudiments of German and Latin, and that they are able to pay fees of 40 to 50 thaler." The problem was structurally embedded in the social and economic realities of the place and the time. "[S]eldom do children of respectable and prosperous parents devote themselves to surgery, and children whose parents are of lesser means . . . prefer to run to Quedlinburg and Halberstadt, where surgeons are satisfied with a smaller fee, and do not really care if an apprentice can read and write properly. If he can do the housework and within three months can give a good shave and help earn the bread he eats, these [surgeons] are content."[148]

Surgeon Schwancke's own sons had been well educated: they were, for example, fluent in three languages. That educational attainment over-qualified them for the position of ordinary surgeon. Both went on to study in Helmstedt. One served six years as senior field surgeon in the Prussian army during the Seven Years' War; in 1768, he was surgeon to the royal orphanage in Potsdam. The other was a physician practicing in Hamburg.[149]

If the work of a surgeon was meager in Blankenburg (with two surgeons sharing a clientele estimated at no more than 140),[150] surgeons and bathmasters also had to maintain eternal vigilance to prevent incursions on their craft. The Pfuscherey of the bathmaster Haupt particularly plagued the surgeon Schlemme. Schlemme complained that Haupt "cause[d] his clients to be unfaithful." The Collegium medicum had examined Haupt and given him permission to practice either in Heimburg or Benzingerode (the first a market town, the second a smaller village in the duchy of Blankenburg), but Haupt did not care to move from Blankenburg.[151]

The conditions of becoming a surgeon or bathmaster were, as we have seen, intimately linked to the existence of a numerus clausus among surgeons and to guild restrictions; after 1747, surgeons also had to pass the examination set by the Collegium medicum. Whereas once cities and towns had more or less freely distributed surgeries and bathhouses to the highest bidder, using the fees as revenue, that right was now restricted and could only be distributed or sold to certified surgeons.[152] This provoked special resentment among the nobility, who viewed their bathhouses as property to be "let out" in the most profitable way.[153] Once more, the imperatives of the Collegium medicum collided with locally established prerogatives. Cities, too, could and did dispute the right to appoint bath-masters with the Collegium, as the city of Blankenburg did several times in the 1780s.[154]

The competition between civil surgeons and barber-surgeons, on the one hand, and military surgeons and medical students, on the other, raged with a querulous intensity over the century. The guild articles of 1716 allowed surgeons and barber-surgeons to monopolize civilian practice. The medical ordinances of 1721 and 1747 likewise deliberately distin-guished between the civil and military states: military medical personnel, whether active, furloughed, or pensioned, were not to treat civilians, "so that each person remains within his proper sphere and that those people whom We pay in Our military" did not injure those who had "a citizen's livelihood and from it must honor their [civic] obligations and pay their taxes." In Braunschweig the surgeons complained repeatedly about the Pfuscherey of soldiers from the local garrison. The medical ordinance allowed military surgeons to treat civilians only in "extraordinary circumstances when someone has a grave and dangerous external wound [and] places special trust in one of the regiment or company surgeons." That was where problems began.[155] Pure and simple illicit practices were equally common, and the Pfuscherey of military practitioners among civilians was a thorn in the side of the civilian surgeons. Similarly, the Pfuscherey of soldiers was common in many other trades; it especially discomforted tailors.[156]

Students, too, stood outside the civil community. Their medical practice was objectionable as much because they were not citizens as because they were still untrained. In many ways, the Pfuscherey of medical students paralleled that of journeymen and apprentices. Of course, it was in Helmstedt, with its university, where the poaching of both students and professors was most noticed and most damaged civilian practitioners. The temptation for students to work clandestinely as surgeons and physicians must have been great. The concentration of such "pfusching" students in Helmstedt was an additional headache to the surgeons and barber-surgeons there. In 1750, for instance, the surgeons in Helmstedt protested the Pfuscherey of the "studiosum Schlagel."[157] Typical also was the protest of two surgeons, Johann Stüber and Johann Butterbrodt, filed with the Collegium medicum in 1760. They complained that the magistrates fobbed them off with only insubstantial promises, and that student Pfuscherey was so egregious as to "force us to make our own inquiries." Their investigations turned up, among others, the dubious activities of the "Candidatus Medicina" Johann Vibrans (who later served as physicus in several places) "who took on a patient with a blow to the lower left arm, which he treated for a week with both internal and external medications."[158]

While the medical practice of students was most visible in Helmstedt, it was occasionally burdensome elsewhere. Medical students who had finished their studies and left the university before taking their degrees often settled in the countryside. They sometimes tried to live from medicine, or often added medical practice to their other pursuits, as did the "Cand. med." Fahrenholz in Langelsheim, who "occasionally" practiced medi-

cine while tutoring, or the "Cand. med." Behrend in Alfeld, who compounded his crime in that he lived outside of the duchy while attracting
patients from Delligsen.[159] Students poached, therefore, both as surgeons
and physicians, although their practice was explicitly forbidden.

Midwives in Braunschweig

Surgeons, barber-surgeons, and bathmasters were male practitioners organized in guilds. Thus it will perhaps surprise no one that they thought
of their craft in guild terms and defended their property and their livelihoods in a discourse common to all guilds. What, then, about other
practitioners, about midwives, for example? Here, too, the same ingredients, the same ideas, the same defenses predominated, and demonstrate
that the concepts of Pfuscherey and corporatism pervaded society and
were not unique to certain sections of it. As women, midwives were not
eligible for guild membership, yet much of their story follows the lines set
out above.

Time and historical indifference have obscured the lives of most midwives in the past. Few enjoyed more than the local esteem of contemporaries, and posterity celebrates a mere handful, among them Justine Siegemund, Louise Bourgeoise, and Mme du Coudray.[160] This long and almost
institutionalized neglect has not quite rendered their biographies inacces-
sible or historically irrelevant. Their lives, their struggles, their ambitions,
their frustrations, and their successes can be recovered, and these experiences reveal much about medical practice, as well as more generally about
the social construction of life, in early modern Europe.[161]

Midwifery has been studied most extensively in England and, for a
later period, in the United States. These geographical emphases have to
some extent, and until very recently, imposed the tyranny of an Anglo-
Saxon model on the history of midwifery. According to this model, the
pivotal moment came when, in the late eighteenth century, midwives and
accoucheurs began the long battle for control in the birthing-room. What
has emerged as a central issue of debate in Anglo-Saxon arenas may,
however, be of limited importance, perhaps even irrelevant, to the experiences of midwives elsewhere. In the German states and cities, different
forces shaped the history of midwifery.[162]

No midwife in Braunschweig acquired the international reputation or
exerted the political and medical clout of a Bourgeoise, a Siegemund, or a
du Coudray, although at least two authored midwifery manuals.[163] These

twin anomalies are not of principal concern here, however. It is rather the everyday and the ordinary that form the substance of this study; that is, the careers of that relatively small number of women who comprised the corps of licensed midwives and their assistants—the evocatively named warming-women (*Wärme-Frauen*)—during the last half of the eighteenth century.

Historians have often discussed midwives and midwifery within the two broader models of professionalization and medicalization. And indeed these models have spawned a rich literature on how the relationships among medicine, state, society, and gender evolved. But the study of professionalism, which focuses on formal education, the coalescence of professional organizations, and the maturation of professional hegemony, and regards these as the loci where professional identities unfolded, proved less useful when historians began to consider "professionalism" in the early modern period and the "professions" females dominated.

One should be skeptical about whether it is profitable to place the history of early modern midwifery *primarily* within the framework of professionalization and medicalization debates. It makes good sense, on the one hand, to ignore the more rigorous standards attributed to nineteenth- and twentieth-century professions when discussing female practitioners of any era (such as lay-midwives of the late twentieth century), and to rely on looser definitions. On the other hand, it remains unclear to what extent midwives understood themselves as professionals by any definition, or, in contrast, viewed themselves as craftworkers or as sisters. Moreover, is the often-discussed tension between "professional" and "sister" in fact anachronistic when applied to the early modern world, in that *neither* label characterizes midwives' conceptions of themselves and their job? It seems more likely that other circumstances molded their lives and their métier, and they were, of course, not alone in being subject to these forces. The defining events that patterned the daily experience of midwifery occurred not only in the midwives' dealings with physicians, with government agencies and with ecclesiastical authorities, but also, perhaps even principally, in their associations with other midwives, with their apprentices and, ultimately, with their patients. By trying to understand these issues and by grappling with the incongruities that arise, we can unearth the basic features of early modern midwifery that scholars have only cursorily considered or dismissed as unimportant or irrelevant.

One articulate inside observer was Anne Horenburg, who was a midwife in Braunschweig at the end of the seventeenth century. In 1700, she published a midwifery text presenting the art of midwifery in the conventional form of a conversation between two sisters. Although Fasbender's magisterial history of obstetrics dismisses the book as "insignificant," it is nonetheless a telling document, for in the preface Frau Horenburg reflected on her life.[164]

She was born in Wolfenbüttel, the daughter of a regimental surgeon named Güldapffel. As a young woman she entered the ducal household as a seamstress, where she fell under the influence of the reigning duchess, who maintained a free apothecary for the poor, providing them, according to Horenburg, with "sage advice" in illness. Horenburg relates how she began "to think more about such things . . . and as Her Highness the Duchess possessed several books on midwifery in her library . . . I studied these and pondered such matters whenever I had time and thus gradually acquired a certain modest perception and knowledge."

Later, Anne married Hans Horenburg, a corporal in the cavalry, "and together we traveled the wide world." The first birth she assisted was that of her landlady in Westphalia, which "turned out so happily that I thereafter no longer felt misgivings about being called to such work and during the war helped deliver many children. It also occurred that occasionally when the midwife made mistakes, I warned her and showed her the right way to proceed, and because of this [the midwives] were often sour with me and told me that it was not fitting for me, a young woman, [to presume] to correct her elders."

After her husband was discharged from the army, they bought a house in Eisleben and lived there for fifteen years. She frequently attended neighbors in childbirth. After she successfully delivered the niece of a certain Dr. Keulings, he suggested to her that she consider becoming a midwife. At first she demurred, arguing that "I am still in my fruitful years, having already borne eight children." She later reconsidered and became midwife to the towns of Eisleben and Mansfeld. When her husband died, she returned to Braunschweig to be with her family. On her mother's urging, she became a midwife by submitting documentation attesting to her previous work in Eisleben and Mansfeld to the city authorities. The city's physicus declared her "competent."

Horenburg had enjoyed no regular instruction in midwifery: she had not attended a school for midwives (such hardly existed around 1700), nor listened to lectures on female anatomy (as midwives were later required to do), nor assisted a mistress-midwife as apprentice. Much of her learning, at least initially, came from reading books. It cannot be claimed, of course, that Horenburg's experience was typical, but it serves as a useful template and as a measure of contrast and comparison with the life stories of the women who later served as midwives in Braunschweig.

Between 1750 and the end of the century, the number of licensed midwives—that is, midwives examined by the Collegium medicum and sworn in by the city magistrates in Braunschweig—rose from five to eight. In 1797, for example, eight were active.[165] Twenty-six of these women can be more closely identified, and the archives yield up information on careers, socioeconomic positions, marital status, ages, and husbands' occupations for all of them, as well as for many of their warming-women. The amount of evidence varies from individual to individual, of course.[166] Yet these materials permit an analysis of the characteristic features of midwifery in eighteenth-century Braunschweig that goes beyond statistical profiles by concentrating on mentalities, illustrating how midwives conceived of their practice and interpreted their roles.

Their composite life history begins with the process of becoming a midwife. The midwifery ordinance of 1757 laid out a course of theoretical and practical instruction, making formal training in female anatomy and physiology compulsory. The professor of obstetrics and gynecology at the Anatomical-Surgical Institute in Braunschweig was responsible for this phase of their education. In addition, prospective midwives were to complete a rather casually designed apprenticeship as warming-women. After the construction of a lying-in facility in 1767, ongoing students honed their skills by delivering babies under a male supervisor's watchful eye.[167] This often added up to little more than extra, unpaid toil for the midwife-to-be, or at least that is how they perceived it. Despite the provision for structured theoretical training, throughout the eighteenth century, the education of a midwife continued to be largely that of learning-by-doing, with an older midwife passing her knowledge on to an apprenticelike assistant. Most instruction was transmitted orally, although the midwifery ordinance of 1757 required that midwives had to be able to read and write, and judging from the archival evidence, all could sign their names. Some were more literate, possessing and apparently consulting midwifery texts. At least one, Clara Catrina von der Mihle, owned a copy of Johan von Hoorn's *Siphra und Pua* (a commonly used manual) and recorded in her own hand the dates of her examination and swearing-in on the back cover.[168]

Until the middle of the eighteenth century, neither the ducal nor the city government prescribed any regular procedure for the selection, train-

ing, and appointment of warming-women: the midwife and her prospective helper struck a mutually satisfying agreement. It appears that
midwives were not legally entitled to any reimbursement for taking on
apprentices, although it is possible they nevertheless received payment.
No law, except custom, compelled a midwife to engage a helper, although many did. In 1755, in an explicit attempt to supervise the education of midwives more closely and to alleviate what was viewed as a
scarcity of trained midwives in the city, the Collegium medicum ordered
"that each midwife in the city of Braunschweig be appointed an assistant
under the name of a warming-woman." City magistrates were to identify
suitable subjects and then report their names to the Collegium for further
scrutiny.[169] The selection of these warming-women, their position in the
hierarchy of midwifery, and their activities (legal or otherwise), created
moments of intense conflict between the Collegium and the midwives,
on the one hand, and between the midwives and their helpers, on the
other.

The city of Braunschweig promised warming-women that although
there were no *emolumenta* connected with their jobs, they were nominated
in spe succedendi—that is, they took a place in line for the position of midwife in the future. Strictly worded regulations forbade warming-women
to deliver babies except in emergencies; neither were they permitted to
carry children to church to be christened.[170] These were common arrangements in early modern cities. The privileges warming-women sa-
vored during the apprenticeship were few; work was hard, hours long,
wages uncertain, prestige nonexistent. Not until 1767 did the government
guarantee midwives an annual wage of 50 thaler. This commitment took
effect only slowly, and as late as 1806, only five of the city's nine practicing
midwives actually drew 50 thaler annually.[171] In addition, of course, midwives collected fees for the specific services they rendered. The midwifery
ordinance of 1757 published detailed fee tables, which calibrated payments according to the difficulty of the birth, the hours of attendance, and
the social status of the mother.[172] Fee tables alone, however, provide a
singularly shaky basis on which to calculate the earnings of midwives and
warming-women. In order to estimate even crudely the "typical" midwife's income, one would also need to know—at very least—how many
women each midwife delivered in a year. What data exist are scanty and
widely strewn. For example, the Collegium medicum reported that 685
women had given birth in Braunschweig during 1789. As there were at
that time nine licensed midwives, this averages out to approximately 76

births for each midwife.[173] This is a worthless statistic: some midwives had more extensive practices than others; older women possibly attended fewer births in a year than did younger, more active ones;[174] personalities and reputations played conspicuous roles in a midwife's popularity as well.[175] Thus the historian cannot compute the earnings of the "average" midwife in Braunschweig unless she or he is satisfied with meaningless numbers that reflect reality only imperfectly. The 50-thaler salary four or five midwives regularly drew after 1767, along with the freedom from some property taxes they traditionally enjoyed, must have compared favorably to what many artisan families lived on.[176] A haze of reciprocal arrangements, family circumstances, and property ownership that is hard to penetrate from the distance of over two centuries, obscures their true economic state from the historian's gaze. Some owned property, others did not; some had inheritances, others had none; some labored alone for their families, others contributed additional money to family economies. Socially, judging by the occupations of their husbands (among them we find lathe turners, tailors, basket makers, stallholders, wheelwrights, weavers, barber-surgeons, journeymen, apprentices, soldiers, and the like), they came from the artisan milieu, although they usually clustered at the lower end of this occupational category, among the poorer and more congested trades, such as tailoring and weaving.[177]

What reverberates throughout this documentation is the sense of need, the sense of misfortune, and the sense of frustration that almost all midwives and prospective midwives wove into the narrative fabric of their petitions and protests. Of course, they were concerned about displaying their cases in the best possible light and in stressing their deservingness over the claims of rivals; thus they, like the other practitioners discussed above, constructed tales they felt would be believed. Yet there is little reason to doubt the general veracity of the facts, especially as they are so often corroborated by other evidence. Women usually chose midwifery (probably as they chose other work) because they had to support themselves or their families. The midwifery ordinances and custom dictated that they had to have passed childbearing age themselves and have borne children. While this rule was not hard-and-fast, few midwives or warming-women were in fact under forty. In 1751, the 44-year-old Christina Altvater reported that she had given birth to thirteen children, of whom eight were young and uneducated. Moreover, she had assisted many "reputable women in travail . . . whereby I acquired the skills necessary for a midwife." Her 60-year-old husband was a citizen of Braunschweig who eked out a pitiful living as a dancing master. But, she continued, as "the [price of] food rises from day to day . . . I [hereby] solicit [*sollicitire*] most humbly the office" of midwife. She was appointed in 1752.[178] While the Collegium medicum and the city magistrates never named women they regarded as unqualified to be midwives, economic arguments frequently swayed them to appoint a poorer woman over one even slightly better off. Furthermore, they often scaled wages to need.[179] This was not sheer altruism on their part; women, especially widows with children, counted among the most frequent recipients of poor relief in early modern cities.

Compared to those of a licensed midwife, however, the anticipated earnings—in wages, gratuities, and gifts—of a warming-woman were negligible. One midwife, Antoinette Becker, reported that despite her best efforts, she had failed to locate any woman willing to take on the job, "because they can expect to earn nothing, and they are scared away by the fact that they must pay Professor Wageler 30 thaler *pro informatione* [that is, for their instruction in midwifery]." She herself had labored as a warming-woman for fourteen years and during all that time had earned no more than 2 or 3 thaler. Two other midwives, likewise unable to locate candidates for warming-women, pointed out that "any woman could do far better as a seamstress." Another midwife, Dorothea Seehausen, agreed, adding that "lying-in women do not want the warming-women around." Not only did mothers fret about the extra costs involved (warming-women were allowed a small fee for their assistance at a birth, and it was customary to tip them and offer them some refreshment during their wait), they also resented the intrusion of strangers into a ritual to which their best friends were summoned—an invitation (or the lack of one) to a birthing carried a significant social message.[180]

. None of this made midwifery seem a particularly attractive option for women. Of the four women the Collegium medicum interviewed in 1764, only one exhibited much enthusiasm for the job. The sole exception was Anna Schrader, wife of a barber-surgeon. She would accept the post only if the city covered the costs of her training "in that I am almost destitute, burdened by a husband who has suffered a stroke, and bereft of all income."[181] A woman could envision little profit and less social prestige accruing from her service as a warming-woman. The cost of instruction was substantial, even though the Collegium decided in 1765 that warming-women need pay only one-third of the specified amount, and public funds would cover the balance. Moreover, this was a benefit enjoyed only briefly; in 1772, the Collegium reversed itself, maintaining that "as midwives in Braunschweig now receive a generous salary and [furthermore] can expect good earnings, the 30-thaler instructional fee is a sound investment for them, and they can no longer demand that the government subsidize their education."[182]

What quickly becomes evident is that warming-women had both motive and opportunity to overstep boundaries. They often waited years for a midwifery post to open up. Frau Becker, perhaps atypically, waited fourteen years, but other warming-women narrated similar tales of trial and tribulation. In 1776, when Frau Heidorn applied for a position that had just fallen vacant, she stressed that "for over five-and-a-half years I have faithfully attended the instruction in the lying-in house, and shied away from neither the costs . . . nor the neglect of my home and family to be present whenever required; all in the expectation of being able to nourish myself and my children eventually by the exercise of this craft, [which I must do] because my husband, a tailor, is almost blind and can no longer work."[183]

The road to a midwife's license could be a long and rocky one. Securing the desired prize necessitated patience, perseverance, and a good deal of luck. In 1774, Dorothea Nußbaum renewed her application for the position her deceased mother-in-law had once held. When she had initially applied in 1772, the Collegium medicum had denied her appeal, advising that she first "acquire a thorough grounding in midwifery," and promising that once she had obtained a certificate from Professor Sommer attesting to her proficiency, she "would be helped." In this hope, "I spared myself neither expense nor effort in achieving the requisite [level of] skill . . . in midwifery." She explained how "in the two years that I was constantly in attendance at the lying-in house, I earned nothing, although I often had to hold myself in readiness for two or three days at a time, while totally ignoring my domestic duties." Furthermore, she insisted, "I shall [soon] be ruined if I continue 'breadless' much longer." This petition, as well as ones she subsequently filed each year from 1775 to 1778, were all rejected. It was not until 1785 that the Collegium finally found a vacancy for her.[184]

Once a position was available, the Collegium medicum consulted its roster of warming-women, and of women who had already passed the midwifery examination, for a suitable replacement. Seniority usually determined the choice, although a candidate was also required to produce on demand a pastor's attestation of the propriety of her conduct, her morals, and her Christian lifestyle.[185] Especially after mid century (and perhaps heartened by the prospect of a 50-thaler salary), warming-women habitually took the midwifery examination once they had completed the theoretical and practical phases of their training. Success in the examination did not, however, bestow on them the right to act as midwives. On the contrary, they were expressly forbidden to do so. This prohibition inevitably resulted in a surplus of trained women for whom no legitimate practice existed. In some instances, the Collegium medicum and the city government agreed to name "supernumeraries," again *in spe succedendi*. They authorized these supernumerary or "extraordinary" midwives to assist women in childbirth but allowed them no salary; they could, however, demand regular fees for their services.[186] It is not hard to imagine that in these circumstances, the relations among licensed midwives, their warming-women, and the supernumeraries were truculent, tense, and not infrequently belligerent.

That friction to a large degree resulted from economic pressures. Warming-women and supernumeraries repeatedly agitated for greater incomes, while midwives reacted hostilely to those who poached on their territory. Complaints about the misconduct of warming-women, supernumeraries, and others arose almost routinely.[187] A fat dossier of grievances signed by all the licensed midwives in Braunschweig in the years 1795–96, and directed against Margaretha Krüger, reveals the complex and consequential issues involved in such accusations: "We see ourselves forced to denounce those midwives from outside Braunschweig as well as some [midwife] candidates, who covertly attend women in childbed; such [actions] greatly damage our incomes, [and] to speak more plainly, snatch the very bread out of our mouths."[188] These terms were, of course, identical to those surgeons, barber-surgeons, bathmasters, and others used when defending their territory against poachers, but there is another lesson to be learned from this.

Frau Krüger personified the early modern quack. In the late 1790s, she lived in the small town of Holzminden and was, in Holzminden, an officially installed midwife who had passed the standard midwifery examination with the grade *sehr gut*. That gave her, of course, no right to practice in the city of Braunschweig. But she did. She was, her detractors asserted, so "cheeky . . . that she peddles her services to people unbidden." When called upon to justify her actions, Frau Krüger conceded that she had in truth delivered several babies in Braunschweig, although "I have only assisted very poor women, from whom the midwives could hardly have received any compensation worth mentioning." Furthermore, she claimed that she had been dispatched as a midwife to Holzminden "in a way completely contrary to my own wishes." The move forced her to sell her house in Braunschweig at a loss. Her husband, a cobbler, had to pay substantial entrance fees to the Shoemakers' Guild in Holzminden. She had only gone to Holzminden in the first place because Professor Sommer had assured her that her earnings as the only midwife there would be ample. Holzminden turned out to be less than a paradise: in a period of six months, she had attended only seven births and thus found herself compelled to hunt about for additional employment, perforce in Braun-schweig.[189] It is crucial to note that nowhere in the midwives' denuncia-tion of Krüger is there any indication that she was unskilled or irresponsi-ble, let alone a menace. The midwives' opposition to her was motivated by ideas of what proper practice was: it involved considerations of money, position, and livelihood in equal measure. Similarly, midwives objected to warming-women who performed emergency baptisms "quite unneces-sarily," thus robbing them of the perquisites they "rightfully enjoyed" from participation in the festive christening ceremony.[190]

As with surgeons, barber-surgeons, and bathmasters, the concept of livelihood again furnishes the essential key to understanding how people constructed and perceived their identities in eighteenth-century Ger-many. Granting the right to exercise a livelihood within the community was a process of entitlement as well as a judgment of proficiency. Most conflicts between midwives and the Collegium medicum crystallized around issues of economic survival and social status that were themselves firmly encased within the early modern concept of livelihood. To assure a living for each midwife, it was felt necessary to divide the market equally (or relatively so) between them and to shield them from the unfair and injurious activities of interlopers—in short, to shield them from quacks like Frau Krüger.[191] For surgeons and bathmasters, both the government and the guilds had much the same motives in mind, although they dis-agreed on how best to assure livelihoods.

While this principle was almost universally accepted, the quotidian execution of it was hotly contested, and it took up much time in the negotiation process that was the essence of governing in the eighteenth century. The midwives, the city government, the warming-women, and the Collegium medicum often harbored quite contradictory notions of what a "sufficient" and a "superfluous" number of midwives might be. The warming-women and supernumeraries, who desperately sought ap-pointments as midwives, insisted that the number of midwives in the city was never enough to supply adequate care to the female population of childbearing age. The Collegium repeatedly denied appeals to increase the number of midwives to more than eight, arguing that eight was "quite enough for a city of 30,000 inhabitants."[192] Midwives, not surprisingly, countered that too many licensed midwives already practiced in Braunschweig, and that overcrowding effectively prevented each of them from securing an adequate living.

The small earnings of the warming-women and the long, sometimes futile wait for a position as a licensed midwife often propelled them into quackery. Neither the Collegium medicum nor the midwives themselves would, however, countenance economic distress as a legitimate excuse for quackery. The midwives pointed out that they, too, had served equally long and equally penurious apprenticeships. Leaping to the offensive, they charged that many warming-women seemed far more preoccupied with lining their pockets than with mastering the rudiments of their craft. Dr. Martini, when dean of the Collegium, also refused to listen to such "nonsense." He contended that like medical students at a university, warming-women should not be reluctant to invest time and money in their futures.[193] Although such encroachment was expressly forbidden and was punished (although mildly), it remained—and had to remain—more or less accepted, to some extent tolerated, and certainly expected in this historical context. As with almost every other kind of medical practitioner, quackery formed an integral part of the life experience of almost all midwives. It was a stage in their craft development. Frequently, even regularly, the entire corps of midwives, or surgeons, or barber-surgeons, or whoever, collectively denounced the quackery of one or another person. Yet these same interlopers almost always themselves became licensed practitioners, and were as quick and as vehement in protesting the quackery of others. Warming-women who became midwives protested the quackery of *their* warming-women and were as zealous in the defense of *their* livelihoods as their own erstwhile critics had been. This conflict defined their existence as much as, if not more than, their training.

Is it possible to conceive of an identity, as done here, almost solely on the basis of discord and competition? Did no sense of craft or gender solidarity emerge? It might be argued that the conflict portrayed here is overstated or illusory, an epiphenomenon of the sources and not a picture of the true state of affairs. This criticism cannot be dismissed out of hand. Harmony tends to occasion little documentation, whereas the mediation of disputes (like the investigation of criminal charges) generates much.

The conflict between midwives and warming-women existed. But perhaps we should view it as a life experience uniting them more than as a bitter controversy dividing them, for almost all the warming-women eventually did become midwives, as did the much-resented Frau Krüger. And no matter what their stance—aggrieved or defiant—they all spoke the same language of livelihood and privilege or of rights and entitlements, and this discourse, and these points of agreement, unequivocally defined them as medical practitioners and members of a group with a common identity.

Rural Midwifery

Outside Braunschweig, Wolfenbüttel, and Helmstedt, other forces helped determine the character of midwifery. In places where only one midwife was active (which was the case in the vast majority of villages), the fear of competition receded, although it never vanished. Here, in the small towns and villages of the duchy, different relationships prevailed.[194]

Several times during the eighteenth century, the government tried to improve the quality of what many viewed as the abysmally low standard of midwifery in the countryside.[195] One writer found midwives "*truly* one of the *greatest* causes . . . of the misery and degeneration of the human race." Another saw midwives as "the very death and destruction of humankind." Physicus Lindemann in Königslutter felt the decline of population there could be attributed "solely to the astonishing ignorance" of the local midwives.[196] The Collegium medicum initiated two formal investigations into the state of midwifery, the first in 1757, and a second, more extensive one in 1784.[197] A comparison of these results for two towns and their surroundings—Eschershausen (a medium-sized market town of about 900 people in 1814) and Seesen (with about 2,000 inhabitants)—shows how little things changed.

Eschershausen in 1757 had one midwife, a 58-year-old widow named Anna Brinckmann. Midwife there since 1754, she had been appointed by the community after being examined and instructed by Physicus Wachsmuth. She had also sworn an oath of office. Two of the four villages near to Eschershausen had their own midwives. They were, respectively, fifty-three and sixty-seven years old. Both had been midwives only for a short period; the first since 1756, the second since 1755. Both were married. Both had been examined and instructed by Wachsmuth. Village authorities had appointed them, and it was to the village or commune that they had sworn their oaths. Like most other midwives, these two had been selected by the women of childbearing age in their community. The village of Holtensen had once had its own midwife, but not any more: "she stepped down as she no longer desired the post." Örlhausen was too small to have a midwife.[198]

In 1784, the report mentioned only one midwife in Eschershausen: a 52-year-old widow, Clare Freÿenberg, who had been appointed in 1777, after the district physicus had examined her. Details of Freÿenberg's life do not, of course, fit each and every midwife practicing in Braunschweig-Wolfenbüttel, but correspond in enough ways to make its retelling useful:

[She had] previously worked in Brinkensen, and usually received about 12 groschen for each lying-in and [an additional] 3 groschen from each godparent. A christening, therefore, not counting the hospitality [given her], yields about 27 to 30 groschen. In each of the past eight years, an average of thirty children have been baptized in Eschershausen and Brinkensen; from these she takes in about 25 thaler. In addition, [she receives] three cords of wood [from the community with a value of] 18 groschen; free pasturage for a cow [worth] 24 groschen; the same for fattening a pig, which generally . . . totals about 12 groschen a year; and freedom from the general taxes and duties for her person [valued at] 18 groschen; a sum of 27 thaler a year.

As the current midwife rents her home and can keep no cow, she does not profit from the 24 groschen pasturage it is worth. She attempts to obtain a little from spinning and the care [she gives] illegitimate mothers. It is hard for her to scrape together the rent for her house and garden, which runs to about 10 thaler a year, [and] which she would like to have in addition [to her other earnings], but it does not seem possible to arrange this [for her].[199]

For Seesen and its eight surrounding villages, the vein of information runs deeper, and the following picture emerges for 1757.[200] Most midwives were older women, with an average age of about fifty-eight; the oldest was seventy, the youngest forty-two. Their health was generally evaluated as good, although the older women tended to be somewhat frail. The number of years as midwife varied greatly, from one to twenty. Many had actually been rather young when first appointed. Marie Hingstin, a 57-year-old widow, had been midwife in Seesen for almost twenty years, and the midwife in Mahlum was about thirty-seven when first selected. The size of a midwifery practice can only be gauged roughly. Reports usually give round numbers, which are surely no more than estimates. The record for Hingstin, which documents 592 deliveries over the course of nineteen years, is an exception.

The vast majority of midwives in Eschershausen and Seesen in 1757 had enjoyed only little, and quite informal, training, despite the provisions of earlier midwifery ordinances.[201] Yet no community mentioned any dissatisfaction. A few midwives had been instructed by relatives, often a mother-in-law or an aunt; only one had received formal instruction from the physicus, and he had examined a pair of them. For each delivery, a midwife tended to get about 9 to 12 mariengulden. As a very rough rule, the smaller the town, the smaller the fee. Only the two midwives in Seesen possessed significant perquisites of office: Hingstin got a wage of 4 thaler and a cartload of wood; her junior associate, the widow Schwalenbier, was also promised a cartload of fuel.[202]

Likewise, few of the midwives in the eighteen villages around Gandersheim drew anything more than the *ordinair*, or fee, they received at birth, which rarely amounted to more than 12 groschen; 9 was more common, and many settled for 6. In some communities, they enjoyed tax relief and, like the other minor officials of the commune such as the swineherd and shepherd, were allowed to fatten a pig at village expense. The midwife in the largish village of Opperhausen (548 inhabitants in 1814) benefited most from these emoluments, although perhaps the extras merely offset the low fee of about 6 groschen a father generally paid for each delivery. Smaller villages, such as Axheim or Orxhausen (with about 200 inhabitants each), had no "proper" midwife; instead, "the women there serve[d] one another in turn." In Bentierode, women in labor called on the midwife from Gandersheim, who took no payment for this because most of the women were her relatives.[203]

In his report on the conditions of midwifery in Seesen and the Harz in 1767, Physicus Müller listed eleven midwives in twelve villages or market towns. Of these, six had been examined. They were all quite old, ranging from forty-three to seventy-five, with an average age of sixty-two.[204] Physicus Spangenberg in Walkenried characterized the midwives in the three most populous villages there (Zorge, Wiede, and Hohengeich) as "all [of them] women in their seventies [who are] finished." Frau Otte in Zorge was "due to age, almost no longer in a position to do what was required of her," although he did not doubt her capabilities. This does not mean, either objectively or subjectively in terms of how the physicus saw it, that these women were unskilled or had been unsuitable for their jobs when they were younger. Indeed, many physici attested to the skill of midwives acquired through their long years in office.

By 1784, little had changed in Seesen. Two midwives still resided in the town proper, a number the magistrates regarded "as quite sufficient for this place." Ilsa Hingstin, aged sixty-six, was senior and had been midwife since 1766. It seems probable that she was the daughter-in-law of the elder Hingstin, who was midwife in 1757. The junior midwife, Rosine Meÿer, was fifty-eight, and at that time had been a midwife for twelve years. Both were "strong and well-loved by all those women they have delivered, and [they] have committed no major errors." Their compensation combined fees and privileges granted by the town. The communal government freed both of them from the major tax, the *Contribution*. Frau Meÿer, who owned a house with brewing rights, and also, as the widow of a member of the shoemaker's guild, carried on her husband's trade through a journeyman, paid taxes on the house itself, and on her profits from the craft. Each woman received fuel from the villagers liable to corvée. The midwives appeared to be content with these arrangements, especially as a fair number of well-to-do persons in the town often gave them higher-than-usual fees.

In the surrounding villages, the lot of midwives had improved only a little. Generally, they now received between 12 and 18 groschen for each delivery, in addition to all the other customary gifts and gratuities. By 1784, many villages had promised to make some additional provision for their midwives, generally in the form of grants of fuel or grain, sometimes housing or a general amnesty from taxes. A major part of the privy council's 1784 initiative to improve midwifery involved trying to persuade villages to treat their midwives with greater generosity. As a result, Dr. Müller recorded, the village of Bornum was ready to extend to its midwife the same allotment of wood a cottager was entitled to, as well as to allow her place for a garden and pasturing rights on the village commons. Schlwecke seemed willing to grant its midwife about one-third of a morgen (i.e., roughly .70 of an acre) as a garden "from surplus land," pasturage, and half the normal wood allotment of a full villager. Several communities volunteered to assume the midwife's rent. Yet these were only plans, and we do not know whether the promises made were kept. Much was determined by the state of communal treasuries. It does seem that the government was interested in improving the lot of midwives, an endeavor physici backed.

Although midwives did not enjoy an enviable lot in life, their position possibly improved late in the century, and their post imparted to them some, admittedly trifling, status. Or did status in the community actually lead to their appointment in the first place? For the most part, the women

of childbearing age picked the village midwife. Civil and religious authorities then confirmed the choice.[205] This was an old process. When the
resident midwife died, the pastor or elder assembled the women and asked
them to designate a new one. In 1749, for example, the women of Hehlen
designated Anne Heinmeyer as their midwife "by a plurality of votes." In
Lelm in 1784, "the majority of the resident, young married women have
agreed to choose the wife of the onetime soldier . . . Levin Hainen,
Catharine Marie née Kanincken, as their future midwife."[206] This method
persisted throughout the eighteenth century and even into the next,
suggesting that the authorities (at least tacitly) agreed that women themselves should have some say in the selection of a midwife. So when Frau
Momberg, midwife to the community of Ahlshausen, died in January
1791, the village pastor orchestrated the selection of her replacement.[207]
Choosing a midwife literally involved a polling, generally oral, of women
in their reproductive years. In Gittelde in 1793, the women approved the
selection of the widow of Peter Einen by a voice vote of fifty-four yeas to
thirty nays. Several years later, three candidates hotly contested the position of midwife to the smaller communities of Badenhausen and Neu-
and Oberhütte near Gittelde, producing a close vote of eighteen for the
widow Mävern, to seventeen for Frau Volbrecht, to thirteen for Frau
Wachsmuth. And in 1798 in Engelade, "all the women there" decided on
the wife of the day laborer Sickfeld as their midwife.[208] Even in larger
cities, a similar process often took place among the women of a neighborhood or parish. In 1746, in Neumarck, a suburb of Helmstedt, thirty-five
young married women asked the magistrates to appoint the "Dutchwoman" (one Maria Henrichs) as their midwife. "We can place our trust
in her, as over the years she has stood by our former midwife and 'caught'
many children, whereby she always remained modest and moderate" in
her demeanor. In 1763, the women in Neumarck made plain "that we
much prefer the widow Gercke [over her two rivals]."[209]

    If we consider the objections raised to women put forth for the post of
midwife, we learn something about the qualities regarded as desirable.
Experience (however acquired) counted, but equally important were
a woman's character and reputation. In Winnigstedt, "the petitioning
wives" objected to the midwife the Collegium medicum had nominated.
The community "will not accept her as [their] midwife and refuses to
call upon her to attend the lying-in of their women, rather they turn to
the wife of the Amt's clerk Schütten." The matrons rejected the widow
Müller because "without the previous knowledge of the community, she

was forced on them." Dr. Pini, the resident physicus, pointed out that the women in Winnigstedt "expressed a great aversion to the widow Müller, are convinced that she is guilty of neglect, and [believe] she has made mistakes in several cases"; she also had a deformed right hand.[210] When the Collegium medicum wanted to install Frau Duvens as midwife in Heßen in 1790, the community complained that they knew this woman all too well "from her many bad sides." Her husband drank heavily and she cohabited with him "in a state of dissension." That was not the worst: "She is herself unclean, her daughter has scabies, and the woman makes . . . [us all] sick with disgust" to have her near.[211] And when the pastor in Bornum proposed a woman named Ahrensens to replace the ancient midwife there, "the entire female community" objected that it was "impossible to place any trust whatsoever in this woman. Her life is anything but blameless. In three years she has only once gone to communion, and she is also unclean. . . . [Moreover] she cannot be suitable . . . in that she is still of an age to bear children and is in fact pregnant."[212]

The selection of the midwife for the village of Zorge near Walkenried in 1737 is, however, a case that demonstrates more precisely the character traits and the conduct village women desired of their midwife. It also shows how village politics were played. In 1737, when Julianne Pfannenschmidt became midwife-designate, the headman of the village, Hans Bischoff, objected. Pfannenschmidt was a woman who could not keep her mouth shut, he insisted, and "she likes to drink and is especially fond of brandy." The deleterious financial consequences that would accompany her appointment were just as serious in his mind: "[S]he hopes thereby . . . to free her house and property from . . . taxes, which, however, [I] in my official capacity cannot condone, because the [number of] 'free houses' in our impoverished region is already too great without another" being created. Reminding the Amtmann in Walkenried "that when a midwife is to be selected, the headman also has the right to express his opinion," he proposed the wife of Conrad Otte. Frau Otte was "sober, quiet, modest, and discreet," and her mother had been midwife in Ellrich. Moreover, "her husband Conrad Otte is a member of the commune and so long as he lives must pay the contribution." With two candidates, a poll was necessary, and about three weeks later, the pastor reported that five women had voted for Pfannenschmidt and thirty-four "and more" for Frau Otte. The pastor certified that the women in Zorge had chosen Otte of their own "free and uncoerced will" and "in their own words, [swore] that they could place their trust in Conrad Otte's wife."[213]

Julianne Pfannenschmidt refused to accept this outcome, however, and pleaded her case with the Amt. Frau Otte "stoops to any means to bring the women of the community over to her side," she said. She also accused Magistrate Fochtmann of favoring Otte, complaining, "[W]hen I tried to present my needs and my case to him, he spoke to me roughly, and would not listen." She charged that the women who had supposedly chosen her rival had not done so freely, and that many who had voted for her did not appear on the list. Several weeks later, sixteen women from Zorge protested the election of Otte by raising questions about the motives of the headman and pastor, as well as about the accuracy of the results they had sent to the magistrates. The women insisted that the vote had never taken place, and that they "knew nothing about it nor had [they] given their support" to Otte. They regarded Otte as unsuitable.

[S]he has not entered a church in two or three years now, and has never attended regularly. She sends her children neither to church nor to school, and one son, who is now fourteen years old, has never been to either place. . . . [W]hen women ask her to be present at their lying-in, and her husband must therefore do without her help, [he] wishes all sorts of evil things on the lying-in women, and it is shameful to have to say the words [he uses].

This plea had no effect; Frau Otte became the midwife in Zorge, where she served for thirty-nine years and delivered well over six hundred children.[214]

Offensive behavior or misconduct often soured a midwife's relationship with her community. In Timmerlahe, "all the local women use [the midwife there] only with the greatest reluctance and have no faith [in her] whatsoever." They maintained that she failed to show the required diligence, and "worse, that [she] handles a laboring woman with little skill and less concern, and instead of trying to raise her spirits with good words, prattles on with silly talk, smokes too much, and drinks brandy."[215] The women in Lauingen evinced even less pleasure with their new midwife, a woman unhappily named Sack, and "revolted" against her. One mother insisted that Sack had stolen a piece of linen from her during her last lying-in. They wanted their old midwife back. Frau Wülfer had been dismissed from office for fornication, yet twenty-two women "now fully agreed" to her reappointment. The pastor in Lauingen admitted that Frau Wülfer was indeed "a worthier subject than the Sack woman . . . if one forgives her first mistake, as apparently the women in Lauingen have done."[216]

Despite this evidence, the position of midwife was, on the whole, not hotly desired. The unattractiveness of the work, its low pay, and the prevailing sense that only poor women took it on, militated against enthusiasm for the post. When the 1784 investigation specifically asked localities to find women willing to learn midwifery, the results were miserable. Most places identified no one at all.[217]

Little changed as the century drew to a close. In 1787, Professor Sommer singled out the lack of livelihood as the foremost reason why the quality of midwifery remained so abysmal, especially in the countryside. He drew on the example of Boffzen, a village of about seven hundred inhabitants with two midwives. About twenty-five births occurred there each year. According to the fee tables, each birth should have yielded 24 mariengulden, but the actual amount rarely added up to half that amount. Sommer calculated that for the work attending a delivery—which included caring for the newborn child, washing the linen, and managing the household until the new mother was up and about—a midwife received only 4 thaler 12 mariengulden a year. And Boffzen offered not even a sliver of free pasture to its midwives. By these standards, the midwives in Braunschweig could regard their lot as considerably better, as could the midwife in Helmstedt, who received 12 thaler and four cords of beech wood.[218]

People closer to local conditions drew comparable conclusions. The physicus in Walkenried had a limited appreciation of midwives' capabilities ("they are fine as long as things go well by themselves"), yet was not unsympathetic to their plight. He deplored the "old and evil custom" of reducing the midwife to "a figure of fun" whom "the common folk" cruelly mocked and scorned. Midwives were also poorly paid, able to keep their heads above water only by "doing whatever they can."[219] Throughout the century, then, midwives in the countryside tended to come from the village's poorest groups; they were often widows or women with invalid husbands who, had they not held the position of midwife, would have almost certainly become dependent on community charity. Not all midwives, however, were so hard-pressed. While some married women were economically distressed, others had husbands who were capable artisans or smallholders. It was very unusual for the wife (or widow) of a more prosperous peasant to become a midwife. The dearth of women willing to train as midwives indicates that almost no one saw midwifery as a life choice. And the general profile of women involved in midwifery—older, poorer, more marginal—did not alter very much or very rapidly even after the new midwifery ordinance of 1803 mandated more training.[220]

If many people remained discontented with midwives' training and abilities, that does not mean disapproval was unanimous or that such women were callous ignoramuses. While, as we have seen, the education of midwives varied a good deal, those in cities and market-towns tended to have had more formal instruction. Some villages sent women to Braunschweig to be educated, although this was expensive and inconvenient.[221] In the 1770s, Amt Harzburg spent over 31 thaler (which included paying a tin founder for a pair of enema syringes) to have two women instructed in Braunschweig. Places like Harzburg were generally unwilling, or perhaps unable, to foot such bills.[222] In smaller localities, the level of formal education was lower, although many women had received at least some guidance from the local physicus and had been examined by him. Still, most midwives drew their knowledge from other sources, as Elisabeth Heine, midwife in Westendorf, explained in 1757. About ten years previously, the former midwife and the prior there, "as well as the district and the community," chose her as midwife. Since then she had successfully delivered over two hundred children. Her instruction came from her own background of bearing eleven children and "having learned this and that from the other midwives." She had read books obtained from Dr. Centner, and "the rest came with time and practice."[223]

Other midwives in the area related similar histories. Eleonora Büdekken in Twieflingen attributed some of her knowledge to having borne five children, some to listening to other people, and some to "reading a book." The widow Drüsen in Saustadt explained that her "knowledge" derived from her own experience of having had five children and three husbands, tuition from the previous midwife in Saustadt, and from "out of a book." Catharine Gackens, midwife to Alversdorf, had delivered seventy-one children in seventeen years. Most of her knowledge had been acquired in her own practice, and "if something happened that I felt unable to handle," she had turned to "the famous midwife in Barnberg, Mother Elisabeth, who died just last year."[224]

Despite the objections many physici and members of Collegium medicum raised, almost no locality complained about its midwives, rating their performance almost uniformly as "good." Their narratives spoke of how much local women cherished their midwife. And most midwives had excellent records and few maternal or child deaths on their consciences. Local authorities seemed little bothered by whether or not a midwife had been examined or sworn to her office, and when the Amt officials of Campen remarked that the midwives in Campen and Wendhausen were not formally instructed, examined, or sworn in, they added that "the [village] elders speak highly of them, and they carry out their office extremely well, and we have heard not the least criticism."[225] Physici themselves by no means categorically denounced midwives. They more frequently protested about a midwife's arrogance, or impertinence, or her unwillingness to bend to their authority.[226] Midwives were rooted in their communities inasmuch as the women of the village had chosen them, and their selection to fill what was, after all, a minor civic post was often the handiest and cheapest way to provide for them.

A Synergy of Quacks

In midwifery, as in surgery, the dynamics of practice and the issue of Pfuscherey make sense only in the context of several larger sets of relationships. Pfuscherey did not only flourish in the larger towns and cities or on the roads and in the marketplaces; in small towns and villages the warfare over rights, privileges, and livelihood raged as fiercely. There was never (or rarely) just one Pfuscher, or, for that matter, a single, isolated accusation of Pfuscherey. Despite its definition by the dictionaries and encyclopedias of the day, and the efforts of governments and guilds to combat it, Pfuscherey was never really an "objective" category. The Pfuscher had no separate identity; he or she could only be defined in association with others, and his or her identity often changed over time. Pfuscherey always depended on the milieu of conflict and competition that characterized much of the self-consciousness of artisans and many medical practitioners. One was, for example, an artisan because one was *not* a Pfuscher.

One such nexus crystallized in Harzburg around the surgeon Nicolai.[227] In 1791, the bathmaster Pape informed the Collegium medicum of the death of one of Nicolai's patients. This triggered an investigation that snowballed into a wider assault on all the Pfuscher in the area. The Collegium fined Nicolai 20 thaler for Pfuscherey and forbade him to practice medicine. This did little to deter him, however, and he maintained his practice into the early years of the next century. He sometimes paid the frequent fines imposed on him, and sometimes not, but always led the authorities on a merry paper chase.

Nicolai was himself quick to denounce the Pfuscherey of others, singling out the apothecary Röhle and the charcoal-burner Schmidt, and accusing "the two together of practicing medicam & chyurgicam." His own defense spurred on a widening investigation and exposed a netherworld of cooperation and denunciation. The physicus in Seesen, Dr. Carl Spohr, cataloged many incidents of Pfuscherey. Most flagrant, of course, was the "surgeon and publican" Nicolai, who "prescribes all sorts of internal medicines and dispenses them himself." The sharpest complaints about Nicolai to reach Spohr had come from the apothecary Röhle, "who tells me [Spohr] that Nicolai's Pfuscherey has grown to such overwhelming proportions that Röhle fears he and his family will ultimately starve." Yet Röhle, "as I [Spohr] know for a fact, [also] gives patients internal and external medications, and visits them like a [proper] physician or surgeon." There also lived in Neustadt "a perfidious Pfuscher," the charcoal-burner Schmidt, "who for years now has quietly been distributing his medicines." Nicolai himself had earlier denounced Schmidt to the Collegium medicum, but "that does not stop him; and he purchases medicines once again from Röhle."[228] Yet Röhle, too, some years later, joined in accusing Schmidt of Pfuscherey, listing for the Collegium's benefit the many patients Schmidt treated, and detailing exactly what Schmidt's Pfuscherey meant to his livelihood. "[T]he charcoal-burner Schmidt sends almost all patients with his slips of paper to the apothecary in Goslar so that his Pfuscherey will remain concealed from me . . . and now comes to me no longer. . . . [M]y business suffers greatly when local patients use a physician in Goslar and have their prescriptions filled there."[229] Röhle whined to Spohr that "things are so desperate with me and my family that we shall soon starve" if no one stopped Schmidt and Nicolai. Röhle also reported that Nicolai "in compounding his medicines buys few simple substances from him." This was a tactical error on Röhle's part, as he thereby admitted complicity in Nicolai's Pfuscherey. Here, too, is another indication of an economic symbiosis among various Pfuscher, which explains in part why they were so ubiquitous and hard to uproot. Röhle's resentment of Nicolai originated in his sense of being cut out of an obviously remunerative business.[230] This collaboration of Pfuscher with apothecaries proved as common as it was mutually beneficial. The apothecary Stolle in Astfeld, for example, profited nicely from his trade with several people accused of surgical and medical Pfuscherey.[231]

Röhle, Schmidt, and Nicolai were not the only Pfuscher in Harzburg. Also to be found there was "a certain pseudosurgeon" named Findler, who "using Nicolai's guild letter, shaves [and] pfusches *externa* and at times *interna* as well." Findler bought all his medicines from peddlers.

These traveling salesmen were themselves a pesky band. Spohr named nine who had "their caches in Goslar, in the surrounding Prussian territory, or hidden away in Harzburg." Although allowed to traverse the duchy with their wares after their boxes had been sealed at the border, they were not permitted to peddle their goods in the duchy itself. But, as Spohr pointed out,

I often see them going around with their boxes only *apparently* sealed—that is, fastened merely with a cord tied about them so loosely that the box can be easily opened without breaking the affixed stamp. [This sort of deceit] obviously requires the complicity of the customs officials at the border. And if I try . . . to have these peddlers arrested, they always defend themselves with [the excuse that] they are only passing through and sell no medicines [here]. From the district authorities I can expect no assistance [in this matter].

The authorities' lack of cooperation, apathy, or outright collusion with Pfuscher frustrated crisp control of abuses. Spohr suggested carrying out an unannounced search of the houses of Nicolai and a peddler named Köhler "in order to [seize and] secure the vast quantities of medicines . . . they both have." But there was little hope of success unless orders were sent directly to Spohr, "for in respect to the surgeon Nicolai, it is to be anticipated that he will otherwise get wind of the plan, and will make other provisions." Much as Spohr feared, Nicolai conveniently absented himself whenever the searchers came to his house, and they refused to break the lock and conduct the investigation by force.[232]

Simple economic motives are by no means irrelevant to comprehending the phenomenon of Pfuscherey, and arguments based on economic necessity or distress swayed the Collegium medicum at times. Even the notorious Nicolai could submit a compelling and by no means ineffectual defense along these lines. He adroitly played on themes that physici, the Collegium, and those who spoke the language of medical reform also used, if to different purposes:

For there is no physician in Harzburg and, because of the poverty of the place, no [physician] can feed himself here, and so it often happens that, as is the custom among the ordinary folk, one neighbor advises another to use home remedies or suggests other medicines, and the results can be tragic.

For these reasons I [always] have some simple medicines in my house, which I have, however, obtained from the local apothecary in order to assist my fellow-man in extremis.[233]

Nicolai drew a rather convincing portrait of the conditions that made his illegal practice understandable and permissible. His observations could have been written by any one of a number of medical reformers who blamed rural poor health and high mortality on just such a synergy of poverty, ignorance, and isolation. Nicolai pointed out that only about one in thirty people could afford to pay a physician; most would be hard pressed to come up with money for the medicines prescribed: "When a doctor from Goslar is asked to come visit a patient [here], the patient must pay 2 thaler for each trip, and therefore it is obvious that only well-off persons can consult a physician." And the "5 or 6 thaler . . . spent in a few days causes a scarcity of bread." No longer able to consult a physician, the patient had to "surrender himself to his fate, and then either a beneficent nature helps him or he dies." Nicolai adopted, and adapted, the language of *bonum publicum*, rather than merely deploying the older language of livelihood to justify his claims. And he was hardly the only one who framed a defense in such terms. The surgeon Beierstadt in Vechelde, for example, excused his treatment of a very poor woman suffering from a lung complaint. She was unable to afford a messenger or go to the city herself because she had to continue working.[234]

What remains unanswerable, however, is to what extent this was a rhetorical strategy consciously espoused to win support? Or was it conviction speaking? The two need not, of course, be mutually exclusive. Where did the language come from? Did it emanate from a changed mentality among a large number of people, or was it learned from specific contacts with local and more distant government authorities? Interestingly enough Nicolai's economic analysis closely parallels that of many medical historians, although both underestimate the willingness and ability of the "common people" to consult physicians. Much of the testimony gathered in Nicolai's case demonstrates that many patients had first consulted a physician, but had then abandoned him, not because of cost, but because the medicines "would not take hold" (*nicht anschlagen wollen*).

Because the cost of consulting a physician was so great, Nicolai argued, people by preference turned to apothecaries, executioners, and the like.[235] The Collegium medicum proved by no means impervious to such a line of argumentation. Although it fined Nicolai for his "medizinische Pfuscherey," it also suggested that: "In consideration of the condition of the district, it would perhaps be some blessing to the inhabitants if the surgeon Nicolai . . . were to be allowed a certain limited *praxis medica interna*."[236] Amt Harzburg had some years earlier come to a very similar conclusion, arguing that if it vigorously suppressed Nicolai's activities, "it is more to be feared that many of the locals will seek help from shepherds and executioners. And the outcome will be worse."[237]

Similarly, in 1747, after fining the bathmaster Albers in Boistedt for his Pfuscherey, and forbidding him to perform "all major surgical operations," the Collegium medicum nevertheless licensed him to let blood, extract teeth, and barber "so as better to earn his living."[238] Three years earlier, when the barber-surgeons in Braunschweig objected to the presence of "the many Pfuscher who presume to shave [customers] not only here but [also] in the surrounding countryside," the enquiries of the Collegium showed that the five men mentioned were in extremis financially. For them, barbering was a stage in an economy of makeshifts that also included agricultural labor and veterinary medicine. Four of the five were demobilized soldiers. Two, despite long service in the ducal army, merited no pensions. Johann Bartels pleaded that he had no means of support and "was forced to try to earn his bread by the thankless task of shaving and barbering peasants." The 30-mark pension Christoph Weeks drew "was too little to live on, so [he too] barbers."[239] Likewise sheer survival dictated the Pfuscherey of a knacker in Calvörde. The Amt pointed out that the knacker was unable to pay a monetary fine because it would "completely ruin him," and ventured that "the income from running the knacker's yard in this place is insufficient to feed him and his family."[240] Thus many knackers turned to Pfuscherey, as to other jobs, to survive, and this remained true well into the nineteenth century.[241]

A physicus in Blankenburg bore witness to the economic distress that helped breed quackery. His discerning, although by no means approving, portrayal of the fate of the average bathmaster shows how want and the need to patch together an income could mold medical practice in rural areas. No matter how ethical a bathmaster was when he first assumed his office:

[S]oon he realizes that he cannot earn enough from the pursuit of his métier to provide decently for himself and his family. His earnings are so small, especially here in the Harz, where poverty crouches in almost every hovel, that he begins to ponder other ways to make money. The opportunity presents itself to him every day. The peasants are accustomed to procure medications from such [men] as he, and the bathmaster quickly learns to be accommodating in order to gain a few extra pennies.[242]

As late as 1818, the position of the country surgeon remained financially precarious. A petition from the surgeons in Gandersheim argued that they simply could not survive unless they were allowed to barber and perform minor surgical operations, such as cupping and setting poultices. The marginalia added to this document by three members of the Collegium medicum *ad votum* did not dispute the facts the surgeons presented, but wondered how barber-surgeons and bathmasters would survive if surgeons were permitted to barber.[243]

All these Pfuscher had their backers and their ties to others in the community. Removing them resembled the process of wresting out a back tooth whose roots entwined with those of other molars; tug on one, shake the others. Extracting Nicolai would disrupt broader communal structures. Nicolai was a taverner in control of a particularly important piece of property in the community and a man who paid substantial rents and taxes.[244] The many-layered identities of men like Nicolai meant that pursuing them for Pfuscherey was not a simple task, but one that could upset several networks of economic, as well as social and cultural, relationships. In the eyes of many locals, a person accused of Pfuscherey by no means counted as a figure of ill-repute, a fact that the Collegium medicum explicitly acknowledged. Despite strongly disapproving the Pfuscherey of the knacker Friedrich in Calvörde, for example, the Collegium regarded his position as unassailable, because "aside from his quackery, the man has a spotless reputation and is highly thought of" in the area.[245] Dr. Müller, physicus in Seesen, while he complained repeatedly about the surgeon Pape, felt that it would be hard to stop him "as his money is indispensable [here] and he understands how to make his debtors into his friends and champions."[246] The Collegium recognized that little could be done to unseat many of those undesirable from a medical point of view, referring specifically to the case of the bathmaster Lütge in Langelsheim. Lütge had incised a tumor on the neck of the pastor's son so ineptly that he sliced a major artery. The child bled to death. Yet it was impossible to banish him from Langelsheim, "as he is established there with his house and lands and thus cannot be gotten rid of entirely."[247]

Such alliances did much to cement the position of a Pfuscher and could complicate the life of a physicus, while fostering the circumstances in which quackery thrived. As the friends, relatives, confidantes, and customers of villagers—as well as property owners, taxpayers, and bearers of diverse communal burdens—quacks enjoyed tangible benefits and considerable shelter. In 1768, when Dr. Müller itemized the "medical infelicities and disorders" in Seesen, he catalogued the many Pfuscher he had uncovered, supplying thumbnail biographies on each. Commonest among the Pfuscher were surgeons like Finck and his son, who "practice[d] internal medicine especially among the lower classes." The most enterprising of the surgeons, and uniquely irksome, was one named Bode, who had signed "a proper contract" with the ducal mining company in the Harz to care for the miners and their dependents. For "treating external and internal cases, complete with medicines," Bode drew an annual salary of 52 thaler. Müller's considerable annoyance stemmed from a personal slight: the company had canceled their agreement with him (for less money!) in Bode's favor. Müller attributed all of Bode's good fortune and his own rotten luck to the "whims and partiality of the mining clerk Hausdörffer," who was Bode's crony and brother-in-law.[248]

The physici and other outsiders could then struggle in vain against such "a generalized conspiracy of silence." A village united in support of a local favorite and against a physicus often made the latter's life miserable. Dr. Freyer, physicus in Holzminden, smarted under the whispering campaign orchestrated by a surgeon in the city. Freyer complained to the Collegium medicum that "although the lies this man spreads do not disturb me directly, indirectly I suffer greatly. He was born here in Holzminden, has a large kinship here, and thus (especially among the so-called 'little people') has unshakable support."[249] Yet physicians, too, not infrequently collaborated with Pfuscher, to reciprocal benefit. Dr. Sandorfÿ in Harzburg, for example, maintained a lucrative connection with the charcoal-burner Heinrich Schmidt, who had been repeatedly accused of Pfuscherey; Sandorfÿ furnished Schmidt with medicines.[250]

It was hardly only physici who faced networks of friendship and partisanship that thwarted them and their ambitions. Nor should one assume that only the "little people" consulted Pfuscher or flocked to their defense. The "rampant quackery" of the saltpeter refiner Jürgens nearly drove the medical society in Wolfenbüttel to distraction. The society's attempts to have his house searched always failed because "one or another member of the city council" warned him. Members of the council consulted Jürgens as well as the feldsher Dreyer in illness, and Dreyer also enjoyed the personal friendship and, one assumes, the protection of Amtmann Breymann. Indeed, the two were co-plaintiffs in a legal case.[251]

Local authorities could help their clients, relatives, and friends, and the "ties that bound" were as wiry as they were convoluted. By 1766, the bathmaster and surgeon Langwell in the town of Lutter am Barenberge had had just about enough of his rival, Tracht. "[H]e currently . . . is treating four patients at once, while I, on the other hand, have nothing to do." Langwell did not attribute this to Tracht's own skills, energy, and personality, or even his cocksure attitude, but to the not-so-secret assistance others furnished. Langwell had learned from a man "whom I do not wish to name right now," that no matter what he did, "whether he sent in ten petitions or ran up to Braunschweig," he would not check Tracht. A concession required money, Langwell was told, and Tracht had cash to burn, having received a hefty sum from his mother as a gift. Moreover, the local Amtmann was a near relative of Tracht's mother "and writes for him," while another Amt official "counseled Tracht in all things and is his good patron and my implacable enemy."[252] It matters hardly at all whether the prejudices and schemes Langwell saw ranged against him had any substance: he could only explain his problems in the terms of connivance, social networking, and reciprocity between clients and kin.

While the mechanism of "insiders versus outsiders" might explain the preference for an indigenous healer over a relative stranger, it does little to elucidate the rivalries between two insiders. There was certainly cooperation among many of the quacks pursued by physici, by guildsmen, or by the Collegium medicum, and local officials who shuffled papers, leaked information, misdirected investigations, allowed them to die of neglect, or adamantly refused to punish a quack whom they perceived to be an otherwise upright member of the community. Still, some quacks enjoyed protection and some did not. All could be pawns in power struggles within villages. This sort of situation almost always resulted in an appeal to outside, putatively higher authorities, to the Collegium or privy council. A flurry of charges and countercharges then flew, sometimes ending (at least temporarily) in the fining or proscribing of one party, who then quickly found himself reinstated (or once again indulged) when his faction regained power. Then his or her rival suffered. One must not be misled into viewing village communities as one big happy family, closed to the outside, and jealously, almost mindlessly, protective of their own. Conflicts within villages were every bit as acrimonious as elsewhere, and perhaps more so. We must not only seek the reasons for preferences and protection in personal affiliations with local notables, although these were undoubtedly important. The brother-in-law of a popular and powerful headman was hardly likely to be molested. Equally important was the extent to which some practitioners adhered more closely than others to a mean of behavior or a method of treatment generally acknowledged as proper and acceptable. To some, of course, this way of selecting medical help and of judging who was or was not a legitimate practitioner might be seen as irrational and illogical, based not on "objective" criteria of worth and a judgment of expertise, but on less tangible cultural values. These decisions had, of course, their own internal logic and rationality, but a further consideration of this point must wait until the final chapter.

Roots and Elective Affinities

So far this chapter has concentrated on those practitioners who possessed some legal right to practice and who fitted, however loosely, into some sort of guild or guildlike structure: apothecaries, surgeons, barber-surgeons, and (if in a less formal way) midwives. These made up a good number of all quacks. What about the others who did not fulfill these criteria? Can their stories be adapted without distortion to the framework of livelihood? Such medical practitioners only rarely emerge from historical limbo, and information on them is always less voluminous than on the others. Yet they too squabbled over livelihood and territory, and they too threatened the security of licensed practitioners. It is hard to know how frequently they were consulted, but much evidence suggests—as we shall see—that patients and their families called on several practitioners in succession or concurrently, squeezing visits to a physician or a surgeon in between trips to the cowherd for herbs, to the executioner for dog fat, and to the goodwife down the road for her teas and tisanes. Some of this story, of course, belongs to the final chapter of this book, but much also belongs here, because it suggests how the worlds of many practitioners overlapped, forming links in those entwined chains of cooperation and competition that defined medical practice—and life—in early modern Europe.

When physici reported on Pfuscherey in their districts, they invariably named all those surgeons, barber-surgeons, bathmasters, apothecaries, and midwives who poached, interloped, and exceeded boundaries. The catalog of Pfuscher did not stop there, however. Georg Spangenberg, whose story introduced this book, also listed a tanner's apprentice, a "baptized Jew," a vagrant *cum* oculist, and a "journeyman blacksmith and Catholic convert." In 1761, Jacob Müller complained about "regimental surgeons, surgeons, bathmasters, [and] apothecaries," but also about "executioners, knackers, shepherds, cobblers, old wives, and similar such people." Near the end of the century, Physicus Spohr counted a whole mob of such Pfuscher, including a horde of traveling medicine peddlers.[253]

Deeply implanted in communal financial and social structures was the executioner.[254] Like the bathhouse, the *Meisterei*, the executioner's home and workplace, was property owned by the commune and was, again like the bathhouse, leased on terms to individuals. Executioners, as members of a dishonorable craft, had no guild. The position was technically not inheritable, although sons often succeeded fathers, and some families built dynasties.[255] The right to bequeath the Meisterei or to divide the job among sons and brothers was sometimes taken for granted. Generally, however, communities publicly auctioned the Meisterei off to the highest bidder.[256] Its possessor was often at one and the same time the executioner and torturer; the knacker, who cleared dead animals off the roads and buried them, or rendered them into fats and other by-products (dog fat was an especially prized curative, which retained its popularity well into the nineteenth century); and the dog catcher, who captured and killed loose dogs, especially during the "dog days" of summer, when rabies was greatly feared.[257]

In Braunschweig, for example, the city contracted with Conrad Funcke for ten years (1781–91) and renewed the contract at least once. The elder Funcke had other sources of income, for when his son succeeded him in 1805, he complained that he lacked subsistence because his father had divided the Nahrung.[258] Such conditions characterized most places in the duchy that employed executioners, or at least a knacker.[259] In the eighteenth century, the proceeds from the job of executioner or knacker rarely sufficed to support a man and his family. The post of knacker and executioner in Calvörde, for instance, generated little income of itself. The man who contracted for it in 1789 was, however, able to supplement his living by buying and selling old horses and "curing among the people living outside the Amt," making him, according to the authorities in Calvörde, an "estimable person." That is, he performed a useful function, added to his livelihood, and paid his rent and the *onera publica*.[260]

Many executioners and knackers engaged in medical Pfuscherey.[261] The connection of the executioner with medicine was a long one, and individual executioners had once received the right to practice as apothecaries, surgeons, or physicians. In 1610, for example, the city of Donauwörth installed its executioner as city physician, and in 1711, Friedrich I named the Berlin executioner, Martin Coblentz, court and body-physician. Other medical practitioners hated the custom, and their objections derived as much from a desire to distance themselves from a dishonorable trade as from fear of the competition or the medical incompetence of the executioner. Increasingly in the seventeenth and eighteenth centuries, various ordinances, medical as well as economic, disallowed executioners any medical practice, although individual concessions continued to be granted. The Collegium medicum, in 1751, while forbidding the executioner in Königslutter to practice medicine, allowed that he as well as all other executioners retained the right to "salve those put to the torture after [their ordeal], to readjust their dislocated limbs, and to treat sick animals."[262]

The executioners and knackers elsewhere in Braunschweig-Wolfenbüttel were little different. In 1758, the Collegium medicum fined the knacker George Unkermann in Braunschweig for administering several drops of a "tinctura macrocosmi" to an apparently dead person in hopes of reviving him, and in 1759 also punished the executioner in Oberlütter for treating ulcerated leg varices. Such practices, however, extended well into the nineteenth century. The knacker Heinze in Neuwallmoden, who "not only engaged in animal doctoring, but also in the treatment of the human animal," was repeatedly denounced to the Collegium, but his Pfuscherey was never halted, and in 1834 his widow still sold her husband's tonics openly.[263] In Schöppenstedt, a four-year campaign against the knacker Rose failed to stop his Pfuscherey. A typical case involved the peasant Alte, who had approached Rose for medicine for his son, who suffered "intolerable pains" in his back and from swollen hands and knees. For 10 groschen, Rose sold him "gummi animal," lamb fat, and hops to apply as unguents and cataplasms. The results were excellent: his father reported that the boy now awoke in the mornings "completely free of his pains, and [was] able to mow all summer without [suffering] a single spasm."[264]

The executioner's right to practice was perhaps cemented in popular belief, although the authorities accepted his special skills and condoned his doings, albeit only under unusual circumstances. The Collegium medicum granted the executioner in Helmstedt, one Johann Scheermesser, a concession for a limited surgical practice, restricted to treating "foreign patients, without distinction," but locals "only when they complain of sprains," in order not to prejudice the business of the resident surgeons.[265] Scheermesser appealed for this right on the basis of his competence and what he called his "inheritance," which he seemed to interpret both in terms of education and the actual endowment of a healing talent by birth. Moreover, as many of his patients were "foreigners," his practice infringed on no citizen's livelihood, and it supplemented his income to the point where he could survive on it.[266]

Not surprisingly, this concession irked the surgeons. In their appeal to the Collegium medicum, they detailed the long history of executioners in

Helmstedt, and highlighted—not only in passing—their own financial distress. They also pointed out that Scheermesser and his brother had been warned in 1726 to desist from all surgical cures, as Scheermesser's father and the previous holder of the position, Hans Schreeden, had been warned before them. The surgeons attributed Scheermesser's preferment to the good will of a municipal official who had backed him, although he "knew little" about the matter. They protested that "rais[ing] the executioner, a coarse ignoramus and idiot in surgery," to their level gravely insulted local surgeons, medical students, and legitimate practitioners. Finally, they accused Scheermesser of failing to observe the restrictions placed on his practice, saying, "as there have been no dislocations and paralyzed limbs here recently, he has taken to other cures, [and as soon as] one gives him a finger's breadth of room, he seizes the whole arm." Scheermesser threatened their livelihoods.[267]

The boundaries between Pfuscherey and legitimate medical practice thus fluctuated, and the distinctions made were almost always artificial. The story of the Krätzers, father and son (like the father-son team of the bathmasters and surgeons Claus in Holzminden around 1800),[268] is an excellent illustration. Peter Krätzer, who had once been the executioner and knacker in Calvörde, observed:

I have now lived . . . [here] for over fifteen years, and earn my living as a horse doctor. Only a small part of my income comes from Calvörde . . . most of my earnings up to now have come from outside. Winning my bread in this way hurts no one, but is an absolute necessity, in that learned doctors disdain to treat animals. . . . Despite this, a few weeks ago in my absence, the local physicus, the apothecary Helper, and the Amtmann violated my home, had the locksmith break open my cupboards, and confiscated my supply of herbs and other drugs.[269]

This unpleasant experience did little to deter Krätzer, and complaints from Calvörde continued to roll in, spearheaded by those from the local apothecary.[270] The privy council admitted that the Pfuscherey involved here was only symptomatic of greater problems prevalent in the district. Krätzer had, after all, mostly treated persons "whom the physicians can scarcely help any more, and thus it seems futile to punish him." If one banished offenders like Krätzer from Calvörde, they merely crossed the border into adjacent territories, "and as the entire Amt is surrounded by Brandenburg lands, it is impossible to prevent [our] people from running after them." The privy council admitted that "in a place like Calvörde, with its geographical peculiarities, one probably could not expect to exert the kind of control one hopes to achieve elsewhere." While the privy council stressed that it was not its intent to tolerate Pfuscherey there, it was all too obviously treading water in Calvörde.[271]

The Krätzer family was deeply rooted in Calvörde, and its generational hold on medical practice continued despite the misadventures of Peter. In 1776, the Collegium medicum fined the new executioner, Georg Krätzer (Peter's son) for medical improprieties. Krätzer laid before the Collegium a story of his life that stressed his services to the duchy and his integral position in his community, as well as his penury and his successes:

I had the honor of serving . . . as musketeer during the last campaigns, to which I sacrificed my health. As I was longer fit for military service, I found it necessary to settle down as the executioner in Calvörde and, like my father before me, to take on the job of knacker.

The earnings from [this position] are . . . so meager that I cannot employ anyone [to help me] and it is impossible for me and my family to live from the [executioner's] income alone.

It is therefore absolutely necessary that whoever is executioner [in Calvörde] be allowed to practice [medicine] on man and beast.

His father had done likewise before him, "draining" patients and money away from Brandenburg lands and into Braunschweig-Wolfenbüttel. Georg Krätzer protested that he (and his father-in-law) had only practiced *extra territorium* and could not understand why this perturbed anyone,

as no one loses anything at all by it. For it is not very probable that people from Brandenburg or from other places who come to see me seeking help would in any way feel themselves compelled to consult a doctor here, as there is no lack of doctors in either Brandenburg or elsewhere. Thus one must accept that such foreign patients are not interested in consulting a doctor, but are seeking my aid and my aid alone, and if they do not find it here, will simply stay away.

Krätzer was fined and his practice prohibited, but the Krätzer medical dynasty continued.[272] In the 1790s, the apothecary in Calvörde complained about this same Georg Krätzer and his son, a doctor of medicine, because they illegally dispensed medicines. Dr. Krätzer admitted his guilt, while pleading extenuating circumstances: he had given medicines away free to the sick poor and prescribed them to be filled by the apothecary in Helmstedt, "in order to revenge myself on the apothecary [in Calvörde] who had advised patients to consult the then-physicus, Dr. Vibrans, [rather than me]."

Of course, executioners did not by any means provide most illicit medical care; equally common was the Pfuscherey of millers, artisans, and women (especially widows), as well as soldiers. Millers, who shared some of the stigma of dishonor with executioners and knackers, seem also to have partaken of their thaumaturgic qualities, although the historian might be better advised to seek their reputation as healers in their role as creditors in villages and as tenants of valuable pieces of village property.[273]

But the list of those involved in quackery rolls on, virtually without end. It includes paperhangers; upholsterers; weavers; cobblers and shoe-makers; tailors and furriers; blacksmiths and farriers; locksmiths, coopers and turners; journeymen and apprentices, as well as masters. In addition, there were grenadiers, dragoons, officers, noncommissioned officers and privates; peasants of various stations; shepherds, cowherds, and goose-herds; administrators of hospitals, saltpeter refineries, iron- and glass-works; pensioners; sextons, pastors and schoolmasters; day laborers, do-mestics, landless laborers, and peddlers.[274] In short, those who might occupy themselves with medical practice of some sort or another beyond the sphere of home medicine or self-medication pretty much reproduced the social structure of town and country in eighteenth-century Germany. While the licensed medical personnel—surgeons, midwives, barber-sur-geons, apothecaries, and the like—were most often accused of encroach-ing, the same sort of economic needs that often drove them to poach, drove executioners to medicate, and drove all the others listed above to treat persons other than their families, although economic necessity was by no means the only compelling, or a sufficient, motive. The language used to represent the activities of these "others" was not, at least on the surface, always as intimately and immediately linked to the guild parlances of encroaching, poaching, and interloping. Yet the underlying concepts were very similar and clearly implied a world of shared burdens and responsibilities, in which people held the community (and government at all levels) responsible for granting and protecting the livelihood of its members. All these fitted into the same general frameworks of language and mentality that circumscribed and described the guildsman's world. In the final chapter of this book, we shall see to what extent the healers' mental worlds and discourses were also those of their patients and fellow citizens.

Not typical, but nonetheless instructive, was the case of a paperhanger and upholsterer from Vorsfelde, one Johann Busch.[275] A letter from the magistrates of the small town of Süpplingenburg first brought Busch to the central government's attention.[276] The prehistory of this letter is tell-

ing. A young woman who worked for a tenant farmer developed a fistula
under her right arm that interfered with her work. Her employer called
on the local feldsher to treat her. Despite lancing the fistula several times,
he was unable to relieve her discomfort, yet requested payment for his
services from poor relief funds. Although small towns like Süpplingenburg had little money to play with, the authorities compliantly assumed
responsibility for assisting the young woman, first paying the surgeon's
fees, then taking further action on her behalf. "We learned that the
paperhanger Busch from Vorsfelde [is able] to cure fistulas simply, and
[that previously] he had thoroughly healed Lieutenant Isenbarth of such
an ailment, although not even the cleverest surgeons had been able to
relieve his distress. [T]hereupon we sent the maid to Busch . . . and
promised to pay him five shillings . . . if he could cure her."

The outcome of their experiment was encouraging: six weeks later the
woman returned to work, her health fully restored. The fortuitous resolution of her case set the magistrates to thinking. Over the years, Busch had
come to enjoy quite a reputation based on his treatments of incurable
fistulas and "cancers." In one instance, Busch had healed a fistula afflicting
a cobbler's son, which several surgeons had been treating for over six years
with no appreciable results. Equally, the magistrates praised Busch's ability
to cure without resorting to the much-feared "cutting." "[S]o we proposed to Busch that, as he has no children other than a small daughter, he
make his secret public and not carry it with him to the grave." Busch was
amenable if the conditions he insisted upon were met. He volunteered to
stand a test of his skill:

[H]e will undertake to cure two or three persons in Braunschweig whom the
Collegium medicum certifies as suffering from fistulas or cancers, after he first
examines them and makes sure that their fistulas have not yet eaten through the
bone into the marrow. Once he cures these persons, he will receive and be
guaranteed both pension and concession; then he will reveal the chemical formula [needed to prepare] his medication.

The whole exchange (here only briefly sketched) shows a hardheaded
capacity to negotiate, as well as Busch's place in what Olwen Hufton
has called an "economy of makeshifts." Paperhanging and upholstering
brought in little, and Busch was forced to patch together several sources of
income to survive, often working as a simple laborer in addition to ex-
ploiting his talents as a healer. He felt, and the magistrates agreed, that if

his skill were to be turned to public benefit, he was entitled to suitable recompense.

The magistrates' petition is dated 12 February 1772. In November the privy council granted Busch his concession, the terms of which suggest that he had indeed gone to Braunschweig, treated several patients, and proved his abilities, at least to the satisfaction of his clients and the privy council.[277] We do not learn whether the Collegium medicum monitored the test Busch proposed. Undoubtedly, the Collegium remained skeptical of Busch's talents, for the privy council issued the concession over its powerful objections. Here, of course, the evidence strongly implies that no tacit agreement (one is tempted to write "plot") had been brewed up between the privy council and the Collegium to promote medical hegemony for physicians. Nor was the privy council willing to bow to the expertise of the Collegium. The privy council, in fact, heeded the testimonials of people representing many social groups, all of whom Busch had healed to their satisfaction. The members of the Collegium fumed in vain.

The outcome of the Busch affair not only infuriated the members of the Collegium medicum. Others felt that the concession Busch received placed their own livelihoods in jeopardy. The Surgeons' Guild howled "foul" at the top of its collective lungs.[278] It was their *right*, its members insisted, to attend all surgical cases without fear of interference from anyone, least of from all quacks like Busch. The privy council stood firm and upheld Busch's position in the face of the combined opposition of the Collegium medicum and of the surgeons—whom Busch referred to as a "cabal" of jealous men. Furthermore, the privy council scolded the surgeons for their avarice and admonished them for a lamentable lack of brotherly love: "[T]hey should allow their suffering fellow beings to seek succor where they might find it, and must not think the exercise of their skills either a right or a monopoly."[279]

Likewise, the master cobbler Friedrich Dreyer was renowned for his ability to cure leg sores. The journeyman draper Georg Ratzkey petitioned the Collegium medicum for permission to let Dreyer bind his eighteen-year-old wound. Several months later, the Collegium medicum's own observer, Dr. Pott, found that the ulcer had been "happily and completely cured." Thereafter others petitioned for the right to use Dreyer, and the Collegium granted many requests.[280]

These cases raise the critically important question of which quacks were pursued and which were not. There existed a group of quacks who were generally left alone, although the Collegium medicum proscribed their practice. Many who took up the practice of medicine, such as pastors and pastors' wives, schoolmasters, gamekeepers, publicans, theology students, and widows, apparently merely added it to their other occupations or undertook it out of feelings of neighborliness and compassion. One finds believable, for instance, the testimony Captain Diez offered in his defense when two surgeons accused him in 1800. Diez had given drops ("consisting of nitro dulci and juniperberry oil") to a friend's wife to relieve her "intermittent fever." He sought no payment, and she had given him nothing. He explained: "I am often asked by friends to undertake surgical cases of a trifling nature; I had no idea that this was illegal and will gladly refrain from doing so in the future." The Collegium voted unanimously to let the matter drop.[281]

Those who believed their territory had been violated, such as the two surgeons who brought the charge against Diez, felt differently; they viewed unpaid treatment as a serious threat. But the Collegium medicum rarely pursued or punished "free cures." A miller from the village of Bettmar, who in the late 1790s treated cancerous sores among his acquaintances (and had done so for many years) "and who never took so much as a penny for it," was simply, and politely, warned off.[282] Other cases were dismissed, or defendants received mild warnings, because no money had changed hands.

Not all those who engaged in medical practice in the friendly spirit of neighborliness or as part of their economy of makeshifts were so considerately handled, however. One-time offenders had little to fear from the Collegium medicum, and even less from local authorities, but many who persisted were caught and punished, if rarely with much severity. The grenadier Lange, for example, had long made medical practice part of his life and livelihood. The legal position was unclear. Lange apparently held a concession from the duke granting him the right to distribute medicines. According to the Collegium, he was "extremely popular" and had won "the trust of rural folk." When several cases came to light in spring 1801, the military authorities decided to let him off with a warning and "forty-eight hours' arrest in the stockade on bread and water . . . in view of his otherwise good, almost irreproachable, conduct." This slap on the wrist hardly caused him to miss a beat. In summer of the same year, the Collegium turned up a woman, this time in the village of Klein Stöckheim near Wolfenbüttel, whom Lange had treated, and who testified to

Lange's repute as a "skilled doctor." Although her husband had refused Lange's treatment and had died, when she herself fell ill with an illness "that had struck almost everyone in Stöckheim with headaches . . . making them completely foolish in the head," Lange visited her and gave her a "mixture." She recovered in a couple of weeks. She paid Lange 8 groschen for each dose and emphasized that, to his credit, he would accept no money for visiting her.[283]

There was no decision against Lange in 1801, and in 1803 he was still practicing. This time a man and his sister-in-law had gone to Braunschweig to consult him. Cases kept cropping up over the next few years, and finally in May 1804, the military authorities, convinced that warnings and mild punishments would avail nothing, had him caned on the parade grounds and threatened him with "pitiless gauntlet-running" if he persisted. But persist he did, and the file ends with him protesting his innocence in 1805 after further incidents came to light.[284]

The Pfuscherey of two schoolmasters in the area of Lutter am Barenberg irritated the bathmaster Johann Hammer.[285] Hammer registered particular distress, inasmuch as both offenders possessed "their own livelihoods." The schoolmaster in Hahausen insisted that he had a ducal concession allowing him to practice his *profession*—bathmaster—alongside his teaching duties. Not only did Hammer lose medical clients to the schoolmasters, they also cut into his barbering trade. Nothing medically illicit fazed the schoolmaster in Bodenstein: he pulled teeth, dressed wounds, distributed medicines ("especially strong purges"), and even barbered, let blood, and cupped "on Sundays . . . for half the [set] fee." There is no evidence that the Collegium medicum or the local authorities did anything, or could do anything, to aid Hammer.[286] These stories could be endless multiplied, but perhaps the best way to see how this kind of Pfuscherey worked is to look at the case of Zacharias Jürgens in Wolfenbüttel.

In 1756, the surgeons in Wolfenbüttel accused Jürgens, who managed the nearby saltpeter works, of dispensing medicines, practicing surgery, and visiting patients "like a proper doctor." When questioned, Jürgens denied that he sold medicines, although he admitted that he practiced "outwards" in Hildesheim, where he had received a concession from the privy councilor and the wife of the territorial administrator of pension funds. He expressed his intention to move to Hildesheim, "because here he suffers constant harassment." However, he neither left nor refrained from practice. A year later, in 1757, the bathmaster Michaels reported that

Jürgens's treatment of a person in Kleines Stöckheim had produced "unfortunate" results; the patient died.[287]

Apparently, though, Jürgens's overall reputation as a healer was excellent. In fact, the privy council ordered the Collegium medicum to test his surgical skills, because his management of several perilous cases indicated that far from being "inexperienced," he was quite adroit.[288] Jürgens refused to submit to the examination, however, explaining that he had not studied surgery *ex professio*, but had rather "racked [his] brains in solitude" pursuing studies in "chymice." He attributed his successes to God's grace, which permitted him to aid those whom "even famous doctors have despaired of saving."[289]

A final incident stresses other aspects of quackery, perhaps most prominently its persistence. There was no truly effective way to root out quackery even when the quacks were sufficiently identified. Take, for instance, the case of that "notorious" quack the widow Asmus. Her husband had been the keeper of fowl for the community of Jerxheim. Her cures won her wide respect. She came to the attention of the Collegium medicum when she treated the son of a peasant in Beierstedt with "a small bottle full of drops," which she sold for 6 groschen. The boy had subsequently died. This was hardly the first time she had been involved in medicine; she had been previously threatened and punished, to no avail. When questioned, people told confused tales or denied they knew the woman. The widow herself, who in 1771 was seventy-nine years old, maintained that she had been sick and bedridden at the time of the alleged incident. She did remember, however, that "a woman, the wife of the tavernkeeper Lohls" came to her and showed her a vessel filled with urine and asked for medicine. Asmus sold her a vial for 6 groschen. Asmus suggested that "it could have been" this other woman who gave the drops to the boy. When the Collegium medicum received this report, its president, von Flögen, felt that the case should be dropped because the evidence was so chaotic and sparse, and "because the accused woman is . . . a drunk and seventy-nine years old and might well give false testimony." In any case, "she'll not be a problem much longer."[290] Little did he realize that almost eight years later, the widow Asmus would still be a thorn in the Collegium's side.

In 1778, the death of another peasant in Hötzum brought Widow Asmus once again under suspicion when the Collegium medicum learned that he had obtained drops "from a woman in Schöningen." Dr. Pott, then secretary of the Collegium, quickly fingered the culprit: it was "probably the Asmus woman . . . one of the most infamous and refractory of all

Pfuschers." The Collegium imposed a 2-thaler fine, which Asmus flatly refused to pay, arguing that a peasant had come to her and only wanted to know "what his brother lacked." And once again the testimony gathered was reluctantly given and inconclusive. The Collegium insisted she pay the fine and ordered the local magistrates in Schöningen to collect it. The authorities later reported back to the Collegium that she had again resisted paying, and that because she was old, sick, lame, and bedridden, one lacked an appropriate *objecto executionu*. The authorities concluded that "as she will never again leave her bed," the best they could do was "to charge the head of the household, the huntsman Asmus, that he must not let any strangers in to see her," and that should effectively end the matter. Von Flögen's postscript to the case imparts a weird sense of déjà vu. Once more he suggested that the case be closed, "as the death of this 90-year-old woman will probably soon make an end of this."[291]

The story of the widow Asmus highlights several of the obstacles the authorities encountered in following up reports of quackery. There was first, of course, the quite sticky problem of ascertaining the true course of events and identifying those involved. Local authorities rarely saw cases of Pfuscherey as crucially important or pressing. It was notoriously difficult to get people to tell a straight story, as the Asmus case reveals. One suspects that deliberate prevarication explains this only in part. One could easily "forget" consulting her, or "dis-remember." But in a world where medical advice flowed from all sides and was not divided cognitively into categories of expert and amateur or "valid" and "false," people indeed tended to lose track of from where and from whom medicines and advice had come. As both advice and medicines passed from hand to hand, it was sometimes next to impossible to determine who the true source of the brew was, not to mention the fact that patients often gulped several medicines at once, or in rapid succession. Even in the close-knit world of the village, there was, as we see here, plenty of opportunity for subterfuge and sneaking around. While the rest of her family was away, neighbors and strangers dropped in to consult the old invalid and went away with her "vials of drops."

These observations return us to the world that nourished quackery and in which medical pluralism flourished. Throughout the eighteenth century, and well into the next, the language of poaching and interloping persisted and it endured because it still suited the world in which people lived. Yet that world was in flux; its older undergirding was slowly being dissolved by the acid of change. The government of Braunschweig-Wolfenbüttel was trying to gain control over the guilds and to transform their corporate structure by reducing their legal powers, although that policy was only imperfectly realized, and the government never mounted—or intended to mount—an all-out attack on the guilds' role as social, economic, or moral institutions. Guilds thus retained much of their integrity, and guildsmen defended their position in the same idioms of rights, privileges, and livelihood as they always had. Characteristically, as the government stood less ready to guarantee their rights and demands, they asserted them more vigorously. Their own solidarity was, however, subverted from within when members broke ranks. Moreover, although guildsmen, the Collegium medicum, and the privy council all condemned Pfuscherey, it remained a clear stage in the working life of many—of guildsmen, medical practitioners, and others alike. While it may be overstating the case to argue that everyone "pfuscht" at one time or another, that seems pretty close to the truth.

One must also understand quackery and medical practice in the context of a world where medical care was judged on several variables. The quack was not just a bathmaster who poached on the surgeons' rights (to take a frequent example): he was a member of a community, perhaps a property-holder, a taxpayer, a debtor or creditor, and connected by ties of blood or marriage to others. This meant that whether we are talking about the quackery that involved overstepping bounds, or the practice of men like Lange and women like Asmus, the obstacles that lay in the way of "rooting out quackery" were formidable. Or rather they were not *obstacles* but integral parts of the world that existed, and until that world disappeared, quackery would continue. While there were clear impediments to the initiatives of government in terms of administrative incompetence and the power of local forces, the real limits emanated from a social and political arrangement that still offered benefits tangibly greater than that of a cozy sense of traditionalism. All healers and all practitioners were tied to their communities by several bonds, and all manner of actions sustained—or ruptured—their links. The "purely medical" counted only partially here. Removing any one quack, for example, or inserting a new presence into a community, meant disturbing, or at least rearranging social, economic, and political structures. Allotments of wood and grain (for example, to midwives) meant sacrifices for someone; punishing a houseowner for quackery could mean that he or she became less able, or completely unable, to pay his or her taxes, or it might mean whittling his or her income away to the point of destitution. Denying a poor surgeon the right to barber could reduce a meager income to virtually nothing. These were calculations local authorities made and stark realities the central government—the privy council and the Collegium medicum—fully recognized. Both hesitated to tamper with circumstances merely in the name of more grandiose projects. In so doing, they were neither lethargic, nor complacent, nor irresponsible; they were simply cautious.

Illness and Society

The diseases people suffered, and either survived or ultimately succumbed to, shaped their perceptions of health and illness, contouring their expectations of life and forming their understanding of the world surrounding them. To understand attitudes toward health and illness, one must first try to discover which diseases mattered—statistically and perceptively—in the eighteenth century. The sources are many and varied, if also cryptic and ambiguous. Inevitably, the manner of collecting information prejudiced the result. While vital statistics are critical here, this chapter is less concerned with ascertaining hard demographic facts than with explicating the experience of illness at both the societal and personal levels. Thus it is to other evidence—impressionistic, anecdotal, and dispersed—that we must turn as well.

Reporting and Classifying Disease

The collection and classification of evidence pertaining to mortality, morbidity, and health have a long history in the Germanies. During the late Middle Ages, municipal governments concerned themselves at least periodically with its accumulation and more fitfully with the allied, more tedious tasks of sorting and storing it. Plague extended what was once almost solely a municipal concern outward to touch areas in the countryside, at first focusing most sharply on border districts. Wars, too, in particular the Thirty Years' War and the Seven Years' War, raised worries about health as troops tramped back and forth across the territory, kindling or threatening to kindle disease. Such events also stimulated the development of more effective means of collecting, collating, and interpreting the particulars obtained. There is an entire history to be written about the administrative nightmares involved in the accumulation of raw data, ranging from deciding who would pay for paper to excuses turning on lame horses and bleeding piles, but it is a tale we must ignore for the moment.[1]

By the 1740s, many governments regularly amassed information on births, deaths, and, if less frequently, on illness, and began to scan it for deeper meanings. Most closely approximating modern statistical compilations were the birth and death records assembled with increasing diligence after the middle of the century. Especially after the Seven Years' War, fears of depopulation and anxiety about the economic torpor that might result animated an attention that quickly moved beyond the crude measurement of rates of growth and decline. These numbers are, of course, hardly as transparent as they may seem: the very means of collection and the categories employed rested on distinctly varied definitions of and presuppositions about human life and death.

Besides exacting a more meticulous registration of births and deaths, the government of Braunschweig-Wolfenbüttel also attempted to gauge morbidity, mandating in 1750 that the sextons and schoolmasters in Blankenburg and Wolfenbüttel report every two weeks on incidents of illness, as well as on births and deaths. This requirement was extended to all parts of the duchy in 1754, and after 1765, a number of local officials, including physici and pastors, were charged with preparing regular analyses of the "increase and decrease of the inhabitants."[2] Political considerations, impressions of landscape and climate, moral judgments, and socioeconomic persuasions determined the content of these documents. Such accounts only seldom exist for the period before 1740, although because of their economic importance, some areas, such as the Weser and Harz districts, as well as the large cities of Braunschweig, Wolfenbüttel, and Helmstedt, were better served. Several government councils reviewed the information thus acquired. The privy council searched for generalized signs of distress; the Collegium medicum noted worrisome outbreaks of disease; and the treasury sought details on the taxability of subjects. These evaluations demonstrate how statistics filtered reality, as well as how statistics, or at least numbers, were beginning to serve in elementary ways as a basis for policy making.[3]

Information on cause of death for the *entire* duchy, unfortunately, appears only very late in the eighteenth century, largely as a result of inability to agree on a practical nosology (that is, a set of terms), but also because of the difficulty of persuading administrators and physici to adhere to the guidelines laid down.[4] For 1795 and 1796, however, we have a listing of causes of death for the entire duchy, with commentary appended by the treasury. This gloss compares the 1795–96 statistics with those of the previous fifteen years.[5] The register lists ten categories: diseases of the head and nerves; diseases of the throat and chest; diseases of the abdomen; diseases of "other parts"; fevers without rashes; fevers with rashes; childhood diseases; female diseases; diseases of the elderly; and violent deaths. Only 1.4 percent of deaths were unclassified. These two mortality lists, although they come late in our period and only cover two years, show the causes of death fairly accurately for the period after the end of the Seven Years' War in 1763. For example, the general breakdown of diseases in these two years reveals a telling order of magnitude, and one that faithfully mirrors what is generally known about early modern mortality. The largest grouping is of diseases of the throat and chest, which accounted for 32.4 percent of deaths in 1795 and 28.6 percent in 1796. Within this aggregate category, the chief killers were "hectic, asthma, and consumption" (*Hektik, Engbrüstigkeit und Schwindsucht*) followed by "pleurisy" (*Seitenstechen in der Brust*) and "coughs of all kinds, including whooping cough" (*Husten aller Art, auch Keichhusten*). Childhood diseases followed, accounting for 20 percent and 19.1 percent of mortality. In fact, this percentage should have been considerably higher, since deaths from smallpox and measles were listed, not as childhood afflictions, but as "fevers with rashes." These fevers mostly killed children and accounted for an additional 254 deaths in 1795 and a whopping 944 deaths in 1796. Likewise, many of the deaths registered under coughs and whooping cough were surely those of children.

Fevers (with and without rashes) made up the third largest group of deaths, although as noted above, many of those who died from "fevers with rashes" were children who succumbed to smallpox or measles, especially in the "smallpox year" of 1796. "The purples" (*Friesel*, another umbrella term, which indicated any disease characterized by an eruption of purplish pustules, and could mean anything from prickly heat, miliaria rubra, or chilblains to more serious cases of erysipelas (sometimes called St. Anthony's fire) and inflammatory fever, counted as the most frequent fevers and together caused 6.8 percent of all deaths in 1795 (52.8% of fever deaths) and 8.8 percent in 1795 (35.6% of fever deaths).[6]

Of the abdominal diseases, diarrhea, dysentery, dropsy, and tympany (*Windsucht*) slew many, although worms, too, caused fifty-five deaths each year (once again, probably mostly of children). Diseases such as gout were serious cripplers for some and annoyances for many more, although seldom fatal. In the category of "diseases of the remaining parts," the broad class of "external ulcers, wounds, cancerous growths, salt rheums, bony tumors, fistulas, and mortification," reaped over a hundred deaths each year (128, or 2.6%, in 1795; 107, or 1.7%, in 1796). The only other major cause of death was old age (433, or 8.8%, in 1795; and 511, or 8.2%, in 1796). At least at the end of the eighteenth century, childbirth does not appear to have been particularly hazardous for women, producing only sixty-nine female deaths in 1795, and seventy-three in 1796. The number of recorded stillbirths was very low. Deaths by accident or through violence were rare; drowning was the most common misadventure. Only one infanticide was recorded in these two years, although this probably refers only to infanticides prosecuted (a very different thing than the number of infanticides).[7] A mere handful of people (nine in two years) committed suicide; there were just two homicides; no one was executed.

These statistics at best only outline actual mortality and morbidity. They are more useful as indicators of what eighteenth-century statisticians knew or thought they knew. In terms of number of deaths per thousand, the picture appears quite a favorable one. In 1795, for Braunschweig-Wolfenbüttel, the birth/death ratio was given as 1,298:1,000; in the smallpox year of 1796, it was a less favorable 1,077:1,000.[8] Not surprisingly, larger cities had less favorable birth/death ratios than did smaller towns and villages. There are, of course, innumerable problems with using these numbers to gauge population and health in late seventeenth- and eighteenth-century Germany. Besides the obvious fact that data from the late eighteenth century did not necessarily reflect earlier conditions, their reliability is also suspect.

There were, in fact, two related problems here: the first was nosographical and a matter of naming and classifying; the second was mechanical and derived from how individuals collected information. While the expectations of government toward the end of the century were high, the means used to gather statistics lacked sophistication. Pastors, schoolmasters, and sextons carried out their duties more dilatorily than diligently and often misassigned cause of death. Still, some diseases were probably noted with a high degree of precision. Few people mistook smallpox; deaths in childbirth and stillbirths were relatively unproblematic. Thus, the categories of disease employed in the eighteenth century, while they do not represent a classification we accept or comprehend today, can be cautiously used to grasp patterns of illness. For example, we know that eighteenth-century nosologists and physicians usually listed what we consider symptoms as diseases (jaundice and dropsy are two good examples) in a way that frustrates retrodiagnosis. "Dropsy" could result from many diseases, and "asthma" (*Engbrüstigkeit*) almost surely refers to more ailments than modern asthma. Chest and lung ailments, fevers, and gastrointestinal conditions in children that resulted in convulsions near death (thus the name: *Jammer*)[9] undoubtedly killed most people.

The oddness of these classifications, at least to the modern eye, highlights a well-known predicament historians face in interpreting mortality and morbidity in the past: with few exceptions, even those terms that seem most transparent (such as smallpox—*Blattern*) can never simply be equated with modern diagnostic categories.[10] More than a decade ago, a joint project at the Free University in Berlin constructed a longitudinal series of mortality data (1715–1874) excerpted from the parish registers of the Dorotheenstadt district in Berlin. By analyzing the changes in terminology over time, Jan Brügelmann, a member of that team, showed that despite the difficulties that such terms and the nosographical logic behind them present to the historian, one could identify the *general* causes of mortality and, by working backwards, actually decipher some of the more obscure and arcane terms (although he himself felt that the historian was restricted to the more modest endeavor of determining terminological shifts by comparing causes of death over time).[11] Jean-Pierre Peter has voiced similar cautions and suggested like ways of dealing with troublesome eighteenth-century terminologies as they appeared in the inquiries conducted by the Société royale de médecine between 1774 and 1794.[12] All good medical historians remain skittish about diagnosing illness in the past. While I accept these limitations as prudent, there remains some difficulty in trying, as I do here, to talk about "patterns and perspectives." One problem is simple, yet intractable. For an English-speaking audience three centuries later, naively reproducing archaic German terms does not seem to me a useful way to communicate. I have therefore chosen to employ reasonable *approximations* for names of diseases and disease-complexes that meant something to eighteenth-century people but are unintelligible or even grotesque within today's totally different system. I can only warn the reader that such labels are imprecise and conjectural.[13]

Diseases of the chest and throat were the most frequent causes of illness and death in the eighteenth century. Often designated by the terms *Brust-*

krankheit, Brustseuche, Brustfieber, Brustbeschwerde, this category included, but was not limited to, influenza, pneumonia, pleurisy, and asthma. *Brust-krankheit* was a description for many illnesses and, as Brügelmann has pointed out, translating it into "a term we can understand today . . . is an almost futile task."[14] Another set of chest diseases, which probably included pulmonary tuberculosis, were subsumed under a plethora of designations. *Schwindsucht* and *Lungensucht* were the most common, but also found here were *Lungenschwindsucht, Schleimschwindsucht, auszehrendes* and *zehrendes Fieber, Zehrfieber, Abzehrung* and *Auszehrung, auszehrende Brust-krankheit* or *Brustfieber*, and *Hektik*. The most common killing disease of the throat was known as *Bräune, häutige Bräune, Croup*, or *böse Hals*, apparently meaning diphtheria in many cases.[15] In other words, when we read the term *Brustkrankheit* (or any of the others, such as *böse Hals* and *Friesel*), it does not imply what modern medicine would consider a distinct disease. While occasionally the circumstances and characterizations of *particular* cases and outbreaks (mortality rates and time of year, for instance) may allow us to venture that we are dealing with pneumonia or influenza, these are nothing more than informed guesses.[16]

Equally important and equally perplexing as a diagnostic category were the fevers.[17] Until just after mid century, the designator *hitziges Fieber*—inflammatory fever—most frequently indicated typhuslike fevers characterized by high temperatures. This omnibus term included typhoid fever and typhus, since the distinction between the first, spread by contaminated food or water, and the second, spread by rickettsiae, was not yet recognized. As the term *hitziges Fieber* began to lose popularity, a series of other names began to replace it: *Faulfieber, Gallenfieber, hitziges Gallenfieber, hitziges Brustfieber, Fleckfieber*, and, at the beginning of the nineteenth century, *Nervenfieber*, or nervous fever, (although *Nervenfieber* is seldom found in the records for Braunschweig-Wolfenbüttel). The eighteenth-century English equivalents for *Faulfieber* and *Gallenfieber* were, respectively, putrid fever and bilious fever; *Fleckfieber* was spotted fever.[18] Besides these "constant" fevers, a host of intermittent fevers—quartan, tertiary, quotidian—indicated the periodicity of fever episodes: malaria figured here. There was also *kaltes Fieber*, known in English as ague or seasoning fever.

Gastrointestinal diseases (with little or no attendant fever) caused the most deaths in children under the age of five in Dorotheenstadt-Berlin, in Braunschweig-Wolfenbüttel, and probably almost everywhere. Such can be found under a truly baffling profusion of names with many local variants: *Jammer, Krämpfe* (cramps), *Ungluck, Konvulsionen* (rarely) and, in some places, including parts of Braunschweig-Wolfenbüttel, the peculiar name of *Schürcke* or *Schäuerchen*. The last two seem to indicate the convulsions that accompanied the terminal stage of infantile diarrheas. In their milder manifestations, they might also be known as *Durchfall* and *Abzehrung*.[19] Also among the gastrointestinal diseases are *Rothe-* and *Weiße-Ruhr*, two diarrheal diseases that must have included bacillary dysentery. Dysentery might also be termed *Durchfall*, that is, diarrhea, although diarrhea could also indicate a milder case of dysentery. Dysentery was, with smallpox (*Blattern*), the most clearly defined epidemic disease in the minds of eighteenth-century people.[20] They knew smallpox as a childhood disease, which they probably accurately diagnosed. *Blattern* therefore corresponds to a modern disease name better than perhaps any other common label, although measles and rubella were sometimes mistaken for smallpox, as were scarlatina and scarlet fever. Moreover, children who died of other causes during smallpox epidemics were often, it seems, listed as smallpox deaths. Plague was a dark memory and a retained fear, but not a reality, in the mortality profile of eighteenth-century Braunschweig-Wolfenbüttel, at least not after 1720.

By the end of the century, and probably considerably earlier, these disease patterns were firmly fixed in the minds of physicians, protodemographers, and government administrators. Writing near the end of the eighteenth century, Christoph Hufeland drew the following picture of expected mortality:

Of each 1,000 people born, 24 die during birth itself; the business of teething disposes of another 50; in the first two years, convulsions and other illness remove another 277; smallpox, which . . . kills at least 1 in 10 [of its victims], carries off another 80 or 90, and measles 10 more. Among women, about 8 die in childbed. Inflammatory fevers cause another 150 [deaths]. Apoplexy [kills] 12, dropsy 41. Therefore, of each 1,000 born, one can expect that only 78 will die of old age, or die in old age. . . . It is apparent enough that at least nine-tenths [of humankind] die before their time and by chance.[21]

Such summaries, of course, by no means provide the only, or even the most useful, information available to us on the occurrence of disease at the time. Moreover, *mortality* statistics only reflect a partial image of the broader experience of disease. And while there is a correlation between morbidity and mortality, the historical relationship has so far resisted attempts to unsnarl it.[22] It seems safe to argue, however, that illness powerfully shaped people's lives, and that not only the diseases that killed were important, but also those afflictions that interfered with ability to work or reproduce, as well as those that caused incapacitating or chronic pain, or conjured up fears and anxieties. Nonlethal afflictions, and accidents, played a crucial role in people's lives, and no study of "experienced illness" can neglect them entirely in favor of the flashier epidemics. While these "lesser" illnesses did not always find their way into mortality or even morbidity records we shall soon see how central they are to understanding health and illness in the eighteenth-century world.

Issues of governance and policy formation informed all these inquiries into illness. At what point did morbidity and mortality become worrisome? How did one determine and link causes? How vigorously should government react? And, finally, how did one calculate what we might today term costs and benefits? Even in the late twentieth century, these questions vex us, and more than two hundred years ago, governments had much less to go on. Statistics, which promised to help sort out increasingly complex socioeconomic realities, were still novelties. But new tools required new expertise. As they grappled with the dilemmas involved, administrators gradually shaped policies, as well as (unintentionally, of course) providing the historian with a colorful, if sometimes distorted, picture of illness and its ascribed meanings.

Epidemics

The easiest diseases to track were epidemic in nature. Here material poured forth in almost diluvian streams and here historians have generally gone fishing.[23] Yet in an age that only partially and incompletely acknowledged the specificity of disease, in which people still thought and acted in terms of humors and miasmas, epidemics could never be cleanly excised from their environments, disengaged from the general constitutions of peoples and places, or even clearly distinguished from milder forms of what were viewed as essentially the same ailments. Dysentery and common diarrhea were often read as gradations of the same disease, for example, and diarrhea was seen as the clement result of an environmental situation that could, if it rankled, spew forth a full-blown epidemic.

The last major outbreak of plague in Braunschweig occurred in 1657, and it had ceased to be an actual menace by 1721, but as it waned in importance, smallpox and dysentery waxed. In the early decades of the eigh-

teenth century, smallpox commanded the medical landscape as plague
had earlier, although it never conjured up quite the same savage images
plague did, perhaps because it was increasingly perceived as a disease of
childhood.[24] Dysentery, which reappeared in varyingly virulent forms
throughout the period, was a wild card. Especially feared was the bloody
flux (*Rothe Ruhr*), which, however, shaded off into lesser "white dysenteries," diarrheas, and "looseness," all imperfectly separated one from another. Dysentery could be epidemic, yet also could break out in more
limited ways, and it tended to resurface seasonally. Dysentery is thus a
sensitive indicator of how observers scaled disease outbreaks. Episodes
ranging from mild to severe, local to ubiquitous, were characterized as
"epidemics," "prevalent diseases," or "worrisome contagions," and sometimes by the graphic, virtually untranslatable term *Menschensterben*. Several
diseases, like dysentery, materialized at different points on the spectrum.

Incidents of undiagnosed illness whose symptoms varied with place
and person, and whose unknown lethality and unexplained means of
propagation were always unnerving, are perhaps even more instructive
historically. Although less terrifying in their manifestations than plague,
for example, epidemics of fever typified the early modern medical landscape, beguiling and bedeviling governments, local officials, physici, and
pastors. The rich profusion of names for them—pulmonary consumption,
influenza, sweating sickness, putrid fever, ague or seasoning fever, petechial or spotted fever, miliary fever, bilious fever, hectic or low fever,
nervous fever, purple fever, scarlet fever—suggests the imprecision of
diagnoses and labels.[25]

The government's often intense and overtly silly preoccupation with
mere sprinklings of disease shows the prominence that disease, and especially contagious disease, had come to assume in governmental calculations by the 1740s. Petitions for remission of taxes and corvée because of
outbreaks of disease reveal several of these linkages. Plague remained the
first diagnosis that popped almost unbidden into the heads of the medical
laity, government officials, and physicians alike when increases in the
number of deaths were unaccounted for. For example, when dysentery
broke out in the 1660s and 1670s in several parts of the duchy, the first,
frightening suspicion was that plague had returned.[26] Dysentery was fear-
some enough, although the death rate never neared that of plague. Bacillary dysentery tended to recur at fairly short intervals, inasmuch as having
had the disease only offered partial and temporary immunity to particular
strains.[27] It also severely debilitated its victims, as a 1661 report from the

Amtmann in Seesen vividly demonstrates. Every village in his district was affected:

[T]here is almost no house where dysentery has not moved in. . . . [As] I passed through one such village on other business, I learned from the headman and other inhabitants there that the children and young people more than the adults were hit by it, to such an extent that today five bodies still have not been buried. . . . Others cannot fulfill their corvée.

One cannot discover where this disease came from, only that the inhabitants believe that it originated in the nearby villages of Grossrhüden and Mechtshausen. . . . [P]eople were still dying there to the extent that on the next day three people [who had died] in Grossrhüden and two in Mechtshausen were yet unburied.[28]

In 1676 and then again in 1678, dysentery scourged the entire Weser district.[29] News from the somewhat larger place of Fürstenberg likewise documented the severity of the epidemic and the issues raised by its appearance. The first whiff of trouble had come from the small village of Eil near Boffzen ten days earlier.

In Eil two or three people have fallen ill with the bloody flux, but they kept this hushed up and did not make immediate report of it. [Thus] in Eil several more became ill, whereby the illness so quickly flared out of control that within ten days, eight people died, among them three aged women, one cottager (still a young man), one girl of fourteen, and three children. Most of the inhabitants lie [ill] in their homes, of which only very few are free [of illness], and little hope of their recovery remains.[30]

As the Amtmann reported, there had been no outbreaks in the Fürstenberg area, but a lumber dealer in Hamm Münden had written several days before to say "that he could not pick up and store the wood he had bought because of the bloody flux, from which his wife and many in the same village suffer."[31]

Within two weeks, conditions had deteriorated rapidly: only two homes in Boffzen were unaffected. "[A]nd through today twenty-six persons, children and several elderly women, have died of it; in each house there are three, four, or as many as five persons sick."[32] Apparently, the outbreak's fury lessened in September and early October, only to strike with renewed force in late October and early November.[33] At this point, the village officials and "the entire community" petitioned the government for remissions, maintaining that the present *plage* had "hurt this community with its small [number of] men greatly . . . and only two or three houses are free of it, and, even worse, about thirty people have died."[34] Their moving description suggests the true dimensions of such a disaster for a tiny community like Boffzen:

[Many have] pawned or sold their possessions, and have fallen deeply into debt. [A]s this illness first hit during last year's harvest, the grain we had [still standing] in the field suffered greatly from mice and other vermin because we could not work. [Moreover], as the Amt ordered that those who were ill should avoid the well, and vice versa, and as the healthy [person] out of fear shunned his neighbors, [there was little help to be had].[35]

Their plea fell on sympathetic ears: the privy council allowed substantial reductions in all taxes and fees owed by the community as a whole and its members as individuals during the outbreak and for one month thereafter.[36]

Widespread, repeated eruptions of dysentery caused similar problems throughout the eighteenth century. About sixty years later, in 1736, dysentery ravaged the entire Weser district, presenting the historian with a more detailed picture of the havoc dysentery could wreak on villages and the concern evoked at higher government levels. From 1736 through 1744, dysentery was a persistent problem, with peaks of occurrence coming in 1736, 1738, and 1743–44. This does not mean, of course, that dysentery was *not* a health problem between the 1670s and the mid 1730s: outbreaks were simply fewer and probably less severe, at least to judge from the extant evidence.[37]

Dysentery returned with a vengeance in 1736. Physicus Blum in Gandersheim, at the time solely responsible for the Weser area, had been requested to survey his district and verify or refute rumors of the disease. In September, he reported from the market town of Greene that dysentery had reappeared there, "and is not only here in this area, but very prevalent throughout the entire district." He quickly polled the pastors serving outlying villages. From Greene, he learned that in some villages, the disease "raged with fair strength" although only a few people had died of it so far. The pastor in Naensen judged the outbreak in Ammensen "rather serious": seven persons had died, four were ill, and "most of the others, who had been afflicted" were now convalescent, having used "nothing but brandy, olive oil, and white bread." In Naensen itself, only one old man and one boy had fallen ill, and both recovered. The stories about the impact of dysentery varied among adjacent villages: in Brunsen and Holtershausen, no illness; in Wenzen, dysentery was "quite common," with seventeen people dying in two weeks, twenty-three still bed-ridden, twenty-four improving, and fifty once again on their feet. Here virtually the entire population had been affected. In Delligsen, "the eleven old people and children who died, did not perish of dysentery, but from other illnesses." Outbreaks of dysentery—autumn's curse—dotted the Weser district.[38] It is, of course, hard to pin down exactly what this "dysentery" was, but contemporaries confidently labeled and quickly classified it. Other diseases, especially fevers, proved more enigmatic. Diagnoses were missing, or experts differed wildly in their estimation of cause, treatment, and impact. If we look, for example, at a series of reports from 1663–1744 on what eighteenth-century observers identified as "[t]hose inflammatory and infectious diseases that are noticed every once in a while," we find incidents of diseases that defy ready categorization but nonetheless contributed to the duchy's disease profile.

In 1682, a peculiar disease raised concern in the village of Wrescherode, near Gandersheim. Here the problem was a rather mysterious illness that had appeared in all eight of the village's houses. A petition from the inhabitants of the village told how practically everyone had had the disease, and how several "grown children" had died, badly setting the village back in its field work "because the disease lasted since the [beginning of the] harvest until now. . . . [T]he corn in the field . . . has rotted and gone bad. . . . [T]he harvest was delayed, and we can reap now only very slowly. [Moreover] summer was late [this year], and if the neighboring villages had not pitied us and helped us with the plowing," things would have been much worse. The village was still in desperate straits:

[T]he emergency forces us to try to sell our grain, which we never would have done otherwise. However, we are tolerated nowhere in the Harz or in neighboring cities, so that we now have no idea what to do next. The Amtmann threatens us with court action [if we do not fulfill] the *onera* we owe . . . especially the contributions from September and October, which we are supposed to deliver with the November contribution, which is a terrible burden on us, and we have no idea where to turn [for help].[39]

Wolfenbüttel's experience with a "malignant fever" in 1758 documents the response of a medium-sized town to an "epidemic outbreak" of fever particularly well.[40] It began in December 1757 and continued through the end of May or beginning of June. The medical society in Wolfenbüttel judged the fever to be contagious, "in that the houses backing on the Oker [River] are almost emptied, and in the other houses those who nursed people during the illness have themselves fallen ill and two of them have died."[41] By March, the municipal government deemed the situation so dangerous that it divided the city into four districts and entrusted each to one of the four physicians in Wolfenbüttel. The privy council then fine-tuned the procedures already set into motion:

The city magistracy . . . should deputize an official to identify those among the inhabitants, be they common citizens, artisans, or landless laborers, who are without means and can consult no physician when they suffer from epidemic diseases [such as] inflammatory chest fevers, erysipelas, and pleurisy and [note] where these are to be found. . . . [They are then] to give immediate notice to the physician of their district, and also if necessary, admonish patients to adhere strictly to his orders. . . . And so that each district *medicus* is aware of the streets belonging to his district, the city magistracy should prepare a specification [of these] for each district and send it to each and every physician.

Similar instructions applied to the medical society and other physicians, who were cautioned to "attend such patients promptly, visit them diligently, and mark their prescriptions with the name of the street in which the patient lives." Physicians also received printed forms on which they were to report each month as to "whether the epidemic grows or shrinks in virulence."[42]

By the first of April, the medical society insisted that the disease had caused "more commotion than its [severity] dictated." Dr. Kayser argued that the lethality of the disease had been grossly exaggerated, and that "the majority of those who died of it, died from lack of [proper] care and regimen." At the end of April, Dr. Hieronymi observed from his practice that the number of cases seemed to be diminishing. However, he also pointed out that "while the Collegium medicum might think that this very short list of those suffering from the *morbus malignis epidemie* is an attempt to conceal the true state of affairs, I deny it. The number of dead and dying was actually quite large, but few patients requested my aid."[43]

The impact of epidemic diseases was especially weighty in the years of war and occupation between 1756 and 1763, when French and allied troops crisscrossed the duchy. Quartered on the populace, they spread typhuslike fevers, dysentery, and venereal diseases. But this does not tell the whole story. The health problems the Seven Years' War generated were multifaceted, and they did not only include diseases carried by troops coming into more or less intimate contact with civilian populations. In the Weser valley in 1761, for example, dead horses posed a threat. The privy council consulted the Collegium medicum for its opinion:

With the presence of the allied army on the Weser River, a large number of horses have died, and several thousands have been left lying between Warburg and Holzminden. [T]he stink of the rotting animals has become so intolerable that the people [living there] have dragged the carcasses to the riverbank and thrown them in. We fear that this might be even more dangerous and menacing than if the dead animals were left [to decompose] in the open air. [Could] eating fish [from the river] that feed on the bodies tragically affect the health of the human beings [who consume them]?[44]

The privy council referred to the experience of some sixty years earlier when, after losing the battle of Helsingborg, the Danish army slaughtered its horses and tossed them into the sea, and then "most probably because of eating the fish that fed on them, a fearful plague arose."[45] The Collegium medicum, however, resolved that eating Weser fish was safe. They argued that allowing the horses to rot in the open would be more likely to "infect the air," suggesting that the remaining carcasses be burned or buried. In the meantime, the local inhabitants should be cautioned to avoid Weser water for brewing or cooking. (Drinking was not mentioned; perhaps it was taken for granted that no one drank water from the Weser!)[46]

Despite these precautions in spring, by summer a "savage epidemic" broke out in the whole Weser valley. It was accompanied by a *dysenteria tam cruenta, quam mucosa,* first diagnosed among Braunschweig's troops in late 1761; by January 1762, it was sweeping through the civilian population as well.[47] The epidemic did not die down, but lasted into the spring, when Physicus Hoffmann reported that

a peculiar [kind of] diarrhea with a number of strange symptoms [has struck] many people here. . . . The reason why such a diarrhea should be epidemic in this region, I can only assume comes from the forced misuse of the six non-naturals [air, diet, rest, exercise, evacuations, and the passions of the mind]. . . . The parishioners in Eschershausen have so filled their cemetery with bodies in these two months [January and February 1761] that there is almost no place left where one can bury another without digging up a partially decomposed corpse. I await warm weather with great trepidation, fearing that once the ground heats up and emits its exhalations, a very dangerous miasma will rise from the holes [in the ground].

As if this mysteriously fatal diarrhea were not problem enough, he reported other, likewise epidemic diseases—smallpox, measles, dropsy.[48]

Interesting also in this context of epidemics was the story of a "vicious fever" in Amt Wickensen in 1802. The fever struck four villages, and the Amt organized a distribution of flour to the needy.[49] Likewise, two years later, in Amt Langelsheim, a "malignant, contagious bilious fever, [accompanied] by a rash and worms in many cases" raged in the nearby village of Wolfshagen. There were sixty patients, and there had been several deaths. (Wolfshagen had 953 inhabitants in 1814.) The Amt had requested the attendance of Dr. Spohr, then physicus in Seesen. Most patients could afford neither medicines nor sufficient food, and "we immediately made the following provisions: all the ill without resources would receive free the medicines prescribed by Dr. Spohr, [as well as] veal broth with pearl barley, or groats or macaroni [?] and what bread was necessary." The same arrangements pertained to convalescents as well. The bill totaled over 405 thaler, which the Amt presented to the privy council and the government paid in full.[50]

Such accounts, often including a lengthy discussion of the course of the disease and its victims, along with details of provision made for their care and a totaling of the resultant costs, proliferated in the eighteenth century. And while the value of the records amassed on contagious disease can hardly be overestimated, the epidemic experience is, by definition, highly unusual. Buried beneath the mounds of documentation are nuggets worth unearthing: strains within the community were thrown into sharp relief by the terror of the times; the hidden realities of power and wealth bubbled to the surface; attitudes, perceptions, and prejudices for once appeared less encrusted by obfuscating layers of civility and normalcy. Yet the epidemic experience always distorts and twists, as well as revealing and clarifying. Peeping into the *Alltag* of health and illness has proven more difficult, and here the epidemic documentation is a less reliable pilot. Different kinds of evidence reveal quotidian experiences more effectively. Records that proceed in chronological order document the flow of life better, and more accurately illuminate the succession of health and illness, and disease after disease, in one locality.

Disease in Everyday Life

Historians and historical demographers have turned to parish registers for several purposes, and above all to reconstruct families and to construct general models of mortality, fertility, and nuptiality. The use of parish registers to determine causes of death, however, presents several problems. First, there is the issue of continuity. It is a stroke of luck when the same person, whether pastor or sexton, stayed in office long enough to compile an unbroken series of observations. If so, one can reasonably assume that he employed about the same words and phrases to describe symptoms. The second problem is the more difficult linguistic one we have already explored: those recording cause of death worked with words and concepts that correspond hardly at all to twentieth-century terms and perceptions. Moreover, they made mistakes. Their information was often only second-hand; they relied heavily on the accounts of relatives and friends. However, as in the reports of the physici, this very imperfection and this subjectivity are themselves valuable to the historian of mentalities. What is recorded in the parish register was, after all, precisely what people believed had killed their relatives, their friends, and their fellow villagers.

Parish registers impart other fascinating bits of information. The very ways they were kept and the completeness of the entries over time track changing valuations of vital statistics. In Braunschweig-Wolfenbüttel, the cause of death was—in general—more regularly recorded after mid century. That was by no means a hard-and-fast rule, however, and there was great inconsistency. For instance, for two places I examined in some detail, the small towns of Walkenried and Bornum (as for other places I surveyed less extensively), the entries for cause of death were primitive and incomplete before the 1740s or 1750s. Much, of course, depended on the individual recorder. The pastor in Kleinrhüden in the 1720s usually, if atypically, noted cause of death, for example, yet one of his successors in the 1770s almost always omitted it. In Bornum only infrequently does one find the cause of death listed before 1750. Oddly enough, the pastor there commented, although vaguely, on the deaths of children (and even some extremely young ones) more often than on those of adults. He often mentioned stillbirths, or that a child had died "of what we call child-fits." Smallpox, too, merited observation, although it was usually in collective form: five children are anonymously recorded as dying between February and May 1724 "of smallpox," for example, and others succumbed in the last week of October 1735 to "the pox." Notable or unusual deaths evoked comment as well, such as the demise of a fifteen-year-old boy on 5 October 1736 due to a "mouth tumor." Protracted bouts of mortal illness tended likewise to elicit notice, as when the wife of Barthold Langen died in 1742 "after a long illness that forced her to keep to her bed for over half-a-year."[51]

From the 1740s through the 1770s, accidental deaths and peculiar circumstances, or cases that allowed a moral conclusion to be drawn, appear to have been thought most worthy of remark: on 19 November, the community buried "the old beer-belly" Johann Eyeling, who, having fallen down in a drunken stupor on the dike, "froze to death"; on 6 January 1752, "a man from Seesen, by the name of Probst" drowned in the local pond; and on 23 March 1770, the local joiner and pond keeper Andreas Körber died "like a Christian" after "a long-endured illness and the painfully attempted cure" of a cancerous growth. These commentaries were parables, warnings, and didactic examples.[52]

All this changed when a new pastor and schoolmaster, Johann Breithaupt, arrived in Bornum in 1776. From then until his death on 1 July 1804 ("of debilitation" and aged ten days less than seventy-one years), Breithaupt conscientiously recorded cause of death, rarely breaking his sober listing in favor of a more moralistic narrative. Information on cause of death is missing for only 4 of the 350 deaths in the twenty-seven years he was in Bornum.[53]

A comparison of Bornum's registers with those of Walkenried underscores the importance of individual initiative and diligence. In Walkenried, from 1704 through 1727, the cause of death is given only sporadically; this pastor was far more likely to ruminate on "conduct." Pastor Kunze and his sexton, who kept the books from 1727 into the 1750s, hardly ever mentioned cause of death, although they did occasionally log special or unusual circumstances. There was, for example, "the very sudden death" of the master brewer on 30 December 1744. The man had, the register tells us, "attended church on the 27th and . . . in the night [of the 30th] had a fit that robbed him of all his senses and sensations, and thus gave up the ghost." Comments on illness were also few; more generally found was extensive information on the burial itself (whether or not a funeral sermon was preached, or if the corpse had been followed by a considerable procession, or buried "without the ringing of bells"), and notes on bereaved parents, orphaned children, and widowed wives, as well as an evaluation of the deceased's behavior—whether or not he or she had led a Christian life and died a "composed" death.[54]

Parish registers tended with the diligence of a Breithaupt can be used to profile causes of death over time or can at least show what diseases, injuries, and accidents people thought killed their contemporaries. Few, however, yield much insight on morbidity, and for that we must rely on other sources. In 1761, Johann Uphoff, schoolmaster to the communities of Hehlen and Daspe, penned the last of the many excerpts he made from the parish registers on mortality. In addition, the morbidity "diaries" Uphoff kept for more than a decade have survived. Happily for the historian, Uphoff's observations were uncommonly comprehensive, and he forwarded them on to the higher authorities with singular dispatch.[55] More typically, in composing mortality tables for his district of Calvörde, Physicus Hinze spoke of the "greatest disorder" and the "inexcusable sloppiness" with which pastors, sextons, and schoolmasters kept records.[56] Reports like those of the schoolmaster in Bornum who preceded Breithaupt were quite routine. While he did indeed produce morbidity reports for six years—1753–54, 1759, 1772–74—only that for 1774 is complete. And while the unnamed schoolmaster usually jotted down something or other in the "Physician Consulted" column, it was almost invariably: "I know nothing about it" or "Used no one." In fact, only once is any physician indicated: in 1774, a 30-year-old woman called upon Dr. Müller from Seesen to treat her "inflammatory disease." It may indeed be that few people turned to physicians or other healers, but the schoolmaster's laxity or desire to avoid unpleasantness are just as probable reasons for these lacunae.[57]

Uphoff, the sexton and schoolmaster in the adjoining communities of Hehlen and Daspe, was thus exceptional. Hehlen was a modest-sized village (673 inhabitants in 1793) snugly nestled on the left bank of the Weser. The place had grown slowly and fitfully over the second half of the century. Its social makeup was unremarkable: mostly peasants, with a sprinkling of artisans and Honorationes. Daspe was much smaller, having only 156 inhabitants in 1814.[58] The diseases and ailments that afflicted these communities are well conveyed by Uphoff's lists when combined with the evaluations of the two physici resident in the area. They allow us to chart the inroads "epidemic" or "rampant" diseases made into such villages, which historians have often ignored or been unable to penetrate, as well as placing the "epidemic experience" in the broader context of other, less lethal events.

Moreover, Uphoff's journals are by no means atypical of how contemporaries perceived and constructed the mental thresholds separating "illness" from "health."[59] Those Uphoff listed as ill were almost invariably bedridden. Ailments and afflictions that did not handicap the ability to perform daily tasks, he judged "minor" or did not acknowledge as "ill" at all. He only occasionally mentioned children among the sick. Missing almost entirely from the *morbidity* records, for example, are smallpox patients. No individual cases appear. Uphoff once merely jotted down that in a two-week period, from 4 to 18 May 1757, he heard no reports of bedridden adults, and "only a few children are ill with the smallpox." Yet over the decade, smallpox killed at least eighteen children.[60] Very few

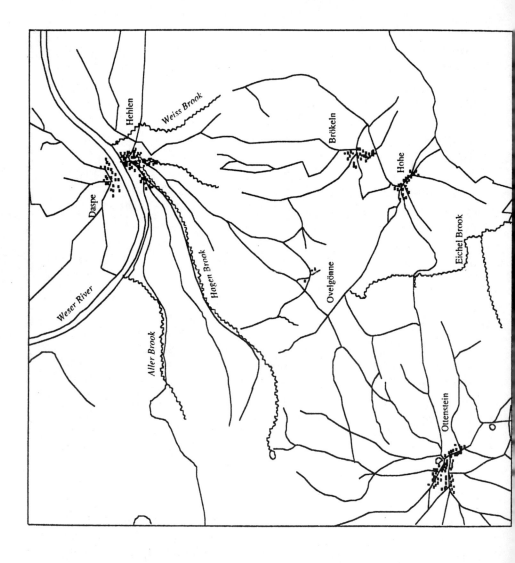

Legend

— Roads

～ Waterways

◯ Ponds

⬛ Houses

under the age of ten wormed their way into the diary. There were only
two: an 8-year-old with a "distended abdomen" and a 7-year-old with
dysentery. Just three children older than ten but under fifteen are listed: an
11-year-old girl "variously diagnosed"; a 12-year-old boy suffering from
"internal tumors"; and a 13-year-old who had been struck by lightning.
During the same period (1751–60), at least 102 children aged ten and
younger (*excluding* stillbirths) died in Hehlen and Daspe.

   The number of deaths varied markedly from year to year. The year
mortality peaked, 1758, shows a high percentage of deaths (35 of a total of
54 deaths, or 64.8%) from illnesses of the chest (variously listed as *Brust-
krankheit, Brust-Seuche, Brust-Beschwerde*). In 1761, Uphoff attributed a
large number of deaths (18 in all) to such chest afflictions. These combined with a number of deaths from diphtheria (*Hals-Schaden*) and infantile diarrhea. There were also a greater number (16) of deaths from unknown causes (or causes not listed) than in previous years. Over the
decade, the biggest killers in Hehlen were, in order of magnitude: chest
afflictions (77/285; 27%); gastrointestinal diseases of children (40/285;
14%); smallpox and measles (22/285; 7.7%); tuberculosis (16/285; 5.6%);
dropsy (15/285; 5.3%); and assorted dysenteries (14/285; 4.9%). The
occurrence of these diseases, and deaths from them, clustered in several
years. Almost half (35/77; 45.5%) of all the deaths from chest afflictions
occurred in 1758, and there were another 18 in 1761. The gastrointestinal
diseases that killed children prevailed mostly in 1753, and again from July
1758 through the end of 1760. Smallpox was a problem in 1753, causing 9
deaths, and again in 1757, when 8 children died of it (some of them possibly of measles). The year 1757, although not as deadly as 1758 or 1761,
was also marked by dysentery and chest diseases. In 1758, the heightened
mortality clearly derived from chest diseases, while the equally great mortality of 1761 had several causes. The smaller peaks of mortality in 1751,
1753, and 1759 can be linked to no one cause; a confluence of several
illnesses was to blame. One can probably accurately, if somewhat vaguely,
link elevated mortality rates after 1756 to worsening economic conditions
during the Seven Years' War and the movement of troops through the
Weser valley. And if Hehlen proper had suffered relatively little in 1752,
areas surrounding the village reeled under what Physicus Struve labeled a
"continuous malignant fever." Deaths for Hehlen and its adjoining villages reached 28 over the eight-week period from 11 January through
8 March; 24 of these Struve attributed to chest conditions.[61]

   In Hehlen, as elsewhere, everyday relationships with diseases took diverse and intricate paths. The epidemic experience, while of great moment in public health, was the exception here, not the rule. Epidemics have so mesmerized historians that we have perhaps come to overvalue their ability to shape mentalities. While epidemics were undoubtedly critical, often skewing mortality and morbidity curves dramatically, a whole series of other ailments, of accidents, and of nuisance afflictions more commonly determined the long-term illness profiles of individuals and communities. In eleven years, only once (and perhaps with less impact a second time) did a single disease elevate death and illness rates in Hehlen. In most years, other diseases molded Hehleners' perceptions of illness and cause of death more decisively.

If we compare the morbidity and mortality lists for Hehlen, we (not very surprisingly) note a certain correspondence between what made people ill and what killed them. But here we must be cautious, as case fatality rates play an important role. Thus in 1757, when many people died of dysentery, there were just as many listed as ill who survived. Some cases held little or no hope of recovery. When the 60-year-old wife of Fritze Schaper fell ill with tumors and dropsy, she suffered for two weeks, appearing twice in the morbidity records. And she died on 18 April from what was listed as consumption. An "apoplectic fit" felled Conrad Böcker, a cottager, on 20 August 1753; thereafter he was epileptic, and he died two weeks later.[62] Dropsies, tumors (including those termed "cancers"), and strokes were mortal in some cases, but often patients experienced episodes and then lived on for years, if in a more or less incapacitated state. A frequent nonlethal (or at least not immediately fatal) consequence of stroke was partial or almost total paralysis, which was perhaps not so grimly regarded when the victim was elderly, such as the almost 80-year-old widow Sanders, whose stroke made her a bedridden invalid.[63] Stroke accompanied by paralysis was another matter entirely in the 21-year-old son of a peasant or a 19-year-old cottager's boy. Intermittent fevers, such as the quartan fever that plagued a 20-year-old on and off for over eighteen months, rarely killed, but in his case, it resulted in eighteen months' inability to work, the need for periodic bed rest, and the cost of medicines and consultations.[64]

Arthritic and rheumatic afflictions show up occasionally in the morbidity pictures, indicating those truly crippled by their ills. For each of these, however, there must have been many others whose stiff joints and shooting pains complicated their lives, frustrating or making impossible basic tasks, whether sowing seed, churning butter, kneading bread, cutting leather, or working metal. The accidents of work took their toll as well: wounds did not heal well or quickly; hernias enlarged and became inflamed or strangulated (with predictably fatal results). The routines of life injured many. The wife of the cottager Johann Sümschlag got caught in the mill wheel while breaking up flax; Johann Hachmeyer died eleven days after taking a whacking great fall from the corn ricks; a ferryman in Hehlen fell off his barge and drowned while transporting passengers across the Weser at dusk.[65] The house and its surrounding farmyard presented grave dangers for children. Tiny people fell down stairs, tumbled into pigsties, cut themselves with knives, poked out eyes with scissors and awls, and burned themselves dreadfully, as did the toddling two-year-old son of Franz Schlüter, who plunged into a kettle of boiling water early in the morning of 18 July 1756 and died the same evening at sunset.[66]

Likewise debilitating, and sometimes even life-threatening, were leg sores and the ulcerated varices that resulted from a combination of injury, stress, and poor nutrition.[67] The records seldom list "cancers" and "internal sores and ulcers" as causes of either morbidity or mortality, but these, like leg ulcers, were a common reason for extensive self-medication or for seeking out more distant medical assistance. People with leg ulcers, fistulas (primarily of spine and anus), like women with "hard" lumps and sores on their breasts were among the most restless searchers for medical aid. Rabies occurred only rarely, or at least it seldom appears in the records, yet it evoked extravagant fears and generated an immense amount of activity on the part of the ducal government.[68]

The record from about the same time (1751–60) for the smaller village of Mahlum, near Seesen in the Harz, strengthens these impressions.[69] Many in Mahlum suffered from a chest or head complaint that might have been influenza or pneumonia in 1753. This was the only disease of any statistical weight that year, skewing the overall distributions of illness and death. And in 1754, of a total of twenty deaths, eleven children died of "the purples." The year 1757, for instance, offers a more "normal" perspective on disease in Mahlum. Then, too, chest afflictions caused illness and death in the wet spring weather of March and April and modified the village's disease profile. Also noteworthy were a handful of smallpox deaths among young children, in what must have been a relatively mild outbreak; many children listed as ill subsequently recovered. Other deaths included two from "tumorous diseases," a stillbirth, a death from wasting (possibly consumption), and one from a seizure, in addition to those who "passed peacefully away," and the usual smattering of unexplained, sudden, or unspecified deaths. Thus, the only illnesses able to distort normal rates of sickness and death were chest ailments, smallpox, and dysentery (although in Mahlum there was no evidence of dysentery either in 1753 or 1754), and that peculiar outbreak of purples in 1754.[70]

The apparently standard profile was reproduced in Walkenried, another small market town (population of 422 in 1814), for a number of years in the 1760s. There were no epidemic outbreaks in 1769, but other elements of a now-familiar configuration appear. Death rates were about what could be expected, and the greatest mortality was among children under ten, as was typical of the entire duchy and most of Europe in the eighteenth century. In Walkenried, 31 of 73 deaths (42.5%) happened before age ten; a typical percentage for a non-smallpox year. Deaths otherwise distributed themselves more or less evenly over the other age cohorts.[71] The principal causes were gastrointestinal in nature (mostly among young children), scarlet fever, dropsy, chest diseases, and "suffocation."[72]

The parish records for Walkenried for 1750 through 1782 flesh out this picture. For more than one-quarter (62 of 238 deaths) of those buried in Walkenried, the cause of death is not given. Over this 33-year period, about 7 people died each year, and six years showed higher mortality (11 or more deaths a year): 1761, 1763–64, 1773, 1777, 1779. For 1773 and 1779, the cause of death was so irregularly noted that it is impossible to draw any conclusions about the grounds for elevated death rates. In 1761, 4 of the 13 died of chest diseases; in 1763 and in 1777, smallpox killed 5; and in 1764, 4 cases of dysentery and 2 cases of what may have been diphtheria inflated death rates. As in other places, chest diseases, fevers, and wasting, as well as in single years, dysentery and smallpox, were the most frequently remarked causes of death. For very young children, with the exception of those who died of smallpox, the cause of death was seldom mentioned, and we find here no evidence of the intestinal diarrheas that carried off so many children elsewhere.[73]

For 1769, the physicus in Walkenried, Georg Spangenberg, appended his own extensive comments to the mortality/morbidity statistics.[74] Although only "very few" epidemic diseases troubled Walkenried, these had been deadly. In the first quarter of the year, whooping cough (*Keichhusten*) was "not so bad," killing only three nursing infants. Scarlatina struck in the second quarter, especially in the settlement of Wiede, where six children, "all those whose throats became malignant," died. In the last quarter of the year, smallpox affected forty-six children, yet only one, an infant of eighteen months, succumbed. For the elderly, those between sixty and eighty years old, "shortness of breath" (*Asthmaticis*) and cachexia were especially bad: sixteen people died of these complaints and attendant dropsy. Terrible accidents claimed the lives of two more. A collapsing wall "smashed" a miner in Hohengeiss, and a 2-year-old child died after pulling a kettle of boiling water down on his head. One case of sudden death was registered: the taverner Baumann was found dead in the woods; the autopsy revealed a *haemorrhagia cerebri*. In another incident, a pregnant woman was bitten by a "mad dog"; happily, she survived.

Bornum offers a more complete picture of perceived causes of death from 1777 through 1803. Over this 27-year period, the major causes of death are unsurprising: chest afflictions (*Brustkrankheit* and all its variants) (21.4%); the peculiarly named *Schäuerchen*—that is, pediatric convulsions (14.9%); wasting, or, in eighteenth-century terms, consumption (11.4%); and smallpox (10%). Following more distantly were tumors and swellings, stillbirths, dysentery, debilitation, purples, childbirth, and single cases of many other ailments and accidents. For years with noticeably heightened death rates (13 deaths was the average), only one, 1798, seems to have been truly epidemical: smallpox carried off 23. In general, however, elevated rates of infant and childhood mortality contributed most to excess mortalities in these years. In other words, the deaths of *more* children raised death rates, although less obviously than in 1798.[75] Infant and childhood mortality was, as everywhere, the greatest contributor to mortality. Of the 350 people who died in Bornum from 1777 to 1803, 181 died before they reached their tenth birthdays; just 10 were over five. All smallpox deaths in these years (35) were among children under ten. Among 52 children who died of convulsions or "fits," only 3 were over five. Stillbirths accounted for 10.5 percent of all infant and child deaths (19 of 181).

The causes of infant mortality hardly astonish anyone familiar with the general demographic history of early modern Europe. But what killed off those who against the odds lived beyond their fifth birthdays? "Old" people, that is those older than sixty, contributed about 19 percent of mortality (67 deaths in all), with the biggest causes of death being chest diseases, debilitation, and "age." They also died of wasting and consumption, and, in isolated instances, from the many things others died of: epilepsy, jaundice, diarrhea. Perhaps more interesting are the diseases that preyed on those in the "prime of life." Of the 58 people who died between the ages of twenty and fifty, women outnumbered men by 41 to 17. Even if one subtracts the number of women who died in childbirth, women were still almost twice as likely to die in their prime as men. (One might argue that using the same age breakdown to identify women and men as "in their prime" is not justified, but women were considerably more likely than men to die even before they reached forty-five, at least in Bornum.) Men and women tended to die of the same things, although only women succumbed to dropsy, jaundice, or stomach cramps. Otherwise the biggest killers in these relatively healthy years were, quite unsurprisingly, wasting and chest diseases.[76]

The patterns identified for Walkenried, for Mahlum, for Hehlen, and for Bornum hold true as well for larger cities, such as Braunschweig and Wolfenbüttel, in years free of epidemics. The year 1765, for instance, was a "nonepidemic" one in Braunschweig (deaths = 891; births = 1,124): only 22 people died of smallpox and 8 of dysentery or diarrhea. Infantile diarrhea (201, or 22.6%) formed the weightiest cause of mortality, distantly followed by the deaths falling into the almost omnifarious category of chest diseases (150, or 16.8%).[77] Thereafter the number of deaths imputed to any single cause dropped off sharply: there were 50 deaths due to tumors and dropsy; 43 stillbirths; 22 due to smallpox; 22 to apoplexy; 15 deaths in childbed; 17 deaths each due to "teething" and old age (a nice balancing of infantile and geriatric mortalities!); 15 deaths to the purples; 30 to "suffocation"; and 11 to inflammatory fever. Other categories amassed only 10 or fewer deaths each.

Disease configurations for the second largest city in the duchy were similar in these years. In 1765 and 1766, Wolfenbüttel's experience almost replicated that of Braunschweig for 1766, *except* that 1766 was a "smallpox year" in Wolfenbüttel. Smallpox (or probably a combination of smallpox, measles, and rubella) accounted for fully one-third (147 of 437, or 33.6%) of mortality. If, however, we set smallpox deaths aside for a moment, we are left with 603 deaths to explain. Only three diseases scored any appreciable mortality (10% or more of total deaths): diseases of the chest (25.7%); wasting (19.9%); and infantile diarrheas (11.6%). With the exceptions of deaths due to tumors or swellings, no single cause of death exceeded 2 percent of the total. The number of deaths from the "big three" remained markedly similar in both years. Deaths from chest afflictions numbered 78 in 1765, 77 in 1766; from wasting, 68 in 1765, 52 in 1766; from infantile diarrheas, 34 in 1765, 37 in 1766. Thus, in Wolfenbüttel, as in Braunschweig, Mahlum, Hehlen, Walkenried, and Bornum, diseases of the chest and infantile diarrheas produced the most fatalities, with wasting running a close third. Time altered little in these patterns for

Wolfenbüttel. A survey in 1785 revealed that the same three diseases still killed most reliably, if they had by then assumed a somewhat different order of magnitude: of a total of 186 deaths, 70 died of wasting (37.6%); 29 of chest diseases (15.6%); and 24 of diarrheas (12.9%). Wolfenbüttel lost population strikingly from the mid to the late eighteenth century, and while the absolute number of deaths decreased, the proportion of deaths to births stayed about the same.[78]

One can—but I shall not—multiply these examples by almost all the villages, market towns, and cities in the duchy. Population size alone served as a poor predictor of patterns, although perhaps if there had been a very large town in Braunschweig-Wolfenbüttel, we might have observed greater urban/rural discontinuity. In years when no murderous epidemics of smallpox raged and when dysentery abated, wasting, mortal lung complaints, and gastrointestinal diseases almost invariably caused most deaths. Smallpox and influenza, and to a lesser extent dysentery, could, however, twist these figures quite dramatically. Smallpox alone might account for a third or more of all deaths in a town or village in epidemic years. Such epidemics struck only periodically: it took time to regenerate the pool of susceptibles, and smallpox rarely ran rampant two years in succession or reappeared with any intensity at intervals of less than two or three years. Hehlen again offers easy proof: in ten years, Uphoff recorded smallpox as a cause of death three times, with four cases in 1751, nine in 1753, and eight in 1757. Of these, only one of the 1753 cases had been born in 1751, and only one of the 1757 cases was alive in 1753. Likewise, in Bornum, from 1776 to 1803, intervals of between two and five years passed between epidemics. Contemporaries spoke of a "divine interval." Small settlements, villages like Hehlen and Mahlum, then, could be hit hard by smallpox, influenza, pneumonia, and dysentery, but here epidemics did their work quickly and then disappeared as the reservoir of susceptibles rapidly drained.

James C. Riley has portrayed this as a world of ten diseases: ascariasis, arteriosclerosis, bacillary dysentery, cholera, influenza, plague, smallpox, sporotrichosis, tuberculosis, and typhoid fever (also typhus?).[79] If we throw out plague and cholera as falling outside the chronological boundaries of this study, we see that the profile for most places in Braunschweig-Wolfenbüttel, while it does not correspond in all its particulars, matches Riley's model pretty well as far as the epidemic and infectious diseases go. The most important causes of death were chest afflictions, gastrointestinal diseases in children, smallpox and measles, tuberculosis, dropsy, dysentery,

diphtheria, and "shortness of breath," or asthma. This list, however, over-
looks a whole range of other illnesses and accidents that were far too
common to be excluded from the disease pattern simply because they
killed less frequently or less reliably.

Explaining Disease

Mortality and morbidity statistics tell us little, however, about how people
experienced their afflictions, or about how observers perceived and represented conditions of health and illness. These are not easy issues to approach. First, one must determine whether people looked at disease and
illness from radically different perspectives, according, for example, to
age, sex, location, or religion, and whether they then defined distinctive
points at which they became "sick." Did they also explain disease causes
and cures differently? Whereas once it was argued that physicians and
nonphysicians held opposite notions about all these matters, that view has
gradually given ground to another, better-supported one: "popular" and
"elite" medicines largely overlapped. This is not the place to review that
debate in full. And this chapter addresses only a part of the subject, while
leaving the more intriguing, if tougher, issue of illness as lived experience
to Chapter 5. Here we shall want to look for a moment at how eighteenth-century physicians tended to interpret diseases and afflictions, and
how they then shaped their therapeutics accordingly.

The physicians whose works are assessed here all belonged to a large
group of men engaged in the eighteenth-century campaign of popular
medical enlightenment. Despite the existence of some hostility to popular medical enlightenment among elites, numerous "popular" books on
health and illness appeared in the eighteenth century. These were purportedly directed at "housefathers," "housemothers," and "all sufferers."[80]
The eighteenth century did not, however, create the genre. All sorts of
predecessors, including almanacs and books on husbandry (*Hausväterliteratur*), had flowed off the presses during the previous two centuries.[81]
While most of these rarely trickled down to the lower levels of society in
their original forms, their more popular manifestations enjoyed greater
publicity. The therapies and theories of disease expressed in them reflected a widely dispersed set of notions about etiology and treatment.
And the number and variety of these works rose appreciably after mid
century.

In Germany, the most influential and celebrated works, at least among
the coterie of the enlightened, were Samuel Tissot's fabulously successful

Anleitung für das Landvolk in Absicht auf seine Gesundheit (published in English as *Advice to the People in General: With Regard to Their Health*) (1763; 2d ed., 1766); Gottfried Bäumler's *Mitleidiger Artzt* (Sympathetic physician) (1736; 3d ed., 1743) and *Präservirender Artzt* (Preventive doctoring) (1738); Ernst Baldinger's monthly *Artzeneien* (Medicine) (1765–67); Johann Unzer's *Der Arzt* (The physician), a periodical that initially appeared from 1759 to 1764, and *Medicinisches Handbuch* (Medical handbook) (1770); and very near the end of the century, Christoph Hufeland's macrobiotic text *Die Kunst das menschliche Leben zu verlängern* (published in English as *The Art of Prolonging Life*) (1797).[82] These writers acknowledged that "the common man" rarely was their audience. They fully intended intermediaries to disseminate their teachings. Many insisted that the most effective advice was always given by word of mouth.[83] Tissot asserted that his *Anleitung* was "by no means addressed to such physicians as are thoroughly accomplished in their professions," and that neither had the title been prompted by any illusion that the book would find its way into the home of every peasant:

Nineteen out of twenty will probably never know of its existence. Many may be unable to read, and still more unable to understand, it, plain and simple as it is. I have principally calculated it for the perusal of intelligent and charitable persons, who live in the country; and who seem to have, as it were, a call from providence, to assist their less intelligent poor neighbors with their advice.[84]

Johann Juncker wrote his *Grundsätze der Volksarzneikunde* (Principles of popular medicine; 1787) to supplement his lectures at the University of Halle and to guide young physicians toward becoming "popular educators." Such popular medicine for Juncker included instruction in dietetics, spiced with enough medical knowledge to cover situations when a physician was not at hand. The other main goal was to teach people to avoid "the clutches of the know-nothings."[85]

The content of these works reflected the state of eighteenth-century medicine. While the "renunciation of authorities" characterized eighteenth-century medical theory, new heroes did not immediately arise to replace the old masters as they were driven from the field. Instead, "every man became his own authority, and there was a proliferation of people offering new medical 'systems.'" Old-style Galenism slowly disappeared, and the idea of the *anima* or psyche as the force "responsible for 'animating' animal and human bodies . . . all but vanished from the discussions of medical men." The modish new term was *mechanism*—that is, "the necessary transfer of motion through a set of physical structures."[86] As it is probably possible to find every conceivable system represented among eighteenth-century medical writers (and practitioners), it is absurd to speak of "the" or of "a" medical theory of the eighteenth century. Yet one finds that several principles won almost universal approbation. "Balance" was seen as the hallmark of health, and the need to stabilize a tottering physiological equilibrium lay at the heart of many therapies. Humoralism persisted, if no longer in Galenic purity. And a sense of the importance of the individual temperament, if less narrowly defined in terms of the four classical temperaments or complexions—sanguine, phlegmatic, choleric, and melancholic—remained a crucial tool in determining predispositions to diseases and selecting appropriately individualized treatments. All these fused with a new Hippocratism—that is, with a revived sense of the environment's power to affect health and cause illness. This last moved from an older, qualitative emphasis on "airs, waters, places" toward the science of large numbers.[87]

Near the end of the century, a growing fascination developed with the role the passions (*Leidenschaften*) played in health and illness. Prominent physician-authors, such as Tissot and Hufeland, concerned themselves especially with this subject in their popular works, advocating a "reasonable lifestyle," unsullied by wild swings of mood and excessive emotions, as a prime means of avoiding illness and preserving health. Hufeland in particular stressed the intimate connection between the moral and the physical sides of life: "[A] human being's physical [capacity] is determined to fit his morally intended purpose [in life]. This relationship forms one of the major contrasts between human and animal natures. Without moral cultivation, an individual stands in continual opposition to his own constitution. On the other hand, only [the moral nature] makes a human being also physically perfect." Others, like Unzer, accepted the power of the imagination to affect physical form. He described, for example, the impact fancy could have on pregnant women, relating how a woman frightened by a mouse bore a child with a mouselike growth on its arm.[88]

Brunonianism, too, won many converts in the Germanies between 1795 and 1815. Its originator, John Brown, postulated that there were, in fact, merely two forms of illness: those that resulted from overstimulation—sthenic illnesses—and those cause by understimulation—asthenic illnesses. Health was a condition of proper—not too much, not too little—stimulus. Among the sthenic illnesses, Brown reckoned all strong inflammations, fevers, smallpox, and measles, as well as manias. The asthenic group included, among others, plague, typhus, apoplexy, amenorrhea, and diarrhea.[89] Thus eighteenth-century medical thought contained bits and pieces of all these "systems," and they were all to be found in discussions of what caused disease and what health was.

Perhaps nothing was so difficult to define as health. Juncker tried to characterize health by indicating what a "healthy body" should be able to accomplish: "to promote the physical and moral well-being of the soul, to preserve one's own existence, to reproduce, and to have the ability to serve . . . self and others."[90] Bäumler defined health as resting "in the smooth functioning of the humors . . . which consumes overabundance, thins what is too viscous, and purges impurities."[91] The appropriate use of the "six non-naturals"—air, diet, rest, exercise, evacuations, and the passions of the mind—alone achieved this order. But, as Georg Hildebrandt, physicus in Braunschweig, pointed out, the totally healthy person "was an unattainable ideal." Few even approached such perfection; most people stood "in the middle, forever suspended between health and illness."[92]

Health was precariously maintained, and easily forfeited. And even if men like Hufeland felt that "we are directly responsible for most illnesses ourselves,"[93] they also acknowledged that some causes of ill health could scarcely be avoided. Inherited illnesses and, to a lesser extent, those produced by the temperaments, were almost inescapable. Others, such as those spawned by the environment, were hard to elude. Likewise intransigent and capricious were contagious diseases. Yet even there, by properly heeding the rules of health, one could mitigate the effects of these unavoidables and, in some cases, shield oneself against them.

These physician-authors delineated the causes of the commonest diseases, ordained rules of regimen, and, most cautiously, proposed treatments. Some deliberately eschewed therapeutic advice. Others, such as Tissot, laid out simple treatments (Tissot proceeded literally "by the numbers").[94] All agreed that a good lifestyle was the most expedient way to maintain and restore health.[95] While accepting that heredity and predispositions to specific diseases were important "causes," all also emphasized an etiology fastened tightly to environment and lifestyle, especially to diet and work. By modifying these, a person could hope to preserve health or regain it. A healthy regimen was predicated on observing the rules of nature: every abuse of nature had to be paid for, and "physical sins bring with them physical pains."[96] Tissot was especially clear here. The commonest diseases of "the people" came from: (1) exhaustion, (2) resting in a cool place after becoming overheated, (3) drinking ice-cold water, (4) shifts in weather patterns, (5) "the common custom in almost all villages of placing the manure heap under the window," and failing to air out rooms thoroughly, (6) gluttony, (7) dietary flaws and spoiled foods, (8) the faulty construction of houses, and (9) inappropriate or excessive drink.[97] This teaching perpetuated and enhanced the doctrine of the non-naturals, which now almost always appeared in combination with emphases on environment and habitat. Some authors singled one or more of these out as most consequential. Juncker, for instance, insisted that if one excluded those illnesses occasioned by "force or unnatural circumstances," all others could be attributed to "dietary indiscretions."[98] Unzer, while by no means neglectful of diet, argued that good health depended above all on the proper functioning of the three evacuations of feces, sweat, urine; this was "simply indispensable" to life.[99]

The commonest proximate cause of disease was for Tissot and Unzer, as for so many others in the eighteenth century, "hampered evacuations." The stoppage or meager flow of sweat, urine, stools, and menstrual blood was sure to cause illness and, if prolonged, even death. "It is easy to see that when such a [proper] evacuation hides itself away, its moistness, which should pass out through the skin, is thrown back on the inner parts and thus tragic results can occur."[100]

Perhaps the easiest way to illustrate how popular medical works addressed these subjects is to look at particular diseases, paying close attention to the language employed. According to Bäumler, for example, one of the commonest illnesses was catarrh. Here he understood a condition where "the watery and phlegmy humors of our bodies . . . become saltier and ropier than they should be." These viscous fluids then clogged up the areas where they were normally found in their more liquid state: lungs, nose, bowels. Such syrupy accumulations produced "slimy diarrheas," "wet coughs," and various forms of "sniffling." The causes were several. Persons who easily succumbed to catarrh had "a spongy flesh," as well as a preternatural sensitivity to outside air, or were elderly.

External cold affects such people [strongly], making their pores contract [so much] that the discharge of harmful sera is inhibited. [This matter then] finds its way into the already weakened lungs, where its sharpness irritates them [and causes] a persistent cough and expectorations. [But] this obstructed sera not only attacks the lungs, it also strikes other parts, for example, the stomach, inducing vomiting, or the glandular parts of the head, resulting in a cold, or the bowels, provoking diarrhea.[101]

The origins of a very different affliction, stroke, could be similarly explicated. It was commonly caused by "an external chill; raw or too warm and humid air; or from too much sitting, violent passions, excessive eating and drinking, [or] by omitting a customary cupping or bloodletting." Furthermore, "the imprudent application of a sulphur salve" to treat scabies only "drives it back" with horrible effect: stroke. Melancholy, described as a "perverse [and] foolish fancy," was caused by something going on, not in the brain, but "in the abdomen, as in the stomach, spleen, mesentery, and their arteries." "Inflammations of the lungs" came on "when a person becomes overheated and then takes a very cold drink, or immediately sits in a draft"; "looseness" when "one overloads the stomach with indigestible and fatty foods, or with unfermented beer, unripe fruit, and other such things." The much-feared dysentery usually occurred in fall, "when the air is most subject to [sudden] changes." During the day "the pores expand too much," whereas at night "the penetrating cold forces them so tightly shut that the essential transpirations" are violently suppressed. Then "this corrupted, sharp moisture" assaults the bowels and stomach and "gnaws at them," producing agony, as well as a brutal diarrhea.[102]

The same sort of reasoning and explanation (with some variations) can be found at the end of the century, for example, in Tissot's work.[103] Here, however, we notice a more pronounced emphasis on the baleful effects of "acrid" or "corrosive" body fluids, as well as a greater stress on proper lifestyle, and especially on the workings of the passions. Like Bäumler, Tissot worried little about a looseness or diarrhea that was not true dysentery, feeling that these only represented the body's attempts to cleanse the system and to restore equilibrium.

They carry off a heap of matter that may have been long amassed and corrupted in the body; which, if not discharged, might have produced some distemper; and, far from weakening the body, such purging . . . render[s] it more strong, light and active.

Such therefore ought by no means to be stopped, nor even speedily checked: they generally cease of themselves, as soon as all the noxious matter is discharged; and . . . require no medicine.[104]

"True" dysentery was far more serious, and was produced when a pernicious atmosphere gripped the body.

The dysentery is often epidemical; beginning sometimes at the end of July, though oftener in August, and going off when the frosts set in. The great preceding heats render the blood and the bile acrid or sharp; and though, during the continuance of the heat, perspiration is kept up, . . . yet as soon as the heat abates, especially in the mornings and evenings, that discharge is diminished; and by how much more viscidity or thickness the humours have acquired, in consequence of the violent heats, the discharge of the sharp humour by perspiration being now checked, it is thrown upon the bowels which it irritates, producing pains in, and evacuations from them.

Dysentery should be dealt with by administering a vomit and abstaining from "flesh-meats." Purges were sometimes imperative. "[T]he purpose of which," Tissot taught, was to "evacuat[e] the offending matter." The worst therapy was to "[stop] the stools by astringents, or by opium. . . . [This is] so mortal . . . as to destroy a multitude of people annually, and . . . throws others into incurable diseases." Retaining such mordant matter in the bowels, "inclos[ed] the wolf in the fold," and further inflamed already irritated organs. This could give rise to "an acute inflammatory cholic . . . mortification and death," or to a "scirrhus, which degenerates into a cancer." If, however, the humor was "repelled elsewhere," it could generate a whole series of dangerous, and perhaps fatal, conditions, among them apoplexy and epilepsy, as well as less serious eye and skin diseases.[105]

Physici in Braunschweig-Wolfenbüttel also worked with such concepts. Physicus Struve, for example, in composing his *historia morbi* on the epidemic of July–August 1757 in Holzminden, told of air filled with "winged mosquitos and horseflies" and tainted with the *effluvius & exhalationibus putrefactivis cadaverum*. A "hot and windless" season and drought multiplied the effects of all these *vis deleteria*. An unusually high consumption of water and a lack of familiar foods had caused a severe "weakness and sensitivity in the primal forces." All these, plus "fear, horror, and grief," had the effect of suppressing the "healing secret excretions," stopped up the liver ducts and permitted the bile and other impurities normally evacuated through the liver to "heap up" in the stomach and intestines, inducing dysentery. The Helmstedt physicus, Johann Lange, highly recommended the regular consumption of sauerkraut and cooked prunes to forestall such accumulations. And when reporting on fever in Thedinghausen, Dr. Marcard linked the "vehemence" of the epidemic to a long stretch of very hot weather, which "enticed the blood to the extremities," weakening the other humors and making digestion difficult. A cold snap then abruptly stopped the transpirations, and the "agitated humors" turned violently *versus interiora*, with predictably evil results.[106]

The same advice permeated the pamphlets the government distributed on the prevention of dysentery and other epidemic diseases. It likewise surfaced in the columns of publications addressed "to the people." The peasant was told, for example, that "what one ate and drank had a great influence on health," and he was specifically warned to live "in a modest and sober manner" and to avoid "overburdening the stomach with too much, or hard, or undercooked foods, or with strong drink." Moreover such "misuse of the gifts of God" made one "unsettled in conscience," and that disaffection could fester and breed "irremediable harm" in the body leading to chronic disease, consumption, or dropsy. To prevent a perilous "ebullience," sour, acidic, and cooling foods—such as wine- or beer-vinegars, lemon juice, whey, buttermilk, and sorrel—were urged on him. If disease nevertheless struck, the patient should be kept in a warm and well-ventilated (never a hot and stuffy) room, and the air purified by steam of vinegar or juniperberry. The patient must eat no meat, eggs, or fish—all of which were likely to contribute to the putrefaction of humors—and should only consume water, thin meat broths, or gruels made of oat grits, barley, rice, millet, or buckwheat, with good bread or rusks. For medicine before the physician arrived, the patient should swallow thirty to forty drops of "mixtur simplex" or red Halle powders, or a blend of crab's eyes, white or refined cream of tartar, and saltpeter. For dysentery, a mild laxative of rhubarb was endorsed. All "cooled and soothed." The "best therapies"—phlebotomy, emetics, laxatives—were to be left to the discretion of physicians, who decided on their applicability "according to each individual's unique constitution."[107]

Hindered flows, irritated organs, gummy, corrupted, and acrid humors were the midwives of illness. Even rheumatism for Tissot most generally arose from "obstructed perspiration, and inflammatory thickness of the blood." Leg ulcers could develop when rheumatism "deposit[s] a sharp humour upon the legs; where it forms vesications, . . . which burst open and form ulcers." Healing leg ulcers too rapidly "would [only] occasion a speedy return of the rheumatic pains." Smallpox, while admittedly a contagion or "poison," came from the "blood being tainted by the venom it has received. . . . [N]ature makes an effort to free herself of it, and to expel it by the skin," causing the rash and sores of smallpox. "Ardent" or "burning" fever was "like all other inflammatory ones . . . produced by the causes which thicken the blood, and increase its motion." These included excessive labor, great heat and "the long continuance of a dry constitution of the air," "inflaming foods," and "excesses of every kind." "[C]orrupt humours, which stagnate in the stomach, the guts, or other bowels of the lower cavity," engendered putrid or bilious fevers.[108] In his *Volksbuch* (Folk book), Heinrich Zerrenner linked dysentery to a "chill . . . that causes the sweat to recede [rapidly] and the pores, which have been opened up by heat and labor, are quickly forced shut by the cold and then the adulterated, sharp, [and] bilious matter . . . suddenly falls [back] on the internal parts, and especially [attacks] the entrails." The cure: "Take a vomit or a purge. That's the thing. When dysentery is about, protect yourself and abstain from all stopping and heating potions."[109] Similarly, Gottfried Bäumler advised people "to avoid drafts and keep as warm as possible. At table, shun all fatty, oily, and sour foods."[110] One could go on and on here, but the point is made, I think. Eighteenth-century physicians tended to construe most disease as arising from some corruption or degeneracy of the humors, which, turning caustic and sharp, needed to be expelled. The treatments recommended were purges, vomits, bleeding, and enemas. In fact, despite the proliferation of medical systems and the battles between their proponents, medical *therapies* were much of a muchness. Banish the inflamed or corrupted material, and all would be well.[111] But mortal complications could set in if the body's own endeavors—its diarrheas, fevers, flows (such as those from leg ulcers, hemorrhoids, nose), and rashes—to correct the unsettled state of the humors were precipitously "stopped" or "driven back." The corrupted humors would then "fall upon" internal organs with dire results. In this context, minor afflictions, such as colds, which were frequent in people whose "perspiration [was] . . . easily checked and restrained," could become dangerous, easily metamorphosing into inflammations of the breast, into pleurisy, or diseases of the throat.[112]

The road to health, then, flowed through skin, bowels, and bladder in the form of regular expulsions of sweat, feces, and urine. A properly balanced regimen best guaranteed such regularity, although many advised the judicious aid of emetics, laxatives, and phlebotomy to correct minor deviations. And while Tissot alerted people to the dangers of the excessive and indiscriminate use of laxatives and emetics, others, like Bäumler, prescribed them for almost every ailment. Ailhaud, too, predicated his system on a single cause of disease—retained feces—and a single curative: his poudre purgative.[113]

Because "inhibiting the transpirations" triggered most illnesses, laxatives and emetics were prescribed heavily for problems other than intestinal ones. For vertigo, too, laxatives and emetics were the cure. Vertigo primarily affected those "who sit too much and [thus] have weak digestions," or those given to "sexual dissipations" and "heavy drinking." Dizziness and tinnitus could also result from the absence of normal blood flows (from hemorrhoids or menstruation), or be caused by consuming "gassy foods." Skin diseases were almost inevitably linked to deficiencies in diet and transpirations. Likewise, because of the close connection between the external integument and the internal organs, scabies was a dangerous disease if improperly treated and "driven inward." Scabies arose from "an impure, brackish blood," which pickled, fatty, or smoked foods could provoke. The recommended cure was a laxative, "so that the salty excessive fluids can be improved and purged." Fever was nothing more than "a healing motion of nature" intended "to stir up the blood" and promote "related evacuations" of sweat, stools, urine, and blood, "thereby freeing the body from the dangers threatening it." Even the "whites," nonvenereal vaginal discharges, were interpreted as attempts by the female body to regain its balance. Bäumler described them as "a sniffling of the womb" that carried "both the viscous and the watery moistness" out of the genitals; it was analogous to a running nose. A woman with the whites either had an "excess of moistness" in her genitals or the blood had "stagnated" there. The cure? Bleeding, physical exercise, and laxatives.[114]

Individuals could prevent or mitigate epidemic diseases by carefully attending to rules of diet and assuring proper expirations and transpirations. Zerrenner's model father, Georg, took just this course during a smallpox epidemic in his village. Frightened for his own children, who had not yet had the pox, Georg set them a good regimen; he allowed them only very little meat, "as the wise physician and pastor . . . had advised him [to do] . . . because flesh makes the humors most susceptible to decay." Instead, he gave them as much fruit to eat as they wished.[115] Likewise, the Collegium medicum argued that even in the case of smallpox, where the contagion itself, as well as very hot weather, could turn mild cases into virulent ones, "a proper diet [could still] preserve most people from illness," whereas a "very bad diet" much increased susceptibility to disease.[116]

Environment

This emphasis on the internal processes of putrefaction, balance, and flows was combined, especially after 1750, with a new stress on the physical surroundings and a reassessment of the effects of climate and the environment on health and illness. James Riley has recently baptized this phenomenon "environmentalism" and sees in it "the origin of a medicine of avoidance and prevention, a medicine that sought to show mankind which disease-conducive circumstances to evade, and to determine what aspects of the environment might be modified to weaken or eliminate their capacity to cause disease."[117] It manifested itself in a series of attempts to accumulate raw data on the environment. Most famous of these was the already-mentioned *enquête* conducted by the Société royale de médecine in France, the purpose of which was to collect observations from physicians on epidemic and epizootic diseases, and on meteorological and climatic conditions. While a huge stockpile of information was thus amassed, it was far too much and far too diffuse to be easily evaluated.[118]

The same star of the "new Hippocratism" guided the writing of the many medical topographies published after about 1750. These works typically reviewed climatic and environmental factors, patterns of illness, and the unique influence of certain localities. The existence of such medical topographies showed that "the medical gaze no longer saw only the suffering body, but had begun to seek causes of illness in the immediately surrounding environment."[119] Are these sources valuable for Braunschweig-Wolfenbüttel? Yes and no. One searches almost in vain in Jan Brügelmann's book, for example, for any mention of a medical topography of Braunschweig-Wolfenbüttel. Although he consulted topographies of the nearby Hannoverian cities of St. Andreasberg, Northeim, and Clausthal, Brügelmann lists only a single report on illnesses in the Oberharz in 1777.[120] In fact, no such extended medical topographies exist for Braunchweig-Wolfenbüttel, with the possible exception of Georg Hildebrandt's valuable set of observations on the smallpox epidemic of 1787 in Braunschweig.[121] If, however, one looks beyond the medical topographies published as books and peruses the pages of more obscure medical journals and the columns of the Braunschweig newspapers, the same kind of environmentalism and the same analysis of medical issues appear.[122] Environmentalist reasoning also figured strongly in the accounts physici, pastors, magistrates, and Amtmänner forwarded to the Collegium medicum after 1765, as well as in their narratives of epidemic conditions. These observations undoubtedly proved valuable for chronicling the emergence of a new outlook on the relationship between health and environment, and, as Brügelmann remarked, for documenting shifts in medical terminologies and in transforming the "medical gaze," as also, as Riley proposed, for verifying the existence of efforts made to modify the physical environment. They are, however, equally replete with information on local government, on the relationships among officials, and on the role of health in the political fora of the eighteenth century.

In 1765, acting on the advice of the Collegium medicum, the privy council distributed a circular to "all physici and magistrates in the cities" specifying that henceforth they should "pay close attention to the obstacles [hindering] marriage and fertility, the neglect of health, and the excesses that contribute to it, and everything else that pertains hereto. [A]t the end of each year, when you prepare your tables of births and deaths, [you should] confer with the magistrate or with his deputies and go through these and [then] report on them separately."[123]

The order specified that such consultations should occur annually, although the documentation shows that only for a few years after 1765 and then again in 1770 and 1785 did this actually happen in more than a small minority of places. Responses in other years were, with some significant exceptions, such as that of the diligent schoolmaster Uphoff, perfunctory or simply absent. We also do not know how, or how meticulously, physici kept such and similar records, since generally only the summaries have survived. Georg Hildebrandt tells how he used an octavo notebook to chronicle smallpox cases during the epidemic of 1787 in Braunschweig. Friedrich Lentin, a well-known eighteenth-century medical topographer, who served as physicus in several places in Hannover, explains how he made the notes he eventually compiled and presented in his published works. On his desk, he always had two tables. On one, he detailed weather conditions and the general state of the environment. On the other, he recorded specific information about individual cases. Significantly, both Lentin and Hildebrandt intended to publish their observations. Not all physici were so fastidious or ambitious, although the writings of some in Braunschweig-Wolfenbüttel, such as August Hinze on Calvörde, demonstrate a good deal of the same scrupulous care in assembling information over time.[124] Even these fragmentary data portray how contemporary physicians and magistrates viewed health and illness in the context of their political and economic, as well as their environmental, surroundings. While their reviews differ greatly in form, content, length, and sophistication, and while some physici and magistrates penned idiosyncratic and bizarre commentaries, most prominently mentioned several points. Ill health and premature death were caused by, in no particular order: the exorbitant costs of medicines and physicians; masturbation and other vices, such as a generalized dissipation; the common man's partiality for "quacks"; alcoholism; an immoderate indulgence in "weakening" or "softening" beverages, such as tea, coffee, and chocolate; tobacco smoking and chewing (both especially offensive among women); epidemics and the inability to monitor and control them. Most reports single out infant mortality as the principal contributor to elevated death rates, blaming in equal measure poor care and upbringing, as well as women's evasion of their "duty" to breastfeed children.[125]

Of course, a list of the principal causes the reports recount hardly does anything to expose the logic behind their interpretations. To understand these, we need to scrutinize individual documents and pull them apart to see how physici and magistrates marshaled their evidence, evaluated it, and placed it within broader contexts of meaning. Especially critical is how they presented their conclusions and their plans to higher authorities and then suggested how the abuses they cataloged might be alleviated. Despite a certain formulaic quality (which is attributable to the strong, and often explicitly acknowledged, influence of Johann Süssmilch's *Die göttliche Verordnung in denen Veränderung des menschlichen Geschlechts* (Divine order in the transformation of the human race) or Johann Peter Frank's *System einer vollständigen medicinischen Polizey* (A system of complete medical police)[126] on many of their physician-writers), and a certain repetitiveness, the narratives remain idiosyncratic enough to illustrate a range rather than unanimity, of opinion and to demonstrate how individual circumstances formed perceptions. Many physici also exploited this opportunity to trumpet their own labors or to emphasize their own allegiance to enlightened reform.

But even the report of the physicus in Wolfenbüttel, Friedrich Topp, a careerist and later a member of the Collegium medicum, was never merely an exercise in political flattery. While Topp sounded the right notes to cement his position with the government clique of enlightenment in Braunschweig, his observations on the health problems in the onetime ducal residence were not merely a rote repetition of the platitudes of enlightened reform.

Topp's commentaries addressed the causes of the "increase and decrease of the number of inhabitants" in Wolfenbüttel over three years, 1772–74.[127] For two of the three years, deaths considerably outweighed births: in 1772 there were 548 deaths, but only 197 births; in 1773, 328 deaths and 157 births. Only in 1774 did near parity return (266 births, 257 deaths). Topp observed that the especially pronounced mortality of 1772 ended a two-year subsistence crisis. Indeed, in 1771 and 1772, ergot poisoning had been a severe problem in neighboring Hannover and Celle, although not in Braunschweig-Wolfenbüttel.[128] Topp identified a "putridlike bilious fever" as the proximate cause of the excessive mortality of 1772, but located the underlying source of that fever in the vagaries of weather. In 1771, excessive rain had caused the rye and wheat seeds to sprout and grow quickly, but just as much had rotted in the fields or bolted; once harvested, the people mixed it with all sorts of weeds or mildewed grain (mold on rye was the cause of ergot poisoning). Grain prices rose, poverty spread, and "worry and grief became the inevitable partners of the lack of a good harvest." Bad times made people "inventive," and the bread they baked from "peas, beans, potatoes, barley, and the moldy rye . . . rarely rose well." Topp had known loaves to be laced with straw and thistles, and all of them were "doughy through and through, which ruined [even] the strongest digestion." "No wonder fever struck here," he commented. "An excessive and corrosive bile destroyed the blood, affected the brain and nerves and quickly demonstrated all the marks of an overwhelming putrefaction. St. Anthony's fire, rashes, petechia, and even carbuncles were its clear signs." Topp concluded that one need look no further for the reasons for the great mortality or for an explanation of low fertility and nuptiality than "[p]overty, ever-increasing poverty: the mother of so many illnesses."

The next year, too, left Topp with the task of deciphering the reasons for a mortality that, while not equal to that of 1772, was still high— although 1773 produced neither a great inflation of prices nor any "dominant raging illness." Topp could only surmise that luxury inculcated greed, and when desires once awakened could not be slaked, there followed a "disgruntlement, which as it eats away at the soul, also consumes the body."

For the final year in this triennium, he had to account for *more favorable* circumstances. Improving economic conditions and a plentiful harvest now allowed the poor to consume better food and with "more inner satisfaction." That produced "a happier mood and healthier humors." So, despite some mild spring fevers and some irregular intermittent ones, which struck in late fall, the general picture was positive, although levels of nuptiality and fertility remained disappointingly low, because of the continued poverty of the region.

Topp hardly stood alone in linking humors, passions, and putrefaction, or in tying economics and illness together. Physicus Hoffmann in Stadtoldendorf opined that health hazards "arose not only from physical, but also from economic causes."[129] And in Holzminden Physicus Struve reported how the *effluvius & exhalationibus putrefactivis cadaverum*, exacerbated by the dog days of late summer had further polluted an air already humming with flying insects. As nasty as these conditions were, they alone bore little blame for the dysentery outbreak. Rather, their combination with "an exceptional thirst quenched with [cold] water," the lack of customary foodstuffs, but also the "violent passions" of fear, horror, and grief propagated by war "suppressed healthful secret excretions, and led to a blockage of the ducts, throwing bile and other filth onto the stomach and other viscera." This witches' brew caused the disease. Struve accepted that mind, body, and environment affected and were affected by one another.[130] Not only physicians thought and wrote in these terms. The Amtmann in Gandersheim, for instance, explained how the inflation of cereal prices and the presence of spoiled grain, like the worries occasioned by fear of dearth, had propagated a putrid fever. And when the magistrates in Wolfenbüttel were faced with accounting for the excessive number of deaths in 1758 and 1759, they confidently referred to the "horrors and alarms" of the French invasion, as well as the many hardships produced by it.[131]

Jason Schulze, physicus in Blankenburg, played on the same themes in 1766, and his remarks nicely illustrate how formula and idiosyncracy combined.[132] On the plus side, Schulze noted that both the city of Blankenburg and the surrounding area had increased in population since 1739. Yet growth over the 27-year period had been only gradual. In Blankenburg itself, births outweighed deaths by a mere 6, although the situation in the principality as a whole was more felicitous: 8,979 births and 7,924 deaths had generated a "surplus" of 1,055 persons. It is in Schulze's evaluation of these seemingly propitious statistics, however, that we catch the workings of his mind and see how he and his contemporaries assessed raw data. Contemporary judgments are, for our purposes, more telling than a "reality" that time has probably irretrievably obscured. Schulze could view the facts he laid out as not betokening auspicious circumstances. He argued that the number of births *would* have been much greater, the number of deaths fewer, and the marriages more, if "circumstances had not stood in the way."

Ranked first by Schulze among the "preventive" causes was "proliferating luxury," followed by the "decline of good morals." Like so many of his contemporaries, he argued that although "lacking all modern agricultural methods, [all] manufactories, [and] countless forms of commerce," the ancient world had nonetheless comfortably sustained a larger and more prolific population. Surely, he reasoned, "the accommodation

of these ancient peoples to plain food in moderate qualities, simple clothing, and less luxurious furnishings" must have been responsible. Again,
like many of his eighteenth-century compatriots, he, too, focused on
infancy, childhood, and the reproductive years of a woman's life. He
sympathized with the mother of the illegitimate child, whom he felt was
less deserving of punishment than the "seducer and deceiver" who led her
astray. But women, too, by their "sins" contributed to sluggish growth of
population or its decline. Women engaged in a "most ruinous vice" when
"in order not to become pregnant so quickly again, they [decide] to nurse
their children too long." Such women deprived the state of more citizens,
while destroying their children's constitutions by suckling them on the
"true poison" of "old and watery milk." They likewise undermined their
own strength: protracted nursing "exhausted" their bodies, rendering
them less capable of bearing children in the future. Added to these flaws
were those of wet-nursing and "chronic indolence, which causes much
infertility."[133]

After venting his spleen on the subject of mothers, Schulze turned to
other topics: Blankenburg's population increase was too slight when one
weighed the many advantages the principality had enjoyed over the preceding generation. Blankenburg lay "in an especially healthy locale . . .
[which] nature endows with salubrious [and] pure water." Likewise,
Blankenburg had been untouched by the epidemics that had slaughtered
thousands elsewhere. And yet Schulze spoke "with the greatest sorrow"
of those people "who according to all the rules of probability should have
survived," but did not. His remedies were general and specific, as well as
common and peculiar. Generally, he advocated control of quackery and a
program of popular medical enlightenment through the improvement of
the medical content of calendars; the publication of popular writings on
matters of health and, more broadly, on morals; and the more intimate
involvement of pastors in composing and disseminating this enlightenment. Schulze estimated that the best way to cultivate health and better
morals, however, was to implant and foster "patriotism." He wished to
instill a feeling of patriotic duty (in the broadly social sense of the phrase in
eighteenth-century Germany) in the common man, to instruct him in
"the civic duties for happiness in this life"—that is, about his obligations to
himself, his family, his society, his community, and the state. This required, Schulze insisted, that men learn "other truths and other responsibilities than merely those Christianity [prescribes]."[134] Many reports
echoed the idea that "moral improvement" would stimulate fertility and

decrease mortality. The magistrates in Holzminden, for instance, when they compared population numbers from 1760 and 1768, confidently attributed a noticeable augmentation of population (from 1,570 inhabitants in 1760 to 2,027 in 1768) to "moral advancement." In dealing with specifics, Schulze was less forthcoming. He added that although Blankenburg had experienced no serious smallpox outbreaks in these years, more children could have been saved had their parents not resorted to "superstitious and harmful practices." While he stopped there, it is clear that he deemed the "proliferation of quacks" especially harmful.[135]

Schulze's combination of variables was only one of many, and similar elements cropped up repeatedly.[136] The mix was often different, and peculiar local circumstances (such as the frequency of mining accidents in the Harz) contributed unusual flavors. The account of Gandersheim portrayed it as "a small place so full of inhabitants" that newcomers could find almost no place to live. The authors of the report found no evidence that "dissipated lifestyles" had deleteriously affected fertility, although "it would contribute much to the increase of the inhabitants if soldiers now garrisoned received their unconditional discharge." The sons of citizens understandably held back from marriage as long as they feared being called to the colors and having to leave their wives and children behind in poverty. This circumstance, of course, directly reflected the impact of the end of the Seven Years' War. The marriage of nubile women was much to be desired, since "it is well known that the female sex is more given to lust than the male." Having no husbands or families encouraged women "in idle moments" to "indulge in the *crimen onanificum masturpatio*," or, if they took lovers and became pregnant, drove them to abortions, which often made them unfit for motherhood later in life. A year later, a high consumption of spirits was singled out as a significant health hazard.[137]

Others preferred other combinations. Johann Schulze, physicus in Calvörde, highlighted the reluctance of locals to use proper medicines and their willingness to flee "good doctors" for quacks. But he also identified broader causes of low fertility in the shortage of housing and resulting high rents, which drove people from Calvörde.[138] In reflecting on the causes of mortality and on fertility in the years 1765–70, the magistrates in Stadtoldendorf noted that births had exceeded deaths, except in 1767, when a bout of "malignant smallpox" killed forty-three children and raised the total number of deaths to sixty (compared to the normal annual rate of between twenty-seven and thirty-two). They trotted out all the wearisome banalities: parents failed to treat their children properly when they fell ill; peasants were far more likely to seek competent medical advice for their animals than for their relatives. However, after listing all the problems generated by poor lifestyle, and after reiterating the inevitable complaints about "plagues of quacks" swarming over the countryside like "locusts," Physicus Hoffmann concluded that neither these nor the "physical condition" of the area bore the most blame for poor health and low fertility. Rather, he censured the adverse political and economic situation: one heard nothing but "complaints" and was overwhelmed by "the miserable life and low incomes" of these people.[139] Physicus Scheibner in Vorsfelde admitted that peasants rarely paid much attention to illness and conducted themselves according to the *principium* that "that whoever is fated to die, will die; and whoever is fated to live, will live," and thus never bothered with medicine and physicians. Yet he also commented that an equally powerful determinant of poor health was the common practice of working children too early and too hard.[140] In the report filed by Georg Spangenberg from Walkenried in 1770, these complaints kept company with others about peddlers of noxious nostrums, the inadequate education of midwives, and the deleterious impact of "repeated fears and alarms."[141]

Thus, while these accounts largely followed the reasoning and replicated the language of more widely publicized medical topographies, and leaned heavily on Süssmilch and Frank, individual circumstances crept in and at times dominated the narrative. And this was inevitable. The logic of medical topography turned on a meticulous observation of local conditions; idiosyncrasy was, in what seems a paradox, actually part of the generalization. Equally obvious is that the authors comprehended health as part of a package of good governance that included, and in truth hinged on, more expansively conceived improvements in social, economic, political, and, especially, moral conditions. Magistrates and physici realized that, for example, the provision of more doctors and the suppression of quackery were only pieces in a larger mosaic; they were almost valueless if not matched by other measures. On the other hand, the recognition that each individual area required different solutions, and that localities often marched to quite different drummers, played through as well. Grandiose plans were well and good, and even necessary, but all must be finely gauged to the peculiarities of a community. Localism did not lock horns with the initiatives of a "centralizing" government, as these tactics themselves were closely attuned to local needs and predicated on local realities.

In 1770, the government requested a similar accounting. Authorities in some places answered perfunctorily, repeating their earlier observations in whole or in part. Others submitted painstakingly designed plans for *local* improvements. A few were strikingly innovative, such as the scheme from Seesen that recommended creating a fund (drawn from tax surpluses) to provide free medical care for all inhabitants of Seesen and not only the needy ones.[142] When the Collegium medicum weighed all the information gathered, its concluding evaluation showed how those at the apex of the medical bureaucracy viewed the problems revealed and regarded the solutions tendered.[143]

The Collegium medicum concentrated on the causes of population decline, which it overwhelmingly attributed to "excess" deaths. It identified the principal causes of death for city and countryside alike as infantile diarrheas, consumption, influenza, pneumonia, dropsy, and smallpox. Most important were consumption and smallpox. None of this especially alarmed or perplexed the Collegium, which observed that these diseases, along with "malignant epidemics," were the chief contributors to deaths everywhere, and especially in populous cities. To reduce deaths from these causes, the magistrates in Braunschweig had suggested that the Collegium prepare an article detailing the evil effects of weaning children too early and feeding them improperly. The Collegium believed, however, that the problem lay elsewhere; children were nursed *too* long rather than not long enough and such protracted nursing was itself a root of consumption. Likewise, the Collegium reacted indifferently to the idea of an article written for popular audiences. Because the common man read little, the best that could be hoped for was that word would filter down from the better classes, or that proper nursing practices would become fashionable. The magistrates in Braunschweig also raised concerns about the brewing of beer and the distillation of spirits. This set the Collegium off on a long, tiresome, and almost silly digression that pusillanimously concluded that something should be done to improve the quality of local beer, although the habit of drinking "green" or immature beer was considered more hazardous to health. Finally, the magistrates commented on the "wrongheaded" care given people suffering from inflammatory illnesses (this was almost certainly an addendum contributed by the physicus). After cataloguing all these ills, the magistrates suggested improvements: reduce costs of medicine and medical care; build a hospital for the poor; promote inoculation; prevent the sale of unripe or rotten fruit and of rye infected with ergot; and take steps to clean up the air and the streets.

All in all, the Collegium rated "these proposals . . . [as] very good," but argued that little could be done. It had, for example, tried its best to make inoculation more general, with limited good results, and had been working on hospital plans for years. The Collegium conducted the whole evaluation with such tepid enthusiasm that it is hard to see much push for change here, or detect the energy radical action required.

When other magistrates in other places repeated some of these messages (many stressed the misuse of wet nurses and the wearing of tight corsets as major causes of child mortality), the Collegium medicum responded lackadaisically that one could indeed attribute "most of the deaths in infancy to the common practice of [using] wet nurses, and a deviation from the [maternal] duty, which nature herself expects of mothers. . . . It is only to be regretted that there is practically nothing to be done to stop this and other abuses." Several localities and cities had also commented on the poor quality of midwifery or the lack of sufficient midwives as a major cause of infant mortality. The Collegium agreed that it was especially necessary to improve midwifery in countryside. Still, "there are many difficulties inherent in achieving this [goal and] they are not easily removed."

Most localities also addressed obstacles to marriage and fertility in extensive detail. Magistrates and physici alike agreed that two things prevented marriage: no livelihood and a love of luxury. For this latter and for similar "moral" flaws, the Collegium medicum saw only few and uncertain solutions: preaching from the pulpit and offering premiums to those who had numerous children, while leaving the development of more stringent penalties for "dissolute living" and the passing of sumptuary legislation to other parts of government.

While one cannot quite characterize the Collegium medicum's position as one of indifference, it hardly seems to have been intent on vigorously pursuing programs of reform, policing, and medicalization.[144] Perhaps this was because the Collegium was already under fire in 1770 for its "highhanded ways" and was being pummeled in the bigger fight between the duke and the estates, or perhaps the Collegium's reticence to act, and its jaded comment that "practically nothing [can] be done to stop this and other practices," reflected its frustration. Was this nothing more than a realistic admission of impotence? Or did it express a distaste for coercion, and fear of its consequences, that permeated eighteenth-century government at many levels?

Legend

Swampy Areas

Waterways

Lakes, Ponds

Roads

Houses

Aue

Eitzum

Rothe Creek

Altenau

Frühlings Brook

Holtorfer Hof

Sambleben

Schliestedt

Küblingen

Schöppenstedt

Sauer Creek

Neindorfer Brook

Bansleben

Altenau

Schöppenstedt

Medicine and Governance

For all the information contained in these reports, which is as vast as it is unwieldy, a crucial element is missing: that of the debate opened up among the groups involved, among physici, magistrates, ducal authorities, and locals themselves. Here it is important to show how medical concerns meshed with or crossed broader affairs of governance. A probe into health conditions in the town of Schöppenstedt in the 1760s details this interplay of social, political, and economic factors with medical ones. A statistical red flag triggered the investigation. A number of alarming events had alerted authorities to what seemed "excessive" mortality. Surprisingly, the death rate in little Schöppenstedt (somewhere between 1,100 and 1,300 inhabitants in 1766) far exceeded that for the much larger and theoretically more insalubrious Braunschweig. The subsequent discussion of the exceptional mortality found in Schöppenstedt confronted many of the questions raised earlier about the occurrence of diseases in a community, the reportage involved, the categories of interpretation brought to bear, and the sociopolitical and socioeconomic circumstances within the community itself.[145] But it was also a discussion of what the role of central and local governments was to be in these and other such instances.

The subject of Schöppenstedt's "health" and "vigor" or its "infirmity" and "debility" was hotly disputed, and although the protagonists deployed the same terms and applied comparable logic and language, conclusions diverged.[146] The year 1766 was by any measure one of appalling mortality. Since 1747, annual mortality in Schöppenstedt had averaged sixty or sixty-one deaths, but in 1766, deaths spiked to a high of ninety-three.[147] Reacting to what they could only view as the "alarming mortality" in Schöppenstedt, the Collegium medicum commissioned Dr. Gottfried Beireis, professor of medicine at the University of Helmstedt, to submit an expert opinion. Beireis looked at Schöppenstedt through a medical-topographical lens, but also through a telescope: he never actually visited the town. Beireis's depiction of Schöppenstedt strictly, even slavishly, emulated the model of most medical topographies. One has the sense that the archetype determined the details of the 36-page account in which Beireis established an intimate linkage between environment and health.[148]

Working from the ancient premise that the main causes of poor health, in Schöppenstedt as elsewhere, lay "in the site of the place," Beireis first appraised climate and locale. Schöppenstedt was, he found, situated in a depression and open only to the dangerously moisture-laden and warm west and south winds. Surrounding hills blocked drying breezes from the north and east, preventing any "proper cleansing of moisture."[149] The resultant, persistent damp

weakens the mechanism of breathing, hinders the preparation of the blood in the lungs, and abruptly stops up the perspiration. [These] are the causes of the almost always fatal chest diseases, which continue unchecked throughout the year there, [and] of the irregular intermittent fevers, especially quartan fevers, of the preponderance of tumors and of dropsy, the last [of which] is almost endemic in Schöppenstedt and the cause of most adult deaths.[150]

Dietary flaws exacerbated topographical infelicities. Beireis blamed the potato—"a thin, gluey, and earthy nutriment, which stops up the gossamer vessels of the liver"—for so much poor health. Common occupations, such as cobbling, weaving, and tailoring, restricted movements of the lower body and "give other opportunities for clogging and hardening the liver." He suspected the water, too, which he found clouded with minuscule particles liable "to stick in the tender little vessels of the liver and of the other viscera, but especially in the glands and ducts, toughening and hardening" them. Added to this was a beer widely reputed to be "the worst in the duchy," which "spoils the very *materia* of the blood and produces flatulence or weakens the stomach," eventually resulting in "a ruined digestion that nurtures chronic and dangerous diseases." One almost needed not mention the universal tendency of the common folk, as pronounced in Schöppenstedt as elsewhere, to turn to quacks and cowherds when ill and run from physicians.[151]

Where Beireis sought and found causes of heightened mortality above all in climate and nutrition, the senior ducal official in Schöppenstedt, Commissioner Schüler, drew other conclusions from the "facts," both as to the exceptionality of mortality and the reasons underlying it. Although he admitted that ninety-three deaths in a single year seemed genuinely shocking and was cause for concern, he also called attention to the fact that thirty-seven of these were children who had died of smallpox. The residual mortality rates were then quite "proportional," and neither excessive consternation nor distress should greet them. More worrisome, in his eyes, loomed the "secret excessive consumption of strong drink, especially spirits" and "the frequency with which young women gulp coffee and smoke tobacco . . . which among pregnant and nursing women cannot have the best influence on their unborn children and nurslings."[152]

The debate on evidence and the significance of that evidence continued. Schüler, responding to Beireis's criticism, argued that the many "fine-sounding" schemes the Helmstedt armchair expert advocated exceeded the financial and technical capabilities of the community and the larger state, while others promised little amelioration. Beireis had singled out the spring flooding of the Altona River as a key contributor to the omnipresent, injurious damp. Schüler insisted that the river overran its banks only seldom and then receded quickly, and that this was, in any case, too minor an incident to warrant expensive projects for damming and dredging. In regard to Beireis's indictment of potatoes, Schüler shot back that some years earlier, the government itself had vigorously promoted potato cultivation in the region. Moreover, few humans consumed potatoes in quantities that could be harmful. Most of the tubers went to fatten animals. As long as grain was cheap, peasants preferred bread to potatoes. When times got tough, and the peasant turned to potatoes perforce, he "dunks them in salt, which is a *digestif*, and is, in the opinion of many physicians, less injurious to health than puddings and dough dishes, which slime up the stomach."[153]

The final salvo in this exchange of reports and interpretations came from Commissioner Funcke in Schöppenstedt. He, too, addressed the three specific points Beireis raised: damp, potatoes, and water supply. Funcke related how much had already been done to correct swampy conditions, pointing in particular to an effort mounted in 1744 by the holder of the Groß-Vahlberg estate, who, in cooperation with local government, drained many of his fields. Other marshy areas Funcke judged less menacing. For example, nearby bogs were much smaller than the regions already tapped. They also lay at some distance from Schöppenstedt. Funcke deemed it highly improbable that miasmas stirred up more than a mile off could carry such lethality with them over the distance to Schöppenstedt.[154]

While Funcke agreed that the health of the people involved in sedentary occupations could be injured by consuming large quantities of potatoes or "any similarly sticky food" on a daily basis, he doubted that the government could do much if anything to modify such "voluntary actions." And before any rash steps were taken, it would be prudent to inspect the evidence more closely to ascertain if "mortality was any larger or smaller" before or since the introduction of the potato. In Schöppenstedt, such an investigation was relatively simple to conduct. Potatoes had been planted there for twenty-two years. Funcke himself had been instrumental in their introduction, having brought with him "a Berliner peck" of seed-potatoes to distribute for planting. He argued that "the most rigorous" scrutiny of the mortality records of the 22-year period would offer no "crystal clear" answer as to whether or not potatoes aggravated mortality. His report repays closer attention, because it illustrates how at least one eighteenth-century administrator "thought statistically" and weighed the prerogatives of health against broader issues of governance.

The absolute number of [deaths] alone can never demonstrate [actual mortality] adequately, because the city has grown very noticeably over the century [and] especially since 1744. When I divide the past sixty years, 1706–65, into twenty-year periods, [I discover that] in the first duodecade, 702 people died, that is, an average of 35 a year. In the second period to 1745, 850, or 42½ each year, perished. . . . In the third duodecade to 1765, 1,158 people, or 58 each year, died. Only [since 1745] have potatoes become a common staple; thus it seems as if they indeed are responsible for our distended mortality! If one considers, however, that in this same *spatio*, more than half again as many people [came to] live here than previously, the relationship with the middle period is about equal, and [thus] potatoes cannot be seen as deadly agents.[155]

One is struck by how crudely Beireis and the Collegium medicum had used their numbers; Funcke easily found the flaws and exploited them. Yet all the participants relied on these statistics to push their points, and it is clear that by the 1760s, all these officials and experts felt comfortable with employing quantitative materials in making and evaluating policy.

In respect to "channeling fresh water supplies into the city," Funcke felt that this was made uneconomic by the high cost (at least 1,000 thaler) and effort involved. Nor would it, he believed, prove especially efficacious in lowering mortality rates.[156] In the end, the privy council, faced with conflicting evidence and interpretations, temporized, and waited to see if the heightened mortality of 1766 would prove to be an aberration, as it did.

When queried three years later about the increase or decrease of the population, the magistrates, after meeting with Physicus Pini, judged the "decline to be very measured."[157] In the two years examined, 1768 and 1769, the number born considerably exceeded the number of deaths: in 1768, forty-one deaths to sixty-four births; in 1769, forty-seven deaths to seventy births. The magistrates therefore concluded "that as long as the [birthrate] in a small city remains at about the ratio of 1:30, most [experts] feel the city will sustain itself, maintain its numbers successfully, and can even expand, without having to "recruit" from outside [its environs]."

The magistrates believed a "more determinant" analysis of deaths was in any case impossible. Mortality could not be attributed to epidemics, which had not occurred, and neither had there been any meaningful influx of aliens.

The report of 1770, therefore, projected a more positive image of Schöppenstedt than the one filed just a few years earlier, although the terms of the discussion were virtually identical. Curiously, *this* account attributed "healthy air" to Schöppenstedt despite its location in a valley; found the ground "neither boggy nor swampy but dry"; and that "[t]hose who are not sedentary in their work, get exercise enough in the city and in the fields." Finally, longevity, not premature death, typified Schöppenstedt: "almost no year passes in which . . . several [persons] do not attain or exceed their seventieth year and some celebrate their ninetieth."[158]

On the negative side, "admittedly the place is not the most fertile [as] . . . very few parents produce six offspring [or more], most stop with the third or fourth, [and] many do not even go that far." In Schöppenstedt, 187 married couples produced only 435 children, an average of fewer than 3 children per couple.[159] The physicus corroborated this unfortunate lack of fertility, observing that "it is nigh on impossible to find couples with 8, 10, or 12 [living] children." The magistrates and Dr. Pini laid the blame squarely on the straitened circumstances of the inhabitants. Yet the argument was not solely economic: it was physiological and psychological as well:

The miseries and worries of many parents depress their courage, sap the strength of their spirit, and leech the vigor from their frames. Both sexes, especially during the harvest, toil beyond their capacities, overheat themselves, and fatigue their bodies. Many live packed together in low, clammy, and dank rooms, which in the winter almost never receive sufficient fresh air. . . . [Too] many young people of both sexes delay for a long time before they [decide to] wed and thus sacrifice the best years for breeding children.

A burden of "too many and too varied taxes" completed a vicious cycle of fertility checks.[160] The uniquely political came more forcefully to the fore during and immediately after the Seven Years' War. Physicus Johann Hoffmann, for example, stressed that in Stadtoldendorf not physical circumstances but political ones had most affected fertility, nuptiality, and morbidity.[161]

Pini, of course, ended with the old complaints: people paid too little attention to their health, avoided him and other physicians, scurried off to quacks, or turned to home remedies when ill. Although he regarded all these as serious handicaps to health and major obstacles to population growth, they were "evil[s] that are not easy to uproot." Thus, he, too, recognized the limits of governmental and programmatic action.

In both Funcke's and Schüler's reports (and to a lesser extent in Pini's as well), the concerns of local administrators rose up against the backdrop of Beireis's testimonial. Funcke and Schüler saw the preservation and the promotion of health as important components of governing, but as only two elements among many others of equal or greater moment. The medical parts needed to be fitted cautiously into other contexts—financial, social, political, personal—widely regarded as equally central to the overall process of governing a community. In short, they all thought in these broader terms, and they much preferred to grapple with day-to-day problems on an ad hoc basis without being shackled to more expansive and more nebulous, if perhaps promising, enterprises. Beireis, Funcke, Schüler, and Pini all shared a discourse in these exchanges. All spoke the same languages: of a medicine caught in the currents of humoralism and environmentalism and of a governing style linked to the specific, the immediate, and the personal. Both languages were malleable; both were inherently impressionistic; both were incapable of accurate measurement and standardization; both could be turned to contradictory purposes. Statistics, too, had had only a limited impact on mentality: people could grasp the significance of series and trends, could understand averages and could calculate mortality rates, but remained less willing to weigh, measure, and test individual difference, or to thrust individual persons or communities onto a procrustean bed of normalization. Thus, the range of attempts at reform, at medicalization, and at disciplining, remained narrow because of the real obstacles to their execution and because of a mental and linguistic inability to shape and express alternatives. Not only was the will to reform basically weak, it seems, but the major groups and individuals involved felt that the possibilities of success were slim and, perhaps more important, that such broadly conceived programs, if introduced on a wide scale, promised too little return and infringed too strongly on local and personal rights.

Choices and Meanings

Health care in the early modern world was woven into a broad communal fabric and the right to aid from the community—in illness as well as indigence—derived from one's membership in a village, parish, neighborhood, or guild. Identity, too, in the eighteenth century was knotted up with position and place, and these together determined an individual's rights. Although new forces strained and attenuated these links in the eighteenth century, they did not snap. Towns and villages had always provided some assistance for strangers and travelers, but this never undercut the basic consequence of "rootedness." As this corporate and communal world began (but only began) to loosen up in the eighteenth century, the system itself started to crack. The greater mobility of people and goods, the troop movements of the Seven Years' War, the growth of population, fresh possibilities for buying and selling, and novel opportunities for styling one's life,[1] tugged at the loose threads in the corporate fabric. Yet what happened was not a sudden break into a brave new world of free market relations or political revolution, but rather the persistence of old structures and old ways of doing things, which, however, increasingly acquired new meanings. We have seen how that happened with the Amtmänner, the physici, sextons, and pastors. Traditional forms and venues were not abandoned. The privy council and the Collegium medicum continued to make individualized decisions and still worked through the old organs, if at the same time pushing new tasks upon them. Medicine and medical care, like medical choice, could not remain unaffected, although they never broke free of the routines of life, even when these routines now moved to new rhythms. Still, if people's logic of choice changed little, they were nonetheless faced with more medical alternatives. What interests us is what happened when people fell ill in a world where seasoned codes persisted and old ways were still honored, yet where many novelties—new men, new forms, and some new techniques (like smallpox inoculation and vaccination)—created special circumstances and allowed uncommon scope for decision making.

Stories of illness form the major evidentiary basis for this chapter. These narratives raise many questions about medical practice and about suffering and healing in early modern times, and this chapter is devoted to answering them. What were the commonest illnesses and afflictions for which people sought aid outside the circle of family and friends? To whom did they then turn? How did people perceive and explain what was happening to them? What did they understand by "health" and "illness"? Was there a split between learned and popular medicine? How commonly did cures involve magic or sympathy? What was the early modern "medical encounter" like? In other words, what did practitioners and their patients do and expect? What role did family members, or distant relatives, friends, and casual observers play in the medical encounter? What treatments and medicines were most frequently applied?[2]

These questions are not original. They have for some time now shaped the research agendas of many medical and social historians. The answers, however, have to a large extent been drawn from the literate classes and from a smaller portion of those who kept diaries or who exchanged views on medicine in their correspondence, or from the case books and notes of physicians.[3] These materials present enormous advantages: they are coherent, often comprehensive, detailed, lively, and, perhaps best of all, accessible. Scholars have sometimes brilliantly exploited such sources in portraying how people perceived health, healing, illness, body, pain, life, and death. What I seek to do here is different, although my findings do not necessarily conflict with those who have used other materials. I am, however, interested in a different group of people, more of them, and from a distinctive perspective. Most of my subjects are obscure or anonymous: at best, we know their names and occupations and perhaps a little more about them. The composite picture, however, is the heart and soul of this analysis. I cannot call on physicians' or surgeons' case books (I have yet to find one for my place and time),[4] but evidence of their practices and of the practices of a whole array of other healers exists abundantly in other documentation: lengthy investigations into "quackery"; stories told by patients and practitioners; parish records; court cases; and government ordinances.

A Host of Choices

Falling ill opened up a host of choices for early modern people. The awareness and definition of illness—when did one stop work, remain in bed, take a home remedy, or consult a healer—was then (as now) neither simple nor straightforward. Especially cruel could be the fate awaiting those who were poor or who lacked ties to a community. These unfortunates might be denied care or be unfeelingly shunted from place to place, as each community tried to dodge responsibility. In 1765, the bathmaster Crusius in Hedwigsburg was unhappily caught in just such an incident: "There was forced on him a fellow from Hildesheim, originally from Ohrum. Lame and hardly able to move, he was so infested with vermin that he had fouled the cloth on which he lay, filling the entire house, yard, and everything about him with his stench." The man had been brought to Crusius's place on a handcart and dumped on his manure heap. (Neither a barbaric nor symbolic act in itself, as the steam from the manure probably prevented him from freezing to death in the raw spring weather.) The commune of Hedwigsburg had tried to ship him back to Ohrum, but Ohrum refused to accept him. Attempts to fob him off on the nearby villages also failed. It was mid April, and the man "has been on my back since Easter," Crusius complained: "I am now at my wit's end." The issue of what to do was debated back and forth for about a week before the problem solved itself: the man had the good grace to die.[5]

Almost every community protected itself from such indigent wanderers and doled out funds for their own poor almost as parsimoniously. Economic realities placed one set of limits on the medical care the very poor and the unattached could expect. Journeymen on the tramp often found themselves in difficulty when they fell ill. While their guild was supposed to assist them in illness, help did not always materialize. In December 1796, the police magistrates in Braunschweig noted the pitiful plight of a journeyman tailor suffering from scabies and swollen feet, shivering with fever. The guild in Braunschweig could not (or would not) pay for his treatment. Until early November, he had been laboring in Lauenberg, but "since he became infested with scabies, he has found no work and has moved from one place to another." He ended up in the poorhouse, although eventually the Prussian branch of his guild sent money. Similarly, in 1801, a journeyman glover named Lieb had to be cared for in the St. Leonhard hospital at public expense. The glovers' guild refused to assist him, arguing that "he has not worked here and is a stranger [to us]."[6]

Braunschweig had several hospital-like institutions for people like Lieb. What were termed hospitals in smaller places, however, were almost always humble houses or rooms that could lodge only a handful of patients. In the late 1740s, the city of Gandersheim designated a small house near the Schutzen-Wall as its hospital: "However, as the good God has been pleased to spare us from illness, the house stands unused [and deserted]." The windows were all out, and during the winter of 1749–50, the ceiling had collapsed. In spring 1750, a soldier and his wife volunteered to repair the house if allowed to rent it cheaply. The wife also declared herself willing "to take in and care for any sick persons."[7]

The ducal government endeavored to improve the care of the abandoned and ill, especially in the countryside, where no guilds and few hospitals or poorhouses existed, and where poor relief funds were limited or absent. In the last third of the century, the government stepped up its campaign to avoid recurrences of the Hedwigsburg cause célèbre. An ordinance of 1770 deprecated such "uncharitable abuses" and sympathetically portrayed the misery of falling ill in a strange place. Communes wishing to "free themselves of the costs of care, or . . . the expense of burial, [and] with no regard for the seriousness of the condition and the severity of the weather ferry the sufferer against his will" out of their village. Placed on wheelbarrows or sleds, they were transported to other villages and unceremoniously tipped out on the outskirts or near the tavern. Many failed to survive such ordeals. The privy council forbade such abuses, and ordered each village and Amt to call on the services of the physicus to examine the person, and to pay for the costs of the physicus's trip and the patient's care. This pertained also to those from outside the duchy, and after 1767, it explicitly applied to Jews as well. Not until after 1795 did the central government make clear how it intended to repay the costs incurred. In the last instance, the state treasury would pay. But such reimbursements remained contested.[8]

Local authorities often brought particular cases to the attention of the government and requested assistance for specific individuals. Very often these men and women had lapsed into mental disorders and could no longer be cared for at home, or posed a danger to themselves, their families, and others in the community.[9] Frequently, local authorities helped people living in difficult family circumstances, as, for instance, in Vechelde in 1802, where they arranged care for the 44-year-old wife of the lodger Johann Schrader. For five years she had been plagued with convulsions, and she could no longer work. Her husband was fifty-eight and seldom employed: "As she can no longer do anything, and contributes nothing to the family economy, she and her husband quarrel, which prevents the beneficent action of medicines and exacerbates her seizures." The physicus and the magistrates felt she would be better off in the hospital in Braunschweig and especially "away from her husband." The privy council arranged for her admission and paid for her care.[10]

Some of the smaller cities and market towns drafted their own, sometimes quite elaborate, projects for medical care. In 1755, the magistrates in Gandersheim floated a plan "for the establishment of a fund to aid the sick poor." The magistrates argued that care was already available for those with contagious diseases. A plague-house on the road between Gandersheim and Rimmerode had been established in the seventeenth century and served as a hostel for elderly persons, "who buy in for 10 thaler, have the use of the garden there, and can live from the alms they are allowed to collect in the city." This foundation had over time accumulated a capital of about 100 thaler; the accrued interest paid for repairs to buildings and the burial of inmates. Yet it alone could not accommodate all the sick poor. The magistrates suggested funneling surplus tax moneys into a cash reservoir for their assistance. While we do not know what came of this plan, it shows how one community thought about solving the problem.[11] And in Holzminden, for example, public funds paid the costs of medicines for workers at the ducal glass manufactory.[12]

What about those who were linked to a community and who were not destitute? What did they do when they fell ill? We can locate one set of answers (if one that social historians have tended to discount) in the learned medical literature of the day. Throughout most of the eighteenth century, the opinion dominated that the people—*das Volk* or *der gemeine Mann*—invariably made unwise and impulsive medical choices. This conviction formed only one stream in the broader current of attitudes toward peasants and, more generally, "the people" that insisted that they were raw in their manners and unthinking in their actions, more akin to the brute beasts of the field than to reasoning humans. Yet this was not the sole viewpoint, and especially after the devastation of the Thirty Years' War, a countercurrent arose that valued the peasant as important in his own right and as a vital element in the growth of state power. Much of this new concern for the peasant sprang from his intimate relationship to agriculture, although governments invested almost equal time and effort in reestablishing guilds and reviving commerce.[13] Pondering the shift from a sense of the peasant as "pariah" to attempts to integrate him into German society as "patriot," John Gagliardo regarded this evolution as "a process inseparable from the major intellectual currents and changes of eighteenth-century Germany."[14] Increasingly, in the last third of the eighteenth century, there were efforts to bring about a peasant enlightenment, principally designed to augment agricultural production and swell state revenues. The advisability of such popular enlightenment was hotly disputed, however, and not everyone agreed on its wisdom or how best to pursue it.[15] The question of popular medical enlightenment therefore depended on to what extent one could, or should, educate the peasant or the common man to care for his own health and that of his family. And here, as we have seen in Chapter 1, opinions diverged.

Medical writers throughout the eighteenth century were almost unanimous in their negative assessment of the ordinary person's reaction to illness and his regard, or rather his *dis*regard, for health. They did not, however, limit their criticism to hoi polloi. They insisted that inappropriate responses to disease and apathy toward health could be found at every level of society, and yet their rhetoric obviously targeted the peasant and the common man.[16]

The majority of mankind, the lowest class of citizen and the peasant, thinks and reasons merely with dim and confused concepts. He believes that a physician needs nothing more than two eyes with which to inspect his disgusting urine and prophesy from it, two hands, a pen, ink, a scrap of paper, on which to smear a couple of Latin words, and finally an ability to mumble a few Latin or Greek phrases. . . . When the "doctor" possesses impudence enough to talk big, trumpet his miraculous cures, and relate much about his heroic deeds, [that is enough for the peasant]. . . . When one of his animals falls ill, he searches for the best possible help. [I]n his own illness, he is satisfied with the first, best quack [to cross his path], or even takes the same medicine prescribed for his ailing horse. His conscience rests easy if he has taken the trouble to use something [no matter] what or from whom, for in his eyes an old hag or an executioner, who detects a great army of evils from [merely] viewing his urine, is as good and as capable a physician as the man who has studied at the most highly acclaimed academies and who has earned the respect of the entire enlightened public.

The human herd was "less happy and more piteous than simple beasts who are led by their instincts" to avoid everything harmful to them.[17]

These authors were to some extent only repeating contemporary platitudes, which distorted, rather than mirrored, reality. Obviously, the picture is self-serving. By deploying a rhetoric that denigrated ignorance and
superstition, they allied themselves with a clique of enlightenment. The
image of the "stone blind," "deaf and dumb," "foolish" ordinary man was
common coin in enlightened circles, and perhaps indeed formed part of
the cognitive reality of many medical men. In the popular medical writings that appeared in ever larger numbers during the last decades of the
eighteenth century, the authors almost invariably concluded that in illness
the actions of the common man could be axiomatically summarized as,
"Do nothing, do too much, do the wrong thing."[18]

This opinion is not only to be found among the famous medical writers of the eighteenth century. It had spread widely among ordinary physici and ducal officials as well. In 1753, Amtmann Cramer in Königslutter
acknowledged that medical practice there was "very slight." The local
people when struck by disease, "apply only household remedies, and
[then] await either their recovery or death without ever seeing a physician."[19] The assessment of physicians, physici, and pastors as to how the
common folk responded to illness during epidemics was identically bleak,
and that appraisal altered hardly at all over the course of the century.
Physicus Wachsmuth grumbled about the problems he faced in combating an outbreak of bloody dysentery in Holzminden in 1741. He had
gone house to house extending his advice and medicines, only to be
brusquely rebuffed. At the same time, he observed that "the great stinginess of so many people [allows them] to think nothing of letting their
children lie ill without using anything," or without consulting a physician.
Or else "too early [in the disease] and at the most inopportune moment
they [employ] stopping and clogging drugs." He admitted that many
could not afford to purchase medicines and thus missed a chance at the
very beginning of illness "to achieve a highly necessary purging of the
sharp biles." They relied instead on "God's will and His mercy."[20]

The problem seemed everywhere the same. Physicus Hoffmann reported from Stadtoldendorf in 1767 that rather than go to a physician or
spend a penny on medicines, "almost everyone . . . lets their sick people
languish in misery, without the least succor and [allows them] to perish
wretchedly." And if desperation finally impelled them to act, they "run to
the apothecary in Alsfeld, or to the executioner in Halle, or to [the
shepherds] Flentge in Hagen or Ziegenbein in Amselsen."[21]

Amtmänner and local officials concurred on the reasons for these troubles. During an outbreak of *febris catarrhalis maligna* in Holzminden, the crotchety Amtmann, Granzien, made much of the impediments in his path. He found the common man "of such a mind, that he prefers to use a foreign quack, shepherd, or cowherd . . . than to let himself be treated free [of charge] by an experienced physician." In Holzminden, the locals ran to "the defrocked reformed minister" in Wöbbel or to someone named Mackensen in nearby Hildesheim.[22] The same complaints sounded in the same language at the end of the century. In Harlingerode, near Harzburg, Superintendent Eggers pinpointed the reason for unnecessary deaths as the prejudices that peasants held against physicians and the blind faith they placed in home remedies: "The peasant always . . . turns first to those who are nearest for home brews and sympathetic cures." In this region, "most of the inhabitants are not so poor that they are unable to afford a physician," but rather those ill-starred twins, prejudice and ignorance, drove them to self-doctoring and "inexperienced Pfuscher."[23]

Pastors complained about Pfuscher as well. Typical was the protest of the pastor in the village of Vallstedt in 1814, who deplored the inordinate confidence his parishioners placed in the widow Hotopp. Her renown was so formidable that not even the tragic death of a 6-year-old child she was treating had shaken the community's faith in her. "The people comfort themselves with the thought that [everyone] has a set course of life, and not even the best physician can help. It also pleases the people that Frau Hotopp takes payment for her medicines alone" and not for advice or visits.[24]

Physicians related comparable stories of how peasants disregarded or spurned their services. During the smallpox epidemic of 1765–66 in Schöppenstedt, Dr. Pini had treated only nine of the thirty-seven children who died. "I would be called only at the very last [moment], when all hope had been abandoned, or [parents] would apply their own concoctions as they saw fit in addition to what I had prescribed." Typical remedies, according to Pini, were dangerously "heating" compounds of bezoar drops, herbal wines, and hard spirits. During the scarlet fever outbreak that raged from August through December 1766, "most of the locals felt it pointless to do anything . . . as at first they observed no dangerous symptoms." Parents believed they had done enough if they administered a few doses of "seizure powders" to their sick children and wrapped a warm cloth about their necks. The result was, according to Pini, the needless death of children from "internal tumors and malignant ulcers." For "cold fever," that is, ague, Pini characterized the local treatment as a "very peculiar thing," consisting of a teaspoonful of white pepper mixed with brandy. Others gulped down "Berlin powders." Pini found that most inhabitants "say that they do not bother much about their own health and that of their families." In illness they usually resorted to home remedies, consulted a bathmaster across the border in Brandenburg, or the cowherd in Röpke. "For children they believe that one cannot usefully give them anything, except powders for a few pennies."[25] When dysentery struck the village of Bornumhausen in 1743, Dr. Blum noted that "most patients conceal their illness until the malignancy is out of control and when they do use medicines refuse to give up their beer and spirits." He attributed such reluctance to admit illness to the prevalent opinion that "the community must assume the costs of medicines, which frightens patients away from seeking treatment," dreading the animosity of their neighbors more than the disease.[26]

In the village of Heyen near the Weser during the more generalized dysentery outbreak of 1757, fifteen people had fallen ill. Of these, exactly *one* had consulted a physician, one a feldsher, and one the executioner Meßing in the village of Halle. The other twelve used nothing at all.[27] And when an "epidemic disease" (typhus?) jumped from the troops to the civilian population in Stadtoldendorf in spring 1761, of the sixty-two people the physicus Dr. Hoffmann listed as ill, just four came to him for treatment. Ten consulted various feldshers and apothecaries; nine saw the shepherd Ziegenbein; fifteen relied on home remedies; and twenty-two denied using anything at all.[28] Physicus Struve in Holzminden complained that during an epidemic among the soldiers and civilians in Holzminden in 1761, he had only cared for a handful. The others stuck to "their noxious and heating potions."[29]

According to these accounts, when patients did see a physician, it was too late, or was done with other, more devious motives in mind. Physicus Müller in Seesen grumbled that during an outbreak of dysentery in 1761, he had treated only three patients, although he felt sure many more were ill. These employed home remedies consisting of "pure astringents, especially French brandy, or they take a bit of mutton fat or broth, which are perhaps the most rational [of their actions]." Of those he saw, "nine out of ten" had been "quacked up" (*gequacksalbert*). These were only taken to him when near death, "in order to shield an illegal healer and to be able to say that the patient had in fact seen a physician."[30]

The mortality lists, of course, conveyed inaccurate information to contemporaries (as they do to historians, for that matter) because of maddening deficiencies in accounting and even fraud. Dr. Spohr charged that schoolmasters did not report reliably on whom patients consulted in illness, and that the magistrates encouraged such deceptions. "Yes, indeed, I know for a fact that some officials . . . in order to avoid inquiries into quackery have given the schoolmasters in their districts explicit directions to leave blank the column as to whom the deceased consulted during his illness." Schoolmasters, "in order to avoid the enmity of officials," failed to ask after the name of the healer who had attended the patient in his or her final days.[31]

Physici, pastors, and Amtmänner often felt themselves to be the victims of a communitywide conspiracy against them. During an outbreak of smallpox in Wolfenbüttel in the early 1770s, Dr. Martini learned of several cases in nearby Wendeburg by word of mouth. The village was supposed to send a horse for him, but he waited in vain for a beast that never arrived. The village objected that as they had not requested Martini's presence, they saw no reason to provide him with valuable animals for his transport. "And if he wants to come at his own cost, then let him come." The trip would be futile though, since most of the children had already "come through" the pox, and those still ill "need[ed] nothing." Furthermore, if any child were forced to take unwanted medicines and then died, it would be as in the hymn: "'For the dead no grass grows, my pious Christian, for everything that lives is mortal,' even if Your Honors see no virtue in this proverb. The community knows that if the doctor runs up bills, we must pay them. He can go back home."[32]

Yet not everyone unequivocally condemned the reaction of the common man in illness. When Physicus Blum in Gandersheim recounted that during an epidemic of what he described as a "contagious catarrhal fever with a rash" in the village of Opperhausen, few admitted being ill and fewer consented to take the medicines he prescribed, the Amt officials emphatically denied his version of events. They pointed out that the village headman—"in his own way a very reasonable fellow"—*had* notified the physicus promptly; Blum's advice *was* heeded; his medicines *were* used. Furthermore, Pastor Ladius had urged his flock to go to the physicus and to follow his instructions.[33]

Here again, we encounter the problems physici had, or thought they had, in dealing with local authorities. Against willful resistance and sullen silence, what recourse was there? Some, like Dr. Johann Martini (later dean of the Collegium medicum) tried to circumvent the obstacles they met with by making a virtue of necessity. When treating smallpox in the village of Küchingen, Martini bent the rules and dispensed medicines himself, although he conceded that such shortcuts had their drawbacks. Martini also requested the pastor to accompany him on his rounds. A father "who had already lost one child . . . still obstinately and pigheadedly maintained that he did not want to thwart Divine will, and [said that] if God wished to take his other three . . . then He would do so, whether he used medicines for them or not." At this the pastor shook his head, saying only: "Prejudice, prejudice, this is nothing but prejudice." The father thereupon broke off his tirade, and allowed himself to be convinced, accepting help for his children, "and [he] came to me later . . . for more advice."[34] One suspects this was an apocryphal or embroidered story, but Martini's conviction that opposition could be overcome with persistence and a little common sense was strong. Still, most physicians firmly believed that people would not consult them of their own free will. Yet privy councilors and the members of the Collegium medicum shied away from urging physicians too forcefully on the disinclined. When the Collegium concluded in 1767 that the cause of the extraordinary mortality in Schöppenstedt over the previous years could mostly be attributed to patients who avoided physicians and relied overwhelmingly on home remedies, it advocated "artful persuasion" over compulsion.[35]

Local governments and municipal authorities avoided force whenever possible, since they feared unnecessarily provoking resistance that might be hard to suppress or overcome. As late as the 1790s, the privy council and the Collegium medicum appeared to be having no great success in obtaining prompt and reliable descriptions of outbreaks of disease in remote localities or in convincing people to consult resident physici. In September 1791, the privy council again reminded pastors and local magistrates of their duties. Municipal officials, such as those in Blankenburg, quickly enumerated the myriad problems the system caused. Pastors misjudged the seriousness of an outbreak, underestimating its significance, or, perhaps worse, "view[ing] it through a magnifying glass and in cases where there is no need for worry, a great alarm goes out, leading to enormous and superfluous expenses." Moreover, little could be done, and little should be done to compel people to consult a physician if they desired not to. Only a prisoner could be coerced against his will. "We doubt that human laws can constrain [a person] to see a physician in whom he has no faith, or even mistrusts, and the district physicus, no matter how skilled he may be, often enjoys the least confidence among the common folk.[36]

The question of trust directs our attention to what really, if anything, divided physicians from the nonmedical laity, and folk medicine from academic. Can it plausibly be contended that not only cost and distance but also manner and mien separated physicians from the vast majority of the population? Did physicians and other healers practice such dissimilar kinds of medicine that the latter were acceptable and the former not? Was there an indigenous or folk medicine with its own logic and structure that itself comprised a system independent of school medicine? Logic perhaps dictates that such a dichotomy existed; reality proves more complex and far more engaging.

The first priority is to determine what physicians actually did in their medical practice during the "medical encounter." The "traditional consultation" as Edward Shorter and others have portrayed it, had four parts: "We may claim," Shorter submits, that "traditional physicians (1) did fairly well in history-taking; (2) virtually omitted any kind of clinical investigation, in the sense of observing and examining the patient; (3) had almost no sense of differential diagnosis; and (4) did—by their own lights—spectacularly at treatment."[37] While Shorter overstates the case for both (1) and (4) (many physicians were cautious, even timorous, in their therapeutics and considerably less impressed with their own and others' cures than Shorter insists), other investigators have agreed that listening to patients' stories—their narratives of illness—rather than conducting physical examinations lay at the heart of the early modern medical consultation or "encounter."[38] Listening to the patient recount his or her ills ranked as the central part of every medical examination, although that history could be taken at a distance in the sense of being relayed by the written or spoken word. Tissot, for instance, felt the patient should be able to respond to the following general questions "when going to the physician for advice":

How old is the patient?

Has he been well before?

What is his previous mode of living?

How long has he been ill?

How did the affliction begin?

Is he feverish?

Is his pulse hard or soft?

Is he restless or still?

Does he have a dry tongue, thirst, an unpleasant taste in his mouth; retching; disgust against food; or desire to eat?

Does he have frequent or infrequent bowel movements?

What are the stools like?

Does he urinate frequently? What is the urine like?

For women, additional questions addressed her menses, and sought to discover if she were pregnant, nursing, or troubled by the "whites." For children, other points took central importance. Besides age, one need to know: How had teething gone? Had the child had smallpox? Worms? A protuberant abdomen?

Similar lists appeared in more popular forms. *Der Bauernfreund in Niedersachsen* (The peasants' friend in Lower Saxony) and Rudolf Becker's more famous *Noth- und Hülfs-Büchlein für Bauersleute* (Book for emergencies), for instance, also specified the questions every patient should be able to answer for his physician.[39]

Still, even if we accept that the patient's narrative and not the physical examination formed the major action in the consultation drama, it is not true that physicians bypassed hands-on examinations entirely. Besides taking the patient's history, the early modern practitioner (especially one in the eighteenth century) usually observed the patient's general appearance, often characterizing it by temperament (sanguine, melancholic, choleric, phlegmatic); felt the pulse, generally recording, not beats per minute,[40] but qualities (full, soft, hard, rapid, weak); and examined the various evacuations (blood, pus, stools, phlegm, and urine), again making mostly qualitative, but also crudely quantitative judgments about thickened blood, "laudable" pus, scanty, turgid, cloudy, or albuminous urine, and the like. Samuel Vogel in his *Das Kranken-Examen* (The medical examination [1796]) painstakingly described a medical encounter that required at least some hands-on experiencing of the patient's body by the attending physician.[41] Joseph Gotthard, at the end of the century, fused the examination and the case history; the second could not be composed in the absence of the first. While Gotthard regarded observation as central to any proper medical examination, touching was critical as well, and he also advocated the use of that newfangled instrument the "fever-stick." Fever could only be accurately gauged by the combination of the "physician's hand laid lightly on the chest," the patient's perception of heat, and the readings of the thermometer.[42] Tissot's many descriptions of illness in his widely published *Advice* make plain that he did more than just note the patient's own words.[43] All five senses, therefore, and not just hearing, played a role in traditional medical consultations and diagnoses.[44]

Writers in the same genre as Tissot took pains to define for their readers the terms doctors employed and how laymen should interpret them. This implies that physicians acknowledged and tried to bridge the gulf distancing them from many of their patients. Gotthard cautioned physicians to converse with patients in the local dialect and to work with expressions "that do not alienate them." They must, for instance, learn to speak of epilepsy as "the curse" or "the evil," and to identify "cholik" and "the mother" as hysteria, and "the holy work" as erysipelas.[45] Baldinger offered detailed instructions on how laymen could judge the quality of the pulse and how to differentiate among "hard, soft, full, slow, strong, [and] rapid" pulses.[46] Bäumler intentionally employed "common and simple" prose, "directed to those for whose benefit I wrote this little book."[47] Authors also couched their advice in parables about fictitious peasants, such as the model couple Georg and Maria invented by Heinrich Zerrenner. In his section on birth and pregnancy, Zerrenner worked a description of obstetrical instruments into an entertaining story:

The women present [at the lying-in] were very curious about what the surgeon had in his satchel, and so to satisfy their inquisitiveness, he went with them into [another room] . . . and showed them the instruments and [explained] how they would be used. When the women saw the great forceps and hooks, they shuddered and cried out: "Oh, oh, oh!" He, however, said: "Children, thank God that today we have not had to use these. God preserve you from it." "Yet we also must be grateful," the pastor added, "that God has given man such powers of invention that he can devise valuable tools and [likewise] endow him with the skill to employ them."[48]

As here, simple explications often shaded off into condescension, and one cannot help but wonder how real-life peasants would have reacted to their fictional kin.

If this was what learned and enlightened medical writers thought about causes of diseases and how the medical encounter should proceed, was there a parallel antagonistic or alternative version? That is, did a folk medicine exist whose precepts and actions deviated from those of the academic physicians, trained and licensed surgeons, and governmental authorities? First, one must admit that *direct* evidence of a vigorous and independent folk culture and medicine is virtually nonexistent in my documentation. Physicians, physici, and pastors alike eloquently attest to the multitude of superstitious practices and the almost unchallenged suzerainty of ignorance, credulity, and error, but they rarely offer specific details. Physicians might bemoan the "absurd treatments" prevalent during outbreaks of fever, smallpox, and dysentery. They might criticize people's failure to observe proper rules of diet and refusal to submit their children to smallpox inoculation. They might shake their heads over the fatalism that produced hardened indifference to illness. Yet almost never do we get much information about what was done.

Folk Medicine

The story of folk medicine has until recently been the concern more of ethnographers and anthropologists than of historians. In Germany, the interest in folk medicine began in the nineteenth century with physicians, mostly those living in rural areas.[49] There were, however, notable eighteenth-century precursors. The Wolfenbüttel physicus Johann Bücking collected and commented on medical proverbs. Pastor Johann Helmuth published a book attacking superstition, in which he inevitably documented many of its practices. And the Calvörde physicus Johann Hoffmann authored numerous articles on herbal remedies.[50]

Despite these early ventures into folk medicine, not until the next century did its study achieve academic stature. Physicians wrote some of the pioneering works.[51] These were followed in the first half of the twentieth century by the more historical contributions of Paul Diepgen and Gustav Jungbauer.[52] Since the 1950s, ethnologists and anthropologists in Germany, working from the interdisciplinary perspective of ethnomedicine, have explored folk medical practices in specific regions.[53] These studies generally assume that there was—and is—a substantial convergence of academic and popular medicines. Usually present is the tendency to decode folk medicine as an anachronistic remnant of an older school medicine. Thus, for example, many popular names for illnesses appear as the linguistic vestiges of an outmoded erudite speech. Practices that came to be denigrated as "superstitious" or "senseless" are interpreted as the tattered remains of a once perfectly respectable academic system. Uroscopy is a frequently cited example: castigated in the eighteenth century as a worthless and deceitful con, in earlier centuries it had been such an accepted part of medicine that iconography symbolized the physician with the urine glass.[54]

Much of the literature on folk medicine written in the middle of the nineteenth century bore these analytical imprints. In 1854, Jonas Goldschmidt, a physician practicing in Oldenburg, published a short volume on folk medicine in Lower Saxony. A good deal of what he describes as the *folk* medicine of the mid nineteenth century reads like the *academic* medicine of the eighteenth. What Goldschmidt characterizes as folk etiology—attributing most illness to a chill or as the end result of a disturbed digestion—would readily have been accepted by many, perhaps by most, physicians in the eighteenth century.[55] Goldschmidt remarks that whereas "as everyone knows," scabies spreads from person to person by contact, folk medicine in the nineteenth century, like academic medicine in the eighteenth, accepted that it was caused by "peccant humors." Moreover, the swift suppression of scabies (or other skin eruptions) by potent salves of sulphur only "drove it inwards" to do far greater damage in the hidden, vulnerable recesses of the body.[56]

Recent historiography, however, has tended to discount a clear division between folk and elite medicines, as well as the idea that folk medicine is the bastard child of a more cultured parent. Writing of sickness and health in seventeenth- and eighteenth-century England, Roy and Dorothy Porter, for example, question the heuristic value of "drawing such hard-and-fast distinctions" between lay and professional medicine, contending that "serious lay/professional divisions postdate our period." Similarly, Lucinda Beier has argued that although "it is possible to identify 'traditional' and 'classical' elements in seventeenth-century medicine, a polarisation between folk and learned medicine simply did not exist. Licensed and unlicensed, educated and unlearned healers shared both theories and therapies among themselves."[57] The anthropologist Françoise Loux has likewise warned against "enclosing folk medicine in too rigid a category." It is important to remember, she insists, that at "each level of transmission between the generations, some new elements are retained, [and] others abandoned." Thus while "some elements of contemporary medicine [are introduced] into popular medicine," the latter has itself "sometimes influenced scholarly medicine."[58]

Certainly those who fulminated against quacks exaggerated the contrasts between their own and quack methods. One distinction that perhaps remains valid, however, lies in the way physicians tended to define themselves in terms of their general learnedness and lifestyle. The physician's judgment derived from the breadth of his education and supposedly distinguished him from the crowd of lesser healers, although neither the therapies he advocated nor his explanations of disease differed greatly from what other healers believed and did.[59]

What role a distinction based on broad educational precepts played in everyday life is debatable. The medical reformers of the eighteenth century themselves went a long way toward constructing something they thought existed: a popular medicine characterized by superstition, ignorance, carelessness, and indifference, and that rested on a whole series of pernicious home remedies and benighted practices. If they generally (although neither inevitably nor uncompromisingly) judged folk medicine harshly, present-day anthropologists and historians have tended to be more sympathetic, depicting a folk medicine with its own logic, integrity, and deep substance, firmly rooted in popular culture, without fully denying the interaction between folk and learned medicine. To some extent, one might therefore argue that folk medicine is a fabrication, and that it never had an autonomous existence, although generations of scholars have successfully reified it. This is not to say, of course, that there were no home remedies or folksy practices around. It is, however, worthwhile to note that as much as professional medicine is a twentieth-century construct forced on early modern times, the notion of a dynamic and autonomous folk medicine may be just as fantastical. Few people in Braunschweig-Wolfenbüttel adhered to one "system" or another, and almost all were medically promiscuous.[60]

Likewise, it is time to generate some disbelief about the prevalence of magical or superstitious cures. Eighteenth-century authors typified the common people as riddled with superstition, willing to accept magical causes of disease and ready to interpret sundry afflictions as manifestations of hexing or possession, for which they sought thaumaturgic relief. Ernst Baldinger, writing in the 1760s, remained convinced that superstitious beliefs reigned supreme. He maintained that terror of witches "kills annually as many people as the mountebanks, quacks, and encroachers [combined]." Franz Gennzinger in his dissertation on "Can the devil cause illness?" cataloged the many ills—epilepsy, St. Vitus' dance, mania, melancholy, catalepsy, nightmares, hysteria, and "the raving madness of women"—once taken for cases of possession and since demonstrated to arise from purely physical causes.[61] Not evil demons, but the imprudence of retiring on a full stomach caused nightmares, just as a disturbed digestion conjured phantasms out of Scrooge's bit of cheese.[62] Such writings reinforced the conviction of enlightened contemporaries and latter-day scholars that superstitions had continued almost unabated throughout the eighteenth century and well into the nineteenth in forms more or less unchanged since pre-Christian times.[63]

Indubitably, superstitious artifacts remained for enlightened observers to uncover in the eighteenth century. The question that needs to be asked is: to what extent and in what spirit did people chant their abracadabras, or rub their warts with the cut side of an onion? Contemporary polemic cannot be taken as proof that superstition was widespread, and such remnants are not prima facie evidence of a greater iceberg of superstitions floating dangerously beneath a superficially secularized and rationalized surface. In fact, belief in magic and possession may have become more alien in the eighteenth century. The number of cures by sympathy and magic, like the number of supposed bewitchments that came to the attention of the authorities in Braunschweig-Wolfenbüttel, was tiny. And is this not in itself some indication of the decline of magic and superstition? As such practices and beliefs became less acceptable, people mentioned them less frequently. Notwithstanding the weight of authoritative testimony to the contrary found, for example, in Hanns Bächtold-Stäubli's *Handwörterbuch des deutschen Aberglaubens* (Dictionary of German superstitions [1936–37]), peasants were beginning to laugh at other peasants who still clung to such notions. It is at least worth contemplating that most people were no longer particularly wedded to superstition and magic either for an explanation of disease or for remedies. Of course, it would be foolish to deny that there might be a very large "dark" number here, and that we shall always be poorly informed about such practices.

Much the same might be argued of religion, although the amount of research that has been done on popular religiosity in seventeenth- and eighteenth-century Germany is too meager to advance many firm opinions.[64] Certainly, the peasants we meet with in Braunschweig-Wolfenbüttel were rarely as fatalistic as scholars have portrayed them. Their often strenuous efforts in seeking their own cures, and their almost herculean exertions to restore the health of their children, hardly show a resignation or a fixation on an afterlife to the neglect of the here and now. Their seeming willingness to accept smallpox inoculation also suggests otherwise, as do their objections to it on grounds of danger (not only as human hubris trying to frustrate God's will).[65]

In sum, then, the documentation hardly supports the idea of an exuberant and robust popular medicine in seventeenth- and eighteenth-century Germany, and neither does it say very much about magical practices and sympathetic medicine. Admittedly, this is in part because of the way the documentation was generated. Face to face with officials, in front of their neighbors, and within the framework of an investigation into quackery, almost no one volunteered information about magical or sympathetic cures, or attributed their problems to spells, curses, or the evil eye. Few said much about the home remedies they undoubtedly used. People were well aware of the rules of the game as it was then being played, and if they consulted magicians, sympathetic healers, or cunning men and women, they carefully avoided mentioning it. This silence acknowledged that such cures were no longer acceptable or fashionable, a recognition that must, I argue, indicate at least some diminution of belief in their efficacy, even if it did not entirely halt their use. In short, few reported undergoing any sort of magical or sympathetic cure. When they sought to clarify why they went to healers like executioners and millers, they phrased their explanations in functionalist and naturalistic terms: it was not the magic that healed, but the salves, the skills, the potions. Patients either realized that to be believed, their stories had to be framed in nonmagical terms, or they themselves had internalized such naturalistic explanations and no longer (or no longer fully) recalled the supernatural or necromantic affinities. For example, the human fat rendered by the executioner and prized as a balm for aching limbs could be used as a cure and its efficacy praised and prized while one only dimly recollected its magical heritage.[66]

Here I am particularly interested in how people described their illness and ailments, as well as the logic behind their selection of practitioners. In several ways it becomes apparent that common beliefs in health and illness were closely linked to school medicine, or rather, that *both* drew on the same stock of knowledge, accepted the same logic, and deployed much the same language. Like many other scholars, the historian Mary Fissell, in looking at medicine in eighteenth-century Bristol, and the ethnographer Elfriede Grabner, in studying folk medicine in eastern Austria, have unearthed a widely accepted set of medical premises, practices, and explanations based on a few broad principles: equilibrium, transference, prayers, blessings, incantations, and sympathy, and it is worth exploring these ideas briefly to see how they worked.

Equilibrium was linked to an older humoral medicine in which health resulted from the delicate balancing of the humors, and disease resulted from imbalances or from the excess of one humor, or from its putrefaction. Treatment rested on a therapeutics of "restoration." To reestablish health, one needed to regain a lost balance or restore a corrupted humor to its former wholesomeness.[67] Johann Krünitz, physician, encyclopedist, and self-proclaimed champion of enlightenment, advocated "spring cures" on just these principles.[68] Adjustments were made either by siphoning off an excess—by letting blood, raising sweats, provoking a vomit—or by using similar techniques to cleanse a humor of its feculence. Drawing off impurities could also be achieved by creating artificial "wounds" through which the tainted matter could disperse. One, for example, set fontanelles (artificial lesions). Similarly, it was dangerous, perhaps even deadly, to let wounds heal up too rapidly, thereby driving the evil humors or impure matter inward and causing them to eat away at the more fragile and vulnerable internal organs. Thus, heroic methods to ban the outward signs of smallpox—its rash and lesions—might only result in the poison assaulting vital organs, with predictably lethal results.[69] Much of this corresponds very closely to what (as we have seen) physicians accepted.

Even the most horrifying treatments could make perfect sense in this system, as did that of a woman who died in childbed in 1750. A man named Mercker treated her:

She was afflicted with a fever [before her lying-in] and had obtained some herbs from Mercker, which she cooked in brown beer to make a draught. Mercker told her to take it for three days in a row . . . [and] then gave her a bottle of drops. . . . A few days later, he cut holes in her leg with a [hot] crossiron and some water flowed out of them. After he made the holes, the woman was unable to walk, and when the holes closed over, Mercker bored fresh ones in [the place of] the old. Finally, it got worse and the wounds became red and blue. When the midwife said that this was gangrene, Mercker answered, "[T]hat's exactly what [I] wanted to achieve," went away, got the ingredients for fomentations . . . smeared something on her feet, applied the poultices, and bound them up. A few days later, Mercker returned and told [her husband] that it was all over with her and shut her eyes. The woman, however, revived and spoke, and did not die until the evening of the same day.[70]

Despite the appalling pain the woman bore and the unhappy outcome, Mercker's treatment was predicated on two widely accepted tenets: creating artificial ways for the "poisons" to drain out of the body and raising fevers in order to drive out "evil humors."

In maintaining health, regaining health, and preventing illness, diet was important and was likewise linked to humoral doctrines. "Heating" diets caused the humors to do something akin to boiling. Salty or fatty foods brought on corruption of the humors; doughy and mealy food stopped the flow of the normal evacuations. Restraint in eating, drinking, sex, indeed, moderation in all things, restored, protected, and healed. As we have seen in Chapter 4, these precepts paralleled what physicians advised in their popular works. Proverbs and popular sayings encapsulated similar beliefs:

Nature is satisfied with little.

Too much is unhealthy.

When food tastes the best, it is time to stop eating.

Excess causes revulsion.

In happy days and days with wine strikes the gout.

Bacchus the father, Venus the mother, anger the midwife, gout the child.

What is good against heat is also good against cold. After eating, one should stand up, or walk a thousand paces.[71]

The Wolfenbüttel physicus Johann Bücking collected these maxims and analyzed their medical content. While Bücking insisted, for instance, that violent exertion directly after dining probably did more harm than good, he could recommend moderate exercise a few hours later: "[W]hen the chyle enters the blood, one can promote sanguification by movement and repeated deep breathing . . . [both of which] accelerate the beating of the heart."[72]

Another obvious example of the congruity between academic and folk medicines came in the realm of herbal remedies. In the eighteenth century, physicians began searching for the reasons why herbal remedies often worked. Dr. Johann Hoffmann, while physicus in Calvörde and in Stadtoldendorf in the 1750s and 1760s, was an eager and knowledgeable botanist, publishing extensively on the subject in the duchy's periodicals.[73] While Hoffmann sought the "scientific" basis for herbs' effects, the prescribed use of many herbal remedies continued to depend on their links to sympathy, analogy, and the doctrine of signs, or signatures. It was thought that "like cured like," in terms either of color or of shapes. For example, yellow-hued herbs and roots, such as white horehound, greater celandine, saffron, and radish were indicated for jaundice. Likewise good for jaundice was yellow broom seed, which was also favored for cases of urine retention, urinary tract stones, gravel, and dropsy. Red plants and roots, such as bloodroot, were applied for all sorts of bloody discharges. Likewise, wrapping smallpox patients in red cloth ("the red cure") and giving them red wine to drink were supposed to be infallible. Shapes and textures worked by the same mechanism; lungwort for lung complaints; maidenhair for baldness; spotted and scaly plants for all sorts of skin rashes and eruptions.[74]

Transference, as its name suggests, shifted a disease, affliction, or growth to something else, as sin could be laden onto a scapegoat. Thus, if one rubbed a piece of meat on warts and buried it in the ground, as the meat rotted away, so, too, the warts would gradually fade. People sometimes turned to the practice of "encircling" to rid themselves of various afflictions. One could, for example, bind a rope around one's waist, then remove it and wrap it around a tree, saying, "Ague, ague, I thee defy; Ague, ague to this tree I thee tie." Or one could transfer fevers to animals by placing them in the patient's bedroom, as Tissot noted as a common practice with sheep for malignant fever.[75] While transference seems to have fallen from favor with physicians in the eighteenth century, many prescribed the herbal remedies discussed above, even if they pooh-poohed the logic of analogy that stood behind them.

A good deal of what we know about home remedies, too, comes from physicians, and much of it was compiled in the nineteenth or early twentieth centuries. Prime examples here are Max Höfler's unsurpassed guide to the names of illnesses, the *Krankheitsnamen-Buch*, and Bächtold-Stäubli's massive *Handwörterbuch des deutschen Aberglaubens*.[76] The sole eighteenth-century work on home remedies in Braunschweig-Wolfenbüttel was written by Johann Lange in 1765.[77] Lange, who served as physicus in Helmstedt from 1758 to 1766, showed himself guardedly sympathetic to folk remedies, which he judged "to work well." Useful for the "hysterical evil" were, in his opinion, the feces of a black cat stirred into spirits, decoctions of garlic and horse dung, dill, chamomile, or cloves. For the ague so common in the marshy area around Wolfenbüttel, Lange praised chelidonium, but also recorded the use of wormwood and theriac, pepper swirled into a glass of whiskey, or a mixture of "a dram of roasted juniper berries, ground to a powder, and [dissolved] in several teaspoons of vinegar." Alum was favored as a suppository for "hysterical women, especially those plagued by constipation," but it also appeared beaten with an egg white in a salve for gangrene and sore eyes. For the chest diseases common in the countryside (known in plattdeutsch as *Bost-Sieckte*), other remedies came into play, which Lange regarded as "not to be dismissed out of hand." In particular, he recommended the juice of young, tender stinging-nettle as effective for consumption. One could go on and on here. A survey of these remedies shows that despite some reliance on the "Filth-Pharmacopoeia" and the mention of a few superstitious cures (such as the one the sister of a pastor mentioned to Lange: she cured her jaundice by "gazing fixedly into a vessel filled with tar"), most home remedies depended on herbs or on medicines available in, and obtained from, the local apothecary, and that the official pharmacopoeia also listed.[78] Therapy was largely based on expelling disease-causing irritants, and thus depended on laxatives, vomitives, and sudorifics, although emollients and soothing solutions, compresses and poultices were used as well. Nothing much distinguished these remedies, or the therapeutic logic behind them, from those of eighteenth-century academic medicine and surgery.

Take a look, for example, at the case of the wife of Ulrich Räuter, who died of "iliac passion"—that is, a bowel obstruction, commonly called "the misery"—in May 1777. During her illness, her husband said, she had "complained merely about severe pains in her gut." She wished to eat, but did not have "an open body," and her abdomen became extremely distended, although she could still "let her water." They purchased no medicines. He had given her chamomile tea to drink, and then he "heated groats in a pan, wrapped them in a cloth, and bound it round her body as hot as she could stand it." When this brought no relief, she sent her husband to the village of Gadenstedt in nearby Hildesheim territory for the bathmaster Hahn, requesting a clyster. Hahn came, administered the clyster, but told her husband to resign himself for there was no hope.[79]

When a young woman in Hessen developed "a large ulcer on her arm . . . and one believed St. Anthony's fire had set in," the father first tried home remedies and then consulted a surgeon named Vögler, whose son, a physician, actually prescribed the treatment. Dr. Vögler explained that "[after listening to] my father's description of the case, I wrote out a prescription for a loosening purgative drink, which was taken only a few times and irregularly [before she died]. Had I been consulted at the beginning, then perhaps an emetic would have lifted the entire illness."[80]

And when a pregnant woman was bitten by a supposedly rabid dog, the local physicus "had the place well-cupped, washed it with vinegar of rue, smeared it with a mercury salve, and gave her pills of sweet mercury, a cathartic, and camphor"[81]—treatments that differed little from what surgeons or laymen would have done.[82]

In fact, physicians, other healers, and patients themselves used very similar language in speaking of illness and therapies. Such a close correspondence is exactly what one would expect if a common fund of medical knowledge and ideas informed them all. In 1770, responding to a complaint the master shoemaker Worthe in Helmstedt brought against the surgeon Wallmann, the Collegium medicum used language that was in no way alien or alienating to a nonmedical laity. Wallmann had previously seen Worthe's stepson for erysipelas on his foot. In a course of treatment lasting over twenty weeks, Wallmann employed external means exclusively. The Collegium judged him negligent, however, in not calling in a physician "to administer a tonic to improve the cachectic humors of the patient." Such was deemed necessary to heighten chances of an external cure and to prevent caries in the bones of the foot. Wallmann had, moreover, "allowed the wound to close too soon." It should have been "kept open so that the wound could clean itself and to allow the caried bones to peel off."[83]

Or take the report of Dr. Nienstedt on a man he visited in his role as physician to the poor in Braunschweig. Nienstedt portrayed his patient as "full-blooded and sturdy" by nature. Now, however, he lay in "an almost unconscious state with half-closed eyes; prostrate; almost delirious; small, very rapid, and weak pulse; profuse sweating; furred tongue; intense pains throughout his body, especially in the legs; a somewhat distended abdomen; and above all a burning heat [*calor mordar*] and great thirst; stool and urine, as far as I could determine, natural." Dr. Nienstedt learned that two weeks previously, the patient had "become overheated and returned home with wet feet," conditions he blamed for the onset of the fever. He ordered a draught of arnica and camphor, as well as blisters to be set on both calves.[84]

Compare these reports in language and logic with the description Dr. Schmidt in Neustadt received from a person requesting his assistance:

A man of forty-five believes that he injured himself [straining to] lift, as from the very beginning of his illness, he has been distressed by a severe spitting of blood, which, however, . . . slowly subsided, to be replaced recently by persistent retching, in the absence of any nausea. He moves his bowels infrequently, only every third day, [and] perceives a heaviness, which hurts into his loins. [On his back] have formed boils, which disappeared when rubbed with a volatile salve but then returned. In the pit of his stomach, he feels as if a mass about the size of a chicken's egg is stuck and seems to be taking root, which he attributes to an inability to pass his wind.

His great appetite for food is undiminished, although [whatever he eats] he does not properly digest, but vomits it forth again. He is sending to you by this messenger [a sample of] his water and hopes that you will at least write to tell him what he lacks, and [trusts?] that it will not be difficult for you to say what best should be ordered for him.[85]

These cases illustrate how lay and academic perceptions and languages overlapped even at the end of the eighteenth century. Popular and academic medicine alike emphasized the importance of regular evacuations; feared what happened when these ceased, or, worse, were suppressed; attempted to restore them by mechanical means (clysters and enemas, for instance) or internal medications (a wide range of purgatives, emetics, and sudorifics of mostly vegetable origin); did not question the linkage between internal afflictions and external signs (such as boils or St. Anthony's fire as the outer signs of inner corruptions); and attempted external cures (such as cupping and blistering) for internal disorders (even rabies).

The rest of this chapter takes a long look at what people did when faced with illness and injury. Did the choice of healers, for instance, vary when confronted with the illnesses of children or women, with chronic afflictions, with injuries, or with infectious diseases?

Firsthand testimony as to what caused people to sicken and die is scarce. One place to look for it is in the parish registers. While the pastors and sextons who filled in cause of death only rarely commented directly on cause of illness, their notations do indicate how people tended to couple disease with other conditions of life, saw some diseases as tied to certain periods in life, or to one or the other sex, and described how bodies worked and wore out. Here, too, they expressed common expectations about the diseases that killed.

Deaths of young children described as "delicate since birth" indicated the importance of constitution. Constitutions weak at birth clung to one throughout life and would often be blamed for deaths in adulthood. Of a 46-year-old forester who died suddenly, the pastor in Walkenried observed that his end shocked no one, because "he was always indisposed [and] never quite right."[86] Robust physiques could be ruined. When a retired forester died in 1775 at about fifty, the pastor commented that "for a while now he has been frail, a feebleness probably attributable to his excessive love of drink." While this may sound like a moral judgment (and, of course, it was), it also shows how people understood the things that could leech vitality from a once-powerful frame. Equally hazardous were the effects of unusual or unusually demanding activities. The Amtmann in Walkenried in 1756 made "an exhausting trip" to Halle and back, doing "fatal damage to his gut." People commonly blamed overexertion for the onset of many chronically debilitating afflictions, of which consumption was the most alarming. When, for instance, the 30-year-old Christian Schottel fell ill with what was called "dropsy of the chest cavity," his mother-in-law, a midwife, explained what she believed had caused this mortal illness: "He was an extremely active, hardworking person, who labored beyond his strength, and this strain . . . was probably also at the bottom of this serious illness."[87] In both cases, the ordinariness of daily life masked hidden dangers that could hurt, maim, and kill. Wars, too, taxed people to the utmost, to the point where health was forever forfeit. When a 60-year-old man died in 1783 from "decay in the belly," the pastor attributed his "sickliness" to his participation in the campaigns of the Seven Years' War.

Every parish register witnessed the misadventures of everyday life. "Unlucky" falls from trees or off walls shattered necks or backs, and bolts of lightning ripped others out of life with frightening suddenness. Where such calamities did not destroy life outright, they rendered people unable to work and dependent on charity. The hospital in Walkenried had its share of those so incapacitated, such as a woman who died in 1773 after spending forty-four years there because of an accident in her youth, or a man who had lived in the hospital since being lamed in the hand by a stroke "and made unable to work" twenty-six years previously. A "very learned and clever" Amtmann died twelve years after suffering an apoplectic fit that "robbed him of his memory and made him incapable of fulfilling his duties." Sudden deaths were common, and the notation that someone had, for instance, been "in two days living and dead," without further comment except the pious hope that they had gone "prepared" to meet their Maker, appears frequently.

Deaths also resulted from long illnesses that slowly, insidiously, siphoned off strength and sapped the will to live. A woman who languished in Walkenried's hospital for seventeen years, "dragging her feeble body about with her," died "sick of life." Leg ulcers could also be perceived as killers. When a 37-year-old forester in Bornum died of dropsy, his demise was attributed to his having an "evil and open" leg ulcer. Another man, just in his mid-thirties, finally succumbed to a 30-year-old "noxious" running sore.

People often teamed mind and body in explaining disease, illness, and death. Deaths of family members and friends jeopardized surviving relatives and acquaintances. When the wife of the Walkenried Amtmann died in 1758, her 58-year-old daughter soon followed her. Although the pastor listed cause of death as a chest disease, he also knew that "the grief of her mother's death contributed much" to her demise. And "the misery her husband caused her" put a woman already doing "poorly" into her grave in 1763. "Vexation," in particular the enmity and spite of her stepmother, contributed to the death of a girl in Hessen in 1798 of a "rheumatic bilious fever." An aunt explained that the stepmother had kept the young woman "on the hop," and that this "constant irritation . . . brought her blood to the boil."[88]

The power of the imagination and of early shocks could also break one's health. The 20-year-old daughter of a day laborer in Walkenried died in 1714 of "a malignant, consuming, [and] incurable rheum" arising from a fright she had received as a young girl: during haying, another child had popped a live frog into her mouth, which stuck in her throat. She was never well again.

Documents discussed in other contexts, such as the diaries kept by Uphoff on the inhabitants of Hehlen in the 1750s, the list of those Dr. Barthold treated in Braunschweig in the early eighteenth century, and parish registers, provide more extensive information about health, illness, and choice, and we shall want to return to these a bit later. First, however, we need to look at epidemic diseases. Physicians and officials agreed that during the epidemics that plagued Braunschweig-Wolfenbüttel in the eighteenth century—smallpox, dysentery, influenza, and fevers—people seldom called upon the services of physicians. This was a grievance almost universally expressed by physicians. But was it true?

The Epidemic Experience

In spring 1758, a "raging epidemic disease" brought much sickness and death to Braunschweig. In February, the magistrates divided the city into five districts, appointing a physician and a monitor for each. In March, the city ordered the monitors to initiate thorough visitations twice weekly and to compose lists of patients, noting their illness, recording the physician or healer, and cataloging the medicines they used.[89] An especially industrious fellow named J. H. Weltschopp served in District C, and his lists reveal who consulted which practitioners in this epidemic year.[90]

Chest diseases and fevers (mostly ardent fever) dominated these months in District C. Of the 111 people ill, 31 (27.9%) suffered from some sort of chest problem, and 59 (53.2%) from fever. Those with chest diseases consulted a physician in 8 cases, or 25.8 percent of the time; 12.9 percent went to other healers, 9.7 percent relied on home remedies, and 51.6 percent did nothing. The last group Weltschopp usually described as "poor" or "poor and can use nothing." For fever, patients turned to physicians 30.5 percent of the time; 6.8 percent went to other healers, 8.5 percent relied on home remedies, and 54.2 percent did nothing.[91]

There is nothing remarkable about this breakdown except that people preferred physicians over other healers by a margin of 2:1 in chest cases and more than 4:1 in cases of fever. In his medical topography of Sigmaringen (1822), F. X. Metzler likewise remarks that while patients rarely consulted physicians for tuberculosis, perceived as a long-term, almost chronic affliction, they often turned to physicians in acute fevers, such as putrid or nervous fevers.[92] Yet these figures are not as transparent as they at first seem: it is possible (even probable) that those who consulted other healers knew that it was forbidden and simply avoided mentioning them, choosing to tell Weltschopp they had used a home remedy or "nothing." Moreover, the number of the latter is suspiciously high. Most probably applied some home remedy. For fever, a common treatment was a fever tea, made of fever-clover, rose hips, elder, chamomile, and linden flowers.[93] Still, a fair number, between one-quarter and one-third of those afflicted, *did* seek a physician's counsel. The poor did not, or perhaps could not (unless they were on relief), but artisans and journeymen did, as did some soldiers and their families. Parents called upon physicians for their children as well as for themselves, and wealthier families often brought a physician to the house to see a servant. Even a simple market woman relied on Dr. Petsch when she diagnosed her own case of the purples.

Although such evidence is too thin to be conclusive, it suggests that while the poor rarely saw a physician (except perhaps one employed by the poor relief), members of other social groups, and especially artisans, often went to physicians during epidemics, as well as in many other instances. Dr. Petsch, for example, treated a tanner for a wasting disease over several months, and a cobbler's son and a clerk for an exanthematic fever, while simultaneously attending the widow of another tanner for "age," and probably arthritis, and her servant for a chest disease. He visited a cabinetmaker for months to mend his broken leg and to set right his generally "sickly state." The other healers who handled chest afflictions and fevers were the feldshers Laue and Knackschmidt, the apothecary Reichmann, the bathmaster Hertz, the councilors Meyer and Reck, and a mysterious Herr Hundemarck.

An outbreak of what Dr. Hieronymi called "that nasty disease, malignant fever" occurred at approximately the same time in Wolfenbüttel. Death rates in Wolfenbüttel for the years 1757 and 1758 rose to abnormal heights. The average for each of the other years in the decade was only 395, but in 1757, 646 died, and in 1758, 660.[94] From January through May 1758, a total of 292 persons died in the Hauptkirche parish of Wolfenbüt-

Causes of Death, Hauptkirche Parish, Wolfenbüttel, January–May 1758

Illness	Number of Deaths
Chest diseases (*Brustkrankheit*)	108
Wasting (*Auszehrung*)	63
Purples (*Friesel*)	22
Fevers of all kinds	17
Convulsions (*Jammer*)	7
Tumors (*Geschwulst*)	20
Chronic, protracted (*langwierige*)	14
Acute, rapid (*schleunige*)	3
Teething	7
Shortness of breath (*Dampf*)	4
Childbirth	2
Not given	25

SOURCE: "Actum Wolfenbüttel d. 17 Mai. 1758 In Societate medica," StAWf, 34N Fb. 1 X 12, fol. 56.

tel: 108 of chest ailments, 63 of wasting, 22 of the purples, and 20 from tumors and dropsies. The category "fever" included several types: "eleven-day," ardent or burning, and spotted (see Table 5.1). Of the 292 who died, 46 (15.8%) had consulted a physician, although the percentage fluctuated according to the illness; for chest and respiratory diseases, it was 21.3 percent, for the purples 27.3 percent, and for all fevers 23.5 percent.

Once again, those who sought the advice of physicians belonged to a range of occupational categories. Twenty-one were artisans or members of artisan families; eleven were local officials, lawyers, or secular and ecclesiastical notables; two were soldiers from the local garrison; two were domestic servants; one was a taverner; another a merchant. This breakdown pretty much paralleled the social composition of this municipal parish, with the exception that day laborers (who were quite numerous) are not at all represented.

Equally instructive is a breakdown by age of those attended by physicians (see Table 5.2). Here, as in other epidemic situations, and as we have previously seen for Hehlen, parents rarely called on physicians to treat children under ten, but adults, even elderly ones, turned far more frequently to physicians than has generally been assumed. Still, there is no dodging the fact that in this epidemic, most of those who died never saw a physician in their last illness. In fact, the administrator of the saltpeter works, Jürgens, treated more patients than any physician. In April and May 1758, Jürgens had fourteen people in his care. While these were

TABLE 2

Age at Death, Hauptkirche Parish, Wolfenbüttel, January–May 1758

Age at Death	Total Number	Number Saw Physician	Percentage Saw Physician
Less than 6 months	14	0	
6 to 11 months	6	0	
1 to 10 years	45	1	2.2
11 to 20 years	11	2	18.2
21 to 30 years	43	9	20.9
31 to 40 years	41	8	19.5
41 to 50 years	52	11	21.2
51 to 60 years	57	6	10.5
61 to 70 years	25	4	16.0
Older than 70 years	13	3	23.1
Unspecified adult	10	2	20.0
Unspecified child	2	0	

SOURCE: "Actum Wolfenbüttel d. 17 Mai. 1758 In Societate medica," StAWf, 34N Fb. 1 X 12, fol. 56.

mostly members of the artisan classes, some lesser municipal officials and even a member or two of the city council did not scruple to seek his advice.[95]

Examination of an outbreak of smallpox in Braunschweig and its surrounding areas in 1768 and 1769 strengthens these impressions. The number of cases in Braunschweig never approached the levels of the severe epidemics of 1761 and 1766, when 435 and 619 people—the vast majority of them children—had died.[96] The epidemic of 1766 attacked several other areas with equal or greater ferocity. In Calvörde, in a population of about 800 (829 in 1774), at least 60 children succumbed to the disease.[97] Thus, while the 66 deaths of children from October 1768 to February 1769 in Braunschweig were not especially numerous, they nonetheless caused some alarm. The Collegium medicum demonstrated no particular disquietude, however, pointing out that the deaths were concentrated almost entirely among the lower classes, and especially among the children of the garrison, 24 of whom had died. Death reaped few victims in the wealthier parts of the city, leading the Collegium to conclude that the smallpox was not really "malignant."[98]

During the outbreak, physicians were consulted in about a quarter of the smallpox cases. Dr. Brückmann, for instance, had only two smallpox patients, although he had inoculated seventeen children in the first three months of 1769. The outbreak continued throughout the spring and early summer, as did efforts to inoculate the children. In March 1769, the phy-

sicians treated thirty-eight patients, of whom five died. In the same period, the sextons noted forty-nine deaths from "natural smallpox," leading
the Collegium medicum to conclude that "very many people either seek
no advice [whatsoever] or only that of feldshers and Pfuscher."[99]

Other epidemics evoked similar responses. During an eruption of putrid fever in early 1772 in Blankenburg, the surgeon Schwancke enjoyed
widespread confidence, and for this Pfuscherey in internal medicine, the
Collegium medicum fined him 20 thaler. In his defense, he insisted that
the local physicians would not have been able to attend to all the patients,
and that, in any case, most patients could afford neither a physician nor his
medicines. Schwancke boasted that none of his patients had died.[100] Blankenburg's city council upheld Schwancke's claims, sending along to the
privy council a thick packet of testimonials in his favor from the city's
Bürgermeister, the Amtmann, the captain, and the pastor of the garrison.[101] In all, of the fifty-four persons he treated for putrid fever, sixteen
wrote on his behalf. The turner Lacht pronounced himself "extremely
satisfied" with Schwancke. The wife and two daughters of the cobbler
Schröder had consulted Schwancke "because she could not afford the
apothecary." Schwancke charged the Schröders, as well as a teamster and
his wife, and many others, only 2 thaler, while the destitute wife of
the linen weaver Becker paid nothing. The farrier Wohltag, whose two
daughters had sickened with "putrid fever and a rash," went to Schwancke
for help because Wohltag trusted him. Four years earlier, he had suffered
from a wasting disease, "which no one had been able to halt despite the
expense of 10 thaler," but that Schwancke cured. A year later, his wife had
an alarming hemorrhage, which Schwancke "happily" quelled. When his
two daughters fell ill, Wohltag confidently turned to Schwancke, and
"after counting in some blacksmith work" he had done for Schwancke, he
paid a little less than 2 thaler. The cowherd Meyerken, his wife, and their
son had all had a combination of what Meyerken termed putrid and
exanthematic fevers in the week before Pentecost. "Because of the present
shortage of work," they had been unable to afford either a doctor or an
apothecary. They asked Schwancke to let blood; he also gave them some
medicines, which cured them, and he charged them only 2 thaler. Schwancke gave Frau Gerber some herbal teas and opened a vein in her arm,
but, "as she was a poor woman," refused to take her money. The teamster
Voigtländer had two daughters ill with putrid fever and the purples,
whom Schwancke likewise restored to health. The master shoemaker
Schauer's son was so low that "his shroud was already sewn" when his

father consulted Schwancke, because he was "a relative of his and [be-cause] his cures had always proved their value." For assisting the city's master miller, Schwancke was given flour worth 2 thaler 2 groschen. When the entire family (husband, wife, and three children) of the linen weaver Esaias fell ill, Schwancke provided the medicines "and asked for recompense neither for them nor for his trouble, rather saying that it was his Christian duty." Schwancke let blood for a smallholder named Schalck and gave him a purge, all for just 8 groschen. He only charged the com-munal forester's wife 16 groschen, while neither the daughter of a soldier nor a soldier's widow paid a penny for Schwancke's assistance. Thus peo-ple turned to Schwancke, not only because he was inexpensive, but be-cause, in their own words, his cures "worked," and because his willingness to treat them did not, in their eyes, depend either on the size of their purses or on their status.

In 1759, an outbreak of what Physicus Blum described as "a malignant or contagious catarrhal fever with a rash" caused forty-seven illnesses and seven deaths in the village of Opperhausen. Blum discovered that "among the deceased there were several who either used nothing at all or had gone to some pettifogging doctor." Blum had ridden to Opperhausen at least twice, but stopped going there when the Amt refused to reimburse his costs.[102] He then dispatched the surgeon Blumenberg as his proxy. Blu-menberg undertook eleven trips to Opperhausen, seeing an average of fifteen patients each time. For example, on 18 January, he visited a Han-noverian soldier tormented by chills and a headache, "[who] refused all medicines, though they cost him nothing." Eleven days later, he attended the schoolmaster's family, dispensing the medicines Blum prescribed. The daughter had suffered for a week with chills and headache, but was now improving, although still a little feverish. The schoolmaster's wife was "very bad," and he did not expect her to live. Their 8-year-old son was confined to his bed, and the schoolmaster's sister-in-law could now get around, but still complained of faintness.[103] While Blum felt that the Amt had consistently failed to assist him, the Amt pointed out that Blumen-berg's report (he had, after all, been far more diligent in visiting patients than Blum!) showed that the villagers only concealed the illnesses of two adults and two children. Some people did not want to use medicines, because they wanted to let the illness "blow itself out" (*ausrasen lassen wollten*), and even these were eventually persuaded to use the medicines urged on them.[104]

When dysentery appeared in the area around Holzminden in late sum-

mer 1757, Physicus Struve was very busy. By August 25, there were
twenty patients in Dehrenthal and thirty-three in Boffzen, in addition to
cases in at least thirty-six families in Holzminden itself. In the tiny village
of Heyen, Struve identified fifteen people with the bloody flux. Almost
all were adults. Of these, twelve used neither medicines nor healer (or at
least said so); one had consulted the executioner in Halle; one, a regimental feldsher, and only a 50-year-old man had used "a little something"
from Dr. Bachmann in Hameln.[105]

A confined outbreak of putrid fever in Ahlshausen shows how one family responded. Pastor Reck observed that the fever was "very pernicious
and contagious" but fortunately had affected only a single household. First
to succumb was the "old mother" (aged fifty-two), who "contrary to my
advice used the medicines prepared by Dr. Behrens in Nordheim." The
son and daughter-in-law then fell ill and were sick for a long time. Both
consulted Dr. Spangenberg in Einbeck. The next victims were the wife's
two unmarried sisters, who had come "from the paternal house to help
out" while the family was ailing. Both had been very seriously ill and
recovered only after swallowing the medicines Spangenberg prescribed.
The wife's parents, who also lived in the house, and "who had just passed
their fiftieth year and seemed [always] to enjoy a rugged good health," died
two weeks later despite Spangenberg's best efforts. A field hand "who
frequented the house" perished next. He had lain bedridden for four
weeks before he died, "much to my [the pastor's] surprise, [and] probably
because of some error in diet."[106]

This discussion of epidemic experiences reveals that while most of
those afflicted did not usually see a physician, a not insignificant number
did. It also appears that certain diseases—fevers and chest diseases most
obviously—tended to send patients of almost all classes to physicians, or to
a physician as well as some other healer. Physicians, then, did not serve
merely as doctors to the rich. Many artisans in Braunschweig, for example, consulted them. Even in the countryside, where admittedly the number of those who turned to physicians during epidemics remained limited, the aid of physicians was never universally scorned.

It is significant, however, that during two of the major recurrent epidemics of the eighteenth century—smallpox and dysentery—the number
of people who saw physicians was always small. Part of this must be
attributed to the sense that physicians had little to offer children with
smallpox and to the rooted feeling that smallpox was "just something
children had to live through" and perhaps formed a critical stage in the

youthful "hardening" process. Parents consulted physicians infrequently for these sorts of childhood diseases, and, as the age breakdown indicates, few children under the age of ten were ever taken to a physician for internal problems.

It was different with children suffering from injuries or congenital deformities. In such cases, many parents sacrificed a great deal of time and money trying to get their children set right again. The Jürgenses had a tiny son with a sore (suspected to be of venereal origin) that had "eaten away all the flesh of the upper lip." For fourteen weeks, his mother carried him from one surgeon and physician to another in Braunschweig, neglected her work, and pawned almost everything, "down to my last shift," searching for a cure. Likewise, the widow Heinemann from Haringen sought everywhere for help for her 8-year-old son, whose "unnatural genitalia made him unfit for marriage." His foreskin did not slide back from the glans, causing him great difficulty in urination. He had already suffered several debilitating infections.[107]

Physicians were also seldom consulted for dysentery, whether the sufferer was an adult or a child. Perhaps this was, again, because patients felt there was little a doctor could do, or that the illness progressed so rapidly to either death or recovery that it left little time for a physician to act and medicines to work. The feeling that a disease must "rage itself out" if it were not to return also contributed to inaction. And it is well to remember that physicians themselves repeatedly cautioned against "stopping" diarrheas too rapidly, thereby reinforcing a wait-and-see attitude. Finally, while patients during such epidemics did not often turn to physicians, they did not frequently turn to other healers either, suggesting that they felt that no one and nothing offered effective help.

Everyday Illnesses

Epidemics were not, however, the stuff of everyday life. What, then, did people do when stricken by the many major and minor nonepidemic illnesses, injuries, and physical annoyances inflicted on them? The medical reports for the village of Bornum give one answer. As no physician resided in the village (although two lived in nearby Seesen), the schoolmaster compiled the reports on illness. His most frequent notations under the heading "physician" were "is unknown to me," "I know nothing about it," and "used nothing." Only once in these five years, in 1774, was a physician called in: Dr. Müller came from Seesen to treat the feverish illness of a 30-year-old man.[108] But Bornum may not offer a true picture, since like many others the schoolmaster in Bornum was a slovenly bookkeeper.

The records maintained by the schoolmaster Uphoff, and discussed at some length in Chapter 4, impart greater insight into the medical choices people made. Over the decade 1751–60, Uphoff listed eighty-one men, women, and children as ill. There were eighty-seven consultations with healers, because several people sought assistance from two or more persons (although no one consulted more than three) or employed a combination of healers, medicines procured from various sources, and home remedies. Most used nothing at all. Thirteen (about 15%) saw a physician.[109] In the 1750s and 1760s, no physician lived in Hehlen, and patients or their representatives traveled to Bodenwerder, Wöbbel in Lippe-Detmold, or Hameln when they wished to have a physician's opinion. Eight persons procured medicines, and perhaps advice as well, from apothecaries in the nearby towns of Bodenwerder and Heyen. Three relied exclusively on home remedies, two purchased medicines from "elsewhere," and two swore by "the medicines of a man by the name of Meßing in Halle near here." Ten turned to either the company feldsher in Bodenwerder or the regimental surgeon in Hameln. Another person tried an unnamed surgeon. One woman had seen an executioner, and four persons consulted a man named Flentje, identified as a shepherd. In forty-three instances, the name of the healer was unknown, or it was remarked that the patient had seen "no doctor" or "used no medicine."

Physicians were, however, called in by a schoolmaster's wife for her *haemorrhagia uteri*; by a cottager for his 8-year-old son, who had a distended abdomen; by a widow for her 20-year-old son with a quartan fever lasting over eighteen months (she had previously been to two different doctors for him); by a laborer for the "variously diagnosed" ailment of his 11-year-old daughter; by another laborer's wife for her apoplexy and for an "obstruction"; by a cottager for his "tumorous fever"; by the wife of a day laborer for hysterics and "wasting fever"; by a prosperous peasant afflicted with a "cancerous sore" on his neck; by the schoolmaster's widow for dropsy; by a cottager's bedridden wife. Thus while the residents of Hehlen and Daspe turned to nearby physicians for all sorts of internal ailments, they were just as likely to see surgeons for these and similar afflictions, including tumorous conditions, fevers, colic, dropsy, suffocation, kidney stones, consumption, and inflamed lungs. Many Hehleners, from the schoolmaster and a quite prosperous farmer to less exalted cottagers, landless peasants, and day laborers, turned at one time or another to a physician. They more regularly consulted surgeons for pains in their joints, ulcerated varices, "heavy spitting of blood," a serious hunting accident (which tore a "collateral artery"), hernias and their attendant "colicky symptoms," and for several other unspecified but apparently grave illnesses. During the dysentery epidemic of 1757, for example, the surgeon in Bodenwerder attended the entire Meyer family. The Meyers procured medicines from the apothecaries in Bodenwerder and from the somewhat more distant town of Heyen.

The shepherd Flentje was almost as busy with patients in Hehlen as any of the surgeons. The cottager listed above requested Flentje's aid for his son's distended abdomen, but he also went to the physician in Bodenwerder. Another cottager called upon Flentje to see his daughter, who was ill with "dropsical fever." And when a respiratory complaint laid low a 53-year-old laborer in 1752, he called upon Flentje for assistance, as did the wife of a cottager also plagued with a dropsy and fever. Twice people obtained medicines from Meßing in Halle. Most people, however, used nothing or relied on providence, the strength of their own constitutions, and home remedies. An old cottager's wife (well over seventy), and ill with dysentery in 1755, "made use of no physician, only some home remedies, among which brandy is supposed to have worked well." Only a single individual went to an executioner for advice, believing that supernatural forces lay behind the illness of her 2-year-old child. She thought him bewitched. The authorities regarded her, however, as "disturbed, very confused, and crazed in her thoughts, and that is probably how she came up with the idea."[110]

Lists of patients kept by practitioners present another way to approach the problem, even if they are less frequent in their occurrence and less complete in their details than one wishes.[111] The practice of Dr. Barthold in Braunschweig in the second decade of the eighteenth century imparts some idea of what diseases prompted people to consult a healer. In 1712–14, Barthold treated a large number of people. Barthold's position was a somewhat ambiguous one, however. While no one doubted that he had studied medicine, he had never taken his doctoral degree, and after the passing of the 1721 medical ordinance, the government therefore forbade him to practice internal medicine.[112] Nonetheless, early in the eighteenth century, he enjoyed considerable popularity, visibly demonstrated in his extensive and varied practice. People from almost every social group called on his services. Artisans formed the majority of his clientele, as he had a contract with the Tailors' Guild. He treated a large number of them, their family members, and their domestic servants. But his practice included people from many different social classes and of all ages and both sexes. While fever cases constituted a large percentage of his clientele, he handled almost every other common ailment, whether mild or severe, from convulsions in children to apoplexy, rheumatism, and dyspepsia. He dealt as well with a small number of surgical cases, including kidney and bladder stones, hernias, eye injuries, and ophthalmic diseases. He did not, to judge from this accounting, doctor either skin conditions or venereal diseases.[113]

Over an eighteen-month period, Barthold saw 329 different patients. Of these, 221 were adults (68.21% of known ages [324]) and 103 (31.8%) were children; 162 were male (59.12% of known sex [274]) and 112 (40.8%) were female. Thus there were among his clients about three adults for every two children and rather more men than women. He did not have an extensive gynecological practice, handling only the occasional case of "vapors." Patients consulted him most often for fevers (129 cases, or about 39.2%) of all kinds—his most frequent diagnosis was "ardent or burning fever"; 59 people (17.9%) sought his help in chest cases; 32 (9.7%) for consumptive disorders, pleurisy, and "suffocation"; 12 for dysentery (3.65%); 7 (2.1%) for head colds. The remaining quarter (27.45%) of his business included scattered instances of epilepsy, rheumatism, arthritis, vertigo, jaundice, dropsy, "hectic," stroke, apoplexy, indigestion, and palpitations (this last only among women), as well as a sprinkling of surgical interventions (16 cases, which included stones and hernias, as well as cataracts). His practice was far more medical than surgical in nature, by a ratio of at least 20:1.

Physicians were, of course, only one variety of eighteenth-century practitioner, and a survey that stopped with these men and their patients would be woefully incomplete. The story of the surgeon Ahrberg in Wetteborn in the first half of the nineteenth century pictures another sort of medical practice and shows that patterns of consultation had changed little over the years (see Table 5.3).[114] In one year, Ahrberg saw at least twenty-two people for diseases usually considered internal, which strictly speaking fell outside his bailiwick. Ahrberg had been actively engaged in medicine since 1801, when the Collegium medicum first appointed him rural surgeon to Wetteborn. Over the years, he had repeatedly petitioned the Collegium for the right to practice internal medicine and had just as often been denied. Yet patients had always consulted Ahrberg for internal complaints. For instance, in 1801, the death of an infant prompted an

TABLE 3
Patients of the Surgeon Ahrberg, 1839

Sex	Age in Years	Illness
M	13	glandular fever (*Drusenentzundung*)
F	1	convulsions (*innere Schäuerchen, Schäuerchen, Krämpfe*)
F	6	brain fever (*Gehirnentzundung*)
F	31	nervous fever (*Nervenfieber*)
M	15	wasting (*Entkräftung, Auszehrung*)
F	40	tumor (*Geschwulst*)
F	45	tumor
F	1	mucous fever (*Schleimfieber*)
F	1	chest disease (*Brustübel*)
F	69	weakness, fright (*Schwäche, Schrecken*)
M	2 months	convulsions
M	42	wasting
M	10	convulsions
M	53	dropsy (*Wassersucht*)
M	53	chest disease
F	68.5	dropsy
F	48	wasting
M	39	liver disease (*Leberkrankheit*)
M	43	chest disease
F	41	hemorrhage (*Blutsturz*)
F	60	chest disease
F	24	nervous fever

SOURCE: StAWf, 111 Neu 3103, case 2.

investigation into Ahrburg's practice. The child's father related that his still unweaned daughter had died of some sort of exanthematic fever, which he called the purples. At the beginning of her illness, he had noticed "small red weals all over her body," which then abruptly disappeared. He turned to the surgeon Ahrberg, explaining that he had called on Ahrberg to treat his 13-year-old daughter for a scalp rash. While Ahrberg was visiting the older daughter, he advised a laxative for the younger. The mixture produced a mild reaction and seemed to relieve the child's distress. Suddenly, however, she took a sharp turn for the worse, and she died eight days later. Ahrberg had also given the older girl a laxative and bound a compress on her head, and her rash had almost cleared up. Fischer said he had known Ahrberg since he was apprenticed to the local surgeon, and that when he visited him in Hilprechtshausen, he often obtained advice and medicines from him. But Ahrberg was not the only healer the father had seen. On the very day she died, Fischer had gone round to the local surgeon and asked him for a vomitive recommended by a neighbor. Two hours later the child died.[115]

Several cases from 1816 further illustrate the dimensions of Ahrberg's practice and the conditions in which patients and their families solicited his assistance. In the summer of 1816, the peasant Steinhof, who had a chest fever, called Dr. Liebrecht to his bedside. There the patient's wife showed Liebrecht a mixture and a salve that Ahrberg had prescribed. The wife attributed her husband's ailments to a severe fall he had taken in the barn a few years previously. Ever since then, he had felt constant, hefty pains under his ribs. When her husband complained of severe discomfort in his right side on a Monday and then again on Wednesday, "I sent my son to Ahrberg in Wetteborn for his advice and to have Ahrberg give him the proper remedies." Ahrberg dispensed an unguent. Then, "about four days later, our workman Illemann had to go to Ahrberg, and he reported to him that my husband, after having smeared the salve on his torso for two days, was spitting up great gobs of bloody phlegm." Ahrberg suggested another salve and the above mixture "to increase the flow of sputum" and end the problem. When neither worked his wife called in Dr. Liebrecht.[116]

The story of the bathmaster and barber-surgeon Ahrens in Stauffenberg demonstrates the range of practice for another licensed healer. In November 1782, the Amt interviewed seven people Ahrens had treated over the past several months.[117] These testimonies and others like them reveal in part why and, just as important, *how* people consulted Ahrens, and reflect, if somewhat less fully, how they perceived their physical troubles. The wife of local official named Wehmeyer, for example, related that

Shortly after Easter . . . Ahrens visited her once, as she was much troubled with a heavy eructation of worms. . . . [He] promised to deliver her from this evil straightaway, and got a white powder from the apothecary in Gittelde [which he mixed with a watery fluid]. . . . The next day he sent the medicine out to her, but as she has a repugnance against all medicines, she could not bring herself to down it. She poured the laxative away, and since then she has not returned to Ahrens.

Between Easter and Pentecost, her daughter had suffered from aches and tightness in the chest, and Ahrens "as if by chance came to her and promised to banish [them] at once." He administered to her a knife-tip full of a white powder. A few days later, he gave her a bottle containing black drops. When her brother asked what they were, Ahrens answered that "the drops must be cooked over a light. If not, the remedy would have no effect." He also handed her "two of these white powders." She, like her mother, threw the medicines away "without concerning herself further with this cure."

The tutor Ludwig Frantz, however, took Ahrens's medicines. He had been attracted to Ahrens "because of his wide repute" and turned to him in this instance because "he sensed much foulness in his body." Ahrens sent him a laxative "made up of small grains," which induced vigorous purging and vomiting. Frantz admitted that "while it was working, he felt intense cramping in his belly, though by evening was quite right again, and has not noticed anything of his previous complaint since then." The widow Sidecum likewise procured a laxative from Ahrens for her husband, who had an intestinal blockage. After taking the medicine, he threw up violently, then died. Ludwig Lagershausen from nearby Gittelde normally only used Ahrens for letting blood, although he also took counsel from Ahrens for his wife, who was tortured by "excruciating pains in her neck." Ahrens got rid of them by "purging her with a white powder . . . which had a moderate effect, and after which his wife felt very well indeed." Lagershausen swore that "at that time almost all the inhabitants of Gittelde consulted Ahrens." Ahrens had also cured the turner Ignatius Helwig of a badly injured hand. Then he treated Helwig's daughter for cessation of her "flowers." Ahrens prescribed a laxative for her, which the girl refused to take. The wife of the goatherd in Gittelde, Frau Baumgarten, had consulted Ahrens for "awful heartburn." He gave her a "fingerlong" vial filled with red drops. She took the dose, felt no improvement, and obtained no other medicines from him.

Of course, one might argue that Ahrberg was a licensed surgeon and Ahrens a licensed barber-surgeon, and that ordinary people might not discern or accept the fine distinctions between those cases surgeons or barber-surgeons were permitted to treat and those reserved to a physician. How did patients then justify their other choices, such as the decision to go to the local executioner or knacker for assistance in illness where presumably the boundaries between licit and illicit practice were more clear-cut?

From about 1770 through about 1810, the knacker Friedrichs in Calvörde carried on a brisk trade in the healing arts. Many people consulted him even in quite serious cases. When an 18-year-old woman fell gravely ill, her father sent to Friedrichs for medicine. When his daughter subsequently died, her father explained what had happened. First he pointed out that other than the pills he had received from Friedrichs, "he had used almost no other medicines during the illness of his daughter." When asked why he had turned to the knacker, he explained:

He had heard from [various] other people that Friedrichs gave out medicines but could not remember who had told him so. He knew that at the time there was no physician in Calvörde. He had not considered the apothecary because he did not know that he was involved in healing. In all his life he had never used one and thought that if anyone requested anything from the apothecary, he must ask for it by name.[118]

Likewise, many people used the executioner Frölich in Ahlfeld. For instance, he was accused of treating two daughters of a man named Jürgen Weiberg (who lived in nearby Greene) for smallpox. One, an infant of twelve months, died. When asked why he had turned to Frölich, Weiberg responded that because of the expense, and because the smallpox seemed not to be dangerous, he had taken the infant neither to Fröhlich nor to a physician, nor had he given the child any medicines. For his other daughter, who was still very weak from her illness, he had consulted two physicians: Dr. Behrens in Nordheim and Dr. Rudelstädter in Gandersheim. He did not deny, however, having used Fröhlich occasionally in the past. "Frölich is often consulted for ague [in the region] and he [Wieberg] had obtained medicines for himself and his brother from Frölich for just this reason." He gauged the action of these medicines as "very effective."[119]

Similarly, when the mortality lists for June 1802 revealed that the cottager Wolf in Badenberg had died of a chest disease under the care of "Chÿrurgius" Fröhlich in Ahlfeld, it spurred another inquiry. Wolf's married daughter testified that "at her father's bidding," she had once gone to Fröhlich for medicines. From her account of her father's condition, Fröhlich diagnosed influenza or pneumonia and sold her a bottle of medicine and a bag of tea for 12 groschen. The man's widow related that during her husband's illness, "they had relied on home remedies and the [advice] of a 'doctor' in Ahlfeld, whom she believed was called Herlig, and who was supposed to be very small of stature." She had never gone to Fröhlich, and neither had her son.[120]

Three cases handled by the blacksmith Möricke from Braunschweig reveal the dynamics of serial consultations and how lay diagnoses influenced the choice of healers. The cottager Julius Krufer went—eventually—to Möricke for help when his 24-year-old daughter developed what he identified as a "treacherous fever" and attributed to overheating. First, he had consulted Dr. Sommer, who medicated her for about three weeks. Under Sommer's care, however, his daughter's health deteriorated so precipitously that "soon she was unable to get up and began to show all the signs of consumption." In his despair, he sought out Möricke, gave him "a true history of her illness," and showed him a sample of the girl's urine. Möricke's medicines worked such a tremendous improvement that only two days later, "when Möricke came to visit, he declared that the illness had been broken" and the danger was past. He then gave the girl a tea and another powder, which "fully restored her." Krufer paid only for the last dose.[121] The plowman Heinrich Kurland also consulted Möricke for his wife, who for seven long years had dragged herself about with crippling arthritic pains. He, too, had initially consulted a physician in Wolfenbüttel, whose six months of treatment produced "absolutely no effect." Then he went to another doctor in Königslutter, and thereafter "[also] used Dr. Niemeyer for a long time, who was able to heal the sores on both her ankles [although] these broke open again." For almost three years, his wife could barely drag herself from her bed and was almost paralyzed with pain and stiffness. All medicines and costs had been fruitless. Finally, and after many people urged him to see Möricke, he did. The smith prescribed powders and tea, and after three weeks, the woman was once again able to move about the house. Her husband felt great confidence in her complete recovery.[122]

Another cottager's family expressed equal satisfaction with Möricke's therapies. The wife related how shortly after harvest home, her husband had begun to labor under a severe chest congestion. She had first consulted the "constable" Lange, who visited him for six weeks and prescribed several medicines. Nonetheless, her husband "became ever more feeble, and everyone believed that he had a consumption, which a hacking cough and the complete depletion of his strength indeed only too clearly portended." About nine weeks before, she had gone to Möricke, who wrote a prescription, which she had filled at the apothecary for 20 groschen. Within three days her husband showed a surprising improvement, and the medicine "so completely revitalized him . . . that he can now get about the farm once again," although he had not yet regained his former vigor. Möricke had also cured their 18–month-old infant, who lay ill for six weeks with a high fever. They had initially called upon the local surgeon. His drops produced no results, except that the child became "so wretched and weak . . . that true consumption was apparent." Möricke administered a powder that worked "a marvelous improvement" in just four days, and for a cost of 2 marks.[123]

While these stories offer, at least in part, some fairly direct indication of why people chose particular healers in certain circumstances, medical choice can also be approached more obliquely by scrutinizing the reaction to the one true triumph of eighteenth-century prophylaxis: smallpox inoculation.

Another Way of Choosing

The introduction of smallpox inoculation and vaccination in the German states has not been studied with the intensity it has elsewhere attracted. Only a few general works and a handful of articles deal with it.[124] In Braunschweig, as elsewhere around mid century, a debate erupted over the advisability of inoculation and its efficacy.[125] On the pro-inoculation side stood the Collegium medicum, the privy council, the editors of Braunschweig's learned journal, many physicians and surgeons, numerous pastors, and a range of prominent persons who moved in the city's enlightened circles. The Collegium medicum first discussed plans for promoting inoculation on a large scale in 1754.[126] On 31 August 1767, the garrison physician, Dr. Topp, carried out an inoculation on the 9-year-old son of Konrad Schmid, professor of theology and Latin at the city's Collegium Carolinum. Inoculation of the two youngest children of the merchant Johann Wilmerding followed in December of that year.

Despite these early initiatives, inoculation in Braunschweig-Wolfenbüttel did not catch on either easily or quickly. Some opposition, here as elsewhere, stemmed from a group of medical men who not unreasonably feared that inoculation might touch off an epidemic of real and deadly smallpox, who doubted the efficacy of the process, and who worried about the transfer of other diseases, especially gonorrhea, syphilis, scurvy, and tumors, from unhealthy donors. Some prejudices against inoculation also existed among laypeople, many of whom viewed inoculation as blasphemous interference with divine law and with nature. Others saw smallpox as the result of original sin, and as an "inborn, rooted, and necessary evil" all children must go through. Perhaps some parents regarded it as a kind of postnatal birth control. Reputedly, in some places, entire communities united in opposition to inoculation, and threatened violence against the introduction of compulsory inoculation. Yet, in fact, it appears that rather than blind prejudice, the major inhibitors were a sense of the danger of the procedure and an inability to think in statistical terms of chances.[127]

In the city of Braunschweig, where deaths from smallpox ranged from

5.5 percent to slightly over 10 percent annually (from 1746 to 1768, about 10%; from 1769 to 1784, 5.5%), smallpox inoculation never took firm hold. Only four attempts to inoculate children en masse were made, and these fell in smallpox years: 1767, twice in 1768, and in 1772. Only 139 were inoculated even in these years, and probably fewer than 350 in the twenty years after 1767. As in the same period about 18,000 children were born in Braunschweig, a total of 350 inoculations hardly represented a resounding triumph for the pro-inoculation faction. After 1780, inoculations continued only when an epidemic threatened, but the numbers inoculated rose considerably. During the 1787 outbreak, about 200 were inoculated (while at least 372 died from June through December).[128]

Two factors in particular account for this lack of success before 1780. First, smallpox epidemics happened only periodically. Second, although the data on smallpox inoculation available in the eighteenth century indicated that the chance of death from inoculation was much less than from "natural" smallpox, people did not, in regard to themselves and their children, reckon in terms of "chances." In the 1780s, many quite enlightened people (by their own definition and judging from their affiliations) felt that the numbers were still too scattered and inconclusive to allow one to make a judicious decision. Rather, as the pro-inoculation observer August Schlözer argued, parents thought in terms of individual children, *their* children. Commenting on the outcome of the May–June 1771 inoculation in Göttingen, when three deaths marred the inoculation of thirty children, Schlözer concluded: "We laymen, for whom the life of one child weighs more heavily than the system, would really like to have more numbers from other places before we resolve that it is better to sacrifice every ninth child on the altar of science than every seventh child on the altar of nature."[129] Still, smallpox in the near environs, or an actual outbreak (or perhaps the memory of the 1766 epidemic that killed 619 in Braunschweig), often canceled apprehensions, or supplanted them with more ghastly ones, encouraging receptivity to inoculation, as the Collegium medicum observed when smallpox reappeared in 1768–69: "[Now] the public is far more aware of inoculation than previously." While the Collegium argued that "many would have done better to have their children inoculated before the natural pox was spreading," it seemed a ripe moment to push ahead with an inoculation campaign. "The common man, here as in other cases, does not decide to do [anything] until a greater danger looms. This seems to be the reason why so many more [people now] than earlier have taken refuge in inoculation." Since the beginning of the smallpox outbreak in late fall 1768, 121 people had been inoculated in the city, and only one had died. Most of the children inoculated by Dr. Brückmann in these days came from the Braunschweig elite: their fathers were city magistrates, advocates, merchants, and army officers; two were Brückmann's own offspring, and another two were the children of the noble Frau von Zastreck.[130]

Elsewhere, inoculations proceeded sometimes with less and sometimes with more facility. In Königslutter, for instance, Dr. Pott inoculated sixteen children on 30 January 1769. Most were the offspring of notables in the town, but several came from lesser circumstances: their fathers were petty officials, an innkeeper, a writing teacher, a tin-founder, a brewer, and a dyer. Of these inoculees, two died, although Dr. Pott assigned blame for these dual misfortunes to complications arising from teething.[131]

If we ask ourselves how vigorous and impassioned opposition to smallpox inoculation was, we come up with two somewhat contradictory answers. Obviously, in terms of numbers, inoculation was pretty much a failure in Braunschweig, but opposition to it was neither violent nor coordinated nor sustained; lack of interest seems to describe parents' reactions best. Parents seemingly did not perceive the direct benefits of inoculation in the way its proponents did. Physicians and surgeons often blamed prejudice, superstition, and indifference for the unenthusiastic response to inoculation. Unfortunately, there is very little testimony from parents either way. One mother did volunteer her child for inoculation, but her motives were mixed. She hoped thereby to get her illegitimate child admitted to the orphanage in Braunschweig. She was possibly also pressured by her employer, the merchant Wilmerding, who had been one of the first in the city to inoculate his children, and who remained a fervent proponent of inoculation. This child, and three others, were successfully inoculated on 30 April 1768.[132]

Such details are rare in the documentation. We know little about what people actually thought about inoculation and why they backed or opposed it, had their children inoculated or did not. The lists of those inoculated remain the best indication of the acceptance of inoculation, especially when they specify the occupations of the children's fathers, and this evidence suggests that while few objected strenuously or vociferously, not many had their children inoculated.

If the introduction of inoculation proceeded with glacial slowness before 1780, and not much faster thereafter, the acceptance of vaccination moved more rapidly,[133] although here, too, doubts lingered. Much the same advocacy and debate about vaccination filled the columns of the newspapers after 1799 as for and against inoculation earlier.[134] Vaccination, which involved inoculation with the mild cowpox, rather than with the possibly lethal smallpox lymph, was much safer. The first vaccinations probably took place in Braunschweig in 1800 on the children of several notables, but the practice only gathered speed a few years later. As with inoculation, examining those vaccinated helps us understand who chose vaccination and how it was popularized. The Amt Campen, for example, in 1805, made detailed provisions for introducing vaccination. The physicus, Dr. Winckelmann, had offered to vaccinate in Windhausen and nearby areas, and the privy council instructed the local authorities to encourage the entire community to participate in this "beneficial discovery." Winckelmann promised to vaccinate each child for 2 groschen, and "if there are any among the poor . . . who wish to have his child or children vaccinated, the costs for these will, if necessary, be covered by poor relief funds." In the thirteen villages of the Amt, parents registered eighty-five children to be vaccinated, and only six at public expense.[135]

Providing cheap or free vaccinations produced good results elsewhere. When smallpox broke out in areas around Gandersheim in early spring 1805, Dr. Harcke donated his services and the requisite lymph. "Thereupon," he reported "several inhabitants resolved to allow their children to be given the cowpox." From 22 March through the end of April, Harcke vaccinated 105 children in and around Gandersheim. The Amt administration had arranged for pastors to preach the benefits of vaccination from their pulpits and, acknowledging that as "the peasant usually seeks to avoid all medical costs, especially in the case when his children still appear to be well," decided that "the best means to win him over to vaccination" was to offer it free."[136]

More interesting were the results of vaccination in Neubrück and Veltenhof, where the parents of 55 children agreed to have them vaccinated at a cost of 2 groschen a child in May 1805. Only the swineherd Christian Fröhlich was unable to pay for the vaccination of his two youngsters. A postscript to the list noted that the number of children would have been much greater had not the surgeon Eggeling already vaccinated 170 children several months previously at a cost of 4 groschen a head. Parents of vaccinees came from almost all the peasant and subpeasant groups. Just two notables took part in 1805: possibly they had allowed Eggling (or someone else) to vaccinate their children earlier. Only three parents refused outright to have their children "poxed."[137] As early as 1801, Johann

Welge, physicus for Harzburg, vaccinated 152 children with little opposition in his district. In some villages, only one or two children remained unvaccinated.[138]

Persuasion often proved unnecessary. In 1802, for example, several inhabitants of the village of Klein Vahlberg approached the physicus Rörhand in Schöppenstedt with the request that he vaccinate their children when smallpox broke out in several homes there. Rörhand was reluctant to do so, as "the vaccination they wish for would not protect their children against [the real] smallpox if they had already been infected—and these people were reasonable enough to understand."[139]

Less immediate in his successes was Dr. Spohr in Seesen. The mortality/morbidity lists from Lutter am Barenberge for 1802 demonstrated the presence of smallpox there, but when he wrote to the Amt asking for information and promising his help, he received no answer. In Seesen itself, "smallpox is everywhere [and] quite severe." He argued that

the worst part [of life] for the physician in the countryside is that he still has to fight tooth and nail against the ingrained prejudices of the countryfolk. [Most firmly fixed] among them [is the misconception] that in [cases of] smallpox, it is not essential to call upon a physician as long as no unusual symptoms appear. It is [they believe] quite enough to keep the patients warm and, when the pox do not want to "show themselves," to give [the patient] plenty of red wine to drink. [They] send to the physician only when it is already too late. Against vaccination there persists a general and unyielding resistance. [The parents] wrongheadedly espouse the opinion that man should not interfere with the will of God by making a child ill without His desiring it.

Still, he eventually accomplished his goal, introducing the procedure in Seesen "even among the lower classes . . . after important figures in the city had their children vaccinated."[140]

Not every physicus agreed that irrational fears or religious obscurantism thwarted the progress of vaccination. In 1816, Dr. Bühring cited the impediments blocking a more comprehensive vaccination. While superstition "indisputably" fueled some opposition, such was only "very seldom" the case in his district. The remaining deterrents Bühring attributed to "the unceasing activity of those living in the Harz." If he sought to vaccinate in summer, "I find the inhabitants seldom at home, for their children are with them" in the fields or forests. Furthermore, parents often wanted to vaccinate their children, but could not watch over them after the vaccination. Illnesses also prevented him from vaccinating the youngsters all at once, so that some always remained untreated. Lack of vaccine was a chronic problem. These logistical bottlenecks, and not the implacable hostility of parents, constituted the main barriers to effecting a broad-based vaccination program.[141]

Thus, at least in some places, the process had spread so widely by 1815 that few unprotected children were still to be found. In Hasselfelde, Physicus Bühring maintained that "only a handful . . . are susceptible to the dangers of smallpox contagion. I stopped vaccinating last autumn because there were no more subjects available. In the many areas that belong to my district, I have [either] vaccinated [all the children] myself, or had them vaccinated by the surgeons, so that here there is no longer any great number to vaccinate."[142]

Another problem, however, began to undercut the progress of the vaccination campaign by 1815–16: the gradually diminishing strength of immunity called the process into question. It eventually, however, led to the procedure of revaccinating at regular intervals. Dr. Spohr ran into resistance to vaccination on just this point in 1815:

[R]umors that inoculated and vaccinated children later get smallpox . . . make a negative impression on the common man. I have had just such an experience in Greene, where I could only with difficulty find two children to vaccinate, despite having with me a list provided by the Amt of over twenty-five unprotected children. The parents protested, what good was vaccination, if the children still got smallpox?

Spohr blamed these rogue outbreaks of smallpox on improperly conducted initial vaccinations:

A self-styled, now deceased, "vaccinating-doctor" from Einbeck traveled around in his carriage with his own son through . . . Greene and Gandersheim about twelve years ago. Many of the peasants' children were vaccinated by him. [H]e well knew that his son had been revaccinated about twenty times so that he could continually have fresh lymph. I was also told that a certain journeyman barber from Einbeck went around with a vial that had in it a clear fluid, with which he vaccinated many children.[143]

But all this equally testified to how readily parents allowed their children to be vaccinated.

Sufferers and Healers

While lists of patients and vaccinees and parish records are valuable guides to medical practice as far as telling us who consulted which healers and for which illnesses, they pass on only inferential evidence about the thought processes behind medical decision making. One may guess that in epidemics, few people consulted physicians, because the effort was felt to be meaningless. Or surmise that they did not use a physician when their children fell ill with smallpox because "it was just something children had to go through." To comprehend their thinking more fully, we must, however, exploit a more suggestive source: narrative accounts of illness and healing. These allow us to venture few generalizations, partly because medical preference always remained a very personal decision. It is a choice from which we can never exclude the workings of a broad range of individual preferences, circumstances, and idiosyncrasies. What can be done, however, is to sketch out how people *tended* to understand their illnesses, how they *tended* to select their healers, and what they *tended* to expect from a healer and from the medical encounter itself, and how all these fitted larger patterns of life. Because I have neither diaries nor correspondence for Braunschweig-Wolfenbüttel in which people reflected at length on health and illness, it is necessary to rely on more fragmentary materials. Especially serviceable here is the testimony taken from people as to why they consulted certain healers in preference to others. This evidence has its problems, because it was almost always collected within the framework of investigations into quackery. Those speaking must inevitably have felt defensive and painfully aware of the need to justify their actions or to protect their friends. Yet eighteenth-century investigative practices were unsophisticated, and information given by witnesses was not yet milled into reality-obscuring uniformity. Thus, despite its ticklishness and its inherent flaws, this documentation can lead us further into the everyday medical world of eighteenth-century Germany. Case histories illustrate best how people judged expectations of cure, how they endured pain, and how they assigned praise or blame for treatments that succeeded or went awry.

In the 1770s, the cobbler Dreyer garnered great fame for his skill in treating a very common complaint: ulcerated leg varices.[144] He used a poultice containing a compound of lead, and in 1780, the privy council granted him the right to treat such afflictions. This meant that prospective patients had to petition the Collegium medicum or the privy council for permission to use Dreyer, as did the teamster Schacht in August 1780. Schacht related how Dreyer's poultice had "liberated me from an evil that I had borne for over seven years." "A man in my position," he explained, "cannot be uncommonly careful of himself, and nothing is easier than for one to wound himself again and again in the same old place."[145] On each of these occasions, Dreyer's plaster had proved its worth. And Dreyer could list a host of other, equally pleased customers.

If Dreyer had limited his practice to the treatment of leg ulcers, he would have been busy enough, but people sought his expertise for other conditions as well. When the shoemaker Hampe had his foot crushed by a falling bell at a foundry, he bound it himself in wine-soaked bandages. When inflammation set in, however, he went to Dreyer. Dreyer described how the toes of the right foot were "totally smashed," the tendons of the fourth and little toes "completely ripped away," and the whole "greatly inflamed." Soon the third toe shriveled and fell off, and pieces of bone began to work their way out of the fourth, although Hampe did not lose it. Dreyer applied his poultice as well as "some liquid of a green color." Yet four months after the accident, the wound still measured well over an inch long and was, Dreyer said, "corrupt."[146]

Despite its popularity and the wide array of uses to which Dreyer put it, the Collegium medicum insisted that his dressing was "no arcanum," and in fact nothing more than a "quite ordinary lead-containing poultice . . . the like of which every apothecary carries." Such preparations were, in its opinion, unable to heal "incurable wounds," and they often "transformed curable ones into those beyond remedy." By indiscriminately applying his poultices, Dreyer "completely stopped up" wounds and "allowed opportunity for inflammation and suppuration to begin." Such had been the unfortunate result when Dreyer had treated a serious head wound; he caused "the pussy matter to be reabsorbed into the blood," upon which a fatal "colliquastive diarrhea" ensued.[147]

And Dreyer's treatment did not satisfy all his clients. The grumblings of the disaffected reveal as much about his practice as the effusive praise his many contented customers lavished on him. In 1780, 37-year-old Conradine Meyer demanded back 6 thaler she had paid Dreyer. For three years she had been suffering from a running sore on her lower leg, and "recently a hard knot about the size of a pea" had appeared on her shin. At first it caused no pain, but when it swelled "to the size of a chicken's egg" and moved round into the calf muscle, she became alarmed and consulted Dr. Heym, who advised herbal packs and cataplasms. Apparently Heym's treatments failed to please her, since she soon deserted him and went to a surgeon, who informed her that "the dressings were too heating" and in place of them prescribed a "cooling" one. He warned her that if the leg did not quickly improve, it must be "cut." When the surgeon's poultice produced no favorable results, and "as she greatly dreaded an operation," she went to Dreyer, because "he cured without any cutting." Dreyer applied his poultice, and within twenty-four hours it had eaten two holes in her leg. He then set another plaster, and on the following day, there were four holes, "which opened up so rapidly that within a week she had a large cavity in her calf, into which she could thrust her whole hand." Terrified of losing the limb, she again showed it to Dreyer, who assured her that it was "nothing to fret about . . . [and] would soon improve." He then advised her "to apply as many plasters as were needed to fill the entire hole."

Two weeks later, the leg was noticeably worse: there was now "a hard white lump anchored in the hole, which within a week became fibrous." Although Dreyer excised this lump, it soon returned. Dreyer lifted it out once more, but the cavity in her leg got no smaller. After twenty-one weeks, she resolved to return to Dreyer no more, and went instead to the hospital surgeon, Eckermann, "who declared the wound incurable and wanted to have nothing to do with it." Since then she had been using home remedies, smearing the leg with salves and applying bran-mash poultices, which sometimes brought temporary improvement. She then appealed to the poor relief in Braunschweig for assistance and, under the care of the surgeon she had consulted earlier and Dr. Reitenmeyer, the leg seemed on the mend. She complained, however, that when she felt "internal paroxysms," the leg also worsened. At this point, she admitted that she "preferred to die" than have Dreyer touch her again. She had withstood "agonies" under his care. Each time he removed an old poultice, "a cloud of steam" rose up out of the wound, and when a new one was set on, it caused "shocking pain."[148]

In the treatment of ulcerated varices and stubborn sores, then, there was little to choose among what surgeons advised, what Dreyer did, and what doctors recommended. Almost all used or prescribed poultices. The Collegium medicum, too, could hardly dispute the *type* of treatment Dreyer applied, although it insisted that Dreyer's poultices were too harsh and, moreover, closed wounds "in an untimely fashion"—that is, before the poisons in them had had a chance to flow out.

The story of the upholsterer Busch offers another look at the medical practice of an eighteenth-century healer. The vast majority of Busch's clients voiced complete contentment. The victualer Koch related how Busch had cured his wife of a leg ulcer she had suffered from for over four years, and that various surgeons had failed to improve. Her testimony fleshed out the story. First, she had consulted a surgeon named Tättner for "a salt rheum" on her leg, but under his care, "it only worsened" by the day. She stopped seeing him and fell back on her own remedies, which were hardly better. Soon the leg was "nothing more than holes," one the size of her hand. Busch cured the leg within a year.[149] Johann Werner, a brass founder, likewise told how Busch had healed his 24-year-old son's chronic leg ulcer, and even produced a testimonial from the city surgeon Joseyli, who had been treating the youth for *ulceribus oedematoris* for more than three years. Joseyli judged the young man's constitution as "on the whole very unsound and cachectic."[150] J. C. Benoit, a language teacher, praised Busch for "extracting a large bone splinter from my thigh, which came from an old break and was festering," by applying external medicines only. When Benoit had fractured the leg, a long, thin sliver of bone became implanted in the flesh of his thigh, causing him frightful, unremitting pain. Benoit consulted the army surgeon Lehn, who operated on the leg "in such a way that it is now useless." Lehn predicted "that the fragment would eventually work itself out." Unconvinced, Benoit turned to Busch, "because he could not sit still for the agony." Busch's treatment eventually expelled the bone fragment from his leg. Lehn insisted that it would have done so anyway. Before seeing Busch, Benoit had also solicited advice from three other surgeons, with no appreciable results.[151]

The leather worker Martin Wendenberg detailed the history of his ailments and likewise related the pitiful tale of his experiences with other healers over the previous two years. In the fall of 1772, "a lump [appeared] on my spine . . . which in time grew much larger." The garrison physician Ralwes and the city surgeon Riesel both diagnosed a "growth" and advised that "it would be best to have it operated on." As Wendenberg rejected the idea of surgery out of hand, Ralwes prescribed medicines instead. "But as they produced no improvement," he discontinued their use and stopped seeing Ralwes and Riesel. Then, after reading in the newspaper "that a certain Busch could cure all cancers and fistulas (which was what he believed the lump to be) without cutting," he showed the mass to Busch, who quickly assured him that it was not cancerous, although he could do nothing until it "ripened and burst." About New Year's Day 1773, the lump, now the size of a human head and filled with purulent matter, broke open. Because Busch had accurately predicted this turn of events, Wendenberg's confidence in him increased. Busch again confirmed that "it presents no danger whatsoever," and irrigated the open wound. After two months under Busch's care, the wound seemed to be improving. The amelioration proved only temporary, however, and the thing soon deteriorated to its old perilous state. At this point, Busch curtailed his visits to Wendenberg, seeing him ever less frequently. Finally, Busch told Wendenberg that he had reached the limits of human help and only providence could aid him now. Wendenberg had not consulted a physician because Busch had told him it was unnecessary, but when the wound rapidly worsened, as inflammation set in, and as Wendenberg sensed "such a tightness in his chest that he thought he would suffocate," he began to look for other assistance. Eight days before Easter, Wendenberg dismissed Busch and returned to Ralwes, at the same time consulting the regimental feldsher Jürgens. On Easter Monday, Jürgens operated, greatly enlarged the existing opening and drained immense quantities of fluid from the mass. The constriction that had so perturbed Wendenberg vanished, but "now all his lower limbs were lame," and "he could taste in his mouth the very [fluid] that had been sprayed into the wound." He no longer entertained any hope of cure.[152]

A case similar to Wendenberg's, although with a happier ending, concerned a Lieutenant Schneebart, then administrator of an estate in Westphalia. Busch had cured his spinal fistula, and for over a year it had neither reappeared nor ruptured. "Busch did for me what not even the most skilled physicians had been able to do, although many have tortured me with their cutting."[153]

Myriad names referred to lumps and growths like those on Schneebart's and Wendenburg's spines. Very frequently, however, both physicians and the medical laity referred to them as swellings or tumors.[154] Such tumorous growths were viewed most often as excrescences of existing tissues and not as tumors as we today think of them. Still, their appearance, especially if sudden, their size, large, and their placement incommodious, always frightened. They could, of course, restrict movement, deform bodies, or threaten life. The commonest treatments aimed at getting the growth to open and empty out its peccant *materia*. Physicians might try medicines with a dispersing effect, while surgeons might propose incising the growth, or, if the patient refused to submit to the scalpel, apply cataplasms and poultices to draw the swelling to a head. A frequent home remedy with the same purpose was a mash poultice. And the terms used—"soften," "disperse," "open"—appeared in a widely diffused discourse on tumorous growths.[155]

People only imperfectly distinguished "cancers" and "cancerous growths" from other masses. The lack of a sensible linguistic distinction meant that early modern people did *not* necessarily regard what they termed "cancers" as incurable. "Cancer" in the early modern world almost always signified an external condition, heralded and manifested by a lump or swelling that persistently resisted excision and grew, often with horrifying speed. Internal cancers were simply unknown, and individual cases can probably be found under the vaguer, more generalized categories of wasting or cachexia. Treatments for cancers, therefore, strongly resembled those for tumors. The logic was almost identical, and those who handled benign lumps served just as frequently as cancer doctors.[156] Busch, for example, produced testimonials from some forty patients whom he had treated over sixteen years for "cancerous growths and fistulas."[157]

These afflictions could be truly appalling and, of course, intractable. Many healers specialized in such grievous cases, where the sufferer assumed that otherwise she or he must abandon hope. In 1751, three men in Braunschweig, a merchant, a brewer, and a saddler, petitioned the Collegium medicum to permit Seligman Joseph, a Jew from Hildesheim, to attend their ulcers and cancers. The merchant suffered from a tumor in his mouth, the brewer from a cancerous growth on his chin, and the poor saddler had "a festering, foul-smelling sore about four fingers wide and just as long on the back of the male member." Although the Collegium opposed granting Joseph even this limited concession, the privy council approved it, stipulating, however, that "the Jew should be explicitly warned that one knows how he has tried to drum up more business here and [seeks] to attract people to him with his deceitful boasts." Dr. Seebode (a member of the Collegium) was thus to supervise the three cases.[158]

Seebode's report on the treatment of the merchant Thies recounts Joseph's procedures in detail: "Behind the tongue, and on the right side near the opposite jawbone, there was a hole about a inch long and so deep that one could insert [the tip of his] little finger [into it]. On both sides of the tongue, near the molars, were several raised and tender places. The tumor was hard through and through. The glands and the blood vessels under the tongue were also involved."[159] Joseph painted the tumor with "a wound tincture, composed of Peruvian balsam dissolved in rectified spirits . . . with the addition of lemon peel." Seebode found in this mixture a white powder, "which seems to be a caustic substance." Joseph continued with this treatment for several weeks with appreciable improvement: the sore although somewhat redder was also smaller. What still remained of the growth, "the Jew detached with brush strokes and tweezers." The ulcers under the tongue were slowly closing. In addition to the tincture, Joseph applied a green salve composed of sublimated lead and a balsam of distilled oils. These he dabbed on with a brush. Soon the entire area under the tongue swelled and the tumor began to advance toward the front teeth; "the flesh of the gums formed a sort of sausage between the lower lip and the jaw, over which the lips were drawn tight as a drumhead." Joseph explained that he wanted the tumor "to work its way out of the mouth," so when he treated the mass he stroked it from back to front. Whenever a bit of flesh loosened or protruded, he extracted it with a pair of tweezers or with scissors. The lump in the front of the mouth sat firmly in the gum, and Joseph attempted to reduce it with a poultice. During the two weeks he applied the packing, the entire area of the lower jaw begin to bulge out to the side, becoming hard and extremely tender. Sheer agony prevented the patient from sleeping at night. Then "the Jew placed on the outside [of the jaw] a compress and sought thereby to bring the painful spot to a head."

Several weeks passed, and the merchant's health deteriorated. The tumor was larger, and three holes had appeared in the soft tissues. "And although much pus flows from the [various] cavities, the tumor continues to grow and [now] prevents the mouth from closing, leaving an opening two fingers wide" between the upper and lower lips. Joseph now tried to banish the swelling using "softening poultices."[160]

Commoner than such truly horrifying and cruelly deforming tumors, but often equally distressing, were breast lumps. Again, people had many names for them. Breast cancers indicated serious, life-threatening conditions, while "breast sore" ran the gamut from tender nipples to mastitis to hard fibroids of impressive size. The line dividing the two categories was imprecisely drawn. Not surprisingly, Busch's competence in treating cancers extended to breast cancers. A. M. Dörrien from Closter St. Crucis related how Busch had cured "a 70-year-old woman of a dangerous cancer on her breast." She had previously consulted two feldshers, who felt a mastectomy was her only hope. As she "so feared" any "cutting," however, she went to Busch.[161] Likewise, when the wife of the locksmith Johann Zackschwendt noticed a discharge from her nipples during her lying-in, her husband first consulted the surgeon Wolfgang, who successfully dried up the flow. When a few weeks later, she discovered a hard lump in her breast, Busch diagnosed it as a cancer and cured it in a few weeks without "cutting."[162]

Fear of "cutting" was, of course, in no way misplaced. Only a few

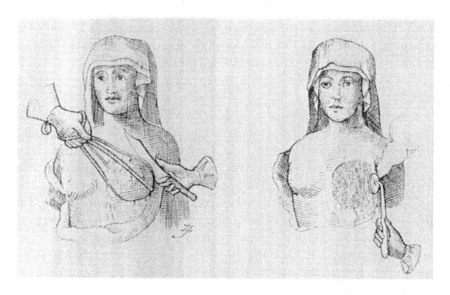

Illustration of a mastectomy procedure. Reproduced with the permission of the Wellcome Institute Library, London.

women could be persuaded to submit to a breast operation, and many understandably preferred Busch precisely because he promised to clear up their breast sores or extirpate their cancers without inflicting the pains and dangers of surgery on them. Often an operation was a success, but the patient died. One such case involved the company feldsher Wendt in Braunschweig. He had "successfully" removed a cancer from the breast of a cook. "It went on so auspiciously that I, with God's help, have a certain hope that I shall see the patient restored [to health] shortly." Dr. Brückmann had advised surgery and regarded the operation as relatively minor, "demanding no particular skill." Unfortunately, within two weeks, "tetanus accompanied by lockjaw" struck the woman, and she died. Brückmann felt this tragic outcome could not be blamed on the operation but "rather could probably be attributed to a chill [she recently] received."[163]

If breast "cancers" were the most grievous of these afflictions, other breast sores and injuries often stubbornly resisted domestic treatments. For mastitis, tenderness, and raw nipples, nursing women often rubbed their breasts with butter or oil, or applied wet compresses combining butter, wax, rose water, and spirits.[164] Busch, too, used poultices to reduce the "scirrhous lumps" Frau Bökel developed in both breasts while suckling her son. Her husband had first consulted Dr. Heyn, whose medicines had no appreciable effect. He then went to Busch, "as the other surgeons charge too much." Busch asked a fee of only 2½ thaler for his attendance, which lasted over four weeks. Similarly, Busch cured the blacksmith Raazener's wife of "a scirrhoid milk gland." Here, too, the couple had first seen a surgeon, who "advocated all manner of things, which were, however, too costly and too troublesome." Busch advised a balm, which did the trick.[165] Likewise, Johann Halme explained how three months after his wife's last confinement, she had fallen ill with a "hectic bilious fever . . . in which a dangerous thing appeared on her breast. She became very weak and [the knot] grew very hard and [the entire breast] was covered with blisters." He first brought Dr. Ralwes in to see his wife, but after five days of his care, they turned to Busch. Under Busch's hand, "the lump ripened in two days, and within ten weeks the entire cure had been accomplished."[166]

As common as breast masses, and somewhat in the same category as lumps and "hardenings," were anal fistulas and hemorrhoids. Home remedies and surgeons' recommendations overlapped here as well. Commonly endorsed were enemas of cold water or water mixed with sugar or mild emollients, compresses made of soothing substances like chamomile, and salves or sitz baths to diminish the pain and itching. After suffering for many years from "a hard tumor on his anus that came from his piles and oozed with a salt rheum," the agent Franz Meyer took his woes to Busch, whose fomentations cured him "thoroughly" in about nine months. Meyer was much relieved, since "for a long time he had not even been able to close his eyes because he itched so badly." A musketeer named Hinrich Dahlen suffered from a rectal fistula that threatened to curtail his military career. Busch brought him round to where "he is now able to carry out his duties without the least 'incommodation.' "[167]

Hemorrhoids were generally thought to arise from a congested "golden vein," resulting from a suppression of the periodic issuance of blood, which supposedly was as necessary to the balance of the humors in men as was regular menstruation in women. Clogged hemorrhoidal flows therefore portended and accompanied more ominous illnesses.[168] In 1750, the bathmaster and barber-surgeon Albers treated another surgeon in Wolfenbüttel, named Brauer. The man had been sick for eleven weeks, and the most notable of his symptoms was that "his hemorrhoids were stopped up." Albers administered medicines including "drops containing opium . . . [and] also rubbing oils and several powders." Brauer soon stopped taking them, however, "because the medicines did not take hold in his case." Ceasing to seek medical help, he thereafter "decline[d] daily with a wasting disease and the hemorrhoids sometimes [bled] freely and sometimes cease[d]."[169] Brauer suffered, in Albers's words, from "constipation of the piles," for which Albers had him drink a draught containing sarsaparilla and cinnamon.[170]

By the same token, abnormal menses also signaled wider corporal disorders, and women often complained of dysmenorrhea and amenorrhea. Elisabeth Erben, a 22-year-old maidservant, consulted the bathmaster Claus because "her monthly courses have been irregular for quite some time." Several people told her that "dangerous consequences" could result from erratic periods, so "she took the idea to be bled from the foot," thus drawing the blood downwards to its proper outlet. After Claus opened a vein, he told her that her blood was "very impure." He gave her a tea to "restore her blood to its former condition." She drank one cup of the tea, but did not continue using it because "it tasted vile."[171]

Of course, the expressed desire of regaining one's menses might be a woman's veiled attempt to break off an unwanted pregnancy. It is hard to tell to what extent women who complained of irregularities in their menstrual cycles may have been consciously or subconsciously seeking abortions. The case of Johanna Hagemeister illustrates this, as well as her own perception of what was happening with and within her body. Johanna Uder, the wife of the executioner's assistant, had supposedly furnished her with an abortifacient. Hagemeister told Uder that she was "uncertain . . . if she were pregnant or not," yet insisted that she "assuredly" had never wished "either to conceal it or [had] the criminal intent . . . to use a medicine to rid herself of the fruit of her womb." Rumor reported Frau Uder to be "very good at correcting *suppressione menstrorum*." Hagemeister showed her urine to Uder, who concluded that she was not pregnant, and that "gas caused the small movements she kept feeling [in her gut]," and that her menses would reappear without fail after taking Uder's potion. For some reason, however, Hagemeister became suspicious and showed the medicine to Dr. Paulus, who analyzed it and found "a powerful, heating abortifacient," which he identified as oil of turpentine.[172]

In 1802, the magistrates in Braunschweig accused the wife of the soldier Knieriem of peddling abortifacients to several women. The apothecary who examined the suspicious compound found it composed of "completely harmless materials." Yet he believed that such basically innocuous ingredients could, "if used at an inopportune moment or in an intemperate manner, provoke extremely injurious reactions." Frau Knieriem maintained her tonic combated heat prostration and "worked excellently when someone who was overheated drank [too] cold a beverage." In 1796, she sold it to the daughter of an ammonia distiller named Schreib. The young woman told how "she had the misfortune to have slept with a tanner's apprentice and been impregnated by him." However, "because she was ignorant of the signs of pregnancy," she believed herself ill. When she began to feel peculiar pains around New Year, she sent her sister to Frau Knieriem "in order to learn from her" what was wrong. After listening to the sister's account, Frau Knieriem diagnosed a "festering" tumor and gave her some medicine. The next day when her "dreadful pains" began, Fräulein Schreib ascribed them to the action of the medicine. "But Frau Knieriem said that the fruit was now dead, and that she should neither take more of the medicine nor allow a physician to see it." Frau Knieriem then supposedly confided to the sister that "if she had come to her sooner, she could have aborted the fetus without any danger, as she had previously done for the daughter of the rope maker Decker, but now, however, it was already too late." The next day the young woman delivered a healthy child.

Although the Collegium medicum found that the drink had apparently "no deleterious effects" on either mother or child, still "it cannot be denied that in this way the forbidden contact between male and female would be made easier, if a maid only knew that it was completely within her power to rid herself of the unpleasant results of her prohibited behavior through the help of such women [as Frau Knieriem]." The magistrates imprisoned Frau Knieriem for three days. And when a young woman later died in Bisperode while giving birth, the authorities suspected an attempted abortion, inasmuch as the young woman had concealed her pregnancy and reportedly taken a drink from "a certain woman [Knieriem], who cooked it up in a new pot."[173]

Women seeking to be rid of their unwanted pregnancies and adults with disabilities and chronic disorders were not the only ones who sought assistance outside the narrow circle of family and friends. Parents often brought their children to Busch, but also to many other healers, including physicians, to alleviate conditions or resolve injuries that incapacitated or disfigured them, even if they did not threaten life. When the ducal coachman Gremmer discovered a suspicious mass in the leg of his 3-year-old son, he first went to Busch, who diagnosed a bone cancer, and cured it in three months. Somewhat later, the same child developed joint evil in his right elbow. The mother took the child to the regimental feldsher, who treated him for about six months "without effect," and then Busch's poultices returned the distended joint to near normal size within a year. In neither case had the parents consulted a physician.[174]

The outcome in the case of a swineherd's 16-year-old son was less felicitous. In 1775, the boy had sustained a severe blow to his knee, and the local pastor advised the father to see Busch. Busch medicated the boy "from Johannis until the summer fair," but his cure "would not take hold." The swineherd then traveled to Braunschweig to consult the hospital surgeon Eckermann, who attended the youth through the end of the year without improvement: "The leg is no better and my son needs a crutch to get around."

Or, take the case of a child with a smashed finger and fractured arm that Busch had failed to help, but that under Eckermann's care "obviously improved," to the point where it was almost completely healed "except for a small opening, and the finger, after a few pieces of corroded bone found their way out, is once again sound."[175]

As many of these cases demonstrate, the distinction between internal and external was by no means a hard and fast one. Serious internal disturbances frequently manifested themselves externally. While physicians maintained their exclusive right to treat some external ailments because they had *internal* causes, surgeons argued their right to internal medicine in order to handle certain *external* problems properly. The mix and the mix-ups were very common. A porter's wife who reputedly "shat herself to death" had taken pills from the bathmaster Albers. Her husband testified that his wife had died of a fever, "and she also had a tumor in her head that had broken through the roof of her mouth." The first surgeon they consulted "wanted to give her nothing and said he could do naught to help her." The husband then heard from several people that the bathmaster in Broistedt, that is, Albers, "had good advice for fever cases, and he had successfully cared for a young girl with fever." Albers prescribed five pills for the woman, telling her to take one a day. Before she took the pills, however, the fever abated, but she took them anyway "and then became worse and the day after taking the fourth pill she went into convulsions and died."[176]

The surgeon Rüland's practice likewise moved across the external/ internal line. The mortality lists revealed that Rüland had been asked to help the wife of the cottager Heinrich Bithaus. Bithaus explained that about the end of November, his wife had without warning lost all mobility in her left hand, the result of what he believed was a stroke. Three days later, he went to the surgeon Rüland and asked him to prescribe something for her. Rüland told him that "his wife's affliction must be cured internally" and gave him a prescription, which Bithaus had filled by an apothecary in Wolfenbüttel. His wife swallowed the medicine for three days in succession with no results, and Bithaus returned to Rüland for additional help. Before she had consumed half of Rüland's second mixture, "she suffered a complete paralysis of her left side from head to toe," and after lying "witless" for an entire day, she expired. Rüland had visited the woman daily and applied a blister of Spanish fly to her paralyzed arm and leg. The widower evidently did not blame Rüland for his wife's demise, because when his second wife was in labor some years later, he called Rüland to her bedside, and yet this wife, too, died.[177]

This final case also raises questions about how people tended to assign guilt for cures that went wrong. The above evidence does not prove that Bithaus regarded the deaths of his two wives with apathy or disinterest; rather, he seems to have recognized that in some instances, such as stroke or childbirth, no one could do much. The surgeon's diligence, persistent attendance, and obvious concern convinced Bithaus that Rüland was properly assiduous and competent. Similarly, the widow of the cottager Christoph Heinstedt felt Rüland bore little if any responsibility for the death of her husband from a chest disease. Upon first falling ill, her husband had gone to see Dr. Bucking in Wolfenbüttel without delay. When the medicines he prescribed had no effect, "her husband lost his trust in this doctor and did not want to take anything more from him," so he went to Rüland. Rüland gave him some medicine. "[A]fter taking it, he felt neither better nor worse," but he subsequently died.[178] About the same time, an infant of some fifteen months expired under Rüland's care. Its mother related that her child had been sickly since birth and had recently suffered so severely from diarrhea that she held little hope of its recovery. A few days before the child died, it had "much internal heat," for which Rüland prescribed beet extract, which seemed to reduce his fever at least temporarily. Clearly, she did not see Rüland as the cause of her child's death.[179]

Nonetheless, it is equally plain that parents did not face the deaths and illnesses of their children with stoic fortitude. They took great pains to alleviate the miseries of their offspring and consulted healers even for very young children, often those just days old. The surgeon Varges in Benneckenstein built up what almost might be called a pediatric specialty, treating numerous children for internal ailments in the 1790s and early 1800s. In 1794, Varges cared for a 2-year-old child with convulsions whose father was the woodcutter Andreas Hahnen. In October 1801, Varges was seeing the infant daughter (aged 4½ months) of the notions merchant Treumann. When the child eventually succumbed to "convulsions and wasting," its mother testified that he was not the only healer she had sought out during her daughter's long illness. She had obtained internal medicines from an apothecary when the child was racked by intense cramps and severely jaundiced. She had asked for advice from Dr. Schulze, physicus for Walkenried, when he briefly visited her village of Hohengeiß. He prescribed a mixture, which reduced the jaundice but intensified the convulsions. She herself had been seeing Varges for a sore on her leg, "and when conferring with him about this external ailment . . . asked his advice" about the girl. He took a look at the child and prescribed a purge for it, "but nothing wanted to help."[180]

The stories of Büsch, Albers, Dreyer, Joseph, Rüland, and Varges illustrate what healers did. All of these men were permitted to practice medicine in some form or another. All of them overstepped boundaries. Those infringements, however, concern us less here than why people turned to them, what they expected from them, and why they judged their cures good or not. We have observed that most frequently, these practitioners handled surgical cases. The conditions that brought them patients were generally chronic or intractable injuries and afflictions that refused to yield to home remedies and also resisted the standard treatments of surgeons and physicians. Many of the ailments mixed internal and external characteristics. Especially frequent were work-related accidents, such as the repeated injuries suffered by the teamster or the crushed foot of the shoemaker. These refused to heal or inflicted great pain, as did the broken thigh that never mended satisfactorily. Infirmities that interfered with the ability to work, such as anal fistulas and hemorrhoids, were common. Ulcerated leg varices appeared so often as to be almost unremarkable, yet they were especially hard to heal owing to a synergy of poor circulation, insufficient nutrition, and repeated injury.[181] Mastitis and many other breast complaints proved notoriously obdurate, and they understandably caused considerable consternation. Just as worrisome were the various fistulas, tumors, and other growths, whose appearance portended an uncomfortable and bleak future. Small fistulas and tumors were awkward and unsightly, but Wendenberg's spinal mass the size of a human head, the growth that broke through the woman's soft palate, and the merchant

Thies's oral tumor were life-threatening dangers, as well as horribly disfiguring. Thus, chronicity, pain, and lack of hope (for children as well as adults) drove people from one healer to another and fed the business of cobblers like Dreyer and upholsterers like Busch, whose cures were perceived as (and probably were) no less effective than those of other practitioners. Of course, what Busch, Dreyer and so many others did deviated hardly at all from "standard" treatments: poultices, fomentations, tinctures, cauterants, balms, and salves were therapeutic standbys in the armamentaria of surgeons and physicians. Dreyer used his "secret" poultice on Frau Meyer, but Dr. Heym had previously prescribed "herbal packs and cataplasms," as did the surgeon she later consulted. Yet Busch, Dreyer, and the others offered something many surgeons did not: they promised to cure without cutting. Frau Meyer, who suffered true martyrdom under Dreyer's care, greatly feared an operation and was drawn to Dreyer because he did not perform surgery. Busch, too, benefited from the terror surgery evoked. Lieutenant Schneebart remarked how Busch cured his spinal fistula without operating, after surgeons had so often "tortured" him. Busch successfully removed the bone splinter from Benoit's leg "using external medicines only," after the surgeon Lehn "lamed me with his butchery." People consulted healers like Busch and Dreyer less frequently for internal afflictions, although surgeons like Albers and Rüland seem to have practiced internal and external medicine indiscriminately, often prescribing medications for internal use as well as applying external physical treatments. Apparently, many surgeons shied away from surgical procedures because their patients resisted them strongly or because they themselves disliked them and dreaded the unhappy outcomes that too often resulted.[182]

The long-term quests of such patients, as they moved from healer to healer, convincingly show that they indeed pursued cures. It has often been argued that early modern people did not really expect healers to banish their ailments completely, hoping rather to find alleviation of pain, to confirm their own diagnoses, or to understand their prognosis. But in the cases analyzed here, it is plain that patients primarily aspired to a restoration of health. They wanted more than palliatives and reassurance, although some may well have settled for and sought both from their healers. Because various treatments refused to "take hold," sufferers moved from one healer to the next. Yet, they often stuck with one treatment and with one person for extended periods. Perhaps what most impresses the observer here is how long people were willing to wait for a cure. Frau

Meyer used several healers and bore with them for a total of over three years. Then she stayed with Dreyer for twenty-one weeks, despite undergoing "agony" each time he set a poultice to her leg. Martin Wendenburg employed a number of surgeons in the two years during which his spinal tumor kept getting bigger before turning to Busch. Busch treated him for at least two months, and then he finally, resignedly, went to another surgeon. It took over a year and a half and the combined efforts of a regimental feldsher and Busch to reduce the elbow of Gremmer's son. Such willingness to hold to treatments that were long and painful indicates something important about the expectations people had. The quest to regain health—to reduce a swollen limb, to heal a stubborn ulcer, to ripen a tumor, or clear up a fistula—was perceived and accepted as a protracted one. Patients did not necessarily anticipate rapid cures (as physicians often accused them of doing), yet the hope of cure was only seldom, and most unwillingly, relinquished.

The Medical Encounter

Each medical treatment produced its own "encounter," a moment and a space of interchange between patient and healer, and of both with a larger public of friends, relatives, acquaintances, and authorities. Some scholars have described this encounter as a theatrical performance possessing its own rituals, rhythms, and dramaturgy. I believe, however, that the medical encounter can best be comprehended as a "play within a play," and one whose gestures and motions make sense only when situated within the greater dramatic settings of community, state, and society. Thus it is to these larger structures that we must look for explanations of medical choice.[183]

The dynamics of the medical encounter could be complicated and draw many people into its plot and action. In Chapter 3, we met the widow Asmus, whose practice the Collegium medicum vainly struggled to halt in the 1790s. The case of Hans Behrens, who died after using Asmus's medicines, begins a discussion of the medical encounter by looking at its opening scene: the form "the way to a healer" took. The encounter was already far advanced when the practitioner and patient first met, whether face-to-face, by letter, or through a messenger. There could well be a prologue to the action: earlier rumors, previous knowledge, the accumulated experience of friends and relatives, or a vague, floating but nevertheless crucial "good reputation."

Behrens's widow and his son explained what happened when the cottager took ill:

He had long been ailing. As he had little money, he would not allow them to obtain medicines from a regular physician, and did not at all want to take anything whatsoever. . . . They asked him if he did not wish to speak once more to his brother, Johann Behrens, a cottager in Sambleben, and he answered, "No." But his son went secretly to his uncle, carrying with him some of the deceased's urine. [The uncle] traveled to Schöningen with the urine and showed it to a woman, who, as far as they could remember, was called the Asmus (and he [the uncle] had already more than once gotten medicines from her that soon fixed him up). She gave him . . . three powders and something in a glass, which was to be dissolved in wine . . . [and] for which he paid 18 groschen. The deceased consumed only two of the powders, and they threw the third out after his death.

Asmus admitted only that "someone" from Sambleben had come to see her, "who, however, asked for no medicine, but only wanted to know what his sick brother in Hötzum lacked." Asmus's daughter-in-law recalled, however, that "the previous year at harvest time," a stranger had come to the house, identified himself as a carpenter, and requested to speak to her mother-in-law. The daughter-in-law could not say if Mother Asmus had handed him anything or not. The man returned eight days later, and the daughter-in-law then denied him access to the old woman's room. The brother of the deceased told a somewhat different story. He said that his brother "had sent his nephew to him, [asking him] to go to Schöningen and procure medicines from Asmus." He then went to her, showed her his brother's urine, and she had ordered her nurse (Asmus was ill and bedridden) to take "a reddish powder" out of the bedroom cupboard for his brother.[184]

The Behrens/Asmus case illustrates how people habitually constructed histories of illness. The story of taking ill and seeking help paced the other cadences of life. People sought healers where they went to market, solicited advice from those who gave it in other instances, and blended health and illness into the familiar pulse of life. In illness, as in social, financial, and political affairs, friends and relatives were the primary consultants and helpers. Behrens's son went with the father's urine to his uncle, and the uncle made the decision about whom to consult: Frau Asmus. Asmus's daughter-in-law identified the visitor, not by name, but as a carpenter who had appeared "at harvest time."

The way to a healer was paved with coincidence, accident, and hearsay. The recommendations of others, which could play a pivotal role, depended on their rank and relationship to the sufferer, as well as on how many of them there were. (As we have seen, Martin Wendenberg sought out a healer because he read about him in the newspaper.) In a typical case, when his son became feverish, the day laborer Otto consulted the miller Claudiz, "because he had recently heard that many people went to Claudiz and let him give them medicines, and thus he did the same." He presented the boy's urine to the miller, who diagnosed "fever and chills" and sold him drops for 10 groschen. While at the mill, Otto had seen there "a number of strangers who also wanted medicines." At first the boy responded well "and could go back into service," but eight days later the fever recurred. His father then turned to Dr. Schmidt in Schöningen and forsook Claudiz.[185]

Participants could misinterpret when and where a medical encounter started and stopped. Partly this was because they did not neatly separate medical events from other day-to-day routines. When the surgeon Beierstedt in Vechelde treated Frau Bargdorf and her son for what Beierstedt called a bilious fever, he gave them "[an] emetic, also a whitish medicine in a small bottle, then a reddish medicine, [and] from the last she was to take one tablespoon every two hours." (Medicines were rarely named: it was "something," or "three powders in a glass," or designated by color—red powders and green liquids were especially popular.) At the same meeting, she told him that her 14-year-old son "had overheated himself, and since then was usually feverish in the afternoons." For him, Beierstedt prescribed another vomit and a "red medicine," which cost 12 groschen. Beierstedt asked 1 thaler for the medicines he had given her "and for an [additional] two bottles [filled] with spirits that she got from him after receiving a blow."[186]

Beierstedt's account followed another story line. Frau Bargdorff came to him complaining of "pain and stiffness in all her joints." He denied diagnosing a fever. He dispensed an emetic and "something to raise a sweat." The last was "a harmless compound" of two grams of camphor dissolved in *spiritus nitri dolcis* and half a dram of *gummi arabicum*. Because she complained that she had lost her appetite, he gave her stomach drops made of *essentia mara* sweetened with syrup. He felt she was suffering from a cold. Her son also had the sniffles and a bad cough, for which Beierstedt advised some licorice dissolved in water and an emetic.[187] Room for misapprehension existed here. Possibly Bargdorff had listed all her ailments, while Beierstedt felt that he was only being consulted for her arthritic symptoms. This is only one indication of how blurry the boundaries dividing the medical encounter from the rest of life were.

Frau Eimke's case provides a better illustration. The journeyman feldsher and bathmaster in Jerxheim, a fellow named Traub, insisted that she had never really asked him to medicate her. Rather she "had spoken to him about a nosebleed on the way to church." He advised her to sniff vinegar and ammonia, and, when the bleeding recurred, suggested a "purifying tea" to thin her blood. He believed she suffered from greensickness (iron-deficiency anemia, or chlorosis) and "a wasting fever," and knew that Dr. Mühlenbein in Schöningen was treating the latter. This medical encounter occurred almost completely within the framework of another social ceremony: going to church.[188]

Hearsay, reputation, and rumor—and not just in medical matters—drew many patients to healers. The son of the schoolmaster Bonhorst in Eitzum had been bothered for over three years with "much discharge from his eyes and sores on them both. . . . [which are] so bad that he cannot see," when his father heard "that a certain person named von Brandstedt worked 'marvels' and was to be found at Kenne's farm." When Bonhorst went to find Brandstedt, about twenty people stood waiting to consult him. Brandstedt promised to "help everyone" but said he had to see the child first. After examining the boy, he pronounced the eye complaint a trifle that one treatment would clear up. He sold the schoolmaster drops to be taken internally and an oil to swab directly on both eyes. These medicines did not, however, have the desired effect; rather, "after he had given the child the medicine a few times, he suffered terrible anxiety, his eyes were as thickly crusted as before, pus flowed from them, and his legs became so swollen and filled with holes, that he let the medicine alone." He then consulted the local physicus.[189]

At that time, Brandstadt had been living in the village of Timmern near Wolfenbüttel for several years. In 1771, the Collegium medicum reported that "the reputation of this man spreads more and more widely among the public and especially among the simple-minded," and that he had acquired the aura of a "miracle worker." "The trust of some people in this 'wonder man' is so great," the Collegium continued, that people were willing to pay him his fee in advance, and "his boasting so deceives them that they believe he can cure them even as they are drawing their last breath."[190] While the Collegium is hardly an impartial witness here, a healer's fame, reputation for good character, and the perception that "all acknowledge his [or her] skill" were thought valid reasons for seeking his or her assistance.

Both medical and surgical problems drew patients to the surgeon Vögler in Jerxheim. One of his clients in 1788, the blacksmith Müller, explained his illness as a bilious fever that had already confined him to his bed for seven weeks. "As he heard so many people both in Gevensleben as well as in Winnigstedt praise the surgeon Vögler as a skillful man," he decided to consult him. Vögler visited him several times and also sent him medicines, but Müller's recovery proceeded very slowly. Each time he felt well enough to climb out of bed, he relapsed. He could not say how much he paid Vögler in all, but each dose of medicines cost between 12 and 18 groschen. Then the pastor recommended he procure a certain powder from Braunschweig, and the use of it "fully returned my health to me."[191]

Or take the story of a cottager in Destedt who said he was afflicted with "stitch in the side" (perhaps pleurisy?). He dispatched his sister-in-law to Braunschweig to obtain medicines for him and gave her some of his urine in a flask. Upon entering Braunschweig, "she approached a man she met on the street, whom she did not otherwise know, and asked where a clever doctor could be found." He answered that "she would do best if she went to a soldier named Lange . . . who had already accomplished many important cures [in the city]." Lange diagnosed a chest inflammation from the urine. At the time, Lange was serving as a soldier in the garrison and had become quite celebrated in the surrounding countryside for his "unfailing successes." A woman from Salzdahlum explained why she went to Lange: "This person is everywhere known as a skillful doctor, and for a long time he has taken on diverse cases in Klein Stöckheim that have all had happy outcomes." Consequently, when her husband fell ill, she scurried off to Lange for medicines, "but as her spouse had a natural disgust for all drugs," he refused to take them. Although her husband died, she later consulted Lange herself when suffering from the disease that "recently raged [here] in Stöckheim . . . [and] people were completely stupid in the head with it." Lange visited her in her home and dosed her with a mixture that quickly restored her health. She paid 8 groschen for the concoction, and "he took nothing for the visit."[192]

Repeatedly, patients praised healers who accepted money only for material things—mixtures, powders, teas—or for physical services—bleeding, cupping, setting blisters—and who refused money for their advice and visits. It seems that while the first were easily seen as requiring monetary recompense (or perhaps payment in kind), medical advice was only more slowly commodified and continued to be seen more as a gift or type of social exchange than a market item. For example, when the medical practice of the hospital administrator Oettinger aroused the wrath of the surgeons' guild, he did not lack for defenders. Several of these, such as the notary Johann Faber, expressed their satisfaction with Oettinger in terms of the effectiveness of his treatments *and* as a function of social reciprocity. Faber explained that "Oettinger was his neighbor and good friend. When he [Faber] was weak and able to earn but little . . . he requested Oettinger to blister him with Spanish fly. He informed Oettinger that . . . he would not be able to pay him. Oettinger accepted this, and also treated him a few months later under similar circumstances." When the Collegium medicum pointed out to Faber that others, licensed surgeons among them, would also have taken him on pro bono, or that the magistrates would have drawn on poor relief funds to pay for his cure, he stuck by his preference for "a friend."[193] Faber and others valued Oettinger as much for his qualities of neighborliness as for his facility in healing. And when the wife of the merchant Habich in Helmstedt injured herself in a fall, her husband consulted a medical student "because he had known him for eight years and was a good companion [of his]."[194]

And those who failed to live up to commonly held expectations might be accused of quackery. The village of Voightsdahlum had long shielded the widow Hagen from prosecution, despite the repeated complaints of the physicus and apothecary, as long as she charged money only for her (by no means inexpensive) teas and herbs. Once she began to demand payment for visiting patients, however, complaints multiplied. Her support sifted away and, quite atypically, several of her neighbors denounced her to the Collegium medicum.[195] In both cases here, medical assistance was apparently not deemed a legitimate part of a commercial or monetary transaction.

Trust once gained was not quickly lost, and even cures that ended unhappily could reinforce faith in a healer. When the 9-year-old daughter of a day laborer fell ill with a diarrhea that continued for more than three weeks, her father requested medicines from Lange. Then, when her older sister "had it in her limbs," the father returned to Lange, whose medicines set her right. When she relapsed into an ardent fever, the father took her urine to Lange, who prescribed another mixture. This did little good, and she soon was troubled with "great pain in her belly and chest." Lange merely "shrugged his shoulders and assured [her father] that it was [the same] malevolent disease that had already killed seventeen people." This time his medicines failed utterly, and the young woman died two days later. The father did not hold Lange accountable for this tragic outcome. He felt that the diagnosis had been accurate, and that little could have been done for her.[196]

A similar story from Niederfreden involved a consumptive woman cursed with a barking cough. Her husband, a cottager, related how his wife's sickness had lasted since Pentecost (it was then late summer or early fall). He believed her illness came from "becoming chilled [while she] bleached the linen cloth" he wove. She had been under Dr. Rudelstädter's care for about three months. When the medicines prescribed remained "completely without effect," her husband turned to an old woman in nearby Oberfreden "whom people endorsed as a clever person, and, as far as he knew, was called the Mittelbacksche woman." She diagnosed consumption and advised a decoction of foxtail. His wife should also "bind a flannel cloth [doused] with camphor on her left side, where she often had sharp pains." These methods produced some improvement, but when his wife continued to hack, "he resolved not to return to the Mittelbacksche again."[197]

The joiner Peters in Bortfeld treated two cases of self-diagnosed ague. The father of a 19-year-old man bought powders from Peters that relieved his son's symptoms. He knew that the inhabitants of Bortfeld often consulted Peters and had heard that several sufferers from fevers had swallowed Peters's powders to good effect. Two of these subsequently denied going to Peters, however. Rather, they had used home remedies. One said he had "helped himself in that he beat a fresh egg in vinegar and then drank it down." This unpalatable brew produced a cure.[198]

These stories show how medical encounters flowed out of wider social and cultural currents. Not surprisingly, people valued and heeded the advice and encouragement of friends and relatives, and these same friends and relatives often served as trusted intermediaries. They, rather than the patient, were often the ones physically present at the medical encounter as bearers of tales or glasses of urine. They mediated, translated, and interpreted from both sides. Not infrequently, they actually picked the healer, or that decision devolved on persons—messengers, maidservants, even passing strangers—who would at first seem extraneous, or only marginal. Geographical realities may in part account for this. Many healers lived far from patients. Another, more speculative answer may lie in the fact that such mediations were givens in the larger transactional world people inhabited: one sent relatives to do business, maidservants and farmhands to shop, relied on hearsay and gossip as ways of learning and of making decisions. Thus a special time of ritual or a special dramaturgy of cure seem not to have existed in most medical encounters; rather, they were set in broader and denser networks that incorporated several kinds of actions and relationships. One might, however, expect to find a larger dramaturgical element in the realm of sympathetic or magical healing.

How Much Magic?

Although there is scant evidence of magical or sympathetic cures, a few cases show how such healers practiced, as well as indicating how people might combine magical or sympathetic cures in serial consultations. The physicus in Stadtoldendorf, admittedly a hostile witness, related the doings of a blind, sympathetic "wonder man" in the village of Lobach near the cloister of Amelunxborn:

A truly extraordinary medicaster has taken up quarters in a tavern [here] . . . and promises to cure with his fabulous method all the people who flock to his door in great numbers. Several years ago he traveled through this area preaching to the people to earn his living. When that failed, the evangelist became a medicaster. . . . The person afflicted must undress. He feels the pulse in the temples, and in the forehead, then he shakes first one arm then the other, stroking the blood from the armpit to the elbow, feels for the pulse there, and also touches the chest cavity. Then [he announces] that the patient has a rheum or catarrh in the head, the chest, or in the abdomen, and at first for this they gave him 1 groschen, yet as his popularity has grown out of all proportion, he now charges 3 groschen. If he tells them what medicines they should use, it costs another 12 groschen. . . . The rich as well as poor . . . go to him for advice.[199]

The razzmatazz of show business constituted part of his method, but his examinations were not so unusual, and the medicines he prescribed were common ones. Nor were his diagnoses bizarre. Physicians, too, blamed rheums and catarrhs for much sickness.

Surgical as well as medical cases could be thought to yield to sympathy. The miller Käseberg in Bettmar "for many years now [has healed] cancers and fistulas with benedictions." He combined sympathetic and physical means, relying on the experience brought him by "long years of study" and his knowledge of herbs. He added that "my income is such that it is not necessary to earn my living with healing," thus exculpating himself of any mercenary motives.[200]

Not all sympathetic healers deployed physical or natural means as part

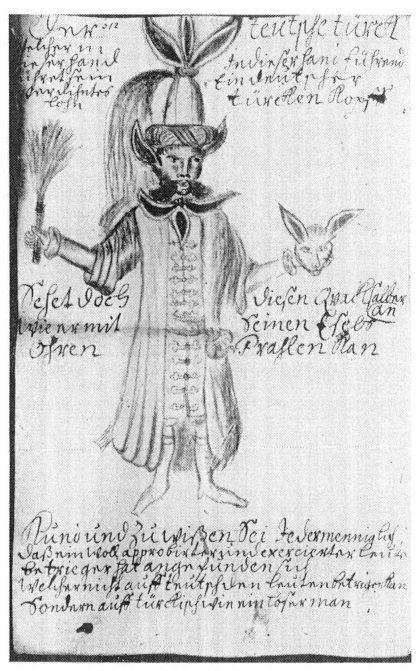

Pencil drawing of a "quack" dressed in Turkish garb, 18th century. StadtB, C II 3, fol. 14. Reproduced with the permission of the Stadtarchiv Braunschweig.

of their therapeutics. Heinrich Kelling in Salder promised "to restore *in integrum* all the feeble-minded and lame, or those afflicted with cancers and other vile afflictions by using two rusty knives and God's help." Kelling regaled his listeners with the marvelous story of how an angel appeared to him and presented him with the blades. One person related that "[t]he sick person, female as well as male, must unclothe himself entirely. . . . Then Kelling begins to swing the old knives in the air, moving nearer and nearer to the patient until he feels either a chill or a flush. This he repeats [with each patient] several times."[201]

Likewise, if less theatrically, the horse doctor Heine practiced his sympathetic cures on man and beast alike. For a chest wound, he employed "no medicines whatsoever, but banished St. Anthony's fire from it by blessing the patient." He handled a running sore on a child's knee sympathetically as well, and when called upon to treat a carbuncle, first opened it with a small knife and then "drove it away by sympathetic means." He also cured a fistula "sympathetically, without any medicines" on a man who had suffered with this affliction for twenty-two years.[202]

Although the number of magical cures that have come to light were few, these several instances show that curing and magic still sometimes fell together, as, for instance, in the case of the horse-doctor Hans Thiele, who stood accused of dosing humans with his equine medicines. He had already sullied his reputation with the authorities, who, a decade earlier, had punished him for "the blasphemous use of God's name as a means to discover who had stolen a fish trap."[203] Yet not all those who peddled their sympathetic cures found a ready audience. A general visitation in the Harz in 1768 turned up "a certain tramp" named von Campen. According to the physicus, the inhabitants used his self-made medications frequently. Yet the report of the Amt Langelsheim on this vagabond presented another picture of his practice, reducing his crime to laughable dimensions by indicating that gullible acceptance was not the only response such "wonder men" evoked. "[He] brags of [having] the knowledge to heal by sympathy. When he hears of someone who is ill, he sends off to them gratis his 'sparigic' balsams, essences, powders, and cataplasms, . . . yet no one believes that such medicines are *probat* [proved], and no one accepts or applies them."[204]

Another form of magical cure—the wearing of amulets—appears to have been less widespread. I have run across only a few instances. Amulets were sometimes sold to help gout, arthritic pains, and dentition. J. H. Sternberg, writing in 1802, listed what children often received to assist them in cutting teeth: the fresh brain of a hare, blood from a cock's comb, "steel filings heated red-hot seven times, and then tempered in human or goat milk," and throat-bands of vipers' teeth.[205] The self-styled court dentist Girault sold an amulet touted as almost miraculous in its ability to ease the pain of teething. His business boomed, apparently because he advertised widely, inserting his bills in the local Braunschweig newspapers as well as in the more distant Hamburg papers.

Healers and patients sometimes combined sympathetic and magical cures with other treatments, and such combinations were far more common than purely magical or sympathetic ones. Frau Kunstche in Esbeck, for example, dispensed medicines as well as casting spells.[206] Patients under the care of physicians and surgeons, and who obediently took the medicines they ordered, might concurrently consult others whose gifts flowed from a more providential source. This common fusion implies that people most often used thaumaturgy to reinforce allopathy, and that few relied on magic alone. The death of a woman in Eich, probably from childbed fever, triggered an investigation when it was rumored that the old-clothes' peddler Reser had performed "a superstitious cure" on her.[207] The testimony of the woman's husband, and of her brother- and sister-in-law, lends perspective on how magical and superstitious cures merged with other medical treatments, as well as on how many medical consultations must have proceeded. It is also a tale that draws together many of the interpretive threads handled separately above. The husband told this story:

His wife, Maria Dederstedt [Osterloh], was delivered of a daughter on 17th June this year and on the 29th of the same month died in her thirty-second year. On the 22d of June, she became desperately ill, complaining of a burning heat in her abdomen, and then began to rave. The wife of the cottager Hennige Brandes gave her some drops, and she, along with the wives of the cottager Hennig Essmann, Sr., and Heinrich Schrader, steeped several herbs together and pressed a juice from them. After swallowing some of this, his wife improved somewhat. The following night, however, she felt much worse, and he went for help to the surgeon Baumgarten, who dispensed two vomitives, which had no effect. He turned then to Dr. Sommer, who prescribed medicines and directed that [blisters of] Spanish fly [be set] and blood let. However, as his wife did not improve, but remained incoherent, he asked his brother, Julius Osterloh, to go fetch the clothing-seller Reser. Reser attended his wife the next evening, the 27th of June, and said that if the illness resulted from a hex, he would soon find it out. Reser shook coals on the shards of a pot and strewed incense on it. Then he paced up and down in the room, sat down for a while at the window, and then from time to time on his wife's bed, all the while mumbling [under his breath]. What he actually said, he [Osterloh] could not hear, as he was so distracted by the condition of his wife that he did not pay much attention to anything that was happening. He did not know if Reser had blessed his wife or blown incense on her. His brother, the cottager Rukemich, the herdsman Warnecke, and several women, as well as some others he does not remember, were also there, and Reser cautioned them to remain very still. After Reser had conducted himself in the above way for about half an hour, he said: "It is not the result of bewitchment."

Osterloh then offered Reser a mettwurst, butter, bread, and some brandy, and after he had eaten, he went away with his brother, and spent the night at his place. As he was leaving, he said that he would send medicines, and would take 1 thaler 6 groschen for his trouble, which Osterloh paid in cash immediately. . . . The next day, the wife of the cottager Heinrich Schrader had to go into the city, and she brought back with her a bottle of drops that she had gotten from Reser. His wife had none of these, as she still was taking the medicines received from Sommer and Baumgarten. She died that [same] night, from the 29th to the 30th. After her death, Osterloh ordered his mother . . . to pitch the drops out in the farmyard.

The deceased woman's sister-in-law also described Reser performance. While her story paralleled that of her brother, she denied that Reser had mentioned anything about magic or cursing in her presence, or that he had either blessed the ill woman or burned incense. She did admit going to the city and getting drops from Reser. She gave the draught to the sister of the swineherd "who was married to the day laborer Meyer in the village and lives on Weberstraße" and who brought the bottle of drops to Borstedt and gave them to Osterloh for his wife.

Osterloh's brother, another swineherd, also had a story to tell. On the day before his sister-in-law died, his brother had given him two pieces of paper, one to take to the local Catholic priest requesting an herb from him and the other a prescription to be filled by the apothecary. As the brother could not read, he was unsure what the two papers contained. He presented the first one to the priest, "who took it through the church and into his garden." When the priest returned, he handed him "a small paper packet with a dried substance in it and said that such grew in his garden." The priest took no money. The brother did not speak to the priest about the illness of his sister-in-law, nor did he request him to say mass for her. He also had no idea who suggested to his brother that he appeal to the priest for aid.[208]

The histories of Frau Osterloh's illness contain important clues to how medical encounters worked. One should perhaps first note here how meticulously people observed and remembered. This story—like many others in this book—is replete with details. People could recount the seemingly most inconsequential particulars—whether, for example, Reser did or did not sit on Frau Osterloh's bed. This impressive ability to recall even tiny events suggests an absorbed interest in, rather than apathy concerning, the health and the sickness of self and others.

If we consider the range of healers and medical advice, we are reminded yet again how wide the circle of available assistance was. Home remedies—in Maria Osterloh's case, drops from a neighbor's wife and herbal potions cooked up by neighbor women—came first. Then her husband consulted a surgeon and a physician, following their advice and trying their medicines, before going to Reser or turning to the Catholic priest. While Reser may have employed some magical means to determine the cause of illness—to ascertain whether or not the woman had been hexed—his treatment was allopathic, not thaumaturgical. His medicines approximated those physicians themselves might have recommended. Moreover, Osterloh's brother did not ask the priest for providential assistance in the form of a mass. The treatments attempted ranged over a wide therapeutic spectrum, and medical boundaries were repeatedly crossed. Surgeon Baumgarten dispensed emetics, and the apothecary gave out unspecified medicines on his own, as, of course, did Reser. Dr. Sommer, while prescribing medicines, also recommended the setting of blisters and letting blood.

Finally, the medical encounter described here in its several phases was public, extended, and tightly woven into the routines of life. The narrative itself melds everyday occurrences with healing acts and blurs the boundaries between them. Osterloh describes the woman's symptoms, the several treatments, and Reser's "performance," but his tale of how he provided food—the simple meal of mettwurst, butter, bread, and some brandy—and how his brother gave Reser a place to sleep, as it was late, is equally integral to the narrative. Several neighbors and relatives were present throughout the several stages of the encounter. And Osterloh relied on acquaintances and his brother to carry messages and medicines back and forth. The whole encounter unfolded within the framework of normal, day-to-day movements. None of this is exceptional. People commonly asked friends on the way to market to stop at the apothecary, to take a flask of urine with them, to pick up an herb or a powder, or to carry stories of illness to healers.

In the end, then, the existing evidence does little to support the idea that magical cures and supernatural means alone were common medical practices. And while we must always credit the possibility that people did not speak (or no longer spoke) freely about such things, and that silence does not indicate the absence of superstitious beliefs and practices, it seems to me just as dubious to argue that they were widespread, when so much of the evidence is obviously biased and self-serving. It is not my desire to deny the existence of magical and sympathetic healing; rather, I argue that scholars have perhaps seriously exaggerated their place in eighteenth-century life and the significance ascribed to them. The vast majority of cures were naturalistic, even if at times a whiff of magic hung about them. And the peasant who brought a sheep into his son's bedroom to transfer the boy's fever to it probably had other people at the bedside as well, among whom it would not be so strange to find a physician.

Meanings

Looking closely at patients' choices, as we have done here, reveals some of the many reasons patients preferred one practitioner to another. It also helps us understand what their perceptions of illness were, how they felt they should be treated, and what expectations they had of being cured. The discussion has emphasized several points. First, and perhaps least controversial, patients hardly distinguished at all among healers. They consulted surgeons, apothecaries, and others for internal ailments. Healers themselves crossed boundaries frequently and almost reflexively. Surgeons, in particular, argued (quite plausibly) that it was difficult for them, and bad medical practice as well, to separate internal and external cures, for some external problems demanded supplementary internal treatment.[209]

Equally apparent, if less widely accepted, is the fact that patients, including those living in rural areas, often used physicians, and not infrequently saw physicians *before* going to other healers. Admittedly, some of this readiness to consult physicians can perhaps be written off as an epiphenomenon of the sources. The evidence is largely drawn from investigations into quackery, and it may well be that those testifying sought to defend themselves or to shield quacks by insisting that they had first consulted a physician or surgeon before turning to other healers, and that they took that last step only when they had been abandoned as incurables. Yet physicians' own accounts, parish registers, and the few morbidity statistics we have also support the idea that people from a wide social spectrum consulted physicians.

The actual medical encounter was a complex affair. Larger forces and local preferences deeply affected its shape and rhythm. Patients almost routinely consulted healers by proxy, sending friends, relatives, or servants to the "doctor" with descriptions of symptoms and more concrete examples of illness, sometimes a stool sample or a glass of urine. Yet many healers visited patients, not only many times, but also over long weeks and months. Knowledge about healers generally spread by hearsay. Reputation was vital (as we have also seen so convincingly demonstrated in the case of the physici) and depended on a variety of factors, among which skill, talent, or "cleverness" in curing was only one. The recommendations of friends and relatives or a vaguer "general acclaim" steered patients to practitioners. Healers often owed their fame and popularity to their ability to cure specific ailments: Busch was good with leg ulcers and breast tumors; Fröhlich with ague; Albers with anal fistulas and hemorrhoids. Men like Dreyer and Busch built their reputations on their handling of maladies that others had been powerless to alleviate. Surgeons, like physicians, were called in for the treatment of external lumps and sores, yet people often abandoned them in favor of the Busches and the Dreyers when faced with the horrors of "cutting." Some, like the poor language teacher Benoit, blamed surgery for worsening their afflictions. People sought cures, but accepted the reality that chronic problems could only be resolved slowly. One is sometimes amazed at the equanimity with which people underwent months and years of painful procedures. Although physicians often accused patients of running off to "quacks" without waiting for their methods to work, much of the evidence suggests that patients did not abandon physicians quickly.

People also *tended* to consult physicians most frequently for fevers and during epidemics of fever or chest diseases, and seldom for smallpox, plague, or dysentery. Many did not turn to any healers in these illnesses, feeling that the disease must simply "run its course" and regarding intervention as vain and possibly lethal. Medical theories that warned of the dangers inherent in abruptly "stopping" diarrhea or allowing wounds to close too rapidly strengthened this attitude. Others turned from one healer to another because the medicines prescribed "did not want to take hold." When the father of a boy suffering from a chest problem turned to the surgeon Nicolai, it was because the medicines of Dr. Sintdorf in

Goslar "would not grip."[210] "Very effective" or "very active" described many medicines. This probably meant that they had some visible result— for example, a laxative "worked well" when it caused several stools to be produced in rapid succession. On the other hand, many patients dreaded the violent action or disliked the bad taste of drugs and avoided or discarded them explicitly for these reasons.

Cost, too, could determine the choice of healer, but this was almost never the sole or primary determinant. It is almost impossible to say that a particular treatment "cost" too much. Patients who raised this complaint often willingly spent totally "unreasonable" sums in pursuit of cures.[211] There seems to have been instead a sense of justified costs working here. Throughout the period, people resented paying for advice or visits alone, while they often disbursed substantial amounts for pills, potions, cataplasms, teas, or tissanes, and paid the surgeon his due for lancing boils, cupping, and letting blood without much complaint.

While the evidence to some extent supports the contention that both the very old and the very young received less medical attention than those in the prime of life, one must be careful not to overstate this or exaggerate its importance. Many of the aged took their chronic sores, aches, pains, and gout to healers in expectation of relief and cure. Stroke brought surgeons and physicians alike to the bedsides of its victims, even elderly and decrepit ones. And families rarely callously neglected the young or the very young. Parents of almost all classes, rural as well as urban, spent a great deal of time and effort in obtaining aid for their children, especially for injuries that jeopardized their ability to work or procreate. Broken legs, enlarged elbows, genital deformities, and eye afflictions sent parents hurrying from one healer to another, often over the course of years. But parents also accepted (for their children and to a large extent for themselves as well) that for some diseases, little could be done, and that the best treatment was to let the disease work itself out. Few parents summoned physicians to treat smallpox, for instance. This should not, however, be facilely interpreted as a stoic acceptance of God's will or parental indifference. That was the propaganda of medical publicists. Adults quickly, and possibly quite accurately, decided whether an outbreak (especially of smallpox) seemed "malignant" or not. If not, they did nothing, which was probably best and was indeed the advice many physicians proffered. Similar thought processes governed their attitudes toward smallpox inoculation and vaccination.

In short, many of the verities about the reaction to illness in early modern times prove less than reliable. The physician was not universally scorned, superstitions and magical cures were not rampant, women, children, and the aged were not invariably slighted. The desire for health was not an artificial goal forced on people by a medicalizing government or a group of physicians on the road to becoming a professional cadre; rather, it was part of their own sensibilities. They pursued it vigorously and felt its lack acutely. If their quest differed from ours, it was because their surroundings were dissimilar, not because they failed to appreciate the value of health or suffered pain any less intensely.

Conclusion

It is now somewhat difficult for me to remember just how I first began research on this book. I have a vague recollection of early forays into the archives in Wolfenbüttel in 1980 and 1981. Armed with a conviction that the documents there would yield up a rich story of popular medical enlightenment, and pretty much convinced that it would support the (then) new ideas about the medicalization of society, I waded in. That initial trip, however, introduced me to a cache of documents that totally recast the project, and that has, over the years, continually challenged me to rethink accepted ideas about the history of medicine, society, and politics. The best days came early as the almost soap-opera-like characters that now people these pages spilled out of the files and onto my desk. And this book, I hope, preserves much of my fascination with these eighteenth-century figures, as well as much of their own individuality and idiosyncrasy, not merely because their stories are so beguiling, but because they are the stuff of the larger history of medicine and society I wanted to write. Indeed, at times the reader may feel that we have strayed far from medicine. I certainly hope so, because in writing about medical history in eighteenth-century Braunschweig-Wolfenbüttel, it has really been my intent to address broader issues in German and European history. And while this little north-German duchy cannot claim the larger historical import of Prussia and Austria, or even Bavaria and Saxony, it does not seem that the rhythms of daily life and local governance were very different there.

This book has taken a somewhat off-center approach to the history of the early modern state and of absolutism. In my analysis of policy making, I have exploited James Vann's argument that the state was not especially future-oriented, and that day-to-day governing consumed almost every moment of privy councilors' time. Ruling in the eighteenth century *was* the business of deciding individual cases and mediating disputes, and privy councilors rarely considered an incident too trivial to discuss seriously. Both the privy council and the Collegium medicum demonstrated a sensitivity to the actualities of life and worked with and within a system of decentralized political authority. While small states may have devoted more attention to single petitions, larger polities also worked reactively. It was not merely a matter of the inability of the central government to enforce its will. Even those at the apices of power did not fully conceive of a governing process that was not multiform. Nor could they offer an alternative vision to replace the one they had inherited. As Vann has pointed out, they had little sense that the future would significantly differ from the past. Governing remained wrapped in a pliant corporatist idiom, which throughout the century proved its innate flexibility by working new words and phrases into its vocabulary and by learning to function within new structures and with new realities.

These essential characteristics of adaptability and suppleness force us to reconsider the relationships that existed between the center and the peripheries, as well as the validity of the insider/outsider mechanism so frequently invoked to explain resistance to the encroaching or intrusive power of the "centralizing, absolutist state." Although they may have differed in social origin, the men at the helm of the ducal government varied little in mind-set from their less exalted brethren, from the city magistrates, the ecclesiastical authorities, and the Amtmänner. Admittedly, this homogeneity was probably more the case in the smaller states. While the ducal government appointed Amtmänner, it does not follow that their candidates unquestionably implemented ducal or ministerial will. Amtmänner often had, or formed, connections in their Ämter, and no Amtmann prospered if continually at loggerheads with the locals, who literally surrounded him.

There were, of course, battles. And much of this book is concerned with conflict. Struggles could be bitter, protracted, and fought on the high ground of morality and theory. But even when they seem most maliciously small-minded, the issues involved were never really inconsequential. Where the physicus sat at public ceremonies, and whether he fattened his pig at communal expense, marked his rank. Whenever and wherever these men and women fought with one another, they did so in terms everyone understood. Much of the time, the language they spoke was corporatist, although toward the end of the eighteenth century, the newer words and phrases of enlightenment—such as *common good, improvement, expedience,* and *reason*—began to appear more frequently. The latter did not, however, push out the former; rather, the two languages merged to form a linguistic arena where both mentalities and both sets of aspirations could be expressed.

In this context, policy emerged from a set of arrangements and accommodations conducted formally and informally at several levels and among several groups. While communities could, of course, defend their own interests against initiatives they felt would work to their disadvantage, and while they could and did bar people from their territories, or make their lives miserable there, they did not personify the state as the enemy. People at almost all levels of society *used* the state to help them in their feuds, and to balance their rights and privileges against those of others who lived much closer to them. This appeal to the several organs of state—whether privy council and councilors, ecclesiastical authorities, the Collegium medicum and its individual members, members of the ruling family, or the Amtmänner—tempered the governing system, making it malleable and responsive, and thus resilient and stable.

Perhaps some scholars would prefer to judge the early modern state as baroquely complex, inefficient, cumbersome, and so layered with competing interests that neither good nor fair government was possible. While one hardly wishes to romanticize the eighteenth-century state, it did, if admittedly not in a democratic manner, permit many viewpoints to be represented and made it possible to respond to local problems without tripping over unbending principles and precedents. Obviously, the eighteenth-century state did not eliminate inequalities—it was not intended to. Nor was it always just. Yet it nonetheless allowed many voices to be sounded and ignored very few of them. Even when and where purportedly "enlightened" reforms were introduced—such as in the creation of a Collegium medicum—the older rules of the game rarely changed.

Enlightenment, therefore, plays a distinctly subordinate role here. I have struggled to avoid terms like *enlightenment* or *enlightened reforms* in favor of showing how splintered the party of humanity could be. Enlightenment in this book means many things. It could be linked to the emerging middle-class lifestyle to which many physici aspired. But enlightenment was also a clique, and itself a form of patronage, which rewarded those who spoke its language well. And at the level of Grub Street, it was often cranky, obscurantist, petty, and bizarre, as liable to provoke laughter, horror, or scorn as admiration.

Clearly, in the eighteenth century, and especially in the later decades of that century, change was afoot. Some autonomous forces, such as population increase and economic acceleration, play a major role in my story. I have not, however, endowed these forces with inexorable power. They were not unaffected by human actions. An economic quickening and the gradual rise of a consumer culture are excellent examples. Consumerism did not merely intrude itself on an unsuspecting or resistant population. Entrepreneurs, often very minor ones such as medicine peddlers, shaped their own versions of consumerism. The availability of more products and more choices, like the existence of more movement and bigger markets, slowly ate away at older ideas of how the economic and social worlds were supposed to work, yet that older world never collapsed into dust. Innovations in production and in marketing took place at several levels, and those who are often portrayed as the victims and the avowed enemies of economic modernization—guildsmen and small producers, for example— often jockeyed adroitly for favorable positions in the newly unfolding consumer world, deploying the traditional languages of interloping and protection where they worked, but moving on to idioms of competition and free market when they served better. Such two-sidedness made the tussles over rights and privileges and over Pfuscherey in the eighteenth century, both in the world of medicine and in the larger socioeconomic universe encircling it, increasingly complicated. The lines of conflict shifted with bewildering rapidity, and participants used at least two languages at once: that of traditional rights and privileges (*Nahrung* and *Hausnotdurft*) and the newer language of free competition and free choice. The word that one day struck the ear with a hated clang might slide sweetly over the tongue on another and in other circumstances. And the client or consumer was equally able to bend language to his or her needs.

When placed in these frameworks, the debates about professionalization and medicalization that have dominated the writing of much medical history over the past few decades turn out to be less relevant. Physicians and physici ranted and raved about superstition and local intransigence, but they themselves were locked into patronage and clientage networks. They rarely acted as budding professionals, and neither, for that matter, did the government—in the form either of the privy council or the Collegium medicum—seek to help them along to a monopoly of power and authority. The initiatives of medicalization remained equally muted and ambiguous. And, on the other side, people did not resist physicians with the vigor we have come to imagine, nor did programs such as vaccination founder on the superstitious hostility of the unenlightened hordes. While it is true that inoculation, for instance, was never a tremendous success, that qualified failure cannot be reduced to the triumph of ignorance, stubbornness, and religious obscurantism alone. An inability to think in terms of chances was perhaps more to blame.

Such strife cannot, therefore, be facilely interpreted as a clash between popular and elite cultures, or, in this context, between folk and academic medicines alone. This book has generally rejected the idea of the split. We have repeatedly seen how much popular and elite medicines overlapped. Indeed, we have discovered little evidence supporting the whole idea of a vibrant and coherent folk medicine carried clandestinely through the centuries by oral tradition. I have tried throughout to avoid partisan politics or special pleading by stressing these complexities. In their reliance on folk remedies, peasants were neither wholly "superstitious minds" nor preternaturally wise, and physicians were neither heroic crusaders nor conniving careerists. Physicians were far more likely to conceive of themselves as clients of the privy council or Collegium medicum or of the party of enlightenment than as members of a profession. Nor was their self-image exclusively medical.

I have also not accepted the idea, so dear to professionalization and medicalization theorists (in regard to the German experience at least), that the state was complicit in promoting *both* the medical hegemony of physicians *and* the medicalization (read: disciplining) of society. While physicians and governments may have drafted plans for improving or medicalizing the population,[1] they were not very forceful in carrying them out. And if we review the reformist literature itself,[2] the schemes of reformers seem curiously insubstantial and sometimes contradictory. In the closing decades of the century, for example, plans were floated in several places, including Braunschweig-Wolfenbüttel, to allow surgeons a limited medical practice in order to improve medical care in rural areas.[3] A close reading of the archival evidence has repeatedly questioned these and other interpretations of medical practice and medical choice in the eighteenth century. Ordinary people were not implacably hostile to physicians, they tended not to rely on magical cures and home remedies alone, and, perhaps most of all, they were not indifferent to health, but desired it greatly. In this regard, they approximated us more than their two centuries' removal in time might suggest.

Archives and Libraries

StAWf   Niedersächsisches Staatsarchiv-Wolfenbüttel
StadtB   Stadtarchiv Braunschweig
StadtH   Stadtarchiv Helmstedt
StadtK   Stadtarchiv Königslutter
HAB   Herzog August Bibliothek-Wolfenbüttel

Publications

AGB   *Archiv für Geschichte des Buchwesens*

AGFK   *Archiv für die Geburtshülfe, Frauenzimmer- und Kinderkrankheiten*

AHR   *American Historical Review*

Annales   *Annales: Economies, Sociétés, Civilisations*

AS   *Archiv für Sozialgeschichte*

AV   *Alphabethisches Verzeichniss der in dem Herzogthum Braunschweig-Lüneburg belegenen Städte, Flecken, Dörfer, Aemter, Stifter, Klöster, etc.* (Braunschweig: Vieweg, 1816)

BA   *Braunschweigische Anzeigen*

BA-GB   *Braunschweigische Anzeigen-Gelehrte Beiträge*

BH   *Braunschweigische Heimat*

BHM   *Bulletin of the History of Medicine*

BJ   *Braunschweigisches Jahrbuch*

BM   *Braunschweigisches Magazin*

CEH   *Central European History*

CM   *Clio Medica*

CMP   *Culture, Medicine and Psychiatry*

FH   *French History*

Hassel/Bege   Georg Hassel and Karl Bege, *Geographisch-statistische Beschreibung der Fürstenthümer Wolfenbüttel und Blanckenburg* (Braunschweig: Vieweg, 1802–3)

HDA   Hanns Bächtold-Stäubli, *Handwörterbuch des deutschen Aberglaubens* (Berlin: Walter de Gruyter, 1936–37)

Hinze   August Hinze, *Lexicon aller Herzogl.[ichen] Braunschweigischen Verordnungen welche die medicinische Polizey betreffen* (Stendal: Franz & Grosse, 1793)

HM   *Hannoverisches Magazin*

HO 1757   "Serenissimi gnädigste Verordnung, das Hebammenwesens betreffend. De dato Braunschweig, vom 18 Febr. 1757"

HO 1803   "Serenissimi Verordnung, das Hebammen-Wesen betreffend" (Braunschweig, 1803)

HR   *Historical Reflections / Réflexions historiques*

HT   *History and Theory*

HW   *Holzmindisches Wochenblatt, 1785–96*

HZ   *Historische Zeitschrift*

JCH   *Journal of Contemporary History*

JEEH   *Journal of European Economic History*

JHM   *Journal of the History of Medicine*

JMH   *Journal of Modern History*

JMP   *Journal of Medicine and Philosophy*

JRCGP   *Journal of the Royal College of General Practitioners*

JSH   *Journal of Social History*

Krünitz   Johann Georg Krünitz, *D. Johann Georg-Krünitz's ökonomisch-technologische Encyklopädie oder allgemeines System der Staats-, Stadt-, Haus-, und Landwirtschaft und der Kunstgeschichte in alphabetischer Ordnung* (Berlin: J. Pauli, 1773–1858)

Lexikon   August Hirsch, E. Gurlt, and A. Werner, eds., *Biographisches Lexikon der hervorragenden Ärzte aller Zeiten und Völker* (Berlin: Urban & Schwarzenberg, 1884–88)

MGG   *Medizin, Gesellschaft und Geschichte*

MH   *Medical History*

MJ   *Medizinhistorisches Journal*

MO 1721   *Hoch-Fürstliche Braunschweig-Wolfenbüttel Medicinal / Ordnung nebst beygefügter Apotheker-Taxa, auf Hoch-Fürstliche Gnädigste Verordnung und Befehl publiciret* (Braunschweig, 1721)

MO 1747   *Serenissimi Reglement und Verordnung das Collegium Medicum in Braunschweig betreffend* (Wolfenbüttel, 1747)

PP   *Past and Present*

RZ   *Rote Zeitung, or Gnädigst Privilegierte Braunschweigische Zeitung für Städte, Flecken und Dörfer insonderheit für die lieben Landleute alt und jung* (Wolfenbüttel, 1787–1858)

SA   *Sudhoffs Archiv*

SH	*Social History*
SHM	*Social History of Medicine*
SM 1747	*Serenissimi Reglement und Verordnung die Societates medicas betreffend de dato Wolfenbüttel den 7. Januarii 1747* (Wolfenbüttel, 1747)
TS	*Theory and Society*
VSWG	*Vierteljahrschrift für Sozial- und Wirtschaftsgeschichte*
Wirth	*Braunschweigische Sammlungen von Oekonomischen Sachen als des einzeln herausgekommenen Wochenblatts der Wirth und die Wirthin* (Braunschweig and Hildesheim, 1756–57)
WMQ	*William and Mary Quarterly*
Zedler	Johann Heinrich Zedler, *Grosses vollständiges Universal-Lexikon, aller Wissenschaften und Künste* (Halle and Leipzig: Zedler, 1732–50)

Introduction

1. StAWf, 111 Neu 1050, "Bericht von denen Umständen des Medicinal-Wesens im Stifft Walkenried," fols. 2–6, 15 May 1747. Here, as elsewhere in this book, translations are mine. I have modernized spellings (especially of place-names) and punctuation.

2. The problems dividing *Alltagsgeschichte* and *Strukturgeschichte* are summarized in David F. Crew, "*Alltagsgeschichte*: A New Social History 'From Below,'" *CEH* 22 (1989): 394–407; see also, Jürgen Kocka, "Sozialgeschichte—Strukturgeschichte—Gesellschaftsgeschichte," *AS* 15 (1975): 43–50.

3. Alf Lüdtke, "Was ist und wer treibt Alltagsgeschichte?" introduction to *Alltagsgeschichte: Zur Rekonstruktion historischer Erfahrung und Lebensweise*, ed. Lüdtke (Frankfurt: Campus, 1989), 9–47; Crew, "*Alltagsgeschichte*," 404–5.

4. "I think we can agree with Roland Barthes, Paul Ricoeur, and Lionel Gossman that shaping choices of language, detail, and order are needed to present an account that seems to both writer and reader true, real, meaningful, and/or explanatory," Natalie Davis observes in *Fiction in the Archives: Pardon Tales and Their Tellers in Sixteenth-Century France* (Stanford, Calif.: Stanford University Press, 1987), 3. People in sixteenth-century France selected incidents, language, and forms of argumentation to compose pardon tales that would influence their audiences and save their skins. Davis makes "the 'fictional' aspects of these documents . . . the center of analysis. I do not mean their feigned elements, but rather using the other and broader sense of the word *fingere*, their forming, shaping, and molding elements: the crafting of a narrative."

5. William H. Sewell, Jr., *Work and Revolution in France: The Language of Labor from the Old Regime to 1848* (Cambridge: Cambridge University Press, 1980), 11.

6. The literature on the professionalization of medicine is too vast to review here. The general tendency has been to accept as a working definition the professionalization model developed by sociologists such as Ernst Greenwood, Morris L. Cogan, Margali Larsen, and Talcott Parsons. In *The Social Transformation of American Medicine: The Rise of a Sovereign Profession and the Making of a Vast Industry* (New York: Basic Books, 1982), Paul Starr (who is, of course, a sociologist himself) follows this line, defining a profession as "an occupation that regulates itself through systematic, required training and collegial discipline; that has a base in technical, specialized knowledge; and that has a service rather than profit orientation, enshrined in its code of ethics" (15). For early modern Europe, definition of the term *professionalism* is much more problematic. See Margaret Pelling, "Medical Practice in Early Modern England: Trade or Profession?" in *The Professions in Early Modern England*, ed. Wilfrid Prest (London: Croom Helm, 1987), 90–128, and Monica Green, "Women's Medi-

cal Practice and Health Care in Medieval Europe: Review Essay," *Signs: Journal of Women in Culture and Society* 14 (1989): 434–73.

7. Müller was first named physicus in Seesen in 1755 or 1757, and then was promoted to first physicus in the Harz district in 1761. On his career as physicus, see StAWf, 111 Neu 1095, 1082, 1101.

8. Evaluation of the character and capacity of "the people" varied, of course. One prevalent tendency was to view them as almost irremediably ignorant and unenlightened. Another stressed the great necessity of popular enlightenment in almost all spheres of life. Everyone agreed that "the people" were less productive, less enlightened, less industrious than they might be. See Harry C. Payne, *The Philosophes and the People* (New Haven, Conn.: Yale University Press, 1976), esp. 1–58; Harvey Chisick, *The Limits of Reform in the Enlightenment: Attitudes Toward the Education of the Lower Classes in Eighteenth-Century France* (Princeton, N.J.: Princeton University Press, 1981), esp. 5–8, 45–75. In *From Pariah to Patriot: The Changing Image of the German Peasant, 1770–1840* (Lexington: University of Kentucky Press, 1969), esp. 24–57, John G. Gagliardo shows how the attitudes toward peasants in Germany began to modify after 1770.

9. Johann Karl Osterhausen, *Ueber medicinische Aufklärung* (Zurich: Geßner, 1798), 394.

10. Daniel Nootnagel, "Vorschlag Aberglauben und Vorurtheile auszurotten," *Deutsches Museum* 1 (1778): 148–55, here 149–50. Similarly, Osterhausen observed that even "learned men" were unable to free themselves of superstition and "[such] men prefer to call the pseudo-physician [*Afterarzt*] rather than the [true] physician . . . and [expect] a man, whom they would otherwise view as crude and ignorant, to restore their lost health" (*Ueber medicinische Aufklärung*, 18).

11. See, e.g., Johann Heinrich Helmuth, *Volkslehre zur Dämpfung des Aberglaubens* (Braunschweig: Waisenhausbuchhandlung, 1786), who calls superstitions an "evil fountain," from which "the saddest results . . . for city people and peasants alike" flow (ix). See also Ute Frevert, *Krankheit als politisches Problem, 1770–1880: Soziale Unterschichten in Preußen zwischen medizinischer Polizei und staatlicher Sozialversicherung* (Göttingen: Vandenhoeck & Ruprecht, 1984), 28–36.

12. StAWf, 2 Alt 11200, fols. 32–33, 5 Apr. 1770.

13. For recent examples, see Matthew Ramsey, *Professional and Popular Medicine in France, 1770–1830: The Social World of Medical Practice* (Cambridge: Cambridge University Press, 1988), and Judith Devlin, *The Superstitious Mind: French Peasants and the Supernatural in the Nineteenth Century* (New Haven, Conn.: Yale University Press 1987). Evelyn Bernette Ackermann offers a more nuanced view:

Much has been written about the peasant mind by scholars who almost delight in revealing its affinity for old structures and its suspicion of anything new. Eugen Weber and Judith Devlin, to name the two most prominent recent examples, chronicle in great detail the tenacity and persistence until the early twentieth century of a solid core of beliefs and activities antithetical to the goals of a rational bourgeoisie. Françoise Loux, in a suggestive and important monograph on child care in the late nineteenth and early twentieth centuries, has modified this view of peasants. Peasant beliefs, she argues, were just as goal-oriented as those of the more officially rational bourgeoisie but seemed different because they were organized according to a different logic. (*Health Care in the Parisian Countryside, 1880–1914* [New Brunswick, N.J.: Rutgers University Press, 1990], 11)

See also, for Germany, Francisca Loetz, *Vom Kranken zum Patienten: "Medikalisierung" und medizinische Vergesellschaftung am Beispiel Badens 1750–1850* (Stuttgart: Franz Steiner, 1993), 88–136.

14. Françoise Loux, *Le Jeune Enfant et son corps dans la société traditionnelle* (Paris: Flammarion, 1978); Ackerman, *Health Care*, 11.

15. Ramsey, *Professional and Popular Medicine*, xi.

16. "Medical Practitioners," in *Health, Medicine and Mortality in the Sixteenth Century*, ed. Charles Webster (Cambridge: Cambridge University Press, 1979), 165–235.

17. As W. F. Bynum and Roy Porter point out in *Medical Fringe and Medical Orthodoxy, 1750–1850* (London: Croom Helm, 1987), 1:

Few medical historians today would argue that regular medicine and fringe medicine have had their own autonomous histories, developing as completely distinct and separate species, the one (in the eyes of its friends) scientific, professional, effective, or (in the eyes of its opponents) monopolistic and authoritarian; the other (according to some) vulgar, cranky and dangerous, or (to others) natural, democratic, harmless. The days of such "saints and sinners" histories are over. Scholars of all stripes agree nowadays that—to a greater or lesser degree—the frontiers between orthodox and unorthodox medicine have been flexible; indeed, the very distinction between the two is one that has been socially constructed. So mobile have been their boundaries, that one age's quackery has often become another's orthodoxy, or vice versa. Thus, plotting the territorial shifts, gains and losses for "proper" and "improper" medicine, is acknowledged to be a task requiring the social historian.

18. See, e.g., Webster and Pelling, "Medical Practitioners"; Ramsey, *Professional and Popular Medicine*.

19. Sabine Sander, *Handwerkschirurgen: Sozialgeschichte einer verdrängten Berufsgruppe* (Göttingen: Vandenhoeck & Ruprecht, 1989). See also Katharine Park, *Doctors and Medicine in Early Renaissance Florence* (Princeton, N.J.: Princeton University Press, 1985); Michael MacDonald, *Mystical Bedlam: Madness, Anxiety, and Healing in Seventeenth-Century England* (Cambridge: Cambridge University Press, 1981); and Ronald Sawyer, "Patients, Healers, and Disease in the Southwest Midlands, 1597–1634" (diss., University of Wisconsin, 1986), which analyzes the medical practice of Richard Napier and reveals the wide social variety of his patients.

20. StAWf, 2 Alt 11628, fols. 26, 40.

21. StAWf, 8 Alt Seesen 3 Nr. 11, fols. 25–26, 29 Nov. 1767.

22. Roy Porter, *Health for Sale: Quackery in England, 1660–1850* (Manchester: Manchester University Press, 1989), esp. 21–59.

23. Ramsey, *Professional and Popular Medicine*, 284–91; Park, *Doctors*, 85–117; Harold J. Cook, *The Decline of the Old Medical Regime in London* (Ithaca, N.Y.: Cornell University Press, 1986), 28–69.

24. On the concept of a moral economy, see E. P. Thompson, "The Moral Economy of the English Crowd in the Eighteenth Century," *PP* 50 (Feb. 1971): 76–136.

25. See Richard M. Titmuss, *The Gift Relationship: From Blood to Social Policy* (London: Allen & Unwin, 1970); Keith Thomas, *Religion and the Decline of Magic: Studies in Popular Beliefs in the Sixteenth and Seventeenth Centuries* (London: Weidenfeld & Nicolson, 1971), 563–64, 553–55, 557–59.

26. Samuel Auguste André David Tissot, *Unterricht für gemeine Leute über deren Gesundheit: Nach der fünften Originalausgabe aus dem französischen übersetzt*, vol. 1: *Sämtliche zur Arztneikunst gehörige Schriften*, trans. Johann Christian Kerstens (Hamburg: Ritter, 1774), 593, 600–601.

27. For example, in 1716, the Barber-Surgeons' and Surgeons' Guild in the city of Braunschweig renewed their complaints about "an interloper" who had settled in Braunschweig; once a military surgeon (felsher) but neither a member of the guild nor a citizen, he openly practiced in the city, prescribing *interna et externa medicamenta* (StadtB, C II 4, fols. 82–83).

28. Apropos of the persistence of corporative language and images well into the nineteenth century, William Sewell refers to "the paradox of corporate language"; there was, he observes, "something distinctly corporative about the working-class world of nineteenth-century France that fit with the continued usage of corporate terms in the workers' language" (*Work and Revolution*, 2–3).

29. In 1741, when another complaint about Pfuscher and Störer reached the privy council, the council responded in similar terms: "The entire corps of barber-surgeons and surgeons has complained to us that regimental and company felshers have done their livelihood [*Nahrung*] great harm, in that these have boldly and without shame taken it upon themselves to barber, let blood, and cure patients among citizens and other nonmilitary persons" (StadtB, CII 4, fol. 198, 23 Mar. 1741).

30. Several fairly recent review articles have testified to this trend. See, e.g., Judith Walzer Leavitt, "Medicine in Context: A Review Essay of the History of Medicine," *AHR* 95 (1990): 1471–84; Randall McGowen, "Identifying Themes in the Social History of Medicine," *JMH* 63 (1991): 81–90; Colin Jones, "Medicine, Madness and Mayhem from the 'Roi Soleil' to the Golden Age of Hysteria (Seventeenth to Late Nineteenth Centuries)," *FII* 4 (1990): 378–88; see also the articles in *Problems and Methods in the History of Medicine*, ed. Roy Porter and Andrew Wear (London: Croom Helm, 1987).

31. Jones, "Medicine," 378.

32. Roy Porter, "Introduction," to *Patients and Practitioners: Lay Perceptions of Medicine in Pre-Industrial Society*, ed. Porter (Cambridge: Cambridge University Press, 1985), 1; see also id., "The Patient's View: Doing Medical History from Below," *TS* 14 (1985): 175–98.

33. Porter, "Introduction," 5. Recent attempts include Porter, *Health for Sale*; Roy Porter and Dorothy Porter, *In Sickness and in Health: The British Experience* (Oxford: Blackwell, 1988); Dorothy Porter and Roy Porter, *Patient's Progress: Doctors and Doctoring in Eighteenth-Century England* (Stanford, Calif.: Stanford University Press, 1989); *Medical Fringe*, ed. Bynum and Porter; Lucinda McCray Beier, *Sufferers and Healers: The Experience of Illness in Seventeenth-Century England* (London: Routledge and Kegan Paul, 1987); Ramsey, *Professional and Popular Medicine*; Ackermann, *Health Care*; Claudia Herzlich and Janine Pierret, *Illness and Self in Society*, trans. Elborg Forster (Baltimore: Johns Hopkins University Press, 1987); Barbara Duden,

Geschichte unter der Haut: Ein Eisenacher Arzt und seine Patientinnen um 1730 (Stuttgart: Klett-Cotta, 1987); Sawyer, "Patients, Healers, and Disease." An early successful attempt to look at people's understanding of disease, in this case, madness, is Michael MacDonald's brilliant *Mystical Bedlam*.

34. Porter and Porter, *Patient's Progress*, vi.

35. Françoise Loux, *Sagesse du corps: La Santé et maladie dans les proverbs françaises* (Paris: G. P. Maisonneuve & Larouse, 1978); Pietro Camporesi, *The Incorruptible Flesh: Bodily Mutation and Mortification in Religion and Folklore* (Cambridge: Cambridge University Press, 1988).

36. MacDonald, *Mystical Bedlam*; Duden, *Geschichte*. Sawyer, "Patients, Healers, and Disease," also relies heavily on the case books of a single healer, but supplements them with other information to widen the scope of his investigation.

37. I am not, of course, suggesting that medical historians have never pointed out how medical history can be used to illuminate larger historical questions. In his *Mystical Bedlam*, for example, Michael MacDonald has offered important new evidence for family history, as Roy Porter has done for the growth of a consumer society, to cite just two cases.

38. I have discussed this more fully in "Confessions of an Archive Junkie," in *Theory, Method, and Practice in Social and Cultural History*, ed. Peter Karsten and John Modell (New York: New York University Press, 1992), 152–80.

39. StAWf, 20 Alt, "Dorf-, Feld- und Wiesenbeschreibungen der Generallandes-vermessung, 1746–1784"; ibid., 25 Alt, "Feld- und Vermessungsbeschreibungen ausserhalb der Generallandesvermessung"; ibid., 22A Alt, "Amtsrechnungen (Korn-, Vieh-, Geld-, Kontributionsregister)" (mid fifteenth century through 1807); ibid., 23 Alt, "Ältere Kontributionsbeschreibungen" (seventeenth century–1806).

40. David Warren Sabean, *Property, Production, and Family in Neckarhausen, 1700–1870* (Cambridge: Cambridge University Press, 1990), esp. 70–87; Sander, *Handwerkschirurgen* (see esp. 110–11 for a discussion of the value of the inventories in determining social and economic structures).

41. James Allan Vann, *The Making of a State: Württemberg, 1593–1793* (Ithaca, N.Y.: Cornell University Press, 1984), esp. 17–23; Thomas Robisheaux, *Rural Society and the Search for Order in Early Modern Germany* (Cambridge: Cambridge University Press, 1989), esp. 1–13. Marc Raeff has presented the other side of the story, that of governments dedicated to a program of modernization, in his *The Well-Ordered Police State: Social and Institutional Change Through Law in the Germanies and Russia, 1600–1800* (New Haven, Conn.: Yale University Press, 1983), esp. 1–10.

42. Two recent surveys of German history are considerably more nuanced and subtle, yet still present a general picture of German backwardness compared to Britain and France. James Sheehan, *German History, 1770–1866* (Oxford: Oxford University Press, 1989), and Hans-Ulrich Wehler, *Deutsche Gesellschaftsgeschichte*, vol. 1: *Vom Feudalismus des Alten Reiches bis zur Defensiven Modernisierung der Reformära, 1700–1815* (Munich: Beck, 1987). I am not, of course, the first person to suggest that Germany's "backwardness" has been overplayed. The "peculiarity" of German history for a later period has been seriously questioned by David Blackbourn and Geoff Eley in *The Peculiarities of German History: Bourgeois Society and Politics in Nineteenth-Century Germany* (Oxford: Oxford University Press, 1984).

43. Sheehan, *German History*, 24–71; Wehler, *Deutsche Gesellschaftsgeschichte*, 1: 218–67. More generally, see *Deutsche Verwaltungsgeschichte*, ed. Kurt G. A. Jeserich, Hans Pohl, and Georg-Christoph von Unruh, vol. 1: *Vom Spätmittelalter bis zum Ende des Reiches* (Stuttgart: Deutsche Verlagsanstalt, 1983).

44. Raeff, *Well-Ordered Police State*; Vann, *Making*; Charles Ingrao, *The Hessian Mercenary State: Ideas, Institutions, and Reform under Frederick II, 1760–1785* (Cambridge: Cambridge University Press, 1987).

45. See, e.g., Reinhart Dorwart, "The Royal College of Medicine and Public Health in Brandenburg-Prussia, 1685–1740," *Medical History* 2 (1958): 13–23; Manfred Stürzbecher, *Beiträge zur Berliner Medizingeschichte: Quellen und Studien zur Geschichte des Gesundheitswesens vom 17. bis zum 19. Jahrhundert* (Berlin: de Gruyter, 1966); id., "Zur Geschichte des Berliner Stadtphysikus im 18. und 19. Jahrhundert," *Medizinische Welt* 1962: 1956–63.

46. James Sheehan has pointed out that we "badly need a study of eighteenth-century German religiosity" (*German History*, 149 n. 8).

47. See also Leon Eisenberg, "Disease and Illness: Distinctions Between Professional and Popular Ideas of Sickness," *CMP* 1 (1977): 9–23; Øivind Larsen, "Die Krankheitsauffassung und ihre historische Interpretation: Ein Auswertungsmodell aufgrund von norwegischen Medizinalberichten aus dem 19. Jahrhundert," in *Mensch und Gesundheit in der Geschichte*, ed. Arthur Imhof (Husum: Matthiesen, 1980), 45–58; Manfred Pflanz, "Der Entschluß, zum Arzt zu gehen," *Hippokrates* 35 (1964): 894–97.

Chapter 1. Medicine, State, and Society

1. The literature on enlightened absolutism is far too extensive to review here. Charles Ingrao has offered an excellent overview in "The Problem of 'Enlightened Absolutism' and the German States," *JMH* 58, suppl. (Dec. 1986): S161–80. See also Eberhard Weis, "Enlightenment and Absolutism in the Holy Roman Empire: Thoughts on Enlightened Absolutism in Germany," ibid., S181–97; and the articles in *Aufklärung, Absolutismus und Bürgertum in Deutschland: Zwölf Aufsätze*, ed. Franklin Kopitzsch (Munich: Nymphenburger, 1976).

2. Max Weber, *Wirtschaft und Gesellschaft*, 2d enlarged ed. (Tübingen: Mohr, 1922).

3. Michel Foucault, *Discipline and Punish: The Birth of the Prison*, trans. Alan Sheridan (New York: Pantheon Books, 1977). Stefan Breuer discusses and compares the various concepts of "social disciplining" in "Sozialdisziplinierung: Problem und Problemverlagerungen eines Konzepts bei Max Weber, Gerhard Oestreich und Michel Foucault," in *Soziale Sicherheit und soziale Disziplinierung*, ed. Christoph Sachße and Florian Tennstedt (Stuttgart: Suhrkamp, 1986), 45–69. For discussions focusing on medicine, see Alfons Labisch, "'Hygiene ist Moral—Moral ist Hygiene—': Soziale Disziplinierung durch Ärzte und Medizin," in *Soziale Sicherheit*, ed. Sachße and Tennstedt, 286–303; Gerd Göckenjan, *Kurieren und Staat machen: Gesundheit und Medizin in der bürgerlichen Welt* (Stuttgart: Suhrkamp, 1985); and *Medizinische Deutungsmacht im sozialen Wandel des 19. und frühen 20. Jahrhunderts*, ed. Alfons Labisch and Reinhard Spree (Bonn: Psychiatrie-Verlag, 1989).

4. Marc Raeff, *The Well-Ordered Police State: Social and Institutional Change Through*

Law in the Germanies and Russia, 1600–1800 (New Haven, Conn.: Yale University Press, 1983).

5. Charles Ingrao, *The Hessian Mercenary State: Ideas, Institutions, and Reform under Frederick II, 1760–1785* (Cambridge: Cambridge University Press, 1987), 3.

6. E.g., Walter Hahn, *Handel und Handelspolitik im Herzogtum Braunschweig-Wolfenbüttel in der Regierungszeit der Herzöge Karl I. und Karl Wilhelm Ferdinand (1735–1806): Ein Beitrag zur Geschichte der deutschen Kleinstaaten des 18. Jahrhunderts* (Braunschweig: Appelhaus, 1931), 12.

7. Hans-Ulrich Wehler, *Deutsche Gesellschaftsgeschichte*, vol. 1: *Vom Feudalismus des Alten Reiches bis zur Defensiven Modernisierung der Reformära, 1700–1815* (Munich: Beck, 1987), esp. 531–46.

8. Ingrao, "Problem of 'Enlightened Absolutism,'" S171–73; id., *Hessian Mercenary State*, 6–8.

9. Raeff, *Police State*, 1–2.

10. Modernity can, of course, be variously defined. In his definition of modernity (ibid., 2–3), Raeff responds to some of the most obvious criticisms of modernity without, however, really questioning its existence, or, for that matter, its desirability:

There are many ways of defining modernity, of course. The most simple-minded is to equate modernity with the present, in contrast to the past. As some have suggested, it may be a sign of arrogance and sociocentrism to claim for the culture of the Western world . . . the distinction of being peculiarly modern. Yet there is no denying that from about the dawn of the sixteenth century (with origins going farther back, of course), Europe embarked on an extraordinary departure from the traditional cultural patterns that one observes in its own past and in most of the world prior to its contact with the West. The most outstanding and characteristic feature of the pattern that makes Western Europe exceptional and that eventually subjected to its sway most societies the world over is an extraordinary dynamism, an entrepreneurial spirit, and the willingness to take risks for results in the distant future. This creative energy and dynamism (some would call it arrogance and aggressiveness) were predicated on an essential assumption: that the resources at man's disposal are greater than perceived, that they may be unlimited, and that it is the task of man's rational and purposeful action to discover, develop, and make use of these resources that lie more or less fallow in the natural state.

11. Breuer, "Sozialdisziplinierung," 45–52.

12. Norbert Elias, *The Civilizing Process*, trans. Edmund Jephcott (Oxford: Blackwell, 1978); id., *The Court Society*, trans. Edmund Jephcott (Oxford: Blackwell, 1983); Gerhard Oestreich, *Geist und Gestalt des frühmodernen Staates: Ausgewählte Aufsätze* (Berlin: Duncker & Humblot, 1969); id., "Policey und Prudentia civilis in der barocken Gesellschaft von Stadt und Staat," in *Barock-Symposium 1974: Stadt-Schule-Universität-Buchwesen und die deutsche Literatur im 17. Jahrhundert*, ed. Albrecht Schöne (Munich: Beck, 1976), 10–21; several works by Foucault, but especially his *Discipline and Punish*; Pierre Bourdieu, *Outline of a Theory of Practice* (New York: Cambridge University Press, 1977).

13. Breuer, "Sozialdisziplinierung," 62–63.

14. Dominick Lacapra, "Is Everyone a *Mentalité* Case? Transference and the Culture Concept," *HT* 20, no. 3 (1984): 296–311.

15. See, e.g., the claims of microhistory. Edward Muir, "Introduction: Observing Trifles," in *Microhistory and the Lost Peoples of Europe: Selections from Quaderni Storici*, ed. Edward Muir and Guido Ruggiero, trans. Eren Branch (Baltimore: Johns Hopkins University Press, 1991), vii–xxviii.

16. In *The Making of a State: Württemberg, 1593–1793* (Ithaca, N.Y.: Cornell University Press, 1984), James Allen Vann has offered a penetrating criticism of such limited approaches to the growth of government and suggested an analysis in which power was "more ambiguously allocated"; see esp. 17–23.

17. Wehler, *Deutsche Gesellschaftsgeschichte*, 1: 229.

18. Vann, *Making of a State*, 22–23. Similarly, Thomas Robisheaux has observed that the "order that emerged came out of conflict, compromise, and, at times, cooperation" (*Rural Society and the Search for Order in Early Modern Germany* [Cambridge: Cambridge University Press, 1989], 11).

19. Wehler admits that the "citizen-state" (*Staatsbürgergesellschaft*) was not "entirely a conscious creation of the early modern state" (*Deutsche Gesellschaftsgeschichte*, 1: 229).

20. Ibid.

21. Wehler, ibid., 235, makes a rather different and by no means invalid point about how governments worked—i.e., in response to the feeling of falling behind the "more modernized" states of western Europe. He points out that in states governed by reform absolutism, "it was not only a matter of conservative or enlightened influences on politics, . . . but a practical government reaction" to the sense of inferiority that spawned a race to catch up.

22. See, e.g., the collection of *Einblattdrucke* in the Herzog August Bibliothek: Walter Petersen, *Verzeichnis der Einblattdrucke und Handschriften aus dem Rechtsleben des Herzogtums Braunschweig-Lüneburg: Ergänzt um den Nachweis weiterer Rechtsquellen*, vol. 1: *1418–1714*; vol. 2: *1714–1807* (Wiesbaden: In Kommission bei Harrasowitz, 1984), and the far more extensive collection of these in StAWf, 40 Slg. Looked at in day-to-day order, two things are striking: (1) the clustering of certain emergency ordinances—e.g., regulations dealing with plague—which then disappear for literally years after the emergency passed, and (2) the variety of topics dealt with in close succession.

23. Peter Albrecht, *Die Förderung des Landesausbaues im Herzogtum Braunschweig-Wolfenbüttel im Spiegel der Verwaltungsakten des 18. Jahrhunderts (1671–1806)* (Braunschweig: Waisenhaus, 1980), has, for example, documented the efforts of the ducal government to promote economic growth. Yet it is clear from Albrecht's analysis that here, too, there were many incongruities, false starts, and contradictions.

24. Exceptionally, Vann, *Making of a State*, and Robisheaux, *Rural Society*, both take special interest in the lower levels of governing. Much can also be learned about village politics from David Warren Sabean, *Power in the Blood: Popular Culture and Village Discourse* (Cambridge: Cambridge University Press, 1984); id., *Property, Production, and Family in Neckarhausen, 1700–1870* (Cambridge: Cambridge University Press, 1990).

25. See Mack Walker, *German Home Towns: Community, State, and General Estate, 1648–1871* (Ithaca, N.Y.: Cornell University Press, 1971); Vann, *Making of a State*, esp. 38–46.

26. "State power did not simply expand in the sixteenth and seventeenth cen-

turies; it was very often drawn into the village by the villagers themselves. State power was also checked, frustrated, often turned to purposes no ruler completely controlled" (Robisheaux, *Rural Society*, 258).

27. A study of the state that stops at the level of ordinances is bound to have many shortcomings. Critics have attacked Raeff's analysis of police ordinances at several points. Dirk Blasius has pointed out the "well-ordered police state" Raeff portrays might well have "exist[ed] only in the minds of a political and bureaucratic elite intent upon its implementation" (review in *JMH* 56 [1984]: 515–17, here 516).

28. The Collegium medicum was renamed the Ober-Sanitäts-Collegium in 1771. To avoid confusion, however, I refer to the body as the Collegium medicum throughout this book.

29. See August Hinze, *Lexicon aller Herzogl. [ichen] Braunschweigischen Verordnungen, welche die medicinische Policey betreffen* (Stendal: Franz & Grosse, 1793).

30. For information on the early history of Wolfenbüttel, I have relied heavily on Hassel/Bege; Joseph König, "Landesgeschichte, einschließlich Recht, Verfassung und Verwaltung," in *Braunschweigische Landesgeschichte im Überblick*, ed. Richard Moderhack, 3d ed. (Braunschweig: Waisenhaus, 1979), 61–109, here esp. 61–77; Günter Scheel, "Kurbraunschweig und die übrigen welfischen Lande," in *Deutsche Verwaltungsgeschichte*, ed. Kurt G. A. Jeserich, Hans Pohl, and Georg-Christoph von Unruh, vol. 1: *Vom Spätmittelalter bis zum Ende des Reiches* (Stuttgart: Deutsche Verlagsanstalt, 1983), 741–63; August Rhamm, *Die Verfassungsgesetze des Herzogthums Braunschweig* (Braunschweig: Friedrich Vieweg & Sohn, 1900); Heinrich Andreas Koch, *Versuch einer pragmatischen Geschichte des Durchlauchtigsten Hauses Braunschweig und Luneburg* (Braunschweig: Fürstliche Waysenhaus-Buchhandlung, 1764); and Wilhelm Havemann, *Geschichte der Lande Braunschweig und Luneburg*, (Göttingen: Dieterichsche Buchhandlung, 1853–57), esp. vol. 3.

31. König, "Landesgeschichte," 77–78, 80, 83; Havemann, *Geschichte*, 173–99, 416–83; Hassel/Bege, 2: 375–76; and Albrecht, *Förderung*, 10–11.

32. The total area of Braunschweig-Wolfenbüttel in 1800 was about 3,690 km², with a periphery of 1,243 km. This relatively large periphery to total area indicates the fragmentation of the state. See Wolfgang Meibeyer, "Die Landesnatur," in *Braunschweigische Landesgeschichte*, ed. Moderhack, 1.

33. Albrecht, *Förderung*, 16–17; Klaus-Walther Ohnesorge, "Die Bevölkerungsentwicklung in der Stadt Wolfenbüttel und ihre Ursachen in der 2. Hälfte des 18. Jahrhunderts (1754–1790)," *BJ* 61 (1980): 37–53.

34. Albrecht, *Förderung*, 16–17.

35. Ibid., 13–14, 17–18.

36. Vann, *Making of a State*; Robisheaux, *Rural Society*.

37. Peter Blickle, *Studien zur geschichtlichen Bedeutung des deutschen Bauernstandes* (Stuttgart: Gustav Fischer, 1989); id., "Untertanen der Frühneuzeit: Zur Rekonstruktion der politischen Kultur und der sozialen Wirklichkeit Deutschlands im 17. Jahrhundert," *VSWG* 70 (1983): 483–522; see also Winfried Schulze, *Bäuerliche Widerstand und feudale Herrschaft in der frühen Neuzeit* (Stuttgart-Bad Cannstatt: Frommann-Holzboog, 1980); and *Aufstände, Revolten, Prozesse: Beiträge zur bäuerlichen Widerstandsbewegungen im frühneuzeitlichen Europa*, ed. Winfried Schulze (Stuttgart: Klett-Cotta, 1983).

38. My discussion here closely follows Günter Scheel's treatment of the administrative history of Braunschweig. The administration of Blankenburg was theoretically separate from that of Braunschweig-Wolfenbüttel, although the structure and competencies of various offices were similar. The privy council, however, was responsible for the general administration of both duchies.

39. *Landtags-Abschied errichtet zu Braunschweig den 9ten April 1770. Imgleichen Gesammter Landschaft des Herzogthums Braunschweig-Lüneburg Wolfenbüttelschen Theils Privilegia und Befugnisse* (Braunschweig: Waisenhausbuchhandlung, 1770), sections on Collegium medicum and its jurisdiction, §§ 28, 55; Scheel, "Kurbraunschweig," 761–62; Albrecht, *Förderung*, 19–20; Wilhelm Schmidt, "Der Braunschweigische Landtag von 1768 bis 1770," *Jahrbuch für Geschichte* 11 (1912): 78–115.

40. Hassel/Bege, 1: 239.

41. Scheel, "Kurbraunschweig," 746–47.

42. MO 1721; MO 1747; Annelise Gerbert, *Öffentliche Gesundheitspflege und staatliches Medizinalwesen in den Städten Braunschweig und Wolfenbüttel im 19. Jahrhundert* (Braunschweig: Selbstverlag des Braunschweigischen Geschichtsvereins, 1983), 14–15; Walter Artelt, "Das medizinische Braunschweig um 1770," *MJ* 1 (1966): 240–60.

43. Carl-August Agena, "Der Amtmann im 17. und 18. Jahrhundert—Ein Beitrag zur Geschichte des Richter- und Beamtentums" (diss., University of Göttingen, 1973), esp. 6–12; John C. Theibault, "Coping with the Thirty Years' War: Villages and Villagers in Hesse-Kassel, 1600–1680" (diss., Johns Hopkins University, 1986), 16–47, 304. For perceptive discussions of local government, see Sabean, *Power*, 1–36, and Vann, *Making of a State*, 38–43, 103–9.

44. The Amtskammerordnung of 1 July 1688 (copy in StAWf, 40 Slg 3268) was the basic ordinance dealing with the development and organization of Amt administration. See Albrecht, *Förderung*, 25–26; Scheel, "Kurbraunschweig," 759–60; Werner Wittich, *Ländliche Verfassung Niedersachsens und Organisation des Amts im 18. Jahrhundert* (Darmstadt: L. C. Wittich'sche Hofbuchdruckerei, 1891); Leopold Friedrich Fredersdorff, *Practische Anleitung zur Land-Polizey aus allgemeinen Grundsätzen mit Hinweis auf die Fürstl. Braunschweigischen Wolfenbüttelschen Landes-Gesetze* (Pyrmont: Helwing, 1800); Thiebault, "Coping," 16–47, 304; Agena, "Amtmann," 36–40.

45. On these sorts of patronage links, see Vann, *Making of a State*; for an excellent study of one physicus and his entanglement in such webs, see Mary Nagle Wessling, "Official Medicine and Customary Medicine in Early Modern Württemberg: The Career of Christoph Friedrich Pichler," *MGG* 9 (1990): 21–44.

46. Agena, "Amtmann," esp. 30–142; Fredersdorff, *Anweisung*; id., *Practische Anleitung*.

47. On the economy in Braunschweig-Wolfenbüttel, see Hassel/Bege, 1: 87–184; Albrecht, *Förderung*; Walther Achilles, "Siedlungs- und Agrargeschichte," in *Braunschweigische Landesgeschichte*, ed. Moderhack, 129–50; and Hans Jürgen Querfurth, "Wirtschafts-und Verkehrsgeschichte," in ibid., 183–87.

48. Wilhelm Bornstedt, *Geschichte des Braunschweigischen Bauerntums: Ein Beitrag zur Rechts-, Sozial- und Kulturalgeschichte der ländlichen Bevölkerung in Südostniedersachsen in der vorindustriellen Zeit* (Braunschweig: Landeskreisverwaltung, 1970), 87.

49. Hassel/Bege, 1: 17–22, 89–106, quotation at 17.

50. Bornstedt, *Geschichte*, 83–89; Albrecht, *Förderung*.

51. As demonstrated for the period after the Seven Years' War in the reports to the privy council, 14 Feb. 1766, StAWf, 40 Slg. 9565. For a specific example, see report from Amt Campen, 1766, in StAWf, 8 Alt Campen Gr. 27 Nr. 23, fols. 18–67.

52. Hassel/Bege, 1: 160–83. On the porcelain factory in Fürstenberg, see Siegfried Ducret, *Fürstenberger Porzellan*, vol. 1: *Geschichte der Fabrik* (Braunschweig: Klinkhardt & Biermann, 1965).

53. Albrecht, *Förderung*, 476–78, 504, 518–29, 538–45.

54. Krünitz, s.v. "Fabrik"; Rudolf Forberger, "Zu den Begriffen 'Manufactur' und 'Fabrik' in technischer und technologischer Sicht," in *Technologischer Wandel im 18. Jahrhundert*, ed. Ulrich Troitzsch (Wolfenbüttel: Herzog August Bibliothek, 1981), 175–87. On manufacturing in Braunschweig-Wolfenbüttel, see Hassel/Bege, 1: 184–205; Albrecht, *Förderung*, 226–370, 475–546.

55. Walther Achilles, *Die steuerliche Belastung der braunschweigischen Landwirtschaft und ihr Beitrag zu den Staatseinnahmen im 17. und 18. Jahrhundert* (Hildesheim: August Lax, 1972), 43; Albrecht, *Förderung*, 350–68. Albrecht counted 158 "Manufacturen und Fabriken" in the ten cities of Braunschweig-Wolfenbüttel, ibid., 475.

56. Hassel/Bege, 1: 189–96; Albrecht, *Förderung*, 538–45; Sabean, *Power*, 10–11.

57. David Sabean, "Aspects of Kinship Behaviour and Property in Rural Western Europe before 1800," in *Family and Inheritance: Rural Society in Western Europe, 1200–1800*, ed. Jack Goody, Joan Thirsk, and E. P. Thompson (Cambridge: Cambridge University Press, 1976), 99. On the relationship between statistical realities and mentality, see James A. Henretta, "Families and Farms: *Mentalité* in Pre-Industrial America," *William and Mary Quarterly*, 3d ser., 35 (1978): 3–32; Sabean, *Property*; and Arthur E. Imhof, *Die verlorenen Welten: Alltagsbewältigung durch unsere Vorfahren—und weshalb wir uns heute so schwer damit tun* (Munich: Beck, 1984).

58. Robert Darnton uses the term *seismic shifts* in "The History of Mentalities: Recent Writings on Revolution, Criminality, and Death in France," in *Structure, Consciousness and History*, ed. Richard H. Brown and Stanford M. Lyman (Cambridge, Mass.: Harvard University Press, 1978), 133.

59. Theibault, "Coping," esp. 16–210; Eric R. Wolf, *Peasants* (Englewood Cliffs, N.J.: Greenwood Press, 1966), esp. 18–59; Sabean, "Aspects," 99–100; Peter Blickle, "Kommunalismus, Parlamentarismus, Republikanismus," in Blickle, *Studien*, 192–93; id., "Der Kommunalismus als Gestaltungsprinzip zwischen Mittelalter und Moderne," in ibid., 69–82.

60. Hassel/Bege, 1: 111, 121–22; Albrecht, *Förderung*, 96.

61. StAWf, 8 Alt Warburg 11, 24 Feb. 1784; on the economic exploitation of forests, see Christa Graefe, *Forstleute: Von den Anfängen einer Behörde und ihren Beamten (Braunschweig-Wolfenbüttel 1530–1607)* (Wiesbaden: Harrassowitz in Kommission, 1989). Reports from other parts of the duchy, right after the Seven Years' War, but also later in the century, indicate that the various communes often proposed changes and innovations that apparently had much widespread support in the commune itself and were not merely schemes Amtmänner concocted. See, e.g., StAWf, 8 Alt Ottenstein 165, 9 Feb. 1766; 8 Alt Campen Gr. 27 Nr. 23, fols. 18–67, 1776; 8 Alt Stauffenberg 31, Feb. 1781. In a general survey of peasant communities, Heide Wunder has pointed out that while peasants have often been seen as slow to "modernize," their

decision to stick with old methods was often very logically calculated and took into account the narrow margin between success and failure. Likewise, some peasants were quick to exploit economic possibilities—e.g., enclosing fields where it was profitable. See Wunder, *Die bäuerliche Gemeinde in Deutschland* (Göttingen: Vandenhoeck & Ruprecht, 1986), 82, 107–8, 113, 137–39.

62. Bornstedt, *Geschichte,* esp. 44, 72–75; Wittich, *Verfassung,* 12–13, 17, 21–22; id., *Die Grundherrschaft in Nordwestdeutschland* (Leipzig: Dunckert & Humblot, 1896); Wilhelm Abel, "Landwirtschaft, 1648–1800," in *Handbuch des deutschen Wirtschafts- und Sozialgeschichte,* ed. Hermann Aubin and Wolfgang Zorn (Stuttgart: Union, 1976–78), 1: 499; Achilles, "Siedlungs- und Agrargeschichte," 142–43; id., *Steuerliche Belastung,* 20; the definitive work on *Meierrecht* is Carl Gesenius, *Das Meyerrecht, mit vorzüglicher Hinsicht auf den Wolfenbuttelschen Theils des Herzogthums Braunschweig-Lüneburg* (Wolfenbüttel: Albrecht, 1801, 1803).

63. Bornstedt, *Geschichte,* 58–63.

64. Ibid., 68–70; Wilhelm Bornstedt, *Chronik von Stöckheim: Siedlungsgeographie, Sozial- und Kulturgeschichte eines braunschweigischen Dorfes* (Stockheim bei Braunschweig: ACO, 1967).

65. Many services were allotted in a set sequence ("in einer bestimmten Reihenfolge"); these full communal members were known as *Reiheleute* and their holdings as *Reihestellen.* See Wittich, *Verfassung,* 57–59.

66. Adolf Hueg, *Dorf und Bauerntum: Eine Fibel als Hilfsbuch zur Niedersächsischen Dorfgeschichtsforschung (Dorffibel)* (Oldenburg: Gerhard Stalling, 1939), 13–14, 18; Ulrike Gleixner, "Hebammen als Amtsfrauen und Gutachterinnen auf dem Land: Eine Fallstudie (Altmark 18. Jahrhundert)," forthcoming in *Frauen in der ländlichen Gesellschaft der Frühen Neuzeit,* ed. Heide Wunder and Christina Vanja. I would like to thank Ulrike Gleixner for providing me with a typescript of her article.

67. Hueg, *Dorf,* 18.

68. Bornstedt, *Geschichte,* 51–57B; Hueg, *Dorf,* 14. Wittich, *Verfassung,* 57–59, 62–63, 67.

69. Hassel/Bege, 1: 84–85, 113; Achilles, *Steuerliche Belastung.*

70. Achilles, *Steuerliche Belastung,* 27, 30–32.

71. Hueg, *Dorf,* 18.

72. For Braunschweig-Wolfenbüttel, see Achilles, *Steuerliche Belastung,* and Albrecht, *Förderung;* on Germany in general, see Wehler, *Deutsche Gesellschaftsgeschichte,* 1: 70, 87–88.

73. Here I rely entirely on Achilles, "Siedlungs- und Agrargeschichte," 144–45.

74. Ibid., 145–46; Walther Achilles, *Vermögensverhältnisse braunschweigischer Bauernhöfe im 17. und 18. Jahrhundert* (Stuttgart: Gustav Fischer, 1965); and Bornstedt, *Chronik.*

75. Achilles, *Steuerliche Belastung.*

76. Sabean, *Property,* 380–86; Hans Medick and David Sabean, "Emotionen und materielle Interessen in Familie und Verwandschaft: Überlegungen zu neuen Wegen und Bereichen einer historischen und sozialanthropologischen Familienforschung," in *Emotionen und materielle Interessen: Sozialanthropologische und historische Beiträge zur Familienforschung,* ed. Medick and Sabean (Göttingen: Vandenhoeck & Ruprecht, 1984), 27–64.

77. Sabean, *Power*, 12–20; id., *Property*, 355–70; Wessling has pointed out that "*Bürgerschaft*, or [the] privilege of citizenship in a town, was not awarded as a matter of course. . . . The physician met obstacles to a career built upon private practice from an unexpected source: the nature of the town itself" ("Medicine and Government," 19–20).

78. Albrecht, *Förderung*, 226; Sheehan, *German History*, 113–18; Wehler, *Deutsche Gesellschaftsgeschichte*, 177–217.

79. Albrecht, *Förderung*, 226.

80. Ibid., 367.

81. Walker, *German Home Towns*, 34–142. Braunschweig had no independent city council after its conquest in 1671, when the old independent council was abolished and replaced with a new one appointed by, and totally dependent on, the ducal government. Thereafter a ducal commission made all important administrative decisions, while the council functioned mostly as a judicial instance. See Richard Moderhack, "Geschichte der Städte," in *Braunschweigische Landesgeschichte*, ed. Moderhack, 159.

82. Albrecht, *Förderung*, 328–61.

83. But see Walker, *German Home Towns*, esp. 73–144.

84. Wehler, *Deutsche Gesellschaftsgeschichte*, 1: 191–92.

85. Anthony Black, *Guilds and Civil Society in European Political Thought from the Twelfth Century to the Present* (Ithaca, N.Y.: Cornell University Press, 1984), 9.

86. James Sheehan has observed that guilds "did not distinguish between occupation and family, economics and politics, the public and the private realms" (*German History*, 108).

87. Black, *Guilds*, 3–31; Walker, *German Home Towns*, 73–107.

88. Wehler, *Deutsche Gesellschaftsgeschichte*, 1: 191–92.

89. Walker, *German Home Towns*, 93–94; especially on the concept of honor and dishonor, see also Rudolf Wissell, *Des alten Handwerks Recht und Gewohnheit*, 2d ed. (Berlin: Colloquium, 1971), 1: 145–273; Werner Danckert, *Unehrliche Leute: Die verfemten Berufe* (Bern: Francke, 1963); Oswald A. Erich and Richard Beitl, *Wörterbuch des deutschen Volkskunde*, 2d ed. (Stuttgart: Alfred Kröner, 1955), s.v. "Handwerk" and "unehrliche Gewerbe"; *HDA*, s.v. "Handwerker" and "unehrlich."

90. Wolfram Fischer, *Handwerksrecht und Handwerkswirtschaft um 1800* (Berlin: Dunker & Humblot, 1955), 26–29, 36; Walker, *German Home Towns*, 93; Sheehan, *German History*, 111–12.

91. Fischer, *Handwerksrecht*, 27–28, 37.

92. Walker, *German Home Towns*, 86, 90–91; Fischer, *Handwerksrecht*, 41, 44.

93. Albrecht, *Förderung*, 229.

94. For a detailed discussion, see ibid., 226–48.

95. The ordinance of September 1692, promulgated in Celle/Hannover, was likewise publicized in Braunschweig-Wolfenbüttel, HAB, Gn Kps 67 (25); "Verordnung und REGELEMENT Wie es . . . der . . . im Gesamthause genommenen Abrede nach/bei denen Aembtern und Gilden der Künstler und Handwerker zu halten," HAB, Einbl. R4: 221, 26 Sept. 1692; the imperial trade edict of 16 Aug. 1731 was made public on 19 Oct. 1731, HAB, Einbl. R1: 38; "Ordnung für die Gilden im Herzothum Braunschweig und Fürstenthum Blankenburg," HAB, Einbl. R4: 1711.

96. Albrecht, *Förderung*, 346–48.

97. Ibid., 236–43, 343–49, 369.

98. Ibid., 325–28; Fischer, *Handwerksrecht*, 45; William H. Sewell, Jr., *Work and Revolution in France: The Language of Labor from the Old Regime to 1848* (Cambridge: Cambridge University Press, 1980). The half-ritualistic "hunting down of encroachers" (*Pfuscherjagd*) was officially done away with in 1805: "Verordnung, wegen Aufhebung des Pfuscherjagens im hiesigen Herzogthum und Fürstentum Blankenburg," HAB, Einbl. R.4: 2591, 12 Nov. 1805. The government's simultaneous attempts to fight encroachment are reflected in ordinances passed on 8 Nov. 1753, HAB, Cod. Guelf. 95, Noviss. 2, fol. 38; 10 Aug. 1756, ibid., fols. 91–92; 11 Feb. 1768 ("Verordnung, den Verkauf der den Fuschern abzunehmenden Handwerks-Geräthschaften und Arbeiten betreffend"), HAB, Einbl. R.4: 1779; 25 Jan. 1802, ibid., Einbl. R.3: 1704; 11 Oct. 1802, ibid., Einbl. R.3: 1718.

99. Fischer, *Handwerksrecht*, 46; Carl-Hans Hauptmeyer, "Aufklärung und bäuerliche Oppositionen im zentralen Niedersachsen des ausgehenden 18. Jahrhunderts," in *Das Volk als Object obrigkeitlichen Handelns*, ed. Rudolf Vierhaus (Tübingen: Max Niemeyer, 1992), 197–201.

100. Walker, *German Home Towns*, 101. Zedler defines "bürgerliche Nahrung" as "in a broad sense, each and every kind of occupation, profession, handwork, trade, commerce, whatever its name, as well as brewing, tavernkeeping, and the like." But in an even wider sense, *Nahrung* also applied to nobles, military, and peasants. Krünitz (1806) defines "Nahrung" as "the very essence of everything by which one gains a living."

101. Renate Blickle, "Nahrung und Eigentum als Kategorien in der ständischen Gesellschaft," in *Ständische Gesellschaft und soziale Mobilität*, ed. Winfried Schulze (Munich: R. Oldenbourg, 1988), 76–77, 82, 85–87.

102. Wehler, *Deutsche Gesellschaftsgeschichte*, 1: 81.

103. Hauptmeyer, "Aufklärung," esp. 201–3.

104. Sabean, *Property*, 61–65.

105. David Sabean, "'Junge Immen im leeren Korb': Beziehungen zwischen Schwägern in einem schwäbischen Dorf," in *Emotionen*, ed. Medick and Sabean, 231–50.

106. Albrecht, *Förderung*, 564.

107. Theodor Penners, "Bevölkerungsgeschichtliche Probleme der Land-Stadtwanderung—untersucht an der ländlichen Abwanderung in die Städte Braunschweig und Wolfenbüttel um die Mitte des 18. Jahrhunderts: Mit einem Übersichtskarte," *BJ* 37 (1956): 57–134; Wolfgang Meibeyer, "Bevölkerungs- und sozialgeographische Differenzierung der Stadt Braunschweig um die Mitte des 18. Jahrhunderts," *BJ* 47 (1966): 125–57.

108. James Allen Vann has observed that "historical change must be explained in terms of tensions between various individuals and groups. . . . the study of human beings working out their conflicts illustrates historical change better than discussions of such abstract forces as religious beliefs, economic ambition, and social cohesion. It is not that these forces are unimportant. They are vital. But they can be grasped in their full complexity only as reflections and aspects of a bargaining process that involves both individuals and corporate bodies" (*Making of a State*, 20–21).

109. Raeff, *Police State*; Reinhold August Dorwart, *The Prussian Welfare State*

Before 1740 (Cambridge, Mass.: Harvard University Press, 1971); id., "The Royal College of Medicine and Public Health of Brandenburg-Prussia, 1685–1740," *MH* 2 (1958): 13–23.

110. Vann, *Making of a State*; Robisheaux, *Rural Society*; and Werner Troßbach, *Sozialbewegung und politische Erfahrung: Bäuerliche Protest in hessischen Territorien, 1648–1806* (Weingarten: Drumlin, 1987) are exceptions. In the realm of medicine, Wessling, "Medicine and Government," is also concerned with these daily interactions, as is, more extensively, Francisca Loetz, *Vom Kranken zum Patienten: "Medikalisierung" und medizinische Vergesellschaftung am Beispiel Badens, 1750–1850* (Stuttgart: Franz Steiner, 1993).

111. MO 1721; MO 1747; and SM 1747. MO 1747 was not, in fact, a comprehensive medical ordinance; rather, it established organs—like the Collegium medicum—to carry out the provisions of the 1721 ordinance.

112. See Alfons Fischer, *Geschichte des Deutschen Gesundheitswesens*, vol. 2: *Von den Anfängen der hygienischen Ortsbeschreibungen bis zur Gründung des Reichsgesundheitsamtes (Das 18. und 19. Jahrhunderts)* (Berlin: Kommissionsverlag F. A. Herbig, 1933), 140–52; and the various works by Manfred Stürzbecher on medical ordinances in the Germanies: "Einige Bemerkungen zur Geschichte der Medizinalgesetzgebung im deutschen Sprachgebiet," *Veröffentlichungen der internationalen Gesellschaft für Geschichte der Pharmazie*, n.s., 24 (1964): 123–32; "Betrachtungen zur Historiographie der Medizinalordnungen," *Öffentlicher Gesundheitsdienst* 25 (1963): 282–88; "Zur Geschichte der Medizinalgesetzgebung im Fürstbistum Münster im 17. und 18. Jahrhundert," *Westfälische Zeitschrift* 114 (1964): 165–91; "Zur Geschichte der brandenburgischen Medizinalgesetzgebung im 17. Jahrhundert," in *Beiträge zur Berliner Medizingeschichte*, ed. Stürzbecher (Berlin: de Gruyter, 1966), 1–66.

113. Ronald Sawyer has pointed out that until recently "historians of healing in early modern England have dealt almost exclusively with the . . . hierarchy of officially recognized practitioners, . . . [but] the pen of Richard Napier and the comments of his patients provide a different picture of officially sanctioned medicine than has hitherto been revealed" ("Patients," 55).

114. The medical ordinances have been principally interpreted as programmatic and legalistic statements. See, e.g., Fischer, *Geschichte*, 140–52; Dorwart, *Prussian Welfare State*; and Raeff, *Police State*, 120–24, 130–32, who remarks (130–31) that medical practice

received official legal status and was subjected to administrative controls. . . . Doctors, of course, had been professionalized during the Renaissance, but now their numbers were expanded and supervised by the authorities. Of still greater significance proved to be the emergence of trained paramedical personnel and the supervision of public health by boards of medical professionals. . . . Medical boards were set up and were entrusted with several important new functions in the professionalization of health care.

For a very different perspective, see Loetz, *Vom Kranken zum Patienten*.

115. MO 1721, preface.
116. MO 1721, Cap. I, § 2.
117. "Unterthänigst entworffener Plan von Errichtung und Einrichtung derer

Collegiorum Medicorum," n.d., probably 1744, in StAWf, 2 Alt 1165, fols. 3–23, quote from fol. 3.

118. MO 1747, §§ 7–9, 13–17, 21–23, 27–29. A copy of this "Revers" ("Q.D.B.V.") can be found in StAWf, 2 Alt 11167, fols. 38–39.

119. Johann Bernhard Martini, *Dispensatorium pharmaceuticum Brunsvicense* (Braunschweig: Orphanotrophen [Waisenhaus Buchhandlung], 1777); "Verordnung, das Hebammenwesen betreffend," HAB Einbl. R 4: 1345, 18 Feb. 1757; "Verordnung, das Hebammen-Wesen betreffend," HAB Einbl. R4: 2544, 10 Apr. 1803.

120. See, e.g., the great mass of material on epidemic diseases in StAWf, 2 Alt 11449–518, and specifically on plague, 2 Alt 11519–607; and in 111 Neu 3135–42 (preventive measures), 3157–58 (ergotism and dysentery), 3226–54 (reports from physicate districts).

121. MO 1747, § 3. One of the earliest suggestions for appointing a *Land-Medicus* to cover the *Ämter* Gandersheim, Seesen, Greene, and Stauffenburg directed his special attention to all "dangerous and contagious diseases" to prevent them from becoming "plagues" (StAWf, 2 Alt 11279, fol. 1, 26 Mar. 1696).

122. SM 1747, §§ 13–15.

123. See the series of contracts and negotiations between the city of Braunschweig and its physici: StadtB, B IV 13c: 1 (1591–1657); B IV 13c: 3 (1608); B IV 13c: 14 (1563–1605).

124. MO 1721.

125. MO 1747, preface.

126. For example, in 1770 the Collegium medicum complained to the privy council "that the local city-magistracy [in Braunschweig] is not cooperative." According to the Collegium, the magistrates were tacitly protecting a quack who was "in fact a *Candidatus theologiae.*" The magistrates refused to answer the queries of the Collegium in the case: StAWf, 2 Alt 11622, fols. 2–3, 22 July 1770.

127. StAWf, 40 Slg. 6370, 29 Aug. 1744. And to avoid such delays, the privy council provided for summary hearings and an "oral process."

128. MO 1747, § 1.

129. StAWf, 111 Neu 9, fol. 2, 26 July 1779; see also "Reskript" from 3 Dec. 1767, in HAB Cod. Guelf. 97 Noviss. 2°, fols. 181–82.

130. For an expression of this, see the clarification of 14 Apr. 1815 in StAWf, 111 Neu 2, vol. 1, fols. 31–32.

131. Ibid., fol. 32.

132. On this reorganization and its meaning, see Rhamm, *Verfassungsgesetze*, 16–18.

133. For a good example of the kind of conflict that arose, see StAWf, 111 Neu 56 on the battle that developed between him and the city magistrates in Helmstedt in 1750 concerning the treatment of a child by a felsher.

134. Karl-Rudolf Döhnel, *Das Anatomisch-Chirurgische Institut in Braunschweig, 1750–1869* (Braunschweig: Waisenhaus, 1957); StAWf, 40 Slg 10079, § 28 of *Landtags-Abschied*, "Serenissimi gnädigste Verordnung, über einige Puncte des Reglements vom 4ten Januar 1747 das Fürstliche Collegium medicum betreffend. De dato Braunschweig, den 26sten April 1770." But the changes and the debate over competencies

continued; see, for one instance, the clarification the privy council issued on 14 Apr. 1815, StAWf, 111 Neu 2, vol. 1, fols. 31–32.

135. Döhnel, *Institut*, 29.

136. StAWf, 2 Alt 11205, "Acta a) die neue Einrichtung des Fürstl. Collegii medici und b) die künftige Einrichtung des Apothekerwesens in Braunschweig betref. 1770"; see esp. the "Pro Memoria" written by Privy Councilor von Flögen, 18 Oct. 1770.

137. StAWf, 2 Alt 11205, "Pro Memoria," 18 Oct. 1770, fols. 19, 21, 28. On Martini's troubles, see ibid. 11316, fols. 26–42, for the controversy between him and Dr. Petsche in 1757–58,; and 11420, fols. 2–3, for the complaints of the midwives in Braunschweig about his arrogance and lack of understanding.

138. For examples, see StAWf, 111 Neu 55, fols. 2–3, 9 June 1750; from 1752, ibid., fols. 17–32. The question of inoculation caused a sharp exchange between von Meibom and Martini in 1768 (StAWf, 2 Alt 11204). Finally, the conversion of Dr. Mühlenbein to homeopathy (among other things) led to conflict in the late 1820s and 1830s; see Andreas Weißmann, "Die Schutzpockenimpfung im Herzogtum Braunschweig-Wolfenbüttel von 1800 bis zum Impfgesetz vom April 1833" (Magisterarbeit, Modern History, Technische Hochschule Braunschweig, 1993), 102–3. I thank Andreas Weißmann for providing me with a copy of his thesis.

139. StAWf, 2 Alt 11193, "Acta die Differenzen des Fürstlichen. Obersanitäts-Collegium mit dem StadtMagistrat hieselbst [Braunschweig] in pto: jurisdictionis betref." includes incidents from 1756 through 1796. On 23 Jan. 1756, the privy council warned the city magistracy and the Collegium medicum "in the future to employ a more courteous tone in your correspondence with each other" (ibid., fol. 15).

140. See, e.g., StAWf, 2 Alt 11193, fols. 23–24, 25–26, 29–31, 41–42, for the complaints the privy council received from magistrates in Braunschweig and from the Collegium medicum in 1756, 1759, 1761, 1770, and 1796; see also 111 Neu 58, fols. 18–22 for the complaint of Collegium medicum about the "misconduct" of magistrates in 1795; ibid. 56, 6, for Helmstedt; and ibid. 57 about magistrates in Blankenburg, from 1792. For examples of lack of cooperation in pursuing quacks, see 2 Alt 11287, fols. 38–40, report of Collegium medicum to privy council, and 2 Alt 11631, fols. 27–28, 10 Aug. 1791, on the case of the cobbler Dreyer in Braunschweig.

141. On publication, see HAB, Einbl. R3: 783, §§ 1–3, 14 Jan. 1749, "Serenissimi Reglement die geschwinder und ordentlicher Ausrichtung der landesherrlichen Befehle betreffend"; StAWf, 2 Alt 11200, fols. 59–60, 20 Dec. 1770. On bookkeeping, see, e.g., StAWf, 8 Alt Seesen 3 Nr. 12, fol. 87, 13 Apr. 1768, and 2 Alt 11359, fol. 55, 14 Oct. 1793.

142. See StAWf, 2 Alt 11205, "Pro Memoria," 18 Oct. 1770, for von Flögen's evaluation of the effectiveness of the Collegium medicum.

143. On appointment of individual members and their salaries, see StAWf, 2 Alt 11165–770; see also Walter Artelt's discussion of the Collegium medicum in "Das medizinische Braunschweig."

144. StAWf, 2 Alt 11166, fols. 63–65.

145. Ibid. 11176, fol. 10.

146. Examples are scattered throughout the records of Collegium medicum; but see esp. StAWf, 2 Alt 11174 and 111 Neu 34–35, 55, and 184–87.

147. StAWf, 2 Alt 11205, fols. 70–72.

148. On the physici in Germany, see Manfred Stürzbecher, "The Physici in German-speaking Countries from the Middle Ages to the Enlightenment," in *The Town and State Physician in Europe from the Middle Ages to the Enlightenment*, ed. Andrew W. Russell (Wolfenbüttel: Herzog August Bibliothek, 1981), 123–40. The first physicus in Helmstedt, the medical licentiate Johann Bosse, was probably appointed in 1652. See Robert Schaper, "Arzt und Apotheker—Das Physikat in Helmstedt," *Aus der Heimat—Für die Heimat*, Sunday suppl. to *Helmstedter Kreisblatt*, 10 Sept. 1966. On Behrens's appointment as physicus, see HAB Cod. Guelf 477, Nov., fols. 724–25, 27 May 1743.

149. StAWf, 111 Neu 3249, fols. 30–33, 51; the severity of the crisis provoked more action from the society later: see ibid., fols. 47–48, 56–57. For von Flögen's comment, see 2 Alt 11205, fol. 27, 18 Oct. 1770. Certainly, the Collegium medicum considered the medical society as it existed in Helmstedt less than ideal. While it was true that the Helmstedt society sent in reports regularly, "they contribute little or nothing to the advancement of medical knowledge" (StAWf, 2 Alt 11338, fols. 9–10, 6 Mar. 1771). Attempts to improve the situation failed. In 1771, the Collegium tried to revive the dying medical society in Wolfenbüttel by installing a new president, but apparently little changed for the better (2 Alt 11348, fols. 27–28, 12 Apr. 1771).

150. Proponents of *Alltagsgeschichte* often refer to this as reading "against the grain." See David Crew, "*Alltagsgeschichte*: A New Social History 'From Below'?" *CEH* 22 (1989): 394–407.

151. MO 1721, Cap. VII, § 1.

152. MO 1747, §§ 34–35. But there is no denying that MO 1747 drew tighter lines around the practice of medicine.

153. MO 1747, § 35; MO 1721, preface, Cap. VII, § 7.

154. In *Work and Revolution*, Sewell points out the persistence of corporatist language well into the nineteenth century.

155. MO 1721, Cap. I, § 1.

156. Ibid.

157. On examination of physicians, see MO 1747, §§ 7–11; for apothecaries, § 14; for civilian surgeons and bathmasters, § 17; military surgeons, § 21; midwives, §§ 27–29.

158. Sewell, *Work and Revolution*. In medicine, most of the work along these lines has been done for France and tied to professionalization. Matthew Ramsey, for example, argues that eighteenth-century Frenchmen "distinguished between a simple *métier* and a liberal profession"—in this case, medicine (*Professional and Popular Medicine in France, 1770–1830: The Social World of Medical Practice* [Cambridge: Cambridge University Press, 1988], 4). That was probably true in Germany as well, but corporatist language did not disappear from the public health field that quickly. On the doctors' self-image, see Thomas H. Broman, "Rethinking Professionalization: Theory, Practice and Professional Ideology in Eighteenth-Century German Medicine," *JMH* 67 (1995): 835–72.

159. MO 1747, §§ 17–19.

160. MO 1747, §§ 19–20. Moreover, this was a far older tradition. For example, in 1651 the provisors of the apothecary guild in the city of Braunschweig complained about the damage being done to their livelihood by the actions of *Störer*. They listed several such interlopers who were especially bothersome and reminded the city government that it bore the "legal and moral" responsibility for combating "with diligence and zeal" such "pestiferous" creatures (StadtB, B IV 13c: 11, 17 Oct. 1651). More than a century later, the surgeons' guild complained in very similar terms about the *Pfuscher* who made their lives miserable (StadtB C VII B7: IV, fols. 22–23, 6 May 1771).

161. MO 1747, § 24.

162. On 13 Dec. 1762, the privy council required all city magistrates to list "the guildsmen [*Professions-Verwandten*] that are lacking." The magistrate in Stadtoldendorf produced the following list of "necessary" persons—nailsmith, wheelwright, roofer—and of "desirable" persons—a skilled surgeon, a turner, hatter, buttonmaker, coppersmith, tinner, tanner, and ropemaker (StAWf, 2 Alt 11347, fol. 35, 22 Dec. 1762).

163. In his study of economic policy and economic development in Braunschweig-Wolfenbüttel, Peter Albrecht suggests a change of this sort over the period 1671–1806 (*Förderung*, 565); and see also id., "Die 'Braunschweigischen Armenanstalten': Ein Beitrag zur städtischen Armenpolitik in der ersten Hälfte des 19. Jahrhunderts (1796–1853)" (Diplomarbeit, University of Hamburg, 1962), 281. Similarly, David Sabean has pointed out that in the eighteenth century "state interest shifted ground . . . away from the issues of property surveillance, measurement, listing, and appropriation to those of production, disencumbering, mobilization, and development" (*Property*, 429–30).

164. E. P. Thompson, "The Moral Economy of the English Crowd in the Eighteenth Century," *PP* 50 (Feb. 1971): 76–136. For a thoughtful critique of Thompson's argument and a review of the historiography on the "moral economy model," see Winifred Barr Rothenberg, *From Market-Places to a Market Economy: The Transformation of Rural Massachusetts, 1750–1850* (Chicago: University of Chicago Press, 1992), 24–55.

165. See Wilfried Reininghaus's suggestions on how to approach the history of guilds from a new perspective. *Gewerbe in der Frühen Neuzeit* (Munich: R. Oldenbourg, 1990), 61–63.

166. In *Health for Sale: Quackery in England, 1660–1850* (Manchester: Manchester University Press, 1989), 21–59, Porter points out that, far from disappearing, quackery flourished, "because of the specific orientation of a commercial capitalist, spectacle-loving, consumer-oriented society, in which the very goal of the quacks—to persuade the public to consume medicine—was expedited by the same forces that explain why the society became more heavily medicine-consuming at large"(55).

167. See, e.g, Neil McKenderick, John Brewer, and J. H. Plumb, *The Birth of a Consumer Society in the Commercialization of Eighteenth Century England* (Bloomington: Indiana University Press, 1982); on France, see Cissie Fairchilds, "The Production and Marketing of Populuxe Goods in Eighteenth-Century France," in *Consumption and the World of Goods*, ed. John Brewer and Roy Porter (London: Routledge, 1993), 228–48.

168. Sometimes, of course, epidemic disease and military conflict were causally

related. For example, extensive measures were taken to prevent outbreaks of epidemic disease in Braunschweig and Wolfenbüttel while they were under French occupation in 1758. See "Acta was wegen der epidemischen Krankheiten in Braunschweig und Wolfenbüttel und deren besorgenden Contagion vorgekommen und verordnet worden," StAWf, 2 Alt 11477, and follow-up files for conditions in Braunschweig in 1758, 2 Alt 11478–481.

169. Erich Keyser, ed., *Niedersächsisches Städtebuch* (Stuttgart: W. Kohlhammer, 1952); id., "Die Pest in Niedersachsen," in *Erlebtes, Erzähltes, Erforschtes: Festgabe für Hans Wohltmann* (Stade: Selbstverlag des Geschichts- und Heimatsvereins, 1954), 108–15; Erich Woehlkens, *Pest und Ruhr im 16. und 17. Jahrhundert: Grundlagen einer statistisch-topographischen Beschreibung der großen Seuchen, insbesondere in der Stadt Uelzen* (Hannover: Niedersächsische Heimatbund, 1954), 151–52, table 12, Nr. 19–20.

170. *Kurzer/ doch nützlicher Bericht/ Wie ein jeder/ bey jetziger grassierenden Seuche/ sich verhalten soll* (Braunschweig, 1657), copy in HAB, Gn Kapsel 55 (8). Perhaps the most famous contemporary discussion of dysentery as a public health problem was Johann Georg Zimmermann, *Von der Ruhr unter dem Volk im Jahr 1765, und denen mit derselben eingedrungenen Vorurtheilen, nebst einigen allgemeinen Aussichten in die Heilung dieser Vorurtheile* (Zurich: Füeßli, 1767).

171. *Kurzer/ doch nützlicher Bericht* (1657); Matthias Ramelov, *Kurtzer Auszug und Unterricht Einiger schlecht- und geringen/ dennoch/ von vornehmsten Medicis, durch die Erfahrung/ zur Vorbewahrung und Heilung der ansteckenden Pest-Seuche bewehrt-befundenen Artzneyen und derselben Gebrauch. Vor das Land und andern gemeinen Volk/ in den kleinen Städten/ Flekken/ und Dörffern/ welche keine Apotheken/ noch Mittel haben kostbare Artzeney/ vielweniger einen Medicum zu gebrauchen/ wie dieselbe sich mit solchen genugen in diesem Auszug gesetzten Mitteln/ und angeführten Gebrauch/ vermittelst Beistand Gottes/ schützen und heilen können: Auf Hochfürstliche-Landesväterlicher Vorsorge/ Und gegebenen gnädigst Befehl/ Alles was in diesem Auszug in Artzneyen und derer Gebrauch enthalten/ und angeführet/ in bloß recht verständlich Teutsch entworffen und eröffnet* (Braunschweig, 1681), copy in HAB, Gn Kapsel 43 (16); *Kurtzer Unterricht/ Wie man sich für der giftigen anklebenden Seuche Der Pestilentz/ Nechst Göttlicher Hülffe und Beystand/ bewahren und fürsehen solle: Und wie dieselbe zu Curiren sey. Auf Verordnung und Befehl der Hohen Landes-Fürstlichen Obrigkeit/ Aufgesetzet* (Wolfenbüttel, 1681), copy in HAB, Einbl. R4: 156.

172. Among others: *Kurzer und nohtwendiger Bericht: Von der Praeservation und Curation der Dysenterie oder Rohten-Ruhr. Zu Nutz und Wolfahrt der Eingesessenen der Fürstlichen Residenz-Stadt Wolfenbüttel/ und des löblichen Fürstenthums Braunschweig-Lüneburg Wolfenbüttelschen Theils Unterthanen/ etc.* (Wolfenbüttel, n.d. [early 1700s]), copy in HAB, Gn 43 (20); Matthias Ramelov, *Der izt grassirenden Kranckheit die Rohte Ruhr genandt Kurze dennoch Außführ- und gründliche Beschreibung: Und zwar 1. Worinn dieselbe Kranckheit eigendlich bestehe. 2. Von dessen Prognostico. 3. Wie man sich vor derselben zum füglichsten praeserviren und schützen könne. Und 4. da irgends einer mit solcher befallen/ zum sichersten zu curiren oder zu heilen sey. Auß Christlicher Vorsorge/ wohlmeinend auffgesetzet/ und in Druck befodert* (Goslar, 1666), copy in HAB, Gn Kapsel 43 (17); *Kurtze Nachricht/ Wie sich In Pest-Zeiten/ und Wann die Rohte Ruhr grassiret/ Die Land-Leute durch geringe Mittel praeserviren und curiren können* (Wolfenbüttel, 1681), copy in HAB, Einbl. R4: 158; *Kurtzer und nohtwendiger Bericht: Von der Praeservation und Curation der*

Dysenterie oder Rohten-Ruhr. Zu Nutz und Wolfahrt der eingesessenen der fürstlichen Residenz-Stadt Wolffenbüttel / und des löblichen Fürstenthums Braunschweig Lüneburg Wolffenbüttelschen Theils. Unterthanen / etc. (Wolfenbüttel, 1718), copy in HAB, Einbl. R4: 565; *Kurtzer und nothwendiger Bericht / Wie man sich gegen die Rothe Ruhr zu praeserviren / und wie solche allenfalls zu curiren* (n.d., n.p., [1719]), copy in HAB, Einbl. R4: 560; as appendix to this, *Unterricht vor die Apotheken / Chirurgos und Bader auf dem Lande / Wie sie die an der vorietzo grassirenden rothen Ruhr darneider liegende Patienten zu tractiren haben* (n.d., n.p., [1719]), copy in HAB, Einbl. R4: 566; *Kurze Anweisung Für die Leute auf dem Lande, Wie dieselben bey der im Schwange gehenden Rohten-Ruhr So wohl für diese Kranckheit sich bewahren als auch in derselben Theils durch Haus- theils durch geringe Artzney-Mittel von denen Apothecken, Sich rahten und helffen können* (Braunschweig, 1736), copy in HAB, Einbl. R4: 697; *Anweisung zur Verhutung und Heilung der jetzt grassirenden gallichten Ruhr* (Helmstedt, 1793), copy in HAB, Q141c Helmst. 4°.

173. "Kritischer Versuch über das Wort Aufklärung, zur endlichen Beylegung der darüber geführten Streitigkeiten," *Deutsche Monatschrift* (1790): 11–44, 205–33, here 19. Specifically on popular enlightenment, see "Bedenklichkeit bei der Verfeinerung und Aufklärung des Landvolks, aus der wirklichen Welt, aus der Lage und dem Charakter des Landmanns abstrahirt; von einem Landprediger," *BM*, 3 Jan. 1789; C. H. F. Käufer, "Ueber die Aufklärung des Landmanns durch Bücher," *BM*, 28 June 1800.

174. See, e.g., "Wie sind neue Verbesserungen und nützliche Vorschläge am leichtesten unter dem Landmann einzuführen?" *BA-GB*, 18 and 21 Oct. 1769.

175. Reinhart Siegert offers an extensive bibliography in his "Aufklärung und Volkslectüre: Exemplarish dargestellt an Rudolph Zacharias Becker und seinem *Noth- und Hülfsbüchlein*," *AGB* 19 (1978): cols. 1253–348; see also Heinz Otto Lichtenberg, *Unterhaltsame Bauernaufklärung: Ein Kapital Volksbildungsgeschichte* (Tübingen: Tübinger Vereinigung für Volkskunde, 1970); Rudolf Schenda, *Volk ohne Buch: Studien zur Sozialgeschichte der populären Lesestoffe, 1770–1910* (Frankfurt am Main: Vittorio Klostermann, 1970).

176. Tissot, *Avis au peuple sur sa santé* (Lausanne: J. Zimmerli, 1761); German ed., *Anleitung für das Landvolk in Absicht auf seine Gesundheit* (Zurich: Heidegger, 1763). I used the 2d rev. and enlarged ed. (Frankfurt a.M., 1766). Zimmerman, *Ruhr*.

177. Friedrich Schlüter, *Immerwährende Gesundheits-Kalender oder Hausbuch zur Kenntniß und Erhaltung der Gesundheit* (Braunschweig: Schulbuchhandlung, 1799).

178. StAWf, 2 Alt 11428, fol. 10, 10 July, 1761.

179. E.g., StAWf, 111 Neu 3426, 7 July 1794.

180. Johann Krügelstein, *Noth- und Hülfsbüchlein in der Ruhr und epidemischen Krankheiten überhaupt* (Ohrduff: n.p., 1803); Bernhard Faust, *Gesundheits-Katechismus zum Gebrauche in den Schulen und beym häuslichen Unterrichte*, 2d ed. (Bückeburg and Leipzig: Kummer, 1794).

181. StAWf, 2 Alt 11189, fols. 17–18, 9 Sept. 1803.

182. *Verbesserter Schreib-Calender / auf das Jahr nach Christi Gerburt [. . .] Wobey der Julianische, Gregorianische und ein besondern Haus-Calender wie auch eine Genealogische Verzeichnis aller jetzt-lebenden Hochst- und Hohen Häuser in Europa. Mit Fleiß gestellet durch Johannem Meyerum. Quedl.Saxon. Mit herzogl. Braunschw. Lüneb. gnädigsten Privilegio* (Braunschweig: F. W. Meyer, 1720).

183. Ludwig Rohner, *Kalendergeschichte und Kalender* (Wiesbaden: Athenaion, 1978), 43–48; Schenda, *Volk*, 279–87; Hartmut Sührig, "Der Braunschweigischer Volkskalender in der Zeit der Spätaufklärung," *BJ* 62 (1981): 87–112, esp. 91–95.

184. "Allgemeine Verhaltungsregeln für Schwangere, Gebährende und Wöchnerinnen auf dem Lande in Absicht ihrer Gesundheit, nebst Vorschriften zur Erhaltung junger Kinder," *Vebesserter Schreib-Calender*, 1786–90.

185. StAWf, 2 Alt 11187, fols. 1–2, 30 Sept. 1784.

186. StAWf, 111 Neu 3426, 7 July 1794.

187. StAWf, 111 Neu 3140, 9 Feb. 1803.

188. John Michael Stroup, "Protestant Churchmen in the German Enlightenment—Mere Tools of Temporal Government?" *Lessing-Yearbook* 10 (1977): 149–89.

189. In *Zur Geschichte des Zeitungslesens in Deutschland am Ende des 18. Jahrhunderts: Mit besonderer Berücksichtigung der gesellschaftlichen Formen des Zeitungslesens* (Leipzig: Stein, 1937), Irene Jentsch concluded that very few peasants subscribed to the *Rote Zeitung* between 1786 and 1788. The majority of subscriptions came from an upper class that included pastors, teachers, cantors, organists, sextons, merchants, army officers, physicians, lawyers, government officials, secretaries, notaries, and women of these groups. Pastors may well either have read it aloud to their flocks or communicated its contents in a more informal manner. Jentsch also suggests a connection between an increase in peasant readership in the 1790s and the change in the character of the *RZ* from a "political-didactic" to an almost exclusively political paper.

190. Johann Helmuth, *Volksnaturlehre zur Dämpfung des Aberglaubens* (Braunschweig: Schulbuchhandlung, 1786).

191. *RZ*, 24 Nov. 1787; Fritz Barnstorf, "Pastor Hermann Braess (1738–1797) der Dettumer Bote und Braunschweigische Hausfreund mit seiner *Roten Zeitung für die lieben Landleute*," *BH* 1966: 128–34; Hanno Schmidt, "Philanthropismus und Volksaufklärung im Herzogthum Braunschweig-Wolfenbüttel in der zweiten Hälfte des 18. Jahrhunderts," in *Volk*, ed. Vierhaus, 189–95.

192. Hermann Braess, "Die Zeitung für die Landleute," *BA-GB*, 22 Mar. 1787.

193. Cf. Fritz Ernst, *Kleinjogg der Musterbauer in Bildern seiner Zeit* (Zurich: Atlantis, 1935); Rudolf Schenda, "Der gezügelte Bauernphilosoph oder: Warum Kleinjogg (und manch anderer Landmann) kein Freund des Lesens war," in *Festschrift für Arnold Niederer zum 65. Geburtstag*, ed. Ueli Gyr (Basel: Schweizerische Gesellschaft für Volkskunde, 1980): 214–28.

194. *Wirth*, 8 Jan. 1757. And this was true of many other, more general popular texts. See, e.g., the treatment of cleanliness ("Wie bei einer ungeschickten, säuischen und unordentlichen Hausfrau immer alles krankelt und elend ist") in Christian Gotthilf Salzmann, *Moralisches Elementarbuch, nebst einer Anleitung zum nützlichen Gebrauch desselben* (Leipzig: Hubert Göbels, 1785), 5–10.

195. Albrecht, *Förderung*, 14; Karl Steinacker, "Das Holzmindische Wochenblatt," *BM* 1903: 37–43.

196. Samuel August Tissot, *Anleitung für das Landvolk in Absicht auf seine Gesundheit*, trans. H. C. Hirzel, 2d ed. (Ausburg and Innsbruck: Wolff, 1766); Rudolf Zacharias Becker, *Noth- und Hülfsbüchlein für Bauersleute, oder lehrreiche Freude- und Trauer-Geschichte des Dorfs Mildheim: Für Junge und Alte beschrieben* (Gotha and Leipzig: Göschen, 1788).

197. See, e.g., the "Health Rules" (*Gesundheits-Regeln*) and the "Rules for Illness" (*Krankheits-Regeln*) published in *Der Bauernfreund in Niedersachsen*, ed. Johann Lorenz Benzler (Lemgo: Meyer, 1755), 337–45 , 353–59, 369–82.

198. See the many complaints registered with the privy council in StAWf, 111 Neu 3138; also Stroup, "Protestant Churchmen."

Chapter 2. The Physici

1. Christian Gruner quoted in Wolfram Kaiser and Arina Völker, *Universität und Physikat in der Frühgeschichte des Amtsarztwesens*, Wissenschaftliche Beiträge der Martin-Luther-Universität Halle-Wittenberg, no. 53 (Halle: Martin-Luther-Universität, 1980), 57.

2. Mary Wessling correctly points out in "Medicine and Government in Early Modern Württemberg" (diss., University of Michigan, 1988), xiii, that "the actual evolution of the office of physicus, and its relation to the medieval office of town physician, must emerge from a holistic treatment of medical culture, with strict attention to its societal nexus." It cannot, as she notes, be derived from studying the many treatises on administrative science or merely by looking at the medical ordinances.

3. Roy Porter and W. F. Bynum, "Introduction," to *Medical Fringe and Medical Orthodoxy, 1750–1850*, ed. Porter and Bynum (London: Croom Helm, 1987), 1.

4. Matthew Ramsey, *Professional and Popular Medicine in France, 1770–1830: The Social World of Medical Practice* (Cambridge: Cambridge University Press, 1988), 1.

5. Ibid.; *Patients and Practitioners: Lay Perceptions of Medicine in Pre-Industrial Society*, ed. Roy Porter (Cambridge: Cambridge University Press, 1985); *Medical Fringe*, ed. Bynum and Porter; Irvine Loudon, *Medical Care and the General Practitioner, 1750–1850* (Oxford: Clarendon Press, 1986); Mary E. Fissell, *Patients, Power, and the Poor in Eighteenth-Century Bristol* (Cambridge: Cambridge University Press, 1991); Ute Frevert, *Krankheit als politisches Problem, 1770–1880: Soziale Unterschichten in Preußen zwischen medizinischer Polizei und staatlicher Sozialversicherung* (Göttingen: Vandenhoeck & Ruprecht, 1984); Wessling, "Medicine and Government."

6. Wessling details the career of one physicus in "Official Medicine and Customary Medicine in Early Modern Württemberg: The Career of Christoph Friedrich Pichler," *MGG* 9 (1990): 21–44.

7. There are, of course, many biographies of individual physici. See, e.g., Dietrich Tutzke, *Christian August Struve (1767–1807): Leben und Werk eines Görlitzer Arztes im Dienste des Humanismus der Aufklärungszeit* (Görlitz: Rat der Stadt Görlitz, 1957); Rudolph Zaunich, *Der Dresdener Stadtphysikus Friedrich August Röber, 1765–1827: Ein sächsischer Gesundheitswissenschaftlicher in der Nachfolge Johann Peter Franks* (Leipzig: Barth, 1966); Alfons Fischer, "Die kulturhistorische Wirksamkeit der Landphysici Gustav Viktor und Gustav Friedrich Jägerschmidt," in Fischer, *Beiträge zur Kulturhygiene des 18. und zu Beginn des 19. Jahrhunderts im deutschen Reiche* (Leipzig: J. A Barth, 1928). While it is not quite fair to describe these and similar works as hagiography, they are seldom especially analytical or critical. Mary Wessling's examination in "Offical and Customary Medicine" of the career of the Württemberg physician Christian Friedrich Pichler is an exception. See also, most recently, Harold J. Cook,

Trials of an Ordinary Doctor: James Groenevelt in Seventeenth-Century London (Baltimore: Johns Hopkins University Press, 1994). On the physici as a group, see Fischer, *Geschichte des deutschen Gesundheitswesens*, 2: 55–57; Kaiser and Völker, *Universität*; Manfred Stürzbecher, "The Physici in German-Speaking Countries from the Middle Ages to the Enlightenment," in *The Town and State Physician in Europe from the Middle Ages to the Enlightenment*, ed. Andrew W. Russell (Wolfenbüttel: Herzog August Bibliothek, 1981), 123–40; *Beiträge zur Berliner Medizingeschichte: Quellen und Studien zur Geschichte des Gesundheitswesens vom 17. bis zum 19. Jahrhundert*, ed. Manfred Stürzbecher (Berlin: de Gruyter, 1966); Werner Piechocki, "Das hallesche Physikat im 18. Jahrhundert," *Wissenschaftliche Beiträge der Martin-Luther-Universität Halle-Wittenberg* 36 (1977): 185–206; Dietrich Tutzke, "Das Budissiner Landphysikat," *SA* 47 (1963): 394–405; and the biographies in Karl Jäck and Ernst Theodor Nauck, *Zur Geschichte des Sanitätswesens im Fürstenberg* (Allensbach-Bodensee: Boltze, 1951). Some older works trace the development of the office of physicus in specific towns. Typical are Werner Bubb, *Das Stadtarztamt zu Basel: Seine Entwicklungsgeschichte vom Jahre 1529 bis zur Gegenwart* (Zurich: Leemann, 1942); Johannes Karcher, *Felix Platter, Lebensbild des Baseler Stadtarztes 1536–1614* (Basel: Helbing & Lichtenhahn, 1949). Also useful are older biographical dictionaries, such as Ernst Gottfried Baldinger and Friedrich Boerner, *Nachrichten von den vornehmsten Lebensumständen und Schriften jeztlebender berühmter Aerzte und Naturforscher in und um Deutschland*, 3 vols. (Wolfenbüttel: Johann Christoph Meissner, 1749–64).

Few people have taken the trouble to deal with the physici as a group and in the social and cultural contexts of their times. Sabine Sander's study of surgeons in Württemberg, *Handwerkschirurgen: Sozialgeschichte einer verdrängten Berufsgruppe* (Göttingen: Vandenhoeck & Ruprecht, 1989), is exemplary for the kind of prosopographical work that needs to be done for physici and physicians. More recently, for the Netherlands, see Frank Huisman, *Stadsbelang en standsbesef: Gezondheitszorg en medisch beroep in Groningen, 1500–1730* (Rotterdam: Erasmus, 1992). Barbara Duden discusses the life of Dr. Storch as physicus in Eisenach, *Geschichte unter der Haut: Ein Eisenacher Arzt und seine Patientinnen um 1730* (Stuttgart: Klett-Cotta, 1987), 67–89.

8. There are some significant exceptions. See, e.g., Michael MacDonald, *Madness, Anxiety, and Healing in Seventeenth-Century England* (Cambridge: Cambridge University Press, 1981); Duden, *Geschichte*; Loudon, *Medical Care*; Hilary Marland, *Medicine and Society in Wakefield and Huddersfield, 1780–1870* (Cambridge: Cambridge University Press, 1987); Huisman, *Stadsbelang*; Roy Porter, *Doctor of Society: Thomas Beddoes and the Sick Trade in Late-Enlightenment England* (London: Routledge, 1992).

9. Of course, the physici were not just private practitioners. By definition, they were employed—or salaried in any case—by the state, and were always expected to find a substantial part of their livelihoods in private practice. Governments therefore viewed their salaries as supplements, intended to cover what the men could *not* earn privately. For instance, physici in poorer districts tended to enjoy bigger salaries than ones centered in larger towns or more prosperous regions. In 1799, for instance, in addition to the seventeen resident physici, at least twenty-six other physicians practiced in the city of Braunschweig. And without counting the physicians who lived outside the duchy but along its borders, there were three others in Wolfenbüttel, five professors of medicine in Helmstedt, and at least ten more scattered around in the

smaller towns of the duchy. "Übersicht des Medizinalwesens der Herzogthums Braunschweig," *Medizinische National-Zeitung für Deutschland* 2, no. 15 (11 Mar. 1799): 237–40; Walter Artelt, "Das medizinische Braunschweig um 1770," *MJ* 1 (1966): 240–60.

10. Generally on the relationship between pastors and the state, see John Michael Stroup, *The Struggle for Identity in the Clerical Estate: Northwest German Protestant Opposition to Absolutist Policy in the Eighteenth Century* (Leiden: Brill, 1984).

11. The lineage is ambiguous, for plague-doctors were often not physicians. Many were surgeons engaged to unburden physicians of the job of treating plague cases and to avoid spreading the contagion into citizens' homes. See, e.g., Nancy G. Siraisi, *Medieval and Early Renaissance Medicine: An Introduction to Knowledge and Practice* (Chicago: Chicago University Press, 1990), 38; Katharine Park, *Doctors and Medicine in Early Renaissance Florence* (Princeton: Princeton University Press, 1985), 87–99; and Ann G. Carmichael, *Plague and the Poor in Renaissance Florence* (Cambridge: Cambridge University Press, 1986), 16–17, 101–7.

12. Zedler, s.v. "Physicus."

13. Krünitz, s.v. "Physikat."

14. Ernst Schwabe, *Anweisung zu den Pflichten und Geschäften eines Stadt- oder Land-Physikus* (Erfurt: Keyser, 1786–87). See also Christian Gruner, *Gedanken von der Arzneiwissenschaft* (Breslau: Kora, 1772), 1: vi–vii, 268–69. Gruner, who was professor of medicine at Jena and editor of the *Almanach für Aerzte und Nichtaerzte*, defines the physicus as a *Staatsarzt* and "the inspector of natural things that can contribute to the preservation or the destruction of health; advisor in finding, selecting, and applying the best means to advance the great good of public health; the competent judge of local illnesses and ravaging epidemics, whether of man or beast." According to him, too, the physicus had to be "more extensively" acquainted with topography, environment, forensics, and veterinary medicine than other physicians. Franz Anton May describes similar duties in his *Stolpertus, ein junger Arzt am Krankenbette*, vol. 4: *Stolpertus der Polizei-Arzt im Gerichtshof der medizinischen Polizeigesetzgebung von einem patriotischen Pfläzer* (Mannheim: Schwan, 1802), 1–5, as do Christian Friedrich Daniel, *Bibliothek der Staats-Arzneikunde oder der gerichtlichen Arzneikunde und medicinischen Polizey von ihrem Anfange bis auf das Iahr 1784* (Halle: Hemmerde, 1785), and Johann Daniel Metzger, *Vermischte medicinische Schriften* (Königsberg: n.p., 1782). See also Fischer, "Wirksamkeit."

15. August Hinze, *Lexicon aller Herzogl.[ichen] Braunschweigischen Verordnungen welche die medicinische Polizey betreffen* (Stendal: Franz & Grosse, 1793). Hinze was physicus in Calvörde from 1790 to 1793.

16. These were called *Land-Physici* in Braunschweig-Wolfenbüttel; in other places they might be known as *Amts-Physici* or *Amts-Ärzte*. At the town level in Württemberg, for example, physici went by the title of *Stadtphysicus*; at the district level, of *Amtsphysicus* (Wessling, "Medicine and Government," 12). In Anhalt, the terms were *Stadtphysicus* and *Landphysicus* (Arina Völker, *Die Entwicklung von Medizinalorganisation und Bevölkerungsversorgung am territorialen Beispiel von Anhalt* [Halle-Wittenberg: Martin-Luther Universität, 1985]).

17. "Specifique Designation von dem, was, laut des gnädigsten Ausschreibens vom 11ten Junii 1770, bey dem zu den Sanitäts-Anstalten gehörigen Cassen, in dem

Michaelis-Quartale a.c. an den Besoldungen abgezogen worden," StAWf, 2 Alt 11205, fols. 70–72, 19 Oct. 1770. See also Wessling, "Medicine and Government"; Kaiser and Völker, *Universität*.

18. StAWf, 111 Neu 63, fol. 3; 2 Alt 11177, fol. 9; Ludwig du Roi, "Leben und Wirken des Leibarztes Johann Philipp du Roi, 1741–1785," in *17. Jahresbericht des Vereins für Naturwissenschaft zu Braunschweig* (Braunschweig, 1913), 187–89.

19. StAWf, 111 Neu 61, fols. 46–67; obituary in *BA-GB*, 6 May 1767.

20. *Lexikon*; StAWf, 2 Alt 11313, fols. 46–53; 2 Alt 11169, fols. 6, 71; 111 Neu 1096, fols. 4, 10.

21. Wessling, "Medicine and Government," 55–103; id., "Offical and Customary Medicine"; Völker, *Entwicklung*. For a nonmedical context, see Anthony J. La Vopa, *Grace, Talent, and Merit: Poor Students, Clerical Careers, and Professional Ideology in Eighteenth-Century Germany* (Cambridge: Cambridge University Press, 1988), 83–110.

22. Friedrich Wilhelm von Hoven, *Lebenserinnerungen*, ed. Hans-Günther Thalheim (Berlin: Rütten & Loening, 1984), 91.

23. Ibid., 95.

24. Ibid., 96–97.

25. Wolfgang Genschorek, *Ernst Ludwig Heim: Das Leben eines Volksarztes* (Leipzig: S. Hirzel, 1985), 70–75; Georg Wilhlem Keßler, *Der alte Heim: Leben und Wirken Ernst Ludwig Heim: Aus hinterlassenen Briefen und Tagebüchern*, 2d enlarged ed. (Leipzig: F. A. Brockhaus, 1846).

26. Irvine Loudon has stressed the importance of horizontal networks. Speaking of conditions in England, Loudon points out that medicine in the eighteenth century "was a small world with a network of masters, pupils, and apprentices keeping in touch to their mutual advantage" (*Medical Care*, 41). While Loudon is not speaking of university-trained physicians, the observation seems as true of them. For the story of another physicus, one who later played a dramatic role in European politics, see Stefan Winkle, *Johann Friedrich Struensee: Arzt—Aufklärer—Staatsmann. Beitrag zur Kultur-, Medizin- und Seuchengeschichte der Aufklärungszeit* (Stuttgart: Gustav Fischer, 1983), esp. 35–88.

27. StAWf, 111 Neu 1132, fols. 34–35, 3 Feb. 1794.

28. See Wessling, "Offical and Customary Medicine."

29. See, e.g., the oath sworn by the Karlsruhe physicus, Gustav Viktor Jägerschmid, in 1724 (reprinted in Fischer, *Beiträge*, 1–2), or those sworn by physici in the various parts of Anhalt in the seventeenth and eighteenth centuries (Völker, *Entwicklung*). The Braunschweig oaths seem very similar to those used in other places. See "Acten in Sachen die Bestellung der Stadt Physici," StadtB, B IV 13c Nr. 1.

30. StAWf, 2 Alt 11312, fols. 16–17, 17 July 1750.

31. StadtB, B IV 13c Nr. 1, fols. 1–2, 7 Aug. 1591.

32. Ibid., fols. 6–26; StadtB, C II 3, fols. 37–39.

33. See StAWf, 34N Fb. 1 XIX 1 and 2 Alt 11306–8 on appointment of physici from 1755 to 1808.

34. The information on the physici in Helmstedt is mostly drawn from two articles by Robert Schaper: "Arzt und Apotheker—Das Physikat in Helmstedt," in *Aus der Heimat—Für die Heimat*, suppl. to *Helmstedter Kreisblatt*, 10 Sept. 1966, and

"Krankenbehandlung der Armen—. . . und die Waisenkinder?" in ibid., 24 Sept. 1966. Additional information on terms of office of Richter, Schmidt, and Siegesbeck in StAWf, 2 Alt 11278, fols. 8–76.

35. "Unvorgreiffliche Gedanken wie die Bestallung eines Landphysici ohngefahr eingerichtet werden könne" (n.d. [probably early 1696]), StAWf, 2 Alt 11277, fols. 14–17. The "Specification der umb Braunschweig nechstgelegenen Fürstl. Ambten, so dem Medico provinciali unvorgreifflich, zu seiner inspection konten angewiesen werden" (n.d. [probably 1696]), ibid., fol. 13, lists the following places: Amt Wolfenbüttel (crossed out by a different pen), Schöningen including Calvörde and Neuhaus, Königslutter, Warberg, Neubrück and Freden, Eich with the surrounding villages, Lichtenberg, Gebhardshagen, Heßen, Voigtsdahlum, Lutter am Barenberge and surrounding area, and "the noble and cloister villages adjoining." This was a very large area.

36. StAWf, 2 Alt 11277, fols. 14–17.

37. Ibid. 11279, fol. 1, 26 Mar. 1696.

38. Ibid., fols. 3, 9. Gandersheim was to pay 30 thaler, Greene 29 thaler 8 groschen, Seesen, 16 thaler 16 groschen, and Stauffenburg, 14 thaler.

39. Conditions of Held's appointment and list of his duties from StAWf, 2 Alt 11295, fols. 26–28, 23 Jan. 1714; "Repartitio über 300 Rthlr welcher der bestellter Land-Medicus Doctor Held Jahrlich haben soll," ibid., fols. 17–18, 8 Feb. 1714; and mandate, StAWf, 40 Slg. 4369, 1 Feb. 1714.

40. Signed "Sämtl. Eingeßene des Gerichts Bettmar," StAWf, 2 Alt 11295, fol. 36, 6 May 1714.

41. Ibid., fol. 51, 22 Jan. 1715.

42. Ibid., fols. 53–55, 58, 66.

43. See Chapter 1.

44. Hieronymi remained as physicus there until his death in 1754 (StAWf, 2 Alt 11306, fols. 2–3, 7).

45. Johann Heinrich Wachsmuth, *Panacea solaris, oder Universal-Gold-Balsam, wodurch Alle Krankheiten des Menschlichen Leibes, so wohl innerliche als äiserliche, besonders Schlag-Fluß, Jammer, Podagra, und alle Arten der Gicht, Stein, Krebs und verstopfte Monaths-Zeiten etc. glücklich durch göttlichen Seegen gehoben worden* (Nordhausen: n.p., 1733); id., *Spiritus vitae catholicus, oder Universal-Lebens-Spiritus, wodurch in Alchymia alles was zum Universal nöthig ist, in Medicina aber in Curirung der Kranckheiten ein grosses kan ausgerichtet werden,* . . . (Nordhausen: n.p., n.d.).

46. See *Geographisch-Statistisch-Topothesische Tabellen Herzogthum Braunschweig-Lüneburg Wolfebüttelschen Antheils. . . . Im Jahr 1803.* Copy in HAB, Einbl. R1: 77.

47. Later this district was divided into four separate physicates: Schöningen, Königslutter, Calvörde, and Vorsfelde (StAWf, 111 Neu 1081, fol. 2). On Centner as physicus, see StAWf, 2 Alt 11312, 11339, 11354; 111 Neu 1081, 1083, 1104, 1110, 2039, 2435; specification of his duties in 111 Neu 1081, fol. 2.

48. At the same time (confusingly to the historian), a district within a district came into being, the Braunschweig district, which excluded the city of Braunschweig but included all the surrounding countryside. Continuity was restored by appointing Dr. Rudolf Behrens, then physicus in Braunschweig, as district physicus. See StAWf, 2 Alt 11313, fols. 7–9.

49. See, e.g., the directions sent to authorities in the Weser and Harz districts: StAWf, 40 Slg. 6168, 14 Mar. 1743, and 111 Neu 1082a, fols. 2–3, 5 Dec. 1743.

50. "Umlauf an Ober und [Unter?] Beamte des Harz Districts wegen des bestellten Land Physici Blumen," StAWf, 111 Neu 1082a, fols. 2–3, 5 Dec. 1743.

51. "Ausschreiben mit der Bekanntgabe der für die Distrikte ernannten Land-Physicus und dessen, was für ihre Inanspruchnahme zu zahlen ist," HAB, Einbl. R3: 786, 29 May 1749.

52. See also "Umlauf an sämmtl. Beamte und Obrigkeit des Harz und Weser Districts betr. die Land-Physios," StAWf, 40 Slg. 6168, 14 Mar. 1743. StAWf, 2 Alt 11304 contains considerable information on these difficulties for the Weser district in the 1730s and 1740s.

53. StAWf, 40 Slg. 7522, 18 Nov. 1751; for documentation on a new series of disputes following this change, see 2 Alt 11350; and for a specific case involving Dr. Spohr during a smallpox outbreak in Münchehof, ibid., fols. 30–35, 14 Nov. 1798; on Struve, 2 Alt 11377, fols. 15–16.

54. In 1808, physicates were found in Blankenburg, Braunschweig, Calvörde, Eschershausen, Gandersheim, Harzburg, Hasselfelde, Helmstedt, Holzminden, Königslutter, Schöningen, Schöppenstedt, Seesen, Vorsfelde, Walkenried, and Wolfenbüttel. See StAWf, 111 Neu 1037, fols. 49–50. Cf. Annelise Gerbert, *Öffentliche Gesundheitspflege und staatliches Medizinalwesen in den Städten Braunschweig und Wolfenbüttel im 19. Jahrhundert* (Braunschweig: Selbstverlag des Braunschweigischen Geschichtsvereins, 1983), 16, who lists the same sixteen men, but erroneously designates Ellrich a district. For a brief period of time, when Hasselfelde had been created and Stadtoldendorf had not yet been dissolved, there were seventeen physicates. Even the government was not quite sure which areas belonged to which physicate, and in 1781, it asked all physici to list all villages and regions under their jurisdiction. See StAWf, 111 Neu 1038, fol. 48, 26 Oct. 1781; "Übersicht des Medizinalwesens," 239.

55. For example, in 1766, Dr. Johann Heinrich Bühring was named adjunct to the aging physicus Dr. Johann Centner (d. 1769) in Schöningen *cum spe succedendi.* Bühring later held several posts as physicus, although never in Schöningen. See StAWf, 111 Neu 1104, fols. 7, 9.

56. StAWf, 2 Alt 11376, fols. 2–6, 36, 42–44, 46–47, 53, 55.

57. Ibid. 11404, fols. 1–11.

58. Ibid., fols. 12–13, 19 Aug. 1782.

59. Ibid., fols. 18–19.

60. Ibid., fols. 20–29; ibid., fol. 45, 25 Nov. 1782.

61. Ibid. 11407, fols. 181–89, 7 Sept. 1797.

62. Ibid., fols. 11–13, 1 Apr. 1798.

63. Ibid., fols. 31–32, 29 May 1798.

64. Ibid., fols. 35–36, 23 Aug. 1798; ibid., fol. 37, 1 Oct. 1798.

65. For Eggers's report, see ibid. 11383, fols. 1–4, 17 July 1794; for deliberations on appointment of physicus 1799–1800, see ibid., fols. 19–20, 22, 25. In 1808, Dr. Welge was still receiving only 30 thaler a year in his capacity as physicus in Harzburg (StAWf, 111 Neu 1037, fols. 49–50).

66. StAWf, 2 Alt 11384, fols. 65–66, 15 June 1794: "Die Bürgerschaft in Stadt Oldendorf unterzeichnete Honoratiores, bitten unterthänigst, daß der Dr. Härtel in Stadt Alfeld, zum Land-Physico in Stadt Oldendorf bestellet werden möge"; ibid.,

fol. 54: Altenburg's letter of 27 June 1794; ibid., 11385, fol. 5: repeated plea on 30 Jan. 1795. Their wish for Härtel was not honored. In March, the privy council confirmed the appointment of Eicke in Eschershausen as physicus in Stadtoldendorf. This was a not totally satisfactory solution as the magistrates in Stadtoldendorf saw it, and later in the year (3 Nov. 1795) they petitioned the privy council to require Eicke to move to Stadtoldendorf, citing the inconvenience of traveling to Eschershausen and the cost of bringing Eicke to Stadtoldendorf when they needed him. Moreover, they felt that people would die because Eicke lived too far away to provide speedy assistance (ibid., fol. 15; repeated 19 June 1796, fols. 21–22). On 12 Sept. 1797, the guilds added their weight to the argument, expressing the desire that physicians be residents, and thus also clients and customers, who would help shoulder the tax burden: "die Gilder und Gemeinheitsmeister zu Stadt Oldendorf wiederholen ihre unterthänigste Bitte dem Stadtphysico Doctori Eicke gnädigste zu befehlen, daß er in Stadt Oldendorf wohnen solle" (ibid., fols. 56–59). But the privy council would not yield and allowed Eicke to stay in Eschershausen. It also pointed out that a physicus was not bound to live in one city. Eicke was, after all, not only responsible to Stadtoldendorf but also served "the interests of a larger public." The privy council went on to reprimand the petitioners for their "unseemly expressions" and to accuse them of "favoring factions" (ibid., fols. 66–67, 14 Nov. 1797).

67. StAWf, 2 Alt 11375, fols. 3–4, 15–16, 20–26. Stolze was appointed on 3 Dec. 1745 (ibid., fol. 6) and removed from office on 19 Aug. 1755 (fol. 26).

68. In *Der Aufstieg der Ärzte im 19. Jahrhundert: Vom gelehrten Stand zum professionellen Experten: Das Beispiel Preußens* (Göttingen: Vandenhoeck & Ruprecht, 1985), 168, Claudia Huerkamp notes that in Prussia in the middle of the nineteenth century, an average of ten candidates presented themselves for each vacant post. For Behrens's estimate, see StAWf, 2 Alt 11317, fol. 6, 15 Jan. 1745.

69. For details of Meyer's examination, see StAWf, 111 Neu 1103, fols. 13–15, 11 Oct. 1766.

70. Petition of 3 Jan. 1766, ibid., fols. 2–3.

71. Ibid., fols. 13–15, 17–19.

72. Ibid., fols. 34–35, 40.

73. StAWf, 111 Neu 1106 (1767) and 1137 (1793–94).

74. StAWf, 2 Alt 11360, fol. 22. Although technically separated from the rest of Braunschweig-Wolfenbüttel in the last half of the eighteenth century, Blankenburg was subject to the same laws and administrative procedures as the rest of the territory. Thus the privy council appointed the physicus.

75. Peter Albrecht, *Die Förderung des Landesausbaues im Herzogtum Braunschweig-Wolfenbüttel im Spiegel der Verwaltungsakten des 18. Jahrhunderts (1671–1806)* (Braunschweig: Waisenhaus, 1980), 13, 19; *Braunschweigsiche Landesgeschichte im Überblick*, ed. Richard Moderhack, 3d ed. (Braunschweig: Waisenhaus, 1979), 151–52. On Blankenburg, see *700 Jahre Blankenburg* (Magdeburg: Städtisches Verkehrsamt [Blankenburg-Harz], 1937); Wilhelm Lüders, "Blankenburg," in Wilhelm Görges, Ferdinand Spehr, and Franz Fühse, *Väterländische Geschichten und Denkwürdigkeiten der Lande Braunschweig und Hannover: Ein Volksbuch*, vol. 1: *Braunschweig* (Braunschweig: Appelhans, 1925), 357–403; Adolf Gerade, "Blankenburg vom Mittelalter bis zum 18. Jahrhundert," *BH* 50 (1964): 33–40.

76. The physicus in Blankenburg in 1762 received 164 thaler; his closest competi-

tors, in terms of salary, were the physici in Wolfenbüttel with 150 thaler and in Holzminden with 116 thaler. Other physici earned between 30 and 95 thaler. In 1808, the physicus in Blankenburg earned 360 thaler, 140 thaler *more* than the next highest paid physicus (in Schöningen). See StAWf, 111 Neu 1037, fol. 35 (1762), ibid., fols. 49–50 (1808).

77. StAWf, 111 Neu 1106, fol. 3; 2 Alt 11357, fols. 8–10.

78. StAWf, 111 Neu 1106, fols. 8–10, 26 June and 3 Sept. 1767. Georgi's conditions of appointment provided him with a salary of 30 thaler annually (2 Alt 11356, fol. 68).

79. StAWf, 111 Neu 1106, fols. 3–4, 22 Jan. 1767.

80. Ibid., fol. 29.

81. Pott's "Pro Memoria" to Collegium medicum, ibid., fols. 32–33, 3 Sept. 1767. On Sandrart, ibid., fols. 53–57, 58 (appointment); more in 2 Alt 11357; 111 Neu 1122 (death).

82. StAWf, 111 Neu 1137, fols. 3–4.

83. Blankenburg to privy council, StAWf, 111 Neu 1137, fols. 3–4, 11 May 1793.

84. Ibid., fol. 23, 15 May 1793.

85. Ibid., fol. 36, 4 June 1793.

86. StAWf, 2 Alt 11370, fol. 38, 18 May 1803.

87. Recommendations of Collegium medicum to privy council, 20 Sept. 1789, ibid. 11377, fols. 38–40.

88. StAWf, 8 Alt Lutter am Barenberge 548, fols. 1, 4, 8–9, 14–16, 14 May, 1 and 28 July, and 4 Aug. 1744.

89. StAWf, 111 Neu 1137, fols. 50–51, 28 June 1793.

90. Ibid., 1129, fol. 8, 22 July 1788.

91. StAWf, ad 111 Neu 1127, fols. 19, 21.

92. StAWf, 111 Neu 1137, fols. 29–30, 1 June 1793.

93. Ibid., fols. 33, 56, 2 June 1793, 27 Aug. 1793.

94. Ibid., fols. 59–60, 31 Dec. 1793.

95. StAWf, 111 Neu 1131, fols. 1–2, 9 May 1789.

96. Ibid., fol. 18, 20 May 1789.

97. Petition signed by notables, 6 Aug. 1789, ibid., fol. 33; also in 2 Alt 11377, fols. 48–49, which lists the twenty-five notables, including Abbot Johann Friedrich Häseler, a pastor, a forester, a customs agent, an Amtmann, a senator, and a major and a captain in the city's militia; from magistrate in Holzminden to Collegium medicum, 6 Aug. 1789, ibid., fols. 34–36.

98. StAWf, 111 Neu 1131, fol. 39, 18 Aug. 1789.

99. From Amt Schöningen, 22 Feb. 1769, StAWf, 2 Alt 11354, fols. 18–19; "Pro Memoria" from Stadtmagistrat in Schöningen, 22 Feb. 1769, ibid., fols. 21–22.

100. Ibid., fols. 16–17, 3 Mar. 1769; ibid., fol. 25, 3 Apr. 1769; ibid., fol. 28, appointment of Scheiber to Schöningen and Bühring to Vorsfelde, 24 Apr. 1769.

101. StAWf, 2 Alt 11384, fol. 46, 26 Apr. 1794.

102. Ibid., 11355, fols. 22–24, 14 Feb. 1791; ibid., fol. 30, 2 Mar. 1791; ibid., fol. 33, 8 Mar. 1791.

103. StAWf, 111 Neu 1114, fols. 3–4, 21 Mar. 1776.

104. Holdefreund's application, 26 Mar. 1776, ibid., fols. 6–7; von Flögen's note,

6 Apr. 1776, ibid., fol. 16 (for more on the adultery and incest cases, see 2 Alt 11332, fols. 32, 35–40; 111 Neu 1105, 1108); May's appointment and confirmation, 6 and 29 May 1776, ibid., fols. 22, 24.

105. Ibid., fols. 26, 28–29, 28 Aug. 1776.

106. Ibid., fols. 38, 41, 8 and 9 Nov. 1776.

107. Ibid., fols. 45–46, 25 Nov. 1776.

108. On appointment of Dehne, ibid., fols. 54–58–59, 62–63, 70, 2 Apr. 1777; May's apointment to Schöppenstedt, ibid., fol. 71, 7 Apr. 1777.

109. Response of the abbess, n.d. (Mar. or Apr. 1761), StAWf, 2 Alt 11382, fols. 15–16; circumstances of Eicke in 1787, StAWf, 111 Neu 1124.

110. StAWf, 2 Alt 11382, fols. 17, 20–21; salaries (1762), 111 Neu 1037, fol. 35.

111. StAWf, 111 Neu 1037, fol. 35 (1762), fols. 49–50 (1808).

112. MO 1747 sketches some of the duties of the physici. On specific responsibilities of the physici in times of epidemics, see StAWf, 40 Slg. 13256, 4 Mar. 1794; in regard to autopsies, ibid., 11983, 1 Dec. 1777.

113. In *Die bäuerliche Gemeinde in Deutschland* (Göttingen: Vandenhoeck & Ruprecht, 1986), 113, Heide Wunder comments on this gradual "opening" in respect to peasant communities.

114. Mary Wessling argues that this kind of situation "made effective functioning in the position [of physicus] nearly impossible" ("Medicine and Government," 22). See also Thomas H. Broman, "Rethinking Professionalization: Theory, Practice and Professional Ideology in Eighteenth-Century German Medicine," *JMH* 67 (1995): 835–72.

115. From Fahrenholtz, 2 July 1756, StAWf, 111 Neu 1090, fols. 23–26; from Pini, 9 Aug. 1759, ibid. 1051, fol. 57.

116. StAWf, 2 Alt 11369, fols. 18–19, 8 Aug. 1753.

117. StAWf, 111 Neu 1129, fol. 4a, 29 June 1788.

118. StAWf, 2 Alt 11305, fols. 5–6, 3 Feb. 1740; Beltz's "Unvorgreiffliches Project, auf was Art und Weise, die Stadt Hasselfelde zu nicht geringen Hoch-Fürstlichen Interesse ohne sonderliche Costen in kurtzer Zeit in Aufnahme und Nahrung zu setzen," ibid., fols. 9–16; decision of privy council, 4 Feb. 1740, ibid., fol. 17.

119. StAWf, 2 Alt 11364, fols. 22–23, 3 Sept. 1794.

120. Krebs's petitions from Oct. and Dec. 1786, ibid. 11359, fols. 2–4; report from Blankenburg, 10 Jan. 1787, ibid., fols. 5–7; approval of privy council, 22 Feb. 1787, ibid., fol. 9.

121. Information on Siegesbeck is taken from ibid. 11278, fols. 21–24, 31–33; StadtH, B VII 11f, vol. 1 (1652–1921); Schaper, "Arzt und Apotheker."

122. StAWf, 2 Alt 11278, fols. 21–22, 9 Jan. 1745. Another example of a longstanding feud between the physicus and local authorities on similar points occurred in Gandersheim; see StAWf, 17 N 2312, fols. 36, 45–47, 52; 17 N 2319.

123. Ibid., fol. 23, 10 Jan. 1743.

124. On Kreyenberg, see Schaper, "Arzt und Apotheker."

125. StAWf, 2 Alt 11278, fol. 23.

126. Quoted in Schaper, "Arzt und Apotheker."

127. Siegesbeck's protest, StAWf, 2 Alt 11278, fol. 24; Cellarius's response, 12 July 1735, ibid., fols. 31–33.

128. See ibid., fols. 57–59, 66–67, 71–73, 75–76 for details from 1736–38.

129. StAWf, 2 Alt 11471 and 11472.

130. StAWf, 2 Alt 11471, fols. 11, 13–15.

131. Collegium medicum on epidemic, 26 June 1756, ibid., fols. 26–28.

132. Ibid., fols. 14–15.

133. Ibid., fols. 19–21, 26–28, 32–37.

134. Granzien's report, 30 Aug. 1756, ibid., fols. 48–52.

135. Privy council to Granzien, 2 Sept. 1756, ibid., fols. 54–55.

136. Granzien's protest, 20 Sept. 1756, ibid., fols. 56–61; privy council's response, ibid., fol. 62.

137. See, e.g., StAWf, 17 N 2312, fols. 36, 45–47, 52–54, Jan.–Feb. 1742, on the operator Meyer,; and 17 N 2319 on the recalcitrance of the apothecary Seitz in 1756.

138. StAWf, 2 Alt 11377, fols. 17–19, 8 Dec. 1764.

139. Report from Rörhand, 29 Oct. 1798, StAWf, 2 Alt 11409, fol. 2.

140. Apfel's petition, 5 Aug. 1783, StAWf, 111 Neu 1119, fol. 8.

141. Meyer's reports to Collegium medicum, 3 June 1767 and 26 Jan. 1768, StAWf, 111 Neu 1107, fols. 19–23, 59–60. In a petition to the Collegium on 16 Feb. 1768, Meyer noted that he had to treat "172 of the municipality's poor without recompense" (ibid., fol. 14). Collegium medicum to magistrates in Helmstedt, 28 Jan. 1768, StadtH, B VII 11a Nr. 3; response of magistrates, 20 Feb. 1768, ibid. See also StAWf, 2 Alt 11362, and Schaper, "Arzt und Apotheker." A similar case was that of Dr. Johann Welge, physicus in Harzburg. His list of complaints, submitted in 1802, virtually reproduces Meyer's. He, too, feuded with the authorities in Harzburg because he resided in Goslar (which the Collegium medicum permitted him to do). The authorities wanted to force him to move to Harzburg, not only to be closer to his clientele, but also to augment the number of taxable citizens in the city (StAWf, 2 Alt 11412). Dr. Schulze's contract in Blankenburg was far more precise both as to his duties and as to exactly what he was to be paid for specific tasks (StAWf, 2 Alt 11357, fol. 3, 7 Nov. 1766).

142. Schaper, "Arzt und Apotheker."

143. From Amt Stauffenberg (Harz), 14 Nov. 1798, StAWf, 2 Alt 11353, fol. 31; response of privy council, 5 Dec. 1798, ibid., fols. 34–35.

144. Information on Müller's career is taken from StAWf, 2 Alt 11381, 11382; 111 Neu 1082, 1095, 1101; 8 Alt Seesen 3 Nr. 11.

145. StAWf, 111 Neu 1095, fols. 72–74, 9 Oct. 1766.

146. Ibid., fols. 91–92, 94–122.

147. StAWf, 8 Alt Seesen 3 Nr. 11, fol. 4.

148. Ibid., fols. 1–2.

149. Müller, "Pro Memoria" to Collegium medicum, 2 Oct. 1766, ibid., fols. 6–7; further report from Müller, 7 Oct. 1766, ibid, fol. 12; report from Stube to Müller, n.d., ibid., fols. 13–14; Müller's report on quackery, 17 Oct. 1766, fols. 161–67.

150. Müller, "Pro Memoria" to Collegium medicum, 2 Oct. 1766, ibid., fols. 2–3.

151. StAWf, 111 Neu 1095, fols. 123–28, 131.

152. The denunciation was signed "M.C." and was not dated. StAWf, 111 Neu 1095, fols. 135–36; see also 2 Alt 11381, fol. 56 and 2 Alt 11382, passim.

153. StAWf, 111 Neu 1095, fols. 135–36.

154. See *Lexikon*, s.v. "Dedekind." Besides his dissertation, Dedekind also wrote a book on smallpox, *Curart der natürlichen Pocken* (Holzminden: Fleckeisen in Helmstedt, 1791) and contributed several articles to *BA-GB*, including "Von Steinen, welche im menschlichen Körper entstehen, und einem sehr großen Steine, welcher einer abgegangen ist" (4 Nov. 1769). On Dedekind's plan for sugar extraction, see Heinz Röhr, *Geschichte der Stadt Königslutter am Elm* (Braunschweig: Hans Oeding, 1981), 112; K. Ulrich, "Die Anfänge der Rübenzuckererzeugung in Königslutter von Dr. med. Dedekind," *BM* (1930).

155. On Holdefreund's case, see StAWf, 2 Alt 11332, fol. 32; 111 Neu 1105, 1108, 1114.

156. Dismissal of Holdefreund, 29 Dec. 1768, StAWf, 111 Neu 1108, fol. 15; appointment of Dedekind, 27 Feb. 1769, ibid., fol. 24.

157. StAWf, 2 Alt 11332, fols. 23–24, 31 Oct. 1774; fols. 26–27, 15 Dec. 1774; fol. 28, 9 Jan. 1775.

158. StAWf, 111 Neu 1102, fol. 24, 4 May 1775.

159. Report of Collegium medicum on Dedekind, StAWf, 2 Alt 11333, fols. 1–3, 29 June 1779; transfer of physici, ibid., fols. 19–20, 29 Dec. 1789; comments on Dedekind, 2 Alt 11377, fol. 38, 20 Sept. 1789; protests against Hellwig, ibid., fols. 44–49 and also in 111 Neu 1131, fols. 34–36.

160. Anonymous, n.d. (probably July 1773), StAWf, 111 Neu 1108, fol. 3; response of Collegium medicum, 2 Aug. 1773, ibid., fol. 2.

161. StAWf, 111 Neu 1131, fol. 60, 1 May 1794; 2 Alt 11392, fols. 20–22.

162. StAWf, 111 Neu 1131, fols. 63–64, 10 June 1794.

163. This was made explicit by the Collegium medicum in 1780, for example, in answering a query from Dr. Siever, physicus in Stadtoldendorf, as to whether he was permitted to handle cases other than in his district. The Collegium replied that like any other licensed physician, he was allowed to practice anywhere in the duchy, as long as he observed normal collegial ethics. See StAWf, 111 Neu 1113, fol. 26, 3 Aug. 1780.

164. Calvörde, 1793–94; Walkenried, 1794–95; Vorsfelde 1795–96; Königslutter, 1796–? (d. 1816). StAWf, 2 Alt 11370, 11364, 11373, 11333, passim.

165. "Übersicht des Medizinalwesens," 237–39.

166. StAWf, 2 Alt 11229, fols. 40–41, 14 July 1758; ibid., fol. 44, 25 July 1758; ibid., fol. 45, 28 Nov. 1758.

167. StAWf, 2 Alt 11396, fol. 2, 10 Nov. 1768.

168. Ibid., fols. 3–4, 21 Nov. 1769.

169. Ibid., fols. 18–19, 22 May 1769.

170. Schüler on Pini's improvement, 12 May 1769, ibid., fols. 14–16; Pini, "Pro Memoria" to magistrates, 16 Mar. 1770, 1 N Schöppenstedt I Nr. 28.

171. StAWf, 1 N Schöppenstedt I Nr. 458, 28 Feb. 1770.

172. The privy council named Dr. May to replace him on 7 Apr. 1777 (StAWf, 111 Neu 1116, fol. 13).

173. Report from Schüler in Schöppenstedt, StAWf, 2 Alt 11396, fols. 57–58, 18 Jan. 1776.

174. StAWf, 2 Alt 11397, fols. 6–7, 15 July 1776.

175. Letter from Pini to privy council, StAWf, 2 Alt 11396, fols. 70–71, 7 Feb. 1776.

176. Opinion of Martini in deliberations of Collegium medicum, StAWf, 111 Neu 1102, fol. 24, 4 May 1775.

177. StAWf, 2 Alt 11396, fols. 47–51, 19 July 1775; letter from Bötticher's widow, ibid., fols. 67–68, 7 Feb. 1776.

178. StAWf, 2 Alt 11396, 11397.

179. See Mary Lindemann, "The Enlightenment Encountered: Medical Practice and Enlightenment in Northern Germany, 1750–1820," in *Medicine in the Enlightenment*, ed. Roy Porter (Amsterdam: Rodopi, 1995): 181–97. I have assembled the details of Loeber's life from StAWf, 1 N Schöppenstedt I Nr. 460; 111 Neu 1132, 1133; 2 Alt 11333, fols. 19–20; 2 Alt 11363, esp. fols. 31–33; 2 Alt 11373, fols. 8–27; 2 Alt 11405; Ratsarchiv Hornburg, Po VI/5.

180. *Lexikon*, s.v. "Loeber, Christian Joseph." Loeber's publications included *De cordis fabrica et functione atque de sanguinis per cor et vasa sanguinea circulatione* (Erfurt: n.p., 1767); *Sendschreiben von wiedergekommenden Pocken nach der Einpfropfung* (Erfurt: n.p., 1767); *Anfangsgründe der Wundarzneykunst* (Langensalza: Schneider, 1770).

181. See Ruth Richardson, *Death, Dissection and the Destitute* (London: Routledge & Kegan Paul, 1987); Fissell, *Patients*, 162–70.

182. See StAWf, 1N Schöppenstedt I Nr. 460, for Loeber's explanation to the magistrates in Schöppenstedt (13 Apr. 1785) and the privy council's decision to allow him to retain the *praeparat* (15 Apr. 1785).

183. For most people the natural world was still an enemy to be subjugated. See Keith Thomas, *Man and the Natural World: Changing Attitudes in England, 1500–1800* (London: Allen Lane, 1983), 25–30.

184. Loeber wrote two works on the old man, Hubrig, who had apparently once been his patient: *Sendschreiben von einer glücklich geheilten Lungenentzündung Hans Hubrigs* (Friedrichstadt: n.p., 1767) and *Freuden Hans Hubrig's: Ein 112jähr.[iger] Greis* (Dresden: n.p., 1778). And see Christoph Wilhelm Hufeland, *Die Kunst das menschlichen Leben zu verlängern* (Jena: Gotthold Ludwig Fiedler, in der akademischen Buchhandlung, 1797); G. R. Gruman, "A History of Ideas about the Prolongation of Life: The Evolution of Prolongevity Hypotheses to 1800," *Transactions of the American Philosophical Society*, n.s., 56 (1966): 3–102. On the negative valuation of old age, for a later period, see Hans-Joachim von Kondratowitz, "The Medicalization of Old Age: Continuity and Change in Germany from the Late Eighteenth to the Early Twentieth Century," in *Life, Death, and the Elderly: Historical Perspectives*, ed. Margaret Pelling and Richard M. Smith (London: Routledge, 1991), 137–38, 140–43.

185. StAWf, 111 Neu 1110, fol. 11, 6 Mar. 1769.

186. Ibid. 1133, fol. 15, 21 Mar. 1790.

187. Louis Spohr lived from 1784 to 1859. Information on his father is taken from Louis Spohr, *Lebenserinnerungen*, ed. Folker Göthel (Tutzing: Hans Schneider, 1968), 1–11; Clive Brown, *Louis Spohr: A Critical Biography* (Cambridge: Cambridge University Press, 1984), 1–22; *Lexikon*; and StAWf, 2 Alt 11382, 111 Neu 1125, 1063.

188. Carl Spohr, *Meditata in casum medico-practicum de vomitu bilioso in gravida* (Altdorf: J. P. Meyer, 1780).

189. StAWf, 2 Alt 11355, fols. 22–24, 30, 33.

190. Thomas Nipperdey, *Deutsche Geschichte, 1800–1866: Bürgerwelt und starker Staat* (Munich: Beck, 1983), 255–71.

191. StAWf, 2 Alt 11378, fol. 36, 7 Apr. 1803.

192. For example, that of the duke of Braunschweig-Wolfenbüttel; see Brown, *Spohr*, 9–10.

193. For Gieseler, see StadtB, C II 3, fol. 18, 23 Feb. 1684; on land for gardens, StAWf, 111 Neu 1109, fol. 4, 7 Nov. 1768.

194. Heinrich Apfel and his father also trained to be apothecaries; see StAWf, 17 N 2309, fols. 56–57, 30 June 1739.

195. StAWf, 2 Alt 11612, fols. 25–28, 9 Oct. 1776; ibid., fol. 40, 4 Nov. 1776.

196. La Vopa, *Grace*, 111–33. In referring to an "underground of enlightenment," I am, of course, borrowing from Robert Darnton, *The Literary Underground of the Old Regime* (Cambridge, Mass: Harvard University Press, 1978).

197. Urban Beltz, "Unvorgreifliches Project, auf was Art und Weise, die Stadt Hasselfelde zu nicht geringen Hoch-Fürstlichen Interesse ohne sonderliche Costen in kurtzer Zeit in Aufnahme und Nahrung zu setzen" (StAWf, 2 Alt 11305, fols. 9–16, probably 1740). See also Pamela H. Smith, *The Business of Alchemy: Science and Culture in the Holy Roman Empire* (Princeton, N.J.: Princeton University Press, 1994), on the significance for the development of commerce and commercial capitalism in the seventeenth century of Johann Joachim Becher, who was trained as a physician and combined science, medicine, alchemy, and commercial enterprises with the life of a courtier.

198. Rohr, *Geschichte*, 112; Ulrich, "Anfänge."

199. On going to Kochstedt, StAWf, 111 Neu 1120.

200. Hoffmann contributed numerous articles on plants and their medicinal uses to *BA-GB*; on du Roi and Siegesbeck, see *Lexikon*.

201. On Brückmann, see Ernst G. Baldinger, *Biographien jetztlebender Ärzte und Naturforscher in und ausser Deutschland* (Jena: Hartung, 1772), 111–20; Johann Meusel *Lexikon der vom Jahre 1750 bis 1800 verstorbenen teutschen Schriftsteller*, 4th ed. (Leipzig: G. Fleischer, der Jungere, 1802–16), 1783: 208–9; 1786: 79; 1788: 50; 1791: 80. On Gesenius, see *Lexikon* and *Versuch einer lepidopterologischen Encyklopadie oder Handbuch für angehende Schmetterlingssammler* (Erfurt: bey Georg Adam Keyser, 1786). Brückmann was also interested in gemstones; see his *Abhandlung von Edelsteinen*, 2d ed. (Braunschweig: Schulbuchhandlung, 1773).

202. See *Lexikon*, s.v. "Holdefreund."

203. On Wageler and Sommer, see *Lexikon*; on Roose, ibid., and Theodor Georg August Roose, *Taschenbuch für gerichtliche Aerzte und Wundärzte bei gesetzmässigen Leichenöffnungen* (Bremen: Wilmans, 1800) with many later editions among his various forensic publications; on Himly and on Hildebrandt, *Lexikon*, and also Hildebrandt, *Lehrbuch der Anatomie des Menschen* (Braunschweig: Schulbuchhandlung, 1789–92); id., *Bemerkungen und Beobachtungen über die Pocken in der Epidemie des Jahres 1787* (Braunschweig: Schulbuchhandlung, 1788); id., *Taschenbuch für die Gesundheit auf das Jahr* . . . (Erlangen: Heyder, 1800, 1801, 1803, 1807, 1812, 1813, 1820).

204. Johann Lange, *Tentamen medico-physicum de remediis Brunsvicensium domesticis* (Braunschweig: Waisenhaus, 1765). See also his *Die heilsamen und hochst wunderbaren Wirkungen des Wasserfenchels*, new ed. (Frankfurt: n.p., 1775).

205. Gerhard Matthias Friedrich Brawe [Brave], *De coctionis atque criseas in febribus impeimentis variisque novis inde oriundis* (Göttingen: n.p., 1768); Johann Jakob Heinrich Bücking, "Etwas über Quartanfieber," *BA-GB*, 25 July 1795; Johann Christian Konrad Dehne, *Versuch einer vollständigen Abhandlung von dem Maiwurme und dessen Anwendung in der Wuth und Wasserschau: Nebst Anmerkungen über die Natur dieser Krankheit, ihrer ansteckenden Eigenschaften und Behandlung* (Leipzig: Weygand, 1788); Carl Heinrich Spohr, "Gedanken über das Ausschneiden des Tollwurms bei Hunden," *BA-GB*, 18 Apr. 1795; Wilhelm Gesenius, *Ueber das epidemische faulichte Gallenfieber in den Jahren 1785 und 1786* (Leipzig: Jacobäer, 1788); August Friedrich Wilhelm Harcke, "Einige Erinnerungen an das Publikum, die Masern betreffend," *BA-GB*, 14 May 1796; Johann Röttger Salomo Holdefreund, *Abhandlung von epidemischen Stickhusten der Kinder* (Helmstedt: Kühnlin, 1775); Friedrich Christian Karl Krebs, "Einige wichtige Ursachen der jetzt so häufigen Lungensucht," *BA-GB*, 22 Nov. 1794; Johann Heinrich Lange, "Von einem besondern Cur des Fleckfiebers," *BA*, 6 May 1758; Joseph Conrad Mümler, "Nachricht von dem jetzt grassirenden Scharlachfieber," *BA-GB*, 4, 8, and 11 Mar. 1786); Johann Philipp du Roi, "Beytrage zu einer leichteren Heilung der Krätze," *BA-GB*, 5 June 1784; Urban Brückmann, "Sichere Methode die Krätze zu heilen," *BA-GB*, 8 Oct. 1783.

206. These are too numerous to mention here. A survey of the *BA* and *BA-GB* produced this list.

207. See Chapter 5, "Another Way of Choosing"; also Peter Albrecht, "Versuche zur Popularsierung der Blatterninokulation in der Stadt Braunschweig von 1754 bis 1780" (manuscript); and Andreas Weißmann, "Die Schutzpockenimpfung im Herzogtum Braunschweig-Wolfenbüttel von 1800 bis zum Impfgesetz vom April 1833" (Magisterarbeit, Modern History, Technischen Hochschule Braunschweig, 1993), esp. 47–70. I thank both authors for making copies of their work available to me.

208. This story is told well by Weißmann, "Schutzpockenimpfung," 98–104. On vaccination, Mühlenbein published "Einige Regeln für ungeübtere Impfärzte bei den Schutzblattern," *BA-GB*, 29 May and 5 June 1802, and "Berichtigung der Kuhpocken-Angelegenheiten zu Oebisfeld," *BM*, 22 Mar. 1802.

209. Marc Raeff, *The Well-Ordered Police State: Social and Institutional Change through Law in the Germanies and Russia* (New Haven, Conn.: Yale University Press, 1983), 179.

210. See, e.g., Frevert, *Krankheit*; Huerkamp, *Aufstieg*.

211. On 20 Sept. 1762, the privy council specified that the ducal treasury was to be responsible only "in subsidium" for what the apothecary fees, or the like, were unable to cover (StAWf, 2 Alt 11389, fol. 11). A good example of the way in which a physicus's salary was pulled together from many different sources can be found in the report of Amt Blankenburg on how it paid Dr. Schulze (ibid. 11357, fols. 1–5, 7 Nov. 1766).

212. For example, Dr. Kipping was 26 when appointed to Vorsfelde (StAWf, 111 Neu 1091a, fol. 3), as was Dr. Ziegler to Walkenried (111 Neu 1115, fols. 10–13); Dr. Fahrenholtz in Königslutter was 27 (111 Neu 1090, fol. 8); Drs. Mühlenbein and Müller, in Schöningen and Seesen respectively, were 28 (111 Neu 1135, fol. 16, and 111 Neu 1095, fols. 14–15); Dr. Stolze in Stadtoldendorf was 29 (2 Alt 11375, fols). 15–16; but Dr. Dehne in Schöningen was a relatively old 36 (111 Neu 1114, fols. 54–58).

Chapter 3. *Quacks, Bread-Thieves, and Interlopers; Friends, Neighbors, and Kin*

1. Jean-Pierre Goubert, the author of the phrase, has emphasized that he speaks of a "medical wasteland" only in the sense of a lack of academic physicians, not of other healers. But as Barbara Duden has observed in *Geschichte unter der Haut: Ein Eisenacher Arzt und seine Patientinnen um 1730* (Stuttgart: Klett-Cotta, 1987), 91 n. 3, the tendency to see the countryside as barren of all medical assistance has persisted.

2. StAWf, 111 Neu 29, fols. 2–3, 31 Dec. 1773. Likewise, in 1769, there were fifteen physicians practicing in Braunschweig; see ibid. 3253, fols. 165–66.

3. "Übersicht des Medizinalwesens der Herzogthums Braunschweig," *Medizinische National-Zeitung für Deutschland* 2, no. 15 (11 Mar. 1799): 237–38.

4. Ibid., 239.

5. On the university in Helmstedt, see Ursula Schelm-Spangenberg, "Schulen und Hochschulen," in *Braunschweigische Landesgeschichte im Überblick*, ed. Richard Moderhack, 3d ed. (Braunschweig: Waisenhaus, 1979), 264–65.

6. StadtH, B VII 9 Nr. 10.

7. Ibid., Nr. 17, 23 Sept. 1805.

8. StAWf, 2 Alt 11322, fols. 6–19; 11356, fol. 15.

9. StAWf, 111 Neu 1057, fols. 1–9, 21 Mar. 1747.

10. "Verzeichniß derer Handwerkern in Gandersheim" (1769), StAWf, 17 N 209, fols. 41–42; "Specificato derjenigen Personen, die sich allhier in der Stadt Gandersheim . . ." (1749), ibid., fols. 1–58; "Summarisches Verzeichniß aller lebenden Personen in der Stadt Gandersheim" (1788 and 1793), 17 N 215, fols. 2–3.

11. "Etat der in der Stadt Gandersheim befindlichen Aerzte, Wundärzte, Apothekern, und Hebammen," StAWf, 17 N 2323, fols. 3–4, 8 Sept. 1814; "Tabellarische Uebersicht . . . am Ende des Jahres 1818," StAWf, 111 Neu 1063, fols. 15–23.

12. See, e.g., "Specification derjenige Fürstl. und Adel. Güter und Gerichte, bey welchen eigene Bader angesetzt sind" (1771), StAWf, 2 Alt 11326, fols. 25–27; "Extract aus den Berichten sämtlicher Fürstl. Aemter, die sich auf dem platten Lande befindlichen Wund-Aerzte und Bader betreffend" (1796), StAWf, 111 Neu, fols. 2–4.

13. StAWf, 8 Alt Lutter am Barenberge 293, fols. 3–5, [7?] Nov. 1682.

14. "Specificatio einiger Patienten welche ich binnen anderthalb biß zwei Jahre allhier in Braunschweig curiret" (n.d. [1714]), in StAWf, 2 Alt 11293, fols. 21–27; on Barthold's relationship with the tailors' guild, see "Actum Braunschweig Neustadter Rath-Hause," 2 Alt 11294, fol. 29, 4 Mar. 1773; ibid., fols. 25–27, 22 Nov. and 4 Mar. 1734.

15. In *Professional and Popular Medicine in France, 1770–1830: The Social World of Medical Practice* (Cambridge: Cambridge University Press, 1988), Matthew Ramsey describes the "complex reality" (p. 18) of the Old Regime's medical system in great detail.

16. MO 1721.

17. StAWf, 40 Slg. 6879; Hinze, 63, 86.

18. Johann Jacob Heinrich Buecking, *Der Arzt und der Afterarzt* (Stendal: Franzen & Grosse, 1789), 7; Mühlenbein quoted StAWf, 111 Neu 3104, case 19, 1 Apr. 1801.

19. Johann Stoll, *Staatswissenschaftliche Untersuchungen und Erfahrungen über das*

Medicinalwesen nach seiner Verfasssung, Gesetzgebung und Verwaltung (Zurich: Orell, 1812–14), 2: 58–59; see also Ernst Gottfried Baldinger, *Artzeneien, eine physicalisch-medicinische Monatschrift, zum Unterricht allen denen welche den Schaden des Quacksalbers nicht kennen* (Leipzig: Martini, 1766–67); id., *Ueber Medizinal-Verfassung: Eine Rede* (Offenbach: Weiß & Brede, 1782).

20. See, e.g., StAWf, 111 Neu 1651–54, 1659–67. These files contain a series of concessions to various oculists, dentists, corn doctors, lithotomists, and the like. See also "Collegii medici Unterthängstes Pro Memoria die für die Bader, Chirurgos und Apotheker auszufertigende Privilegia betref.," StAWf, 2 Alt 11324, fols. 32–34, 11 Nov. 1747.

21. MO 1721; MO 1747; StAWf, 40 Slg. 13249 (20 Jan. 1794); 111 Neu 2 (vols. 1–2); Hinze, 3–12, 30–33, 39–43, 97–106, 114–19, 126, 142–45, 155, 161, 238.

22. Ramsey defines encroachment as the "infringement by one occupation on the domain of a neighboring occupation" (*Professional and Popular Medicine*, 388).

23. MO 1721, Cap. V §§ 5, 6, 8. The surgeons argued that it was infeasible, and in some cases actually dangerous for their patients, for them not to be allowed to dispense internal medicines in some surgical cases. But the Collegium medicum would not budge and warned the surgeons that they had a choice: either adhere to the terms of their oaths or give up their practices. See petition of surgeons of 17 May 1748, StAWf, 2 Alt 11282, fols. 54–59; and responses of the Collegium of 6 July and 17 Aug. 1748, ibid., fols. 60–84.

24. Zedler defines an *Operateur* as "in surgery, one who undertakes a surgical operation; generally, however, someone like a lithotomist is so designated."

25. MO 1721, Cap. VIII § 2.

26. MO 1721, Cap. VII, §§ 1, 4 7; Hinze, 155, 238.

27. MO 1747; Hinze, 155, 238; 4 Oct. 1791, StAWf, 111 Neu 1451.

28. Zedler defines an *Oculiste* or *Augenarzt* as "a doctor, who knows just how to alleviate eye problems; either with internal or external medicines, or by a surgical operation." He goes on to point out that "today there are in Europe many skillful oculists whose experience allows them to cure cataracts . . . and many other [eye] afflictions."

29. On the traveling oculists, see Julius Hirschberg, *Geschichte der Augenheilkunde im Mittelalter und in der Neuzeit*, vol. 13 of *Handbuch der gesamten Augenheilkunde*, ed. Alfred Graefe and Theodor Saemisch, 2d rev. ed. (Leipzig: W. Engelmann, 1898); Georg Bartisch, *"Ophthalmodoyleia," das ist "Augendienst": Neuer und wohlgegründeter Bericht von Ursachen und Erkenntniss aller Gebrechen, Schäden und Mängel der Augen und des Gesichts* (Dresden: Stöckel, 1583; reprint, Stuttgart: Medicina rara, 1977) and Wolfgang Straub, "The First German Textbook of Ophthamology 'Augendienst' by G. Bartisch, 1583," in *History of Ophthamology*, vol. 1 (Dordrecht: Kluwer, 1988), 104–11; on Hilmer, see Hirschberg, *Geschichte*, 502.

30. Schmidt to Rat (Braunschweig), 28 June 1653, StadtB, B IV 13c Nr. 16; Jill Kohl and Mary Lindemann, "Augustus in tenebris," in *Barocker Lust-Spiegel: Studien zur Literatur des Barock. Festschrift für Blake Lee Spahr*, ed. Martin Bircher, Jörg-Ulrich Fechner, and Gerd Hillen (Amsterdam: Rodophi, 1984), 187–204.

31. On traveling practitioners in general, see Christian Probst, *Fahrende Heiler und Heilmittelhändler: Medizin von Marktplatz und Landstraße* (Rosenheim: Rosenheimer

Verlaghaus Alfred Förg, 1992); Frank Huisman, "Intinerant Medical Practitioners in the Dutch Republic: The Case of Groningen," *Tractrix* 1 (1989): 63–83; and id., "Gevestigden en buitenstaanders op de medische markt: De marginalisierung van reizende meesters in achttiende-eeuws Groningen," in *Grenzen van genezing: Gezondheid, ziekte en genezen in Nederland, zestiende tot begin twintigste eeuw,* ed. Willem de Blécourt, Willem Frihoff, and Marijke Gijswijt-Hofstra (Hilversum: Verloren, 1993), 115–54. The distinction, however, dates at least from the eighteenth century. In *Anleitung für das Landvolk in Absicht auf seine Gesundheit,* 2d ed. (Augsburg and Innsbruck: Wolff, 1766), 592, Samuel Tissot, for example, divided "quacks" into two types: traveling quacks and village doctors. Johann Christian Stark constructed an entire hierarchy of quacks and charlatans, *Versuch einer wahren und falschen Politik der Aerzte, zu Vorlesungen bestimmt* (Jena: Voigt, 1784). And see Krünitz, s.v. "Pfuscher."

32. StAWf, 2 Alt 11288, fol. 2, 24 July 1788. Among other things, Seiffert advertised (under the device "Soli deo gloria") a "worm cake," "a yellow anondyne poultice" recommended for headaches and pains in the back, side, and pelvic areas, and a "wonder gland or Lapis Medicamentesa" for toothache. Ibid., fols. 6–7.

33. See Köring's case in StAWf, 111 Neu 1652, case 6 (1750). This file includes a copy of his advertisement entitled "Ubi vinum est vendible, ibi suspensa opus est hedera"; on Meyer, see StAWf, 17 N 2312, fol. 45, 17 Feb. 1742.

34. StAWf, 111 Neu 1651, 18 Oct. 1723.

35. MO 1721, Cap. VII § 1; quoted in Hinze, 153.

36. From 1779 in StAWf, 111 Neu 1654, case 6; 2 Alt 11290, fols. 1–12.

37. See, e.g., the advertisements and flyers of Johann Georg Eckstein for his "Universal-Balsam" and his "Rothfarben Gülden-Balsam" from the 1790s, StAWf, 111 Neu 1651; on Knupf, see StadtB, C VII S42, fols. 177–78.

38. Ernst Schubert, *Arme Leute, Bettler und Gauner im Franken des 18. Jahrhunderts* (Neustadt a.d. Aisch: Kommissions-Verlag Degener, 1983), 234–321; Carsten Küther, *Menschen auf der Straße: Vagierende Unterschichten in Bayern, Franken und Schwaben in der zweiten Hälfte des 18. Jahrhunderts* (Göttingen: Vandenhoeck & Ruprecht, 1983), 40–45.

39. StadtB, C II 3, fol. 3, 31 Aug. 1688.

40. For instance, Johann Siegreich paid 5 thaler 33 mariengroschen for the concession granted him on 11 Apr. 1782; see StAWf, 111 Neu 1654, case 25.

41. "Avertisement," copy in StAWf, 111 Neu 1651.

42. Petition from 8 Aug. 1786; Fredersdorf's testimonial, 27 Aug. 1784, both in StAWf, 111 Neu 1654, case 21.

43. Ibid., 5 Aug. 1785.

44. StAWf, 111 Neu 1667, 14 Feb. 1798.

45. See flyers and advertisements in StAWf, 111 Neu 1651–54, 1659–67, and advertisements in BA.

46. Roy Porter, *Health for Sale: Quackery in England, 1660–1850* (Manchester: Manchester University Press, 1989), esp. 21–59; Lucas's advertisement in StAWf, 111 Neu 1654, case 16.

47. StAWf, 2 Alt 11274, fols. 16–17, 15 Nov. 1647.

48. Ibid., fol. 26, 3 Dec. 1660.

49. Ibid., fol. 27.

50. StAWf, 2 Alt 11280, 16 Feb. 1697, 1 Mar. 1697, and 12 Apr. 1701.

51. StAWf, 111 Neu 1654, case 24; 2 Alt 11320, fols. 2–3, 9; on Siegreich, 111 Neu 1654, case 25.

52. StAWf, 2 Alt 11320, fol. 10, 20 Aug. 1756.

53. Ibid., fols. 17, 21, 3 and 9 Feb. 1764; 111 Neu 1654, 9 July 1764.

54. StAWf, 2 Alt 11320, fols. 30–31, 15 July 1770.

55. Mack Walker, *German Home Towns: Community, State, and General Estate, 1648–1871* (Ithaca, N.Y.: Cornell University Press, 1971), 101. Zedler defines *bürgerliche Nahrung* as "in a broad sense, each and every kind of . . . work, profession, handwork, commerce, trade, and transportation, as well as distilling, brewing, [and] keeping a tavern." Traditionally, a "bürgerliche Nahrung" applied only to burghers in a city and their activities. In a wider sense, the concept of "Nahrung" also pertains to nobles, military men, and peasants. Krünitz equates "Nahrung" with what one does to earn a living, and with "Gewerbe"—that is, with trade, business, and occupation.

56. Renate Blickle, "Nahrung und Eigentum als Kategorien in der ständischen Gesellschaft," in *Ständische Gesellschaft und soziale Mobilität,* ed. Winfried Schulze (Munich: R. Oldenbourg, 1988), 76–77, 82, 85–87.

57. MO 1721; MO 1747, Cap. III ("Was denen ordinariren und privilegirten Apotheckern/ auch denen Gesellen und Jungen obliege"), which included a "Taxa medicamentorum."

58. StAWf, 40 Slg. 3599, 2 Apr. 1696. In 1651, the apothecaries protested inroads on their practice by "interlopers," pointing out that citizens in their citizen's oath promised not to deal in apothecary wares. "Verordnet. Provisiores zur Apotheker der Stadt Braunschweig," 17 Oct. 1651, StadtB, B IV 13c: 11. See also decision of 4 May 1713, 40 Slg. 4329, repeated on 8 Apr. 1730, 40 Slg. 5305; similar decisions on 24 Aug. 1765, 40 Slg. 9489; 24 Aug. 1767, 40 Slg. 9762; 30 May 1768, 40 Slg. 9880; 20 Oct. 1785, 40 Slg. 12632; 11 May 1786, 40 Slg. 12670; 22 Dec. 1786, 40 Slg. 12714[b]; 3 Apr. 1810, 40 Slg. 15382.

59. See, e.g., the file on "Der Kampf gegen die Winkelapotheken, 1643–1651" in StadtB, B IV 13c: 11.

60. StAWf, 40 Slg. 4329, 4 May 1713. On traveling medicine men, see Probst, *Fahrende Heiler.*

61. StadtH, B VII Nr. 3, 7 Jan. 1745.

62. Probst, *Fahrende Heiler,* 58–171.

63. For a list pertaining to apothecaries, see *Helmstädter Apotheken Taxi Und Verzeichniß Aller Medicamenten So in der Fürstlichen Julius-Universität Und E.E. Rahts Apotheken daselbst vorhanden/ Nebenst vorgesetzter Apotheken Ordnung/ Jedermänniglichen zur nachrichtung und besten in druck gegeben* (Helmstedt: Henning Müller, 1663).

64. A good critical review of the medicalization and professionalization literature can be found in Francisca Loetz, *Vom Kranken zum Patienten: "Medikalisierung" und medizinische Vergesellschaftung am Beispiel Badens, 1750–1850* (Stuttgart: Franz Steiner, 1993), 19–56.

65. Porter, *Health,* 55. The importance of economics in fringe and orthodox practice is now well documented. See, e.g., the various essays in *Medical Fringe and Medical Orthodoxy, 1750–1850,* ed. W. F. Bynum and Roy Porter (London: Croom Helm, 1987).

66. Mary E. Fissell, *Patients, Power, and the Poor in Eighteenth-Century Bristol* (Cambridge: Cambridge University Press, 1991), 37.

67. Ramsey, *Professional and Popular Medicine*, 284–91.

68. For examples of *Pfuscherey* among shoemakers and cobblers (1779 and 1781), coopers (1783), lathe-turners (1789), and wheel- and cartwrights (1801), see StAWf, 9 Alt Wendhausen 70.

69. Zedler, s.v. "Pfuscher," "Pfuscher (medizinische)," "Bönhasen," and "Nahrungs-Störerey."

70. See complaints of 9, 17, and 28 June and 7 Aug. 1795, in StAWf, 111 Neu 58, fols. 1–6, 8. For another case, from 1794, see 111 Neu 3112, case 154.

71. This was part of an initiative to protect urban guildsmen. See ordinances of 29 Apr. 1749, StAWf, 40 Slg. 7172; 23 Sept. 1749, 40 Slg. 7215; 11 Feb. 1768, 40 Slg. 9842; 18 Apr. 1782, 40 Slg. 12337ª. The term *Pfuscher* continues to appear in context of artisan work at least as late as 1805 in Braunschweig-Wolfenbüttel: "Verordnung, wegen Aufhebung des Pfuscherjagens im hiesigen Hzt. und Fürstentum Blankenburg," 12 Nov. 1805, HAB, Einbl. R2: 1858.

72. StAWf, 10 Alt Hehlen 31, 20 Oct. 1751.

73. *Den grossen Unterschied zwischen rechtschaffener Medicorum und derer Quacksalber medicinischen Wissenschafften und Curen: Kurtz und deutlich beschrieben* (Görlitz, 1716 [?]), 49.

74. William H. Sewell, Jr., *Work and Revolution in France: The Language of Labor from the Old Regime to 1848* (Cambridge: Cambridge University Press, 1980).

75. Krünitz, vols. 112 (1809) and 119 (1811), s.v. "Pfuscher" and "Quacksalber." Compare the definition of "After" (*Afterarzt*). Krünitz, 2d ed. (1783), vol. 2, notes that the use of the word was very common, especially among artisans. It meant "something that was not as good, or . . . in combination with other words, the same as 'behind,' 'after,' 'below'."

76. See Roy Porter, "Before the Fringe: 'Quackery' and the Eighteenth-Century Medical Market," in *Studies in the History of Alternative Medicine*, ed. Roger Cooter (New York: St. Martin's Press, 1988), 1–26.

77. StadtB, C II 4, fols. 82–83.

78. After 1747, all disputes concerning the activities of "quacks" were to be forwarded to the Collegium medicum for its decision (Hinze, 86). Oettinger's story is case 151 in StAWf, 111 Neu 3112, petition dated 9 Aug. 1803.

79. StAWf, 111 Neu 3112, case 151.

80. StadtH, B VII 12 Nr. 2, 24 June 1749.

81. Sewell, *Work and Revolution*, 2–3. This tradition persisted longer in Germany than in western Europe; see Wolfram Fischer, *Handwerksrecht und Handwerkswirtschaft um 1800* (Berlin: Dunker & Humblot, 1955), 18.

82. StAWf, 111 Neu 3112, case 151ᴵᴵ, 23 July 1817.

83. Zedler, s.v. "Pfuscherey." This is the sense in which the terms *Pfuscher* and *Pfuscherey* were used in describing medical "interloping" in the eighteenth century. See examples of how the term *Pfuscher*, or *Fuscher*, was used in Braunschweig-Wolfenbüttel in StAWf 40 Slg. 7172, 7215, 9842, 12337a. By contrast, the word *Empiricus* connoted lack of adherence to a "method." Zedler, s.v. "Empiricii," describes an *empiricus* as someone in medicine who "uses his own arcana, compositions, chemical

preparations and the like . . . and thereby scorns the Hippocratic and Galenic or other academic principles."

84. "Acta verschiedene Pfuscher in den Beamtern Winnigstedt und Voights-dahlum betref. 1764," StAWf, 111 Neu 3102.

85. The surgeons here, like others who penned similar denunciations, constructed stories they felt would be believed. This does not mean they lied or deliberately constructed half-truths (although they were, of course, perfectly capable of duplicity on occasion). Rather, they selected incidents, language, and forms of argumentation that would influence their audience. They could be quite adept in manipulating these elements and modifying them as needed. See Natalie Davis, *Fiction in the Archives: Pardon Tales and Their Tellers in Sixteenth-Century France* (Stanford, Calif.: Stanford University Press, 1987), 3.

86. The most work in this direction has been done for England, see Porter, *Health*, 36–39, 42–43; Dorothy Porter and Roy Porter, *Patient's Progress: Doctors and Doctoring in Eighteenth-Century England* (Stanford, Calif.: Stanford University Press, 1989), 33–52. For perspectives on the number of new products introduced (especially in the Germanies), see Wolfgang Schneider, *Lexikon zu Arzneimittelgeschichte*, vol. 4: *Geheimmittel und Spezialitäten* (Frankfurt am Main: Govi, 1969); Bernhard Nathan Gottlieb Schreger, *Kritisches Dispensatorium der geheimen, spezifischen und universellen Heilmittle die nach ihren Erfindern, ihren Wirkungen, oder nach denen Krankheiten, in denen sie empfohlen werden, benennt worden* (Leipzig: Weygand, 1795); Heinz Peickert, *Geheimmittel im deutschen Arzneiverkehr: Ein Beitrag zur Wirtschaftsgeschichte der Pharmazie und zur Arzneispezialitätenfrage* (Leipzig: Edelmann, 1932).

87. Wolfram Kaiser and Werner Piechocki, "Anfänge einer pharmazeutischen Industrie in Halle und ihre Begründer," *Münchener Medizinische Wochenschrift* 109 (1967): 143–49; id., "Die pharmazeutische Industrie von Halle in der zweiten Hälfte des 18. Jahrhunderts," ibid., 110 (1968): 420–30; Renate Wilson and Hans Joachim Poeckern, "Pietism and Medical Care in Colonial Georgia," *MGG* 9 (1990): 99–126.

88. Schreger, *Kritisches Dispensatorium*, 68–69; Maurice Bouvet, *Histoire de la pharmacie en France des origines à nos jours* (Paris: Editions Occitania, 1937); id., "Un Exemple de publicité médico-pharmaceutique par brochures au XVIII\u1d49 siècle: Le 'remède universel' au 'poudre d'Ailhaud,'" *La Pharmacie française* 26 (May 1922): 193–207; Ramsey, *Professional and Popular Medicine*, 177–78.

89. Jean Ailhaud, *Traité de l'origine des maladies et de l'usage de la poudre purgative. . . . Avec un recueil de plusieurs guérisons apérées par ce remède* (Avignon: J. Rousset, 1742); two different German versions, *Universal-Arzney oder Abhandlung von dem Ursprunge der Krankheiten und dem Gebrauche des abführenden Pulvers* (Strasbourg: Lorenz, 1765); *Kurzer Auszug des Systems der Herren von Ailhaud über den Ursprung der Krankheiten* (Strasbourg: Christmann & Levrault, 1766); and also *Kurzer Auszug der merkwürdigsten Genesungen so durch die Ailhaudschen Pulver gewirket worden, aus den dreien Theilen der deutschen Genesungs-Briefe gezogen* (Strasbourg: Lorenz, 1768).

90. Bouvet, "Un Exemple," 206–7; Fielding H. Garrison, *An Introduction to the History of Medicine*, 4th rev., enlarged ed. (Philadelphia: W. B. Saunders, 1929), 388.

91. Schreger lists a number of specifics, including, for instance, Hoffmann's "great pills," "pox-pills," "life-elixir," and "balsam pills" (*Kritisches Dispensatorium*, 38–40, 103–4, 156). For example, Stahl produced and marketed a "balsamic blood-purifying

pill," a nerve tonic, a wound balsam, and stomach pills (ibid., 271, 278, 290–91, 315–17). Unzer produced a powder that bore his name: "das Unzersche Freßpulver" (ibid., 100). Johann Heinrich Wachsmuth, *Panacea solaris, oder Universal-Gold-Balsam, wodurch Alle Krankheiten des Menschlichen Leibes, so wohl innerlich als äuserliche, besonders Schalg-Fluß, Jammer, Podagra, und alle Arten der Gicht, Stein, Krebs und verstopfte Monath-Zeiten etc. glücklich durch gottlichen Seegen gehoben worden* (Nordhausen: n.p., 1733) and *Spiritus vitae catholicus, oder Universal-Lebens-Spiritus, wodurch in Alchymia alles was zum Universal nöthig ist, in Medicina aber in Curirung der Kranckheiten ein grosses kan ausgerichtet werden* (Nordhausen: n.p., n.d.), copies in StAWf, 2 Alt 11300, fols. 48–64, 65–68.

92. Roy Porter offers an excellent discussion of proprietary medicines in his *Health*, esp. 35–55. J. Harvey Young's *The Toadstool Millionaires* (Princeton, N.J.: Princeton University Press, 1961), from which I have borrowed the expression, uses "toadstool millionaires" to designate quacks in the sense of frauds and deceivers, rather than medical entrepreneurs.

93. Matthew Ramsey, "Traditional Medicine and Medical Enlightenment: The Regulation of Secret Remedies in the Ancien Régime," in *La Médicalisation de la société française, 1770–1830*, ed. Jean-Pierre Goubert (Waterloo, Ont.: Historical Reflections Press, 1982), 215–32.

94. "In the history of the mass promotion and distribution of manufactures in the early Industrial Revolution, an innovatory role was played by proprietary medicine vendors. Quack medicines were among the very first standardised, nationally marketed, brand-name products," Roy Porter notes (*Health*, 46). See also P. S. Brown, "The Vendors of Medicine Advertised in Eighteenth-Century Bath Newspapers," *MH* 19 (1975): 352–69; id., "Medicines Advertised in Eighteenth-Century Bath Newspapers," ibid., 20 (1976): 152–68; C. Y. Ferdinand, "Selling It to the Provinces: News and Commerce Round Eighteenth-Century Salisbury," in *Consumption and the World of Goods*, ed. John Brewer and Roy Porter (New York: Routledge, 1993), 396–400.

95. Schreger lists a whole series of these, including specifics against cancer ("Des Grafen von Arundel Spezifika wider den Krebs"), for venereal diseases (such as "Miro's, jetzt Schifferts Arcan wider die Lustseuche"), and for rabies, including the powder made from the oil beetle, and the Prussian remedy, likewise using the beetle, but also the "Hungarian specific for hydrophobia" (*Kritisches Dispensatorium*, 23–25, 36–37, 43, 290–91). For a list of the Halle medications, see ibid., 232–43.

96. Bouvet, "Un Exemple," 196–98; "Nachricht an das Publikum: Die Würkung des Ailhaudischen Pulvers betreffend," *BA-GB*, 11 and 14 Jan. 1769; for debates on its composition, see, e.g., the contributions to the *Kölnische gemeinnützige Anzeigen aus dem Reiche der Gelehrsamkeit von einer Gesellschaft Literaturfreund* (Cologne, 1778), 65–66, 272, 404–5, 454–57, 501–5, 714–16, 757–59 and, in Braunschweig-Wolfenbüttel, Carl G. Wageler's analysis of 19 Nov. 1768, StAWf, 2 Alt 11696, fols. 1–2; Beireis's analysis of 24 Mar. 1768, 2 Alt 11694, fols. 46–49.

97. The study of consumerism and consumer culture has focused overwhelmingly on the nineteenth and twentieth centuries. For earlier centuries, Neil McKendrick, John Brewer, and J. H. Plumb's pioneering work *The Birth of Consumer Society: The Commercialization of Eighteenth-Century England* (Bloomington: Indiana University Press, 1982) is crucial. Recently, considerably more interest has been devoted to

the seventeenth and eighteenth centuries; see, e.g., *Consumption*, ed. Brewer and Porter, which, however, includes no article on Germany. Germany still seems to be terra incognita as far as students of consumer culture in early modern times are concerned, despite a long-term interest of the *Volkskundler* in *Wohnkultur* and the recent investigations into *Alltagsgeschichte*. See, however, Ruth-E. Mohrmann, *Alltagswelt im Land Braunschweig: Stadtische und ländliche Wohnkultur vom 16. bis zum frühen 20. Jahrhundert* (Münster: F. Coppenrath, 1990), which offers a real bonanza of information, if little sustained analysis. The best work so far on medical consumerism is Porter, *Health*.

    98. Hinze, s.v. "Medicamenten"; MO 1747, § 7.

    99. Ibid.; StAWf, 2 Alt 11286, fols. 35–38, 45–47, 16 Oct. and 9 Nov. 1773; 2 Alt 11391, fols. 18–19, 21 Oct. 1776.

    100. StAWf, 2 Alt 11184, fols. 12, 14, 22 Dec. 1758 and 2 Feb. 1759.

    101. "Nachricht an das Publikum: das Sal mirabile Glauberi oder Glaubersche Wundersalz, sonderlich dasjenige, welches allhier zu Braunschweig in der Gravenhorstschen Fabrik verfertiget wird, betreffend," *BA-GB*, 28 Jan., 1, 4, and 8 Feb. 1769; "Etwas von dem medicinischen Gebrauche und Nutzen des Salis mirabilis Glauberi, oder Glauberischen Wundersalzes. Mit Approbation des Herzogl. Braunsch. Lüne. Collegii Medici," *BA-GB*, 21 Feb. 1770. The Gravenhorst brothers moved in the circle of enlightened and influential men in Braunscheig. They were also promoters of inoculation; see their "Nachricht von der Einimpfung der Blattern an vier Kindern," *BA-GB*, 8, 11, 15 and 25 Apr. 1772. Their factory also manufactured ammonium chloride (household ammonia), which found a good market among artisans, Peter Albrecht, *Die Förderung des Landesausbaues im Herzogtum Braunschweig-Wolfenbüttel im Spiegel der Verwaltungsakten des 18. Jahrhunderts (1671–1806)* (Braunschweig: Waisenhaus, 1980), 485, 494; "Fernere Nachricht an das Publikum, das Braunschweigische Salmiak betreffend," *BA-GB*, 21, 25, and 28 Mar. 1772.

    102. Charles Ingrao, "The Problem of 'Enlightened Absolutism' and the German States," *JMH* suppl. 58 (1986): S176–77; Hans-Joachim Braun, "Economic Theory and Policy in Germany, 1750–1800," *JEEH* 4 (1975): 313–15.

    103. StAWf, 2 Alt 11317, fols. 5–6, 15 Jan. 1745.

    104. Albrecht, *Förderung*, 565.

    105. Winifred B. Rothenberg has argued that in the case of colonial New England, the putative resistance to capitalist development is untestable and probably wrong. She points out that much of the debate about the emergence of a market economy, and about the transition from pre-capitalism to capitalism in New England, "has been formulated as the assault of instrumental, self-seeking, commercial values on the mentalité of a 'moral economy' " (*From Market-Places to a Market Economy: The Transformation of Rural Massachusetts, 1750–1850* [Chicago: University of Chicago Press, 1992], 51–55, 242–44).

    106. Unless otherwise noted, all information on Ailhaud's remedy in Braunschweig-Wolfenbüttel is taken from StAWf, 2 Alt 11694–97; StadtB, C VII S20, vol. X; and StadtH, B VII Nr. 1. A similar case involved the sale of Goslar vitriol in 1752; see "Unterthänigstes Pro Memoria den Verkauf des Goslarischen Vitriols betreffend," StAWf, 2 Alt 11181, fols. 30–40, 23 Oct. 1752.

    107. Urban F. B. Brückmann, "Beantwortung der Aufgabe, ob das seit einiger

Zeit bekannt gewordene Pulver des Hrn. Ailhaud beÿ verschiedenen in Krankheiten Hülfe geleistet, oder Schaden gethan habe?" *BA*, no. 40 (17 May 1755).

108. StadtH, B VII 11a Nr. 2, 31 Oct., 10 and 24 Nov., 9 Dec. 1747, 5, 10, and 11 Jan., and 31 May 1748.

109. Ibid., 2 Jan. 1750. For earlier examples of how the government tried to use such lists to draw boundaries between grocers and apothecaries, see "Aus dem Protocol vom 30 [August?] An. 1628 und [1]591. den Kramern und Zucker Bäckern gebieret die Materialien, So auff die Apotheke gehören, nicht feil zu haben," StadtB, B IV 13c Nr. 11, 21 Dec. 1643. See also the conflict fought on the same terms between the apothecaries and the merchant Hummel thirty years later (StadtB, B VII 11a Nr. 4).

110. See StAWf, 8 Alt Thedinghausen 227, 25 Apr. 1759; or similar complaints about the apothecary Zincke in Pabstdorf, who sold spirits, StAWf, 8 Alt Hessen 7, fols. 35–36, 15 Nov. 1792.

111. See StAWf, 2 Alt 11281, fols. 16–17, 20–21, 26–29, for 6, 7, 24 and 27 Sept. 1742; or the similar conflict that arose concerning the liquor trade of the apothecary in Heßen and Pabstdorf in the 1790s, StAWf, 8 Alt Hessen 7, fols. 35–36, 44, 55, for 15 Nov. 1792, 12 Sept. 1793, 12 Sept. 1797.

112. StAWf, 2 Alt 11694, fols. 12–15, 15 Dec. 1767.

113. "Magistrat zu Helmstedt berichtet, wegen des Gebrauchs der ailhaudschen Pulver," StadtH, B VII 11 Nr. 1, 22 Mar. 1770.

114. Mary Lindemann, "Aufklärung and the Health of the People: Volksschriften and Medical Advice in Braunschweig-Wolfenbüttel, 1756–1803," in *Das Volk als Objekt obrigkeitlichen Handelns*, ed. Rudolf Vierhaus (Tübingen: Max Niemeyer, 1992), 101–20; see also Robert Heller, "'Priest-Doctors' as a Rural Health Service in the Age of Enlightenment," *MH* 19 (1975): 361–83.

115. "Serenissimi gnädigste Verordnung die Einschleppung der verbotenen fremden Medicin betr.," StAWf, 40 Slg. 9818, 21 Dec. 1769.

116. StAWf, 2 Alt 11285, pp. 4–5, 11–12, 14–15, 6 and 29 Aug. 1759, 24 Apr. 1763. See also the story of the grocer Francke in 1767, who sold a variety of products, including ammonium chloride purchased wholesale from the Gravenhorst factory in Braunschweig (2 Alt 11616).

117. The best treatment of economic policies in Braunschweig-Wolfenbüttel is Albrecht, *Förderung*; see esp. his conclusions, 565.

118. E. P. Thompson, "The Moral Economy of the English Crowd in the Eighteenth Century," *PP* 50 (1971): 76–136.

119. Anthony Black has argued that alternatives to "guilded thinking" always existed, which he calls the ideas of "civil society" (*Guilds and Civil Society in European Political Thought from the Twelfth Century to the Present* [Ithaca, N.Y.: Cornell University Press, 1984], 12–43).

120. See Cissie Fairchilds, "The Production and Marketing of Populuxe Goods in Eighteenth-Century France," in *Consumption*, ed. Brewer and Porter, 228–248.

121. Merely distinguishing among these practitioners is a daunting task. The names were often applied in a confusing and capricious manner: bathmasters were often called barber-surgeons, while barber-surgeons frequently insisted on the title of surgeon, and so on. The more modern term *Wundarzt* became common only in the

eighteenth century. Speaking of "Chirurgorum oder Wundaerzte," MO 1721 suggests that the latter term was still unfamiliar enough to require further elucidation.

122. StAWf, 40 Slg. 13871, 29 Oct. 1801.

123. HAB Cod. Guelf. 478, Nov. fol. 313, 5 Apr. 1746; StAWf, 40 Slg. 9435, 1 Apr. 1765; 40 Slg. 9919, 26 Sept. 1768; "Declaration wegen Aufhebung des Unterschiedes zwischen Chirurgis und Badern," StAWf, 40 Slg. 10031, 6 Dec. 1769; HAB, Einbl. R4: 1812; StAWf, 40 Slg. 11677, 30 Jan. 1775.

124. "Prozeß der Braunschweiger Barbiere und Chirurgen vor dem Reichskammergericht 1635 bis 1688," StAWf, 2 Alt 12711; "Weitere Auseinandersetzungen 1686–1738," 2 Alt 11271–72; "Gewerbe-Akten vor 1750: Bader und Barbiere," StadtB, C II 4. See also Karl-Rudolf Döhnel, *Das Anatomisch-Chirurgische Institut in Braunschweig, 1750–1869* (Braunschweig: Waisenhaus, 1957), 10–11; Annelise Gerbert, *Öffentliche Gesundheitspflege und staatliches Medizinalwesen in den Städten Braunschweig und Wolfenbüttel im 19. Jahrhundert* (Braunschweig: Selbstverlag des Braunschweigischen Geschichtsvereins, 1983), 5–8; Albrecht, *Förderung*, 319; Franz Fuhse, "Die Bader und Barbiere in der Stadt Braunschweig während des 16. Jahrhunderts," in *Unsere Heimat Niedersachsen*, ed. Rudolf Benze (Braunschweig: Westermann, 1924), 30–36. Jarndyce *v.* Jarndyce is an interminable lawsuit in Charles Dickens's novel *Bleak House* (1852).

125. "Ordnung und Privilegia der Barbiere und Chirurgorum in Braunschweig de dato Braunschweig d. 27ᵗᵉⁿ Febr: 1716," StAWf, 40 Slg. 4519.

126. Fuhse, "Bader und Barbiere"; Döhnel, *Institut*, 10–11, 21, 30–31; Gerbert, *Gesundheitspflege*, 5–6.

127. Döhnel, *Institut*, 21.

128. MO 1721 (Cap. V, § 1) specified that the guild certified the surgeons and bathmasters "by means of a public examination and masterpiece." MO 1747 (§ 17) specified that they had to be examined by the Collegium medicum. And this merely repeated what had already been done on 8 Mar. 1745, StAWf (40 Slg. 6480). Fees and procedures were set on 4 Jan. 1747 (40 Slg. 6881). The necessity of doing a masterpiece was done away with in 1752 as a "useless exercise" (StAWf, Barbiere, 2 Alt vorl 12410).

129. Döhnel, *Institut*, 21–22;

130. StAWf, 40 Slg. 13249, 20 Jan. 1794.

131. StadtH, B VII 11k Nr. 1, 18 Nov. 1749, 19 Aug. 1754, 31 Aug. 1754.

132. Ibid., 20 and 21 July, 4 Aug., 21 Sept., 26 Oct. 1767, 18 Dec. 1768, 7 Feb., and 29 Mar. 1769.

133. StadtK, St. VIII, 1, 18 Mar. 1726.

134. In 1747, the privy council prohibited the nobility from distributing "Privilegia privata" to bathmasters (StAWf, 2 Alt 11324, fols. 3–4, 30 May 1747).

135. See Schneider's petition to magistrates in Königslutter, 3 [?] June 1762, StadtK, St. VIII, 1; request refused, ibid., 11 June 1762.

136. Ibid., 8 Feb. and 6 May 1762. In 1769, the artisans in the city included one bathmaster, with two apprentices; one barber-surgeon, with one apprentice; and one apothecary (Wilfried Kraus, "Untersuchungen zur Geschichte der Stadt Königslutter im 18. Jahrhundert" [Hausarbeit, Braunschweig, 1967], 37).

137. StAWf, 2 Alt 11292, fols. 120–21, 15 Apr. 1767; StadtK, St. VIII, 1, for 6 and 21 Oct. and 1 Nov. 1784.

138. StadtK, St. VIII, 1, for 8 Mar. 1791.

139. Ibid., 6 June and 14 Nov. 1793, 19 Feb. and 4 Dec. 1794.

140. Ibid., 7 and 19 Dec. 1796, 11 Jan., 6 Feb., and 24 May 1797.

141. See "Acta die med. Pfuscherey des Chirurgus Rühland und des Sohn des verstorbenen Chirurgus Fischer zu Königslutter betreffend," from 1817–27, StAWf, 111 Neu 3113, case 170. For similar stories, see StAWf, 1 N Schöppenstedt I Nr. 457–458; 1 N Schöppenstedt I Nr. 457, fols. 9–10, 20 Oct. and 1 Nov. 1773. For the leasing of the bathhouse in Helmstedt, see StadtH, B VII 11k Nr. 1.

142. StAWf, 8 Alt Seesen 3 Nr. 15, fols. 10–11, 13 May 1758; 8 Alt Seesen 3 Nr. 14.

143. Ibid., fols. 18–19, 3 Dec. 1754.

144. StAWf, 8 Alt Seesen Nr. 15, fols. 46–47, 18 July 1775.

145. On the stigma of theft, see James R. Farr, *Hands of Honor: Artisans and Their World in Dijon, 1550–1650* (Ithaca, N.Y.: Cornell University Press, 1988), 163–64.

146. In the last half of the eighteenth century, concessions to surgeons in the countryside (*Land-Chirurgen*) were generally only granted for a period of six years; they had to be renewed periodically (StAWf, 2 Alt 11328, fol. 8).

147. The government forbade nonguild surgeons and bathmasters to accept apprentices, 26 Sept. 1768, HAB, Einbl. R3: 1120.

148. "An Fürstl. Regierung alhier," StAWf, 11 N Blankenburg 4, 2 Dec. 1768.

149. Ibid.

150. Ibid.

151. StAWf, 11 N Blankenburg 3, 8 July 1772.

152. MO 1747, § 17; StAWf, 40 Slg. 9435, 1 Apr. 1765.

153. They had been prohibited from doing so since 1747 StAWf (2 Alt 11324, fols. 3–4, 30 May 1747).

154. Concerning the surgeons Schuster and Langehals, see StAWf, 11 N Blankenburg 7, 18 Feb. and 5 Mar. 1783; concerning the surgeon Reuter, see ibid., 9 Sept., 6 Oct. 1786, and 1 Nov. 1786, 30 Jan. 1787, 26 Mar. 1788; for an example of Reuter's continued Pfuscherey, see StAWf, 11 N Blankenburg 9, 11 Aug. 1794.

155. "Ordnung und Privilegia der Barbiere und Chirurgorum in Braunschweig," 27 Feb. 1716, in StAWf, 40 Slg. 4519, Tit. XII; MO 1721, Cap. V. § 8; MO 1747, §§ 24–25. Such strictures were repeated throughout the eighteenth century; see, for instance, "Acta die Curiren der Regiments und Compagnie Feldschers p.p. bey bürgerlichen Personen betref.," 1752–68, StAWf, 2 Alt 11366; for 1769–74, 2 Alt 11398, passim; "Abermalige Vorstellung des Amts hiesiger Stadts-Wundärzte keinen der hiesigen Militar Wundärzte concessiones zum practiciren unter der Bürgerschaft zu ertheilen," 2 Jan. 1787, 2 Alt 11368, fols. 2–4; and 20 Jan. 1794, 40 Slg. 13249. For an example of the complaints raised by the surgeons, see "Ambt-Chirurgi in Br[aunschweig] abermals wegen ihrer über einige Compagnie-Feldscher und Soldate habende Beschwerde," 16 Mar. 1745, StAWf, 2 Alt 11282, fols. 9–14. Mediating between surgeons and military surgeons took up a great amount of the Collegium medicum's time, see disputes and petitions in 2 Alt 11340–41, 11366–68, 11390, 11398.

156. HAB Einbl. R2: 658 (26 June 1719); Einbl. R2: 868 (19 May 1741); StAWf, 40 Slg. 12140 (8 Oct. 1779); 12364 (26 Sept. 1782); 12704 (19 Oct. 1786); 13249 (24

Jan. 1794); 13314 (13 Oct. 1794); Albrecht, *Förderung*, 326–28. On the problems city surgeons had in obtaining an adequate livelihood, see esp. their complaints in StAWf, 2 Alt 11282, fols. 9–14, 16 Mar. 1745; StadtB, C VII B7: IV, fols. 3–7, 18 July 1778; ibid., fols. 22–23, 6 May 1771.

157. StAWf, 2 Alt 11283, fols. 12, 15, 29 Aug. and 20 Sept. 1750. But this was an old story. For various complaints about how students harmed the Nahrung of surgeons, see StadtH, B VII 24 (3) Nrs. 1–4 (1646–90, 1703–33, 1734–73, 1775–1808); similarly, for bathmasters, StadtH, B VII 24 (2) Nrs. 1–2 (1722–70).

158. StadtH, B VII 11a Nr. 3, 8 and 10 May 1760. Note, too, the Pfuscherey of the medical students Schlägel in 1750 (StadtH, B VII 11a Nr. 2, 14 Oct. 1750) and Sandorfy in 1801 (StAWf, 2 Alt 11290, fol. 6).

159. StAWf, 111 Neu 3106, case 57 (Fahrenholz), n.d., 1800; 2 Alt 11395, fol. 12 (Behrend), 16 Aug. 1768.

160. Siegemund, Bourgeois, and du Coundray were all authors: Justine Siegemund, *Die König.[liche] Preußische und Chur-Brandenb. Hof-Wehe-Mutter* (Leipzig: Johann Friedrich Braun, 1715); Louise Bourgeois, *Observations diverses sur la stérilité, perte de fruict, foecondité, accouchements et maladies des femmes et enfants nouveaux naiz. Amplement traitees et heursement practiquées* (Paris: A. Saugrain, 1609); Angélique Marguerite Le Bousier du Coudray, *Abrégé de l'art des accouchements* (Paris: Widow of Delaquette, 1759; reprint, Paris: Editions Roger DaCosta, 1976).

161. It is impossible to review here the extensive historical literature on midwives. For a good orientation, see *The Art of Midwifery*, ed. Hilary Marland (London: Routledge, 1993). For a recent study of a midwife in eighteenth-century England, see Isobel Grundy, "Sarah Stone: Enlightenment Midwife," in *Medicine in the Enlightenment*, ed. Roy Porter (Amsterdam: Rodopi, 1995), 128–44. On Germany, one should mention Elseluise Haberling, *Beiträge zur Geschichte des Hebammenstands* (Osterwieck: Staude, 1940); Georg Burkhard, *Die deutschen Hebammenordnungen von ihren ersten Anfängen bis auf die Neuzeit* (Leipzig: W. Engelmann, 1912); F. C. Wille, *Über Stand und Ausbildung der Hebammen im 17. und 18. Jahrhundert in Chur-Brandenburg* (Berlin: Ebering, 1934); Dietrich Tutzke, "Über statistische Untersuchungen als Beitrag zur Geschichte des Hebammenwesens im ausgehenden 18. Jahrhundert," *Centaurus* 4 (1965): 351–59; id., "Zur materiellen Lage der Niederlausitzer Hebammen im 18. Jahrhundert," *SA* 45 (1961): 334–40; id., "Die Entwicklung des Hebammenwesens in der Oberlausitz bis zum Beginn des 19. Jahrhunderts," *Oberlausitzer Forschung* (1961): 284–306; Brigette Menssen and A.-M. Taube, "Hebammen und Hebammenwesen in Oldenburg in der zweiten Hälfte des 18. und zu Beginn des 19. Jahrhunderts," in *Regionalgeschichte: Probleme und Beispiele*, Ernst Hinrichs and W. Norden (Hildesheim: Lax, 1980); Merry Wiesner, "Early Modern Midwifery: A Case Study," *International Journal of Women's Studies* 6 (1983): 26–43; Ulrike Gleixner, "Hebammen als Amtsfrauen und Gutachterinnen auf dem Land: Eine Fallstudie (Altmark 18. Jahrhundert)," in *Frauen in der ländlichen Gesellschaft der Frühen Neuzeit*, ed. Heide Wunder and Christina Vanja (forthcoming). I thank Ulrike Gleixner for providing me with a manuscript copy of her article.

On midwives in Braunschweig, there is some important older literature, especially Adolph Friedrich Nolde, *Notizen zur Kultur-Geschichte der Geburtshilfe in dem Herzogthum Braunschweig* (Erfurt: Hennings, 1807). "Das Collegium Anatomico Chirurgicum und die Accouchir-Anstalt in Braunschweig," in *Zum Aufbau der Hebammen-schulen in Niedersachsen im 18. und 19. Jahrhundert von Dokumenten, Darstellungen und Instrumenten in der Wandelhalle des Niedersächsischen Landtags vom 23. September–16. Oktober 1981*, exhibition catalog (Hannover: Niedersächsische Sozialminister, 1981), 17–21, was very useful.

162. For example, the conflict between men and women midwives was muted in Germany, and, for the most part, midwives continued to deliver babies throughout the eighteenth and nineteenth centuries. Physicians did attempt to gain control of the education of midwives in attempts to improve their training, but they never really tried to muscle them out of the business entirely. There were, of course, male physicians and surgeons in increasing numbers who delivered babies.

163. Anne Horenburg, *Wohlgemeynender und Nöhtiger Unterricht der Heeb-Amme* (Hannover and Wolfenbüttel, 1700). Christian Franz Paullini recommended the book to all midwives as "a useful little work" (*Das Hoch-und-Wohl-gelahrte Teutsche Frauen-Zimmer Nochmals mit mercklichem Zusatz vorgestellet* [Frankfurt and Leipzig: J. C. Stößel, 1705], 74). The midwifery manual written by Elisabethe Margarethe von Keil (also Reil), who died in 1699, is also favorably mentioned by Paullini (ibid., 81). Keil's husband was a physician who practiced in Celle in the late seventeenth century. Case books of midwifery practices are also quite rare. Most famous now, of course, is that of Martha Ballard as treated by Laurel Thatcher Ulrich, *A Midwife's Tale: The Life of Martha Ballard, Based on Her Diary, 1785–1812* (New York: Knopf, 1990). Another well-known case book is Catharina Geertruida Schrader, *"Mother and Child Were Saved": The Memoirs (1693–1740) of the Frisian Midwife Catharina Schrader*, trans. and annotated by Hilary Marland, with essays by M. J. van Lieburg and G. J. Klooster-mann (Amsterdam: Rodophi, 1987); and Willem Frijhoff, "Vrouw Schraders beroepsjournal: Overwegingen bij een publikatie over arbeidspraktijk in het ver-leden," *Tijdschrift voor de geschiedenis der geneeskunde, natuurwetenschappen, wiskunde en techniek* 8, 1 (1985): 27–38.

164. Heinrich Fasbender, *Geschichte der Geburtshilfe* (Jena: Gustav Fischer, 1906; reprint, Hildesheim: Olms, 1964), 146; Horenburg, *Unterricht*, Vorbericht.

165. There were five midwives in 1755, six in 1759, and five in 1764 (StadtB, C VII S20, vol. VII, fols. 238, 281, 293).

166. From the following sources: StadtB, C VII S20, vol. VII; StAWf, 2 Alt 11416–20; 111 Neu 1757, 1764, 1768, 1797.

167. HO 1757, §§ 3–4; StAWf 40 Slg. 11250; Döhnel, *Institut*, 25–28, 34–36; "Das Collegium Anatomico-Chirurgicum und die Accouchir-Anstalt in Braun-schweig," 17–21; Hinze, 69–70. Lectures for midwives were often advertised in the newspaper, see, e.g., J. C. Sommer's advertisement in *BA*, 7 Oct. 1767. Between 1767 and 1792, 1,185 children were born in the Lying-In Ward, of which 120 died after birth (mortality = 10.1%); there were fifty stillbirths (4.2%) and only 11 maternal deaths (Hinze, 87).

168. Von der Mihle was appointed midwife in Braunschweig in 1739, as she recorded in the back of her copy of Johan von Hoorn's *Die Zwo um ihrer Gottesfurcht und Treue willen von GOTT wohlbelohnte Weh-Mütter Siphra und Pua* (2d ed.; Stockholm and Leipzig: bey Gottfried Kiesewettern, 1737), which can be found in HAB under call number Mr143.

169. Procedures for choosing and appointing warming-women are described in StadtB, C VII S20, vol. VII, fol. 289. The appointment of warming-women became standard practice for the entire duchy in HO 1757 (§§ 3, 19); StAWf, III Neu 1727. Among medical reformers, there was almost universal agreement that midwifery was in a miserable state in the eighteenth century. In his influential and widely read *Gedanken über Hebammen und Hebammenschulen auf dem Lande* (Frankfurt am Main: Andreä, 1784), 5, Bernhard Christoph Faust maintained that "midwives are *certainly* among those most responsible for the destruction of the health and the vitality and therefore also [among the principal causes of] the misery and decay of the human race." Likewise Krünitz, s.v. "Heb-Amme"; Johann Christoph von Ettner, *Des getreuen Eckarths unvorsichtige Heb-Amme* (Leipzig: J. Fr. Braun, 1715); J. D. F. Brunner, *Entdeckung der Irrthümer und Bosheiten der Hebammen* (Solingen, 1740); Johann Peter Frank, *System einer vollständigen medicinischen Polizey* (Mannheim: Schwan, 1779), 1: 609–78; and August Hinze, "Vorschläge zur Verbesserung des Hebammenwesens, insonderheit der Hebammen des platten Landes," *BM*, 16 Apr. 1791. One result of all this bad publicity was an attempt to improve midwifery through better education and through stricter supervision and control. These initatives led to a new series of midwifery ordinances passed in quick succession after mid century. Among other places, we find new midwifery ordinances in Augsburg (1750), Nuremburg (1755), Strasbourg (1757), Holstein (1767), and Basel (1770). See Alfons Fischer, *Geschichte des Deutschen Gesundheitswesens*, vol. 2: *Von den Anfängen der hygienischen Ortsbeschreibungen bis zur Gründung des Reichsgesundheitsamtes (Das 18. und 19. Jahrhunderts)* (Berlin: Kommissionsverlag F. A. Herbig, 1933), 234–35.

170. HO 1757, § 1, forbade anyone "other than [properly] appointed and certified midwives to assume the duties of a midwife, except in emergencies." This was repeated many times. The order of 7 May 1772 grounded this prohibition explicitly in the need to protect the livelihoods and incomes of the licensed midwives in the city (StadtB, C VII S20, vol. VII, fol. 219).

171. The edict of 24 June 1767, StAWf, III Neu 1757, fol. 164, provided an annual salary of 50 thaler out of city funds for each midwife to be appointed *in the future*. Salaries were introduced gradually. For example, in 1777, the Collegium medicum distributed "salary improvements" to two midwives, raising one woman's salary to the stipulated 50 thaler, while the other received 25 thaler (StAWf, III Neu 1764). Nolde noted that in 1765, each midwife received 5 thaler 29 mariengulden in salary plus some tax advantages (*Notizen*, 103–04). By 1806, of the nine midwives in the city, the five senior practitioners each received 50 thaler, the next two 25, the eighth 8 mariengulden, and the ninth, a supernumerary, nothing.

172. HO 1757, §§ 21–22.

173. "Summarischer Auszug aus den Listen der Gebohrenen, Gestorbenen und Copulirten de 1789 a) Von den Städten, b) vom platten Lande," StAWf, 2 Alt 11417, fol. 30.

174. But not necessarily, as other rhythms often governed a midwife's life and, thus, her practice. See Ulrich, *Midwife's Tale*, 339, and Schrader, *Mother and Child Were Saved*, 6–21.

175. The extent of each one's practice is impossible to calculate, since we have neither case books nor (with scattered exceptions) monthly lists registering births. In

spring 1797, however, the Collegium medicum and city magistrates requested midwives to send in lists of babies they had recently delivered. The authorities were searching for the mother of a murdered infant. These "reports" (which must be very like the monthly reports midwives filed or were supposed to file) are mere slips of paper. From them, one can pull together a very rough calculation of the relative size of each midwife's practice. The midwife Voges delivered four children in three weeks (thus, at the same rate every three weeks, 69/year); Becker two children in five weeks (21/year); Bollmann six children in ten weeks (31/year); Goetze thirteen children in twelve weeks (56/year); Zoebebier ten in seven weeks (74/year); Niederhütter eighteen in eight weeks (117/year); Nußbaum sixteen in eleven weeks (76/year). See StadtB, C VII S20, vol. VII, fols. 51–72. For midwives' repeat practices in seventeenth-century London, see Doreen Evenden, "Mothers and Their Midwives in Seventeenth-Century London," in *Art of Midwifery*, ed. Marland, 9–26.

176. Nolde, *Notizen*, 104; StadtB, C VII S20 vol. VII, fols. 347, 383.

177. The husbands' occupations are compiled from the files listed in n. 166 above. See the similar findings of Menssen and Taube, "Hebammen und Hebammenwesen," and Tutzke, "Über statistische Untersuchungen."

178. StAWf, 111 Neu 1757, fols. 19–20, 8 Nov. 1751.

179. See, e.g., a decision reached in 1777, StAWf, 111 Neu 1764.

180. StadtB, C VII S20, vol. VII, fols. 235, 238, 246; StAWf, 2 Alt 11420, fol. 2.

181. StadtB, C VII S20, vol. VII, fols. 239–41.

182. Cited in Nolde, *Notizen*, 99, 103.

183. StadtB, C VII S20, vol. VII, fol. 216.

184. Ibid., fols. 136–60, quotation from fols. 137–38; for more on Nußbaum, StAWf, see 111 Neu 1797 and 1757.

185. I have reconstructed the sequence of events from the files listed in n. 166. For examples of decisions made and procedures followed between 1750 and 1800, see StadtB, C VII S20, vol. VII, and StAWf, 111 Neu 1757, passim.

186. Dorothea Elisabeth Seehausen petitioned for the status of supernumerary in 1755, an appointment she received in October of that year. In 1756, an official midwife's post opened up, and she was selected to fill it (StAWf, 111 Neu 1757, fols. 34–36, 40). Similarly, Christiane Henriette Margaretha Backhaus was appointed "extraordinnaire" in 1784 (ibid., fol. 255).

187. See, e.g., "Acta die Hebammen-Pfuscherey der Peitschen, Heidorn, Leitloffen und Nußbaum hieselbst betref. 1773," in ibid., fol. 2; for renewed complaints about these same women, see ibid., fols. 13–14.

188. "Acta die Beschwerde der hiesigen Heb-Ammen gegen die Hebammen Candidata Krügern betrf," StadtB, C VII S20, vol. VII, various complaints from 1795–1800.

189. Ibid., fols. 79–86.

190. Complaint submitted on 12 June 1798, ibid., fols. 33–36.

191. HO 1757, § 20.

192. See, e.g., the decision of the Collegium medicum from 10 Apr. 1779, StadtB, C VII S20, vol. VII, fol. 133.

193. StAWf, 111 Neu 1797, fol. 7, 20 Nov. 1773.

194. The best history of midwifery in Braunschweig-Wolfenbüttel is also the

oldest: Nolde, *Notizen*. In 1806, Nolde was appointed professor of obstetrics at the Anatomical-Surgical Institute in Braunschweig.

195. See, e.g., "Fiscal Zincken, das Hebammen Wesen auf dem Land, betref.," 22 Dec. 1768, StAWf, 2 Alt 11415, fols. 1–5; "Verbesserung des Hebammenwesens auf dem Lande," 1784, 2 Alt 11433. The government ordered a general survey of all midwives in the duchy in 1784 as preparation for a reform of midwifery, providing a printed "Formular zu der von den Obrigkeiten auszufülenden Tabelle," 40 Slg. 12567 and ad 12567. See also "Gedancken über des Hofraths Sommer Vorschläge, die Verbesserung des Hebammen Wesens auf dem platten Land betref.," 14 Dec. 1785, 2 Alt 11416, fols. 25–41; "Fürstl. Ober-Sanitats-Collegium berichtet unterthängist des Hebammenwesens besonders auf dem Lande," 16 Nov. 1787, 2 Alt 11417, fols. 7–15; and Hinze, "Vorschläge."

196. Faust, *Gedanken über Hebammen*, 5, 15; Physicus Lindemann's assessment, 26 Jan. 1766, StAWf, 2 Alt 11198, fol. 25. Attacks on midwives as the primary cause of death and depopulation were common in the late seventeenth and eighteenth centuries, see Ettner, *Unvorsichtige Heb-Amme*; Johann Peter Süssmilch, *Die göttliche Verordnung in denen Veränderung des menschlichen Geschlechts*, 4th ed. (Berlin: Buchhandlung der Realschule, 1775–76), 1: 188, 3: 106–8; Frank, *System*, 1: 609–78.

197. The quantity of material here, especially from 1784, is almost overwhelming; see StAWf, 2 Alt 11435–42. Below I discuss Seesen and Eschershausen extensively, but I also base my conclusions on material drawn more generally from the 1784 reports and on a more detailed analysis of reports on Wendessen in StAWf, 10 Alt Wendessen 16; Scheppau in 10 Alt Scheppau 1; Langelsheim in 8 Alt Langelsheim 94; and Hohengeiß in 5 Blankenburg (Walkenried) 21.

198. "Bericht die Hebammen den Kirch-Spiel Eschershausen betreffend," StAWf, 111 Neu 1729, fols. 54–56, 5 Feb. 1757.

199. StAWf, 2 Alt 11429, fols. 35–36, 20 Dec. 1784.

200. The eight villages were (with population figures for 1814 in parentheses): Bornum (492); Engelade (294); Herrhausen (507); Jerze (153); Klein Rhüden (677); Mahlum (362); Schlewecke (443). *AV*; "Tabularischer Auszug aus den Gerichte von denen Hebammen in den zwei Aemtern, Seesen und Langelsheim," 10 Apr. 1757, StAWf, 111 Neu 1729, fols. 133–34; 28 Dec. 1784, 8 Alt Seesen 3 Nr. 5; 8 Jan. 1785, 2 Alt 11429, fols. 45–46.

201. "Unterricht vor die Heb-Ammen oder Bade-Mütter in der Stadt Braunschweig sampt deren Eyde," 1686, StAWf, 40 Slg. 3219; MO 1721; MO 1747 §§ 26–33.

202. StAWf, 111 Neu 1729, fols. 133–34, 8 Apr. 1757.

203. "Nachricht wegen der Hebammen in dem Fürstl. Amt Gandersheim," n.d. (1761), StAWf, 111 Neu 1730, fols. 100–101.

204. Müller's report cited in Nolde, *Notizen*, 71.

205. This is how Dr. Müller described the process of midwife selection (ibid.). After being chosen by the women of Königslutter in 1656, for instance, Catharina Blumm was charged with a *juramento* by the city council (StadtK, St. 1, 5, 28 Apr. 1656).

206. StAWf, 10 Alt Hehlen 5, 28 Feb. 1749;, 8 Alt Königslutter 152, fol. 38, 22 Dec. 1784.

207. StAWf, 8 Alt Stauffenberg 648, 25 Jan. 1791.

208. Ibid., 27 Feb. 1793; "Specificatio einer Stimmen Samlunge der Frauen von der neuen angesetzten Bademutter in Badenhausen, Neue und Oberhütte hier zu sich gemeldet, betreffend," ibid., 19 Apr. 1801; 8 Alt Seesen 3 Nr. 16, fol. 16, 17 May 1798. Cf. the selection of the midwife Packmann [Sackmann?] in Münchehof, 15 Feb. 1806, 8 Alt Stauffenburg 652, where forty-two women voted.

209. StadtH, B VII 11 Nr. 3, 10 June 1746 and 20 Oct. 1763. For other examples, see how midwives were appointed in the villages of Rieseberg, StAWf, 8 Alt Königslutter 152, fol. 6; Schlewecke, 8 Alt Seesen 3 Nr. 6, fols. 31–32, 14 May 1768; Kissenbrück, 10 Alt Hedwigsburg 46, 16 Mar. 1790; Ahlshausen, 8 Alt Stauffenberg 648, 25 Jan. 1791.

210. StAWf, 8 Alt Winnigstedt 7, 18 Nov. 1777.

211. StAWf, 2 Alt 11444, fols. 5–6, 20 Feb. 1790.

212. StAWf, 8 Alt Seesen 3 Nr. 6, fol. 67, 3 Mar. 1790.

213. StAWf, 5 Blankenburg (Walkenried) 20, 3 and 22 July 1737.

214. Ibid., 27 Nov. 1737, 23 Dec. 1771, and 15 Nov. 1776.

215. StAWf, 8 Alt Eich 483, vol. 1, fol. 49, 24 Jan. 1777.

216. StAWf, 8 Alt Königslutter 152, fol. 22, 18 Jan. 1782.

217. See results of the 1784 survey in StAWf, 2 Alt 11435–42. The authorities in Hohengeiß, Langelsheim, and Wendessen (to cite just three examples) found no one, although the community of Scheppau could name one person not "too disinclined" to take job. StAWf, 5 Blankenburg (Walkenried) 21, 22 Dec. 1784;, 8 Alt Langelsheim 94, fol. 17; 10 Alt Wendessen 16, 9 Jan. 1785; 10 Alt Scheppau, 22 Nov. 1784.

218. Quoted in Nolde, *Notizen*, 78–79; see also Hinze, "Vorschläge." On wages of the midwife in Helmstedt, StadtH, B VII 11k Nr. 2, 25 Sept. 1784 and 9 May 1785.

219. StAWf, 2 Alt 11200, fol. 54, 20 Jan. 1770; for more reports in a similar vein, here on midwives in Walkenried, see StAWf, 5 Alt Blankenburg (Walkenried) Nr. 21.

220. HO 1803; reports on midwifery in the countryside early in the nineteenth century in StAWf, 12A Neu 13 Nr. 235.

221. The French government solved the problem by appointing a traveling teacher, Madame du Coudray. See Nina Gelbart, "Midwife to a Nation: Mme du Coudray Serves France," in *Art*, ed. Marland, 131–51.

222. StAWf, 2 Alt 11424, fol. 12, 15 Apr. 1770.

223. StAWf, 111 Neu 1729, fol. 81, 25 Feb. 1757.

224. Ibid.

225. Ibid., fol. 26, 23 Feb. 1757. There were, of course, some complaints about neglect or malpractice. See, e.g., the complaint the Amt and Dr. Büscher from Zellerfeld lodged against Sophie Henriette Wietzen, "who forced the lying-in women too early and too forcefully to labor" (111 Neu 3124, 30 Dec. 1757). Or the complaint about a mistake made by a midwife that was thought to have resulted in a stillborn child in Amt Achim in 1803 (111 Neu 3110, case 146). Still, the number of these complaints was tiny when compared to the far greater mass of materials concerning Pfuscherey—that is, poaching.

226. See, e.g., Physicus Blum's complaint about Frau Sievers, StAWf, 17 N 2312, fol. 4, 29 Oct. 1746.

227. StAWf, 111 Neu 3111, cases 150[I-IV].

228. StAWf, 111 Neu 3111, case 150^I, 25 Apr. 1792.

229. Ibid., 27 Feb. 1794.

230. Ibid., 25 Apr. 1792, ibid.

231. StAWf 111 Neu 3106, case 56; also similar cases in 111 Neu 3107, case 79; 3114, cases 178 and 181; 3115, case 206.

232. StAWf, 111 Neu 3111, case 150^I, 25 Apr. 1792.

233. Ibid., 21 Aug. 1792.

234. Ibid., 10 Feb. 1792; 111 Neu 33104, case 23^I, 13 Feb. 1805.

235. StAWf, 111 Neu 3111, case 150^I, 10 Feb. 1792.

236. Ibid., May 1793.

237. Ibid., 16 Oct. 1787, ibid.

238. StAWf, 111 Neu 3103, case 8, 13 May 1747.

239. StAWf, 111 Neu 3100, 23 Nov. 1747.

240. StAWf, 111 Neu 3106, case 61^I, 17 Dec. 1794.

241. See the case of the knacker in Schöppenstedt from 1814 to 1818, StAWf, 111 Neu 3113, case 168.

242. StAWf, 2 Alt 11199, fol. 23, 8 Mar. 1766.

243. StAWf, 111 Neu 1584.

244. StAWf, 111 Neu 3111, cases 150^I–150^{IV} describe Nicolai's Pfuscherey from 1787 to 1803.

245. StAWf, 111 Neu 3106, case 61^I, 13 Sept. 1787.

246. StAWf, 111 Neu 1052, fols. 26–30, Jan. 1767; see also 111 Neu 1095, fol. 79, 9 Oct. 1766. For other examples, see the position of the surgeon Blumenberg in Gandersheim, who owned two houses there and needed to be allowed to practice surgery in order to fulfill his civic obligations (17 N 2307, fols. 35–36, 20 Dec. 1761); or the cooperation between the surgeon Ahrberg, his helper Schrader, and Schrader's father, the schoolmaster (111 Neu 3103, case 2 [c. 1836]).

247. StAWf, 2 Alt 11610, fols. 14–15, 26 May 1755.

248. "Anzeige einiger Unordnungen in Medicinal Wesen, durch Fuschereÿen im Seesenschen Physicats Theils des Harzdistricts," StAWf, 2 Alt 11285, fols. 45–49, 8 Dec. 1768; 111 Neu 1095, fols. 94–122. Another case involved the factor employed at the ironworks in Delligsen. This man, named Milli, had established a network involving the workers at the ironworks and men in the nearby market town of Ahlfeld. Milli was very friendly with two members of the city council in Ahlfeld: Dr. Sander and the town apothecary. Milli sent for Sander to treat the workers and had the prescriptions filled by the apothecary in Ahlfeld. He then paid costs from the workers' contributions and from the ironworks' funds. See StAWf, 2 Alt 11395, fols. 2, 4–5, 7, 9, and 18, for 16 Apr., 30 June, 20 July, 9 Aug., and 17 Nov. 1768.

249. StAWf, 111 Neu 3104, case 20, 13 Sept. 1805.

250. StAWf, 111 Neu 3114, case 181, 23 June 1804 and 9 Feb. 1806.

251. StAWf, 111 Neu 3249, fols. 53–55, 17 June 1758.

252. StAWf, 8 Alt Lutter am Barenberg 33, fol. 14, 7 Apr. 1766.

253. StAWf, 111 Neu 1050, fols. 6–7, 15 May 1747; ibid., 3111, case 150^I, 25 Apr. 1792.

254. On the position of executioners in folklore and society, see Werner Danckert, *Unehrliche Leute: Die verfemten Berufe* (Bern: Francke, 1963); Otto Beneke, *Von unehrlichen Leuten: Culturhistorische Studien und Geschichten aus vergangenen Tage deutscher*

Gewerbe und Dienst, mit besonderer Rücksicht auf Hamburg, 2d rev. ed. (Berlin: Hertz, 1889); Albrecht Keller, *Der Scharfrichter in der deutschen Kulturgeschichte* (Bonn: K. Schroeder, 1921; reprint, Hildesheim: Olms, 1968); Johann Glenzdorf and Fritz Treichel, *Henker, Schinder und arme Sünder,* 2 vols. (Bader Münder am Deister: Wilhelm Rost, 1970). On the medical practice of executioners, see Wolfgang Oppelt, *Über die "Unehrlichkeit" des Scharfrichters: Unter bevorzugter Verwendung von Ansbacher Quellen* (Langfeld: Antiquariat Traute Gottschalk, 1976), 376–87; Gustav Jungbauer, *Deutsche Volksmedizin: Ein Grundriß* (Berlin: Walter de Gruyter, 1934), 68, 162; Max Höfler, *Volksmedizin und Aberglaube in Oberbayerns Gegenwart und Vergangenheit* (Munich: Otto Galler, 1893), 62–63.

255. For two hundred years, Möllers were executioners in Husum, Pickels in Kiel, and Raches in Trier (Glenzdorf and Treichel, *Henker,* 1: 47). On contracts between communities and executioners/knackers, see, e.g., for Campen, "Acta die Abdeckerey und desfals ertheilte Privilegia betrf., 1670–1792," StAWf, 8 Alt Campen Gr. 17 Nr. 1; for Seesen, 8 Alt Seesen 16 Nr. 1 (1667–1721) and Nr. 4 (1756–1768).

256. See, e.g., the advertising of the Braunschweig *Nachtrichterei* (another name for the *Meisterei*), which appeared in several newspapers both in and outside of the duchy, specifying that the post would be leased to "whoever bid the most, or otherwise offered the most advantageous terms" (*Hannoverische Anzeigen,* 20 Nov. 1780, col. 1535).

257. See "Zum abzustellenden Verkauf des Hundefetts durch den Scharfrichter betrcf.," StAWf, 2 Alt 11189, fol. 14, 17 June 1803; *HDA,* s.v. "Hund"; Krünitz, s.v. "Scharfrichter."

258. Contract with Conrad Johann August Wilhelm Funcke, StadtB, C VII A8, fols. 133–38, 16 Feb. 1781; contract with his son, Georg Friedrich August Conrad Funcke, 1805, ibid., fols. 248–255; petition of son for monetary assistance from government, July 1806, ibid., fols. 257–60. On this Funcke family, see Glenzdorf and Treichel, *Henker,* 1: 339.

259. Krünitz, 2d ed. (1782), vol. 1, s.v. "Abdecker," defined the knacker as responsible for the removal of dead animals; see also Glenzdorf and Treichel, *Henker,* 1: 116–30. For specific illustrations: in Seesen, StAWf, 8 Alt Sessen 16 Nrs. 1 & 4; in Helmstedt, StadtH, B V 22, Nrs. 1–5; in Campen, StAWf, 8 Alt Campen Gr. 17 Nr. 1; in Stauffenberg, StAWf, 8 Alt Stauffenberg 390–91.

260. StAWf, 2 Alt 11505, fol. 2, 23 Nov. 1791.

261. Glenzdorf and Treichel, *Henker,* 1: 116; Oppelt, *Unehrlichkeit,* 377. For some cases other than the ones discussed more extensively below, see the practice of the executioner in Braak (near Eschershausen) in the middle of the century, who enjoyed "a good reputation" (StAWf, 2 Alt 11488, fols. 18–24); or that of the executioner Sachse in Seesen in the 1760s and 1770s (StAWf, 8 Alt Seesen 3 Nr., fols. 40–42). Sachse had petitioned the Collegium medicum to be allowed to sell the "arcana" that executioners "inherited from their fathers and fathers' fathers," but the Collegium refused (2 Alt 11326, fol. 34, 14 Feb. 1771).

262. Oppelt, *Unehrlichkeit,* 378–79; Glenzdorf and Treichel, *Henker,* 1: 104–15; StAWf, 2 Alt 11283, fols. 37–38, 15 Apr. and 27 Oct. 1751.

263. StAWf, 2 Alt 11284, fols. 16–17, 27 May 1758; ibid, fol. 27, 13 Feb. 1759; 111 Neu 3107, case 87, 26 Nov. 1819; for 1834, see 111 Neu 3107, case 88.

264. StAWf, 111 Neu 3113, case 168, 6 June 1814, 25 Aug. and 2 Nov. 1818.

265. This had been granted him on 6 June 1737; see his petition of 16 Jan. 1739, StAWf, 2 Alt 11608, fols. 39–42.

266. StAWf, 2 Alt 11608, fols. 11–12, 26 Aug. 1736.

267. Ibid., fols. 19–24, 20 Oct. 1738.

268. StAWf, 111 Neu 3105, cases 41–42.

269. StAWf, 2 Alt 11612, pp. 2–3, 2 July 1758; the Collegium medicum authorized the search on 28 Nov. 1758 (ibid., fol. 18).

270. E.g., ibid., fol. 21, 8 Dec. 1758.

271. Ibid., 23 Jan. 1759.

272. Ibid., fols. 25–28, 9 Oct. 1776; ibid., fol. 40, 4 Nov. 1776.

273. See, e.g., the cases of the miller Claudiz in Fallersleben (1799), StAWf, 111 Neu 3105, case 40; the miller Käseberg in Bettmar (1800–1801), ibid., 3108, case 102; and the miller Meyer in Bahrberge near Gandersheim (1818), ibid., 3110, case 137.

274. I have assembled this list from several files in StAWf, but the same cast of characters appeared in all the documents I examined. For particular examples of artisans involved in medicine, see 2 Alt 11627–29 (upholsterer); 2 Alt 11630–33 (journeymen draper, cobbler, blacksmith); 111 Neu 3104, case 19 (cobbler) and case 26 (master tailor); ibid., 3105, case 54 (blacksmith), case 57 (farrier), case 59 (locksmith); ibid., 3108, case 98 (shoemaker); ibid., 3109, case 128 (tailor); ibid., 3110, case 140 (blacksmith); ibid., 3112, case 157 (turner); ibid., 3114, cases 181–82 (charcoalburner); 17 N 2310 (master tailor). For various other occupations 2 Alt 11284 (shepherd); 2 Alt 11611 (saltpeter works manager); 111 Neu 3104, case 28 (peasant), case 45 (*Pensionaire*), case 48 (captain); ibid., 3105 (noncommissioned officer); ibid., 3106, case 72 (émigré); ibid., 3107, case 81 (day laborer), case 83 (administrator) case 95 (*Einwohner*); ibid., 3108, case 105 (soldier); ibid., 3109, case 121 (grenadier), case 123 (sexton), case 124 (*Provisor*), case 126 (pastor), case 131 ("erstwhile dragoon"); ibid., 3110, case 144 (sexton); ibid., 3112, case 151 (hospital administrator), case 155, cases 158–60 (cowherds); ibid., 3113, case 166 (clothing peddler); ibid., 3114, case 176 (policeman); case 180 (retired peasant), cases 190 and 193 (lodger); 8 Alt Lutter am Barenberg 28 and 8 Alt Thedinghausen 226 (schoolmasters); 10 Alt Hehlen 27 (cottager). For cases involving women, and over half of them widows, see 2 Alt 11611; 111 Neu 3103, case 11; ibid., 3104, cases 29–30; ibid., 3107, cases 84, 90, 96; ibid., 3108, cases 106 and 111; ibid., 3110, cases 139 and 146; ibid., 3115, cases 198–99; 111 Neu 3116, case 210.

275. Busch's case is recorded in StAWf, 2 Alt 11627–28. Walter Artelt discusses Busch in "Das medizinische Braunschweig," 246.

276. StAWf, 2 Alt 11627, fols. 2–5, 12 Feb. 1772.

277. Ibid., fol. 11, 30 Nov. 1772; Olwen H. Hufton, *The Poor of Eighteenth-Century France, 1750–1789* (Oxford: Clarendon Press, 1974), 15.

278. Ibid., fol. 12, 28 Dec. 1772.

279. Ibid.

280. Ibid., 11630, fols. 2–7, 11, 14, for 10 and 17 Oct. 1775, 27 July and 14 Oct. 1776; more petitions and concessions in 2 Alt 11630–31. The treatment of another person, Conradine Heinriette Meÿer, was not as successful. See Chapter 5, pp. 338–39.

281. StAWf, 111 Neu 3105, case 48.

282. The Collegium medicum investigated him in 1800; see ibid., 3108, case 102.

283. Ibid., 3109, case 121, 23 Aug. and 18 Sept. 1800, 10 Apr. and 3 July 1801.

284. Ibid., 2 July 1803, 12 May 1804.

285. For another example, see the case against the schoolmaster Wolf in Wester-wick in 1802, StAWf, 8 Alt Thedinghausen 226.

286. StAWf, 8 Alt Lutter am Barenberge 28, fol. 10, for 11 Jan. 1759.

287. StAWf, 2 Alt 11611, fols. 3, 13–14, for 12 Oct. 1756, 25 Feb. 1757, 11 May 1757, 26 Nov. 1757, 17 Dec. 1757. For more on Jürgens' activities, see StAWf, 111 Neu 3249, fols. 47, 56–57, 69, 73, 74–76.

288. StAWf, 2 Alt 11611, fol. 25.

289. Ibid., fols. 27–28, for 25 Nov. 1758.

290. StAWf, 111 Neu 3103, case 11, 5 Dec. 1771, 10 Jan. 1772, 22 July 1772.

291. Ibid., 30 Nov. and 18 Dec. 1778, 21 and 24 Jan. 1779, 18 Feb. and 17 and 19 Mar. 1779. A similar case involved the wife of a Lieutenant Oppermann, who was active from 1744 through at least the early 1770s. See three reports of the Collegium medicum, StAWf, 2 Alt 11626, fols. 2–6, 11–12, 16–17, and passim, 30 Oct. 1772, 25 Jan. 1776, and 29 Mar. 1776.

Chapter 4. Illness and Society

1. See, e.g., the response of the Consistorium to the privy council's orders of 4 Nov. 1750, StAWf, 2 Alt 11459, fols. 39–40.

2. "An Consistorum zu Wolfenbüttel und zu Blankenburg, die Einsiedlung intus gedachten Listen betref.," StAWf, 2 Alt 11459, fol. 37, 24 Oct. 1750; StAWf, 40 Slg. 7774, 2 Apr. 1754; repeated and strengthened, 40 Slg. 11556, 25 Oct. 1773; "Acta die Untersuchung der Liste der Gebornen und Gestorbenen und da daher entstehenden Vermehrung und Verminderung der Einwohner betr." (1765–86), in StAWf, 2 Alt 11198–203.

3. For an especially good example, see the report of the treasury on "den Ausfall der Geburts- und Sterbe-Listen von den Jahren 1795. und 1796.," StAWf, 111 Neu 3349, fols. 2–11, 19 June 1797; tabular summary, fols. 12–16.

4. See the nosology proposed in 1794 by Dr. Hensler to the Collegium medicum (StAWf, 111 Neu, vol. 2), which eventually adopted a similar set of categories (ibid. 3349, fols. 16–17, 23–24).

5. "Verzeichniß der im Jahr 1796 [1795] in den sämmtlichen Herzoglich[en] Braunschweigischen Landen Gestorbenen nach den Krankheiten," StAWf, 111 Neu 3349, fols. 16–17 (1796), 23–24 (1795).

6. *Friesel* is an especially difficult term, (1) because it included so many varied illnesses, and (2) because people tended to refer to it as *Frais*, which, however, as the *HDA* points out, is more usually another term for *Krampf* (cramp, convulsions). See *HDA*, 5: 372, s.v. "Krampf." I use "the purples" as a translation for Friesel to indicate general symptoms of purplish spots or purple-colored swellings. In Switzerland, Friesel was often known as "the violet" (ibid.). St. Anthony's Fire could also be ergotism, which was often also called Friesel.

7. Historians may well have consistently overestimated the number of infanticides in the eighteenth century. See Otto Ulbricht, *Kindsmord und Aufklärung in Deutschland* (Munich: R. Oldenbourg, 1990), 174–216.

8. StAWf, 111 Neu 3349, fols. 4, 8.

9. Such convulsions were also often called *Krampf* or *Frais* (a form of cramp). *Frais* and *Jammer* included convulsive conditions in children. See *HDA*, 5: 372–76, s.v. "Krampf"; 2: 1724–30, s.v. "Frais." *Jammer* could also be used to denote epilepsy, but it and *Gichter* were also frequently used in the sense of eclampsia or other convulsions. See ibid., 2: 1168–78, s.v. "Fallsucht"; 3: 839–41.

10. The difficulties involved in dealing with archaic medical terminologies are nicely laid out in Jean-Pierre Peter, "Disease and the Sick at the End of the Eighteenth Century," *Biology of Man in History: Selections from the Annales: Economies, Sociétés, Civilisations*, ed. Robert Forster and Orest Ranum, trans. Elborg Forster and Patricia Ranum (Baltimore: Johns Hopkins University Press, 1975), 81–124. In "Causes of Death as Historical Problem" (paper presented at a conference on the History of the Registration of Causes of Death, 11–14 Nov. 1993, Indiana University, Bloomington), Guenter Risse has identified five major problems involved in studying cause of death in the past: (1) the shifting ecology of disease; (2) the shifting definitions of health and disease; (3) the shifting definition of death and its causes; (4) the shifting construction of death records; and (5) the shifting use of death records and statistics. See also Jean-Noël Biraben, "Histoire des classifications de causes de décès et de maladies aux XVIIIᵉ–XIXᵉ siècles," in *Mensch und Gesundheit in der Geschichte / Les Hommes et la santé dans l'histoire*, ed. Arthur E. Imhof (Husum: Matthiesen, 1980): 23–34; Jan Brügelmann, *Der Blick des Arztes auf die Krankheit im Alltag, 1779–1850: Medizinische Topographien als Quelle für die Sozialgeschichte der Gesundheitswesens* (Berlin: Freie Universität, 1982), esp. 243–47; Michael Stolberg, "Patientenschaft und Krankheitsspektrum in ländlichen Arztpraxen des 19. Jahrhunderts," *MJ* 28, no. 1 (1993): 3–27.

11. Brügelmann, *Blick*, 243–85. For more consideration of the methodological problems involved in evaluating the Dorotheenstadt records, see Arthur E. Imhof, "Methodological Problems in Modern Urban History Writing: Graphic Representations of Urban Mortality, 1750–1850," in *Problems and Methods in the History of Medicine*, ed. Roy Porter and Andrew Wear (London: Croom Helm, 1987), 101–32, esp. 115–22.

12. Jean-Pierre Peter, "Kranke und Krankheiten am Ende des 18. Jahrhunderts (aufgrund einer Untersuchung der Königlich-Medizinischen-Gesellschaft, 1774–1794)," in *Biologie des Menschen in der Geschichte* ed. Arthur Imhof, 274–326 (Munich: Beck, 1981).

13. I have used several reference works to assist me in this task. The starting point for anyone grappling with archaic German medical terminologies is Max Höfler, *Deutsches Krankheitsnamen-Buch* (Munich: Piloty & Loehle, 1899; reprint, Hildesheim: Georg Olms, 1970). Philipp Andreas Nemnich, *Lexicon nosologicum polyglotton omnium morborum, symptomatum vitiorumque et affectionum propria nomina decem diversis linguis explicata continens* (Hamburg: C. Müller, 1801), is equally valuable for translating eighteenth-century German terms into their eighteenth-century English equivalents. Two other useful eighteenth-century nosologies are Christian Gottlieb Selle, *Rudimenta pyretologiae methodicae* ([Mediolani]: B. Cominus, 1787), and *Onomatologia medico-practica Encyklopädisches Handbuch für ausübende Aerzte in alphbestischer Ordnung ausgearbeitet von einer Gesellschaft von Aerzten*, ed. Friedrich August Weber (Nuremberg: Raspe, 1783–86).

14. Brügelmann, *Blick*, 250.

15. Ibid., 237, 250.

16. For a good discussion of how difficult it is to draw these sorts of conclusions, see the discussion of seasonal morbidity in Jean-Pierre Goubert, *Malades et médicins en Bretagne, 1770–1790* (Paris: Librairie C. Klincksieck, 1974), 271–76; on the basis of mortality rates, see Monika Höhl, "Pest in Hildesheim in Spätmittelalter und früher Neuzeit (1350–1658)" (Staatsexam, University of Bielefeld, 1987).

17. See the various articles in *Theories of Fever from Antiquity to the Enlightenment*, ed. W. F. Bynum and V. Nutton (London: Wellcome Institute for the History of Medicine, 1981), esp. Johanna Geyer-Kordesch, "Fevers and Other Fundamentals: Dutch and German Medical Explanations, c. 1680–1730," 99–120.

18. Brügelmann, *Blick*, 271–74.

19. Ibid., 100, 100 n. 70, 278–85.

20. On dysentery, see Johann Georg Zimmermann, *Von der Ruhr unter dem Volke im Jahr 1765, und denen mit derselben eingedrungenen Vorurtheilen, nebst einigen allgemeinen Aussichten in die Heilung dieser Vorurtheile* (Zurich: Füeßli, 1767); Erich Woehlkens, *Pest und Ruhr im 16. und 17. Jahrhundert: Grundlagen einer statistisch-topographischen Beschreibung der großen Seuchen, insondere in der Stadt Uelzen* (Hannover: Niedersächsisches Heimatsbund, 1954).

21. Christoph Wilhelm Hufeland, *Die Kunst das menschlichen Leben zu verlängern* (Jena: Gotthold Ludwig Fiedler, in der akademischen Buchhandlung, 1797), 365–66.

22. James C. Riley, *Sickness, Recovery and Death: A History and Forecast of Ill Health* (Iowa City: University of Iowa Press, 1989), 47–61, 115–27.

23. It is impossible to list even a fraction of the works on the history of epidemics. Diseases such as plague and cholera have mesmerized historians, and the study of them has produced a number of truly outstanding historical works. For some orientation, see Guenter B. Risse, "Epidemics and Medicine: The Influence of Disease on Medical Thought and Practice," *BHM* 53 (1979): 505–19, and Charles E. Rosenberg, *Explaining Epidemics and Other Studies in the History of Medicine* (Cambridge: Cambridge University Press, 1992).

24. Donald Hopkins, *Princes and Peasants: Smallpox in History* (Chicago: University of Chicago Press, 1983); Neithard Bulst, "Vier Jahrhunderte Pest in niedersächsischen Städten: Vom Schwarzen Tod (1349–51) bis in die erste Hälfte des 18. Jahrhunderts," in *Stadt im Wandel: Kunst und Kultur des Bürgertums in Norddeutschland, 1150–1650*, ed. Cord Meckseper (Stuttgart–Bad Cannstatt: Edition Cantz, 1985), 251–70.

25. On fevers, see *Theories*, ed. Bynum and Nutton.

26. See, e.g., reports in StAWf, 2 Alt 11451, esp. the response of the privy council to rumors of the appearance of a "catching disease" around Fürstenburg that suggested that plague was to be found in the neighboring towns of Corvey and Paderborn, and that it would "be necessary to set up better precautions on the frontiers" (ibid., fol. 21, 30 Aug. 1676). The Amt Fürstenberg quickly responded that it was dysentery, not plague, in Paderborn and Corvey, and that the number of deaths had, moreover, been greatly exaggerated (ibid., fols. 22–23, 9 Sept. 1676).

27. Fatality for bacillary dysentery ranged between 10 and 25 percent; for plague, up to 60 percent (Riley, *Sickness*, 111).

28. StAWf, 2 Alt 11451, fol. 2, 27 Dec. 1661.
29. StAWf, 2 Alt 11451, passim.
30. Ibid., fol. 24, 8 Aug. 1678.
31. Ibid., fols. 24–25.
32. Ibid., fols. 28–29, 24 Aug. 1678.
33. Ibid., fol. 30, 11 Nov. 1678.
34. Ibid., fol. 32.
35. Ibid., fols. 32–33.
36. Ibid., fols. 34–35, 9 Nov. 1678. "Kurtzer Unterricht/ Einiger wolbewherten geringen Mittel/ derer sich die Land-Leute bey grassirender Rohten und Weissen Ruhr/ ohn anwendung grosser Kosten/ nützlich gebrauchen können" (n.p., n.d. c. 1678) and "Kürtzer und nohtwendiger Bericht: Von der Praeservation und Curation der Dysenterie oder Rohten-Ruhr. Zu Nutz und Wolfahrt der Eingesessenen der Fürstlichen Residentz-Stadt Wolfenbüttel/ und des löblichen Fürstenthums Braunschweig. Lüneburg Wolfenbüttelschen Theils Unterthanen/ etc." (Wolfenbüttel: n.p., n.d. [c. 1678]). Copies in StAWf, 2 Alt 11451, fols. 37–38, 41–47.
37. See, e.g., StAWf, 2 Alt 11452.
38. Neither dysentery nor influenza in the early modern period has attracted much historical attention, but see Woehlkens, *Pest und Ruhr.* Important contemporary accounts include Zimmermann, *Ruhr* and Johann Daniel Metzger, *Beytrage zur Geschichte der Frühlings-Epidemie im Jahre 1782* (Königsberg and Leipzig: Hartung, 1782).
39. StAWf, 2 Alt 11454, fols. 10–16.
40. "Acta die Epidemie zu Wolfenbüttel betr. 1758," StAWf, 111 Neu 3249, fols. 25–77.
41. Ibid., fol. 32.
42. Ibid., fols. 37–40, 30 Mar. 1758.
43. Ibid., fols. 47–48, 1 and 30 Apr. 1758.
44. StAWf, 2 Alt 11483, fol. 3, 20 May 1761.
45. Ibid.
46. Ibid., fols. 5–6, 22 Mar. 1761; postscript to above report, ibid., fol. 8, 26 Mar. 1761; orders of privy council to authorities in Weser district, ibid., fol. 9, 31 Mar. 1761.
47. StAWf, 111 Neu 3226, fol. 63, 12 Dec. 1761; "Acta die Epidemie in den Weser-District bey den Braunschweigischen Trouppen betr. 1761," ibid., fols. 75–204.
48. Ibid., fol. 71, 21 Feb. 1762.
49. "Verzeichniß der Unterthanen . . . welchem am 12. April 1802 Brotkorn Unterstützung von Amtswegen zugetheilt ist," StAWf, 2 Alt 11465, fols. 24–25, 14 Apr. 1802.
50. Ibid., fols. 29–34.
51. Parish register, Bornum, StAWf, 1 Kb 192 (burials).
52. Ibid., 1 Kb 193 (burials and marriages).
53. Ibid. (burials for the period 1748–1810 recorded on pp. 386–536).
54. Parish registers, Walkenried, StAWf, 1 Kb 1223 (burials, 1667–1752); 1 Kb 1224 (burials, 1752–1814).
55. "Verzeichniße der Gebornen, Kranken, und Gestorbenen," 1751–61, StAWf,

10 Hehlen 6–16. I have used Uphoff's records for 1751–60. His entries for 1761 are vague and uncharacteristically brief. For example, between 1 Mar. and 1 Apr., he merely noted: "There are a number of persons ill here; but it appears that with God's help they will recover." The final year of Uphoff's recordkeeping was 1761; he died on 28 May 1762 of "a wasting disease," after serving about fifteen years as schoolmaster (parish register, Hehlen, StAWf, 1 Kb 559 [burials]). Uphoff's superior in Hehlen, Pastor Henke, testified to Uphoff's diligence, as did Physicus Wachsmuth, who referred to Uphoff's lists as "well prepared." Henke's report, StAWf, 111 Neu 1051, vol. 1, fols. 25–27, here fol. 25, 19 Jan. 1755; Wachsmuth note, ibid., fol. 37, 23 Jan. 1755.

56. "Tabellarische Verzeichniß der Getauften, Getrauten, Zwillinge, und gestorbenen Wochnerinnen von 1751 bis 1788 eingeschlossen, nach den Kirchenbüchern des calvördischen Physikats-Distrikts, wozu ausser der Landstadt Calvörde, die Dörfer Uthmäden, Zabbenitz, Wellstorf, Bexenbrock, Powleib, Lossewitz und Hünerdorf gehören," AGFK 3 (1789): 285.

57. "Medicinal Berichte des Dorfs Bornum," in StAWf, 8 Alt Seesen 3 Nr. 8.

58. Population figures for 1793 are taken from Hassel/Bege, 2: 361–63; for 1756–79 from StAWf, 10 Hehlen 17. Social breakdown is from the population lists for 1777–83, 10 Alt Hehlen 23.

59. Øivind Larsen, "Die Krankheitsauffassung und ihre historische Interpretation: Ein Auswertungsmodell aufgrund von norwegischen Medizinalberichten aus dem 19. Jahrhundert," in Mensch und Gesundheit, ed. Imhof 45–58; id., "Eighteenth-Century Diseases, Diagnostic Trends and Mortality," Scandinavian Population Studies 5 (1979): 38–54.

60. StAWf, 10 Hehlen 17. I have counted four cases of "Maßeln" (measles?) in 1757 as smallpox cases because smallpox was a problem in that year and there is good reason to suspect a misdiagnosis here.

61. StAWf, 10 Alt Hehlen 16.

62. Ibid. 6, fols. 8, 10; ibid. 8, fols. 18–19.

63. Ibid. 11, fol. 27.

64. Ibid. 6, fol. 2.

65. Ibid. 7, fol. 21; ibid. 6, fol. 5; ibid. 8, fol. 27.

66. Ibid. 11, fol. 16; in Bornum the nine-month-old daughter of the swineherd was so badly mauled by a pig that she died (parish register, Bornum, StAWf, 1 Kb 193 [burials], 25 Oct. 1757).

67. Irvine Loudon, "Leg Ulcers in the Eighteenth and Early Nineteenth Century," JRCGP 31 (1981): 263–73; 32 (1982): 301–9.

68. The government passed many ordinances on rabies in the eighteenth century. Most touched on controlling dogs and on preventing rabies by removing the "Tollwurm" (that is, the tendon under the tongue). The first of these was promulgated on 18 Sept. 1745, StAWf, 40 Slg. 6594; for specific places, StAWf, 8 Alt Seesen 8 Nr. 6 (1746–91); 8 Alt Eich 484 (1745–1801).

69. Mahlum had a population of 362 in 1814 (AV); StAWf, 8 Alt Seesen Gr. 3 Nr. 7, fols. 1–249, 17 Jan. 1751–1 June 1760; parish registers, Mahlum, StAWf, 1 Kb 849, 851 (burials, 1751–60).

70. "Medicinal Berichte des Dorfes Mahlum, 1751–1760," in StAWf, 8 Alt Seesen 3 Nr. 7; parish register, Mahlum, StAWf, 1 Kb 851 (burials, 1752–1806).

71. StAWf, 2 Alt 11200, fol. 52; parish registers, Walkenried, StAWf, 1 Kb 1223–24 (burials).

72. Ibid. See also Riley, *Sickness*, 125; John E. Knodel, *Demographic Behavior in the Past: A Study of Fourteen German Village Populations in the Eighteenth and Nineteenth Century* (Cambridge: Cambridge University Press, 1988), 35–69. Cf. W. R. Lee, *Population Growth, Economic Development and Social Change in Bavaria, 1750–1850* (New York: Arno Press, 1977), 52–106, on infant mortality rates in Bavaria.

73. Parish register, Walkenried, StAWf, 1 Kb 1224 (burials, 1752–1814).

74. StAWf, 2 Alt 11200, fols. 53–55, 20 Jan. 1770.

75. In 1785, the six children who died of convulsions and the three who died of the purples (erysipelas?) made up nine of the twenty-five deaths; in 1788, four smallpox deaths, two from convulsions (all six of them very young children) and three stillbirths contributed nine of a total of twenty-six deaths; and in 1793, of twenty-one deaths, six were of children with smallpox and five of children who died of convulsions.

76. Bornum had 492 inhabitants in 1814 (*AV*); parish register, Bornum, 1777–1803, StAWf, 1 Kb 193 (marriages and deaths, 1748–1810).

77. Report of Physicus von Hagen, StAWf, 2 Alt 11198, fol. 33, 3 Feb. 1766; cf. similar figures for 1759, when there were only seven deaths from smallpox and four from measles, but when consumption and chest diseases caused 320 of a total of 922 deaths (or 34.7%) and what was probably infantile convulsions killed 213 (or 23.1%). Mortality among children under ten (mostly, as von Hagen observes, from convulsions) comprised 43.6 percent (or 402 of all 922 deaths). Christian Thedel Heinrich von Hagen, "Todtenregister der Stadt Braunschweig vom Jahre 1759," *BA*, 30 Jan. 1760. For smallpox deaths, see also "Der bisherige Verlust der Stadt Braunschweig, durch die Blattern oder sogenannten Kinderpocken," *BA-GB*, 18 and 22 July 1767.

78. Causes of death for 1765, StAWf, 2 Alt 11198, fol. 44; for 1766, StAWf, 34N Fb. 1 X 12; "General-Liste der Gebornen und Gestorbenen zu Wolfenbüttel von 1752. bis 1765 incl." (n.d. [1766]), ibid.; for 1785, StAWf, 2 Alt 11202, fol. 56.

79. Riley, *Sickness*, 109–14.

80. Alfons Fischer, *Geschichte des Deutschen Gesundheitswesens*, vol. 2: *Von den Anfängen der hygienischen Ortsbeschreibungen bis zur Gründung des Reichsgesundheitsamtes (Das 18. und 19. Jahrhunderts)* (Berlin: Kommissionsverlag F. A. Herbig, 1933), 152–61.

81. Otto Brunner, "Hausväterliteratur," in *Handwörterbuch der Sozialwissenschaften*, 5th ed. (Stuttgart: Gustav Fischer, 1956–65); Fritz Hartmann "Hausvater und Hausmutter als Hausarzt in der Frühen Neuzeit," in *Staat und Gesellschaft in Mittelalter und Früher Neuzeit: Gedenkschrift für J. Leuschner*, ed. Katharina Colberg, Hans-Heinrich Nolte, and Herbert Obenaus (Göttingen: Vandenhoeck & Ruprecht, 1983), 151–75; Hartmut Sührig, *Die Entwicklung der niedersächsischen Kalender im 17. Jahrhundert* (Göttingen: Buchhändler-Vereinigung, 1976). Many works were modeled on *Kluger Haus-Vater, verständige Haus-Mutter, vollkommener Land-Medicus* (Leipzig: Groschuff, 1698), published under Johann Joachim Becher's name, which went through many editions. It appeared well into the eighteenth century.

Discussion of lay medical advice has become a mini-industry. Particularly useful for early modern times are Paul Slack, "Mirrors of Health and Treasures of Poor Men:

The Use of Vernacular Medical Literature in Tudor England," in *Health, Medicine and Mortality in the Sixteenth Century*, ed. Charles Webster (Cambridge: Cambridge University Press, 1979), 237–73; Roy Porter, "Lay Medical Knowledge in the Eighteenth Century: *The Gentleman's Magazine*," *MH* 29 (1985): 138–68; G. S. Rousseau, "John Wesley's *Primitive Physic*," *Harvard Library Bulletin* 16 (1968): 242–56; William Coleman, "Health and Hygiene in the *Encyclopédie*: A Medical Doctrine for the Bourgeoisie," *JHM* 29 (1974): 399–421; Charles Rosenberg, "Medical Text and Social Context: William Buchan's *Domestic Medicine*," *BHM* 57 (1983): 22–42; Ginnie Smith, "Prescribing the Rules of Health: Self-Help and Advice in the Late Eighteenth Century," in *Patients and Practitioners: Lay Perceptions of Medicine in Pre-Industrial Society*, ed. Roy Porter (Cambridge: Cambridge University Press, 1985), 249–82; and my own " 'Aufklärung' and the Health of the People: 'Volksschriften' and Medical Advice in Braunschweig-Wolfenbüttel, 1756–1803," in *Das Volk als Objekt obrigkeitlichen Handelns*, Rudolf Vierhaus (Tübingen: Max Niemeyer, 1992), 101–20.

82. Gottfried Samuel Bäumler, *Mitleidiger Artzt, welcher überhaupt Alle Arme Krancke insonderheit aber Die abgelegene Land-Leute gründlich und aufrichtig lehret / wie Sie mit Gemeinen Hauß-Mitteln und anderen nicht allzukostbaren Artzeneyen sich selbst curiren können* (Strasbourg: Joh. Reinhold Dulßecker der Aeltere, 1736, 1743); id., *Präservirender Artzt; oder gründliche Anweisung wie sich der Mensch . . . bey guter Gesundheit erhalten . . . könne* (Strasbourg: Joh. Reinhold Dulßecker der Aeltere, 1738); Samuel August André David Tissot, *Anleitung für das Landvolk in Absicht auf seine Gesundheit*, 2d ed. (Augsburg and Innsbruck: Wolff, 1766); Ernst Gottfried Baldinger, *Artzeneien, eine physikalisch-medicinische Monatschrift* (Langensalza: Martini, 1766–67); Johann August Unzer, *Der Arzt* (Hamburg: n.p., 1759–64), and *Medicinisches Handbuch* (Lüneburg and Hamburg: G. C. Berth, 1770); Christoph Wilhelm Hufeland, *Die Kunst das menschliche Leben zu verlängern* (Jena: Gotthold Ludwige Fiedler, in der akademischen Buchhandlung, 1797). There are many lesser-known works of regional importance. See, e.g., Lebrecht Friedrich Benjamin Lentin, *Beobachtungen der epidemischen und einiger sporadischer Krankheyten am Oberharz vom Jahre 1777 bis incl. 1782* (Leipzig and Dessau: Buchhandlung der Gelehrten, 1783); Johann Friedrich Zückert, *Von den wahren Mitteln, die Entvölkerung eines Landes in epidemischen Zeiten zu verhüten* (Berlin: Mylius, 1773)

83. As did Zimmermann, *Ruhr*, 173.

84. Samuel August André David Tissot, *Advice to the People in general with Regard to their Health . . .* , trans. J. Kirkpatrick (Boston: Mein & Fleeming, 1767), 12–13. For more on Tissot and his influence, see Antoinette Emch-Dériaz, *Tissot: Physician of the Enlightenment* (New York: P. Lang, 1992).

85. Johann Christian Wilhelm Juncker, *Grundsätze der Volksarzneikunde: Zur bequemeren Benutzung des mündlichen Vortrages seinen Herren Zuhören entworffen* (Halle: Waisenhaus, 1787), 3, 7, 9–13.

86. Andrew Cunningham and Roger French, *The Medical Enlightenment of the Eighteenth Century* (Cambridge: Cambridge University Press, 1990), introduction, 2. See also Karl E. Rothschuh, *Konzepte der Medizin in Vergangenheit und Gegenwart* (Stuttgart: Hippocrates, 1978), 336; Erwin H. Ackerknecht, *Geschichte der Medizin*, 4th rev. ed. (Stuttgart: Ferdinard Enke, 1979), 113–26. Animism was not, however, dead. In the eighteenth century, it was represented by Georg Ernst Stahl and several of

his disciples, among them Johannes Juncker and Georg Philipp Nenter; see Rothschuh, *Konzepte*, 293–305, and Johanna Geyer-Kordesch, "Passions and the Ghost in the Machine: Or What Not to Ask about Science in Seventeenth- and Eighteenth-Century Germany," in *The Medical Revolution of the Seventeenth Century*, ed. Roger French and Andrew Wear (Cambridge: Cambridge University Press, 1989), 145–63.

87. James C. Riley, *The Eighteenth-Century Campaign to Avoid Disease* (New York: St. Martin's Press, 1987), 1–30; also traced by Brügelmann, *Blick*.

88. Rothschuh, *Konzepte*, 308–9; Hufeland, *Kunst*, xii–xiii.

89. Although little of this doctrine appears in Hufeland, *Kunst*, he later discussed and accepted much of Brunonianism. See Rothschuh, *Konzepte*, 342–52, 330–36.

90. Juncker, *Grundsätze*, 15.

91. Bäumler, *Präservirender Arzt*, 542.

92. Antoinette Emch-Dériaz, "The Non-Naturals Made Easy," in *The Popularization of Medicine, 1650–1850*, ed. Roy Porter (London: Routledge, 1992), 134–59; L. J. Rather, "The 'Six Things Non-Natural': A Note on the Origins and Fate of a Doctrine and a Phrase," *CM* 3 (1968): 337–47; James C. Riley, "The Medicine of the Environment in Eighteenth-Century Germany," *CM* 18 (1963): 167–78; Peter Niebyl, "The Non-Naturals," *BHM* 43 (1971): 486–92; Georg Hildebrandt, *Taschenbuch für die Gesundheit auf das Jahr 1801* (Erlangen: Heyder, 1800), preface.

93. Hufeland, *Kunst*, 364.

94. Tissot, *Advice*.

95. Baldinger, *Artzeneien*, 2: 6–7.

96. Ibid., 82; similarly Zückert, *Mitteln*, esp. 12–20.

97. Tissot, *Advice*, 23–34; similar list in Hufeland, *Kunst*, 639.

98. Juncker, *Grundsätze*, 20–21.

99. Unzer, *Arzt*, 1: 65.

100. Tissot, *Anleitung*, 31.

101. Bäumler, *Mitleidiger Arzt*, 54–55.

102. Ibid., 170, 192, 245, 289, 292.

103. In *The Philosophy of Medicine: The Early Eighteenth Century* (Cambridge, Mass.: Harvard University Press, 1978), 232, Lester S. King points out a possible problem with the approach I take here: "It might be interesting to go over a whole series of diseases, especially various infections and fevers, and study the ways in which various authors of the eighteenth century dealt with the causes of these conditions. Such an exposition, however, might get bogged down in details which, although of great antiquarian interest, would not provide significantly greater insight into the basic thought modes of the eighteenth century."

104. Tissot, *Advice*, 251.

105. Ibid., 253, 255–56, 261.

106. StAWf, 111 Neu 3226, fols. 213–16, 21 Aug. 1757; Johann Heinrich Lange, *Briefe über verschiedene Gegenstände der Naturgeschichte und Arzneykunst* (Lüneburg and Leipzig: Johann Friedrich Wilhelm Lemke, 1775), 91; StAWf, 2 Alt 11461, fols. 5–7, 27 Aug. 1750.

107. "Unterricht wie sich die Leute auf dem Lande bey grassierenden Krankheiten zu verhalten haben" (n.d. [probably Sept. 1761]), StAWf, 2 Alt 11486, fols. 22–25; similarly in the "Gesundheits-Unterricht für die Landleute," composed by the

Collegium medicum and published in installments in the *Verbesserter Schreib-Calender* between 1769 and 1790, as well as in the various articles on health and illness in *Gnädigst Privilegierte Braunschweigische Zeitung für Städte, Flecken und Dörfer insonderheit für die lieben Landleute alt und jung*, known as the *Rote Zeitung* and in *Der Bauernfreund in Niedersachsen*. See Lindemann, "Aufklärung."

108. Tissot, *Advice*, 135, 138, 163–64, 184, 187.

109. Heinrich Gottlieb Zerrenner, *Volksbuch: Ein faßlicher Unterricht in nüzlichen Erkenntnissen und Sachen mittelst einer zusammenhängenden Erzehlung für Landleute um sie verständig, gut, wohlhabend, zufriedener und für die Gesellschaft brauchbarer zu machen* (Magdeburg: Scheidhauerschen Buchhandlung, 1787), 2: 211, 127, 220.

110. Bäumler, *Mitleidiger Artzt*, 292.

111. Ackerknecht, *Geschichte*, 126. Therapies changed slowly. Surveying medieval and early Renaissance medicine in *Medieval and Early Renaissance Medicine: An Introduction to Knowledge and Practice* (Chicago: Chicago University Press, 1990), 97, Nancy G. Siraisi points out that it is not appropriate "to look for radical conceptual changes or large increments of new knowledge in the work of *medici* who . . . perceived their task in regard to anatomy and physiology as one of understanding, interpreting, and passing on an existing tradition of learning. Indeed, certain basic physiological concepts and associated therapeutic methods—notably humoral theory and the practice of bloodletting to get rid of bad humors—had a continuous life extending from Greek antiquity into the nineteenth century."

112. Tissot, *Advice*, 133–35, 138, 164–65, 183–87, 106.

113. Tissot, *Anleitung*, 60; Bäumler, *Mitleidiger Artzt*, passim; Jean Ailhaud, *Universal-Arzeney; oder Abhandlung von dem Ursprunge der Krankheiten und dem Gebrauche des abführenden Pulvers* (Strasbourg: Lorenz, 1765).

114. Bäumler, *Mitleidiger Artzt*, 153–57, 395–96, 12, 488–90. Johann Storch would probably have agreed. Barbara Duden, *Geschichte unter der Haut: Ein Eisenacher Arzt seine Patientinnen um 1730* (Stuttgart: Klett-Cotta, 1984), 154.

115. Zerrenner, *Volksbuch*, 325–26.

116. "Über die große Mortalität der Pocken und die Mittel dieselben zu verhüten," StAWf, 111 Neu 3366, 18 Jan. 1788.

117. Riley, *Campaign*, x.

118. Ibid., 47–48. For more detailed discussion of the *enquête*, see Peter, "Disease"; id., "Kranke und Krankheiten"; and Biraben, "Historie."

119. Brügelmann, *Blick*, 78.

120. J. W. G. Klinge, "Einige physisch-medicinische Bemerkungen über die Gegend und das Klima der Kurhannoverischen freyen Bergstadt St. Andreasberg, so wie auch über die Lebensweise und Krankheiten der Bewohner derselben," *Journal der Arzneykunde und practischen Wundarzneykunst* 6 (1798): 880–904; Lebrecht Friedrich Benjamin Lentin, *Denkwürdigkeiten, betreffend Luftbeschaffenheit, Lebensart, Gesundheit und Krankheit der Einwohner Clausthals, in den Jahren 1774 bis 1777* (Hannover, 1800); id., *Beobachtung*; Johann Philipp Rüling, *Physisch-medicinisch-ökonomisch Beschreibung der zum Fürstenthum Göttingen gehörigen Stadt Northeim und ihrer umliegenden Gegend* (Göttingen: Vandenhök & Ruprecht, 1779).

121. Georg Friedrich Hildebrandt was appointed professor of anatomy at the Anatomical-Surgical Institute in Braunschweig in 1786. Among his several publica-

tions was *Bemerkungen und Beobachtungen über die Pocken in der Epidemie des Jahres 1787* (Braunschweig: Schulbuchhandlung, 1788).

122. See, e.g., the topography of Calvörde composed by Pastor Helmuth, "Beschreibung des Amts Kalvörde: Ein Beitrag zur Topographie des Fürstenthums Wolfenbüttels," *BM*, 13 Oct., 24 Nov., and 1 Dec. 1798.

123. Circular of 3 May 1765, copy in StAWf, 2 Alt 11198, fol. 1.

124. Hildebrandt, *Bemerkungen*, Vorbericht; Lentin, *Beobachtung*, xxv–xxvi; August Hinze, "Fünfzehnjährige Liste der am Leben gebliebenen und verstorbenen Wöchnerinnen des calvördischen Physikats-Districts von den Jahren 1776 bis 1790, und siebenjährige Liste aller Wöchnerinnen der Stadt Braunschweig in den Jahren 1781 bis 1787," *AGFK* 2 (1788): 512–18.

125. Gathered from reports on "Vermehrung und Verminderung," StAWf, 2 Alt 11198–202 and 111 Neu 1053.

126. Johann Peter Süssmilch, *Die göttliche Verordnung in denen Veränderung des menschlichen Geschlechts*, 4th ed. (Berlin: Buchhandlung der Realschule, 1775–76); Johann Peter Frank, *System einer vollständigen medicinischen Polizey* (Mannheim: C. F. Schwan, 1779–1827). See also the "Fürstl. Finanz-Collegium den Ausfall der Geburts- und Sterbe-Listen von den Jahren 1795. und 1796. betr.," which explicitly refers to Süßmilch as a model. StAWf, 111 Neu 3349, fols. 2–26.

127. StAWf, 34 N Fb. 1 X 12, 21 Jan. 1773, 1 Feb. 1774, and 9 Feb. 1775.

128. Johann Ernst Wichmann, *Beytrag zur Geschichte der Kriebelkrankheit im Jahre 1770* (Leipzig and Celle: Gsellius, 1771); Lebrecht Friedrich Benjamin Lenten, *Beobachtungen einiger Krankheiten* (Göttingen: Vandenhoeck, 1774), 1–33. For a modern account of ergotism that, despite its exaggeration, offers some valuable information on incidence and perceptions, see Mary Kilbourne Matossian, *Poisons of the Past: Molds, Epidemics, and History* (New Haven, Conn.: Yale University Press, 1989).

129. StAWf, 2 Alt 11198, fols. 18–19, 10 Jan. 1766.

130. "Consignatio historia morbi per mensem Julium & Augustum a.h. euntis 1757. epidemice grassantis," StAWf, 111 Neu 3226, fols. 213–16, 21 Aug. 1757.

131. StAWf, 2 Alt 11463, fols. 5–6, 2 Apr. 1774; "des Magistrats zu Wolfenb. unterthänigste Bericht die Tabelle der gebohrnen und gestorbenen daselbst betref.," StAWf, 34N Fb. 1 X 12, 27 Jan. 1766 and further reports from 5 Feb. 1767 and 24 Jan. 1773.

132. StAWf, 2 Alt 11199, fols. 6–27, 8 Mar. 1766.

133. Ibid., fols. 10, 16–17.

134. Ibid., fols. 19, 23–25. It should also be noted that Schulze wrote presciently and with understanding of the ways in which quackery developed, especially in poor areas. For example, he saw how easily a rural surgeon, hard pressed by his own poverty and the poverty of his clients, could be trapped into quackery by the simple need of making his living. On popular medical enlightenment, see Chapter 1. On patriotism in this context, see Rudolf Vierhaus, "'Patriotismus': Begriff und Realität einer moralisch-politischen Haltung," in *Deutsche patriotische und gemeinnützige Gesellschaften*, ed. Vierhaus (Wolfenbüttel: Herzog August Bibliothek, 1980), 96–109.

135. StAWf, 2 Alt 11200, fols. 14, 20–21, 18 Mar. 1770.

136. Cf., e.g., the report of the magistrates on Wolfenbüttel, StAWf, 34N Fb. 1 X 12, 27 Jan. 1766.

137. StAWf, 2 Alt 11198, fols. 8–9, 7 Sept. 1765; ibid. 11199, fol. 1, 14 Feb. 1766.

138. Ibid. 11198, fols. 10–11, 2 Oct. 1765.

139. Magistrates' report, ibid. 11200, fols. 16–31, 25 Mar. 1770; report from Hoffmann, ibid. 11198, fols. 18–19, 10 Jan. 1766.

140. Ibid. 11198, fols. 50–51, 12 Feb. 1766.

141. Ibid. 11200, fols. 53–55, 20 Jan. 1770.

142. Ibid., fols. 58–64, 20 Dec. 1770.

143. Ibid. 11201, fols. 47–52, 17 July 1771; draft copy with some interesting marginalia in StAWf, 111 Neu 1053.

144. Francisca Loetz comes to similar conclusions about government initiatives in Baden, *Vom Kranken zum Patienten: "Medikalisierung" und medizinische Vergesellschaftung am Beispiel Badens, 1750–1850* (Stuttgart: Franz Steiner, 1993), 253–316.

145. StAWf, 2 Alt 11473, fols. 7, 14.

146. Ibid., fols. 14, 48; "Der Magistrat zu Scheppenstedt von der Vermehrung oder Verminderung der Einwohner zu Scheppenstedt," StAWf, 1N Schöppenstedt I Nr. 28, 19 Mar. 1770.

147. StAWf, 2 Alt 11473, fols. 14, 28; StAWf, 1N Schöppenstedt I Nr. 28, 19 Mar. 1770.

148. Beireis's report, StAWf, 2 Alt 11473, 6 May 1767, esp. fols. 9–14. On medical topographies, see Brügelmann, *Blick*; and see Geneviève Miller, "Airs, Waters, and Places in History," *JHM* 17 (1962): 129–38.

149. StAWf, 2 Alt 11472, fol. 9.

150. Ibid., fol. 1.

151. Ibid., fols. 11–14.

152. StAWf, 2 Alt 11473, fols. 30–32, 18 May 1767.

153. Ibid., fols. 50–53.

154. "Verschiedene den Gesundheits-Zustandt der hiesigen Einwohner betreffend Verkehrungen," ibid., fols. 54–59, 5 July 1767.

155. Ibid., fols. 55–57, 61–62, 5 July and 9 Oct. 1767.

156. Ibid., fol. 63, 15 Oct. 1767.

157. "Der Magistrat zu Scheppenstedt von der Vermehrung oder Verminderung der Einwohner zu Scheppenstedt," StAWf, 1N Schöppenstedt I Nr. 28, 19 Mar. 1770.

158. Ibid.

159. Ibid.

160. Report of Dr. Pini, ibid., 16 Mar. 1770.

161. StAWf, 2 Alt 11198, fols. 18–19, 10 Jan. 1766.

Chapter 5. Choices and Meanings

1. Peter Albrecht, "The Extraordinary Life of a Retired Sexton on the Brink of Poverty: Friedrich Wilhelm Hirsemann (1741–1802)," *CEH* 27 (1994): 185–204; Robert Darnton, *The Literary Underground of the Old Regime* (Cambridge, Mass.: Harvard University Press, 1982).

2. For a similar agenda and assessment, see Francisca Loetz, "Histoire des mentalités und Medizingeschichte: Wege zu einer Sozialgeschichte der Medizin," *MJ* 27 (1992): 283–84.

3. See, e.g., *Patients and Practitioners: Lay Perceptions of Medicine in Pre-Industrial Society*, ed. Roy Porter (Cambridge: Cambridge University Press, 1985); Roy Porter and Dorothy Porter, *In Sickness and in Health: The British Experience 1650–1850* (New York: Basil Blackwell, 1988); Dorothy Porter and Roy Porter, *Patient's Progress: Doctors and Doctoring in Eighteenth-Century England* (Stanford, Calif.: Stanford University Press, 1989); Lucinda McCray Beier, *Sufferers and Healers: The Experience of Illness in Seventeenth-Century England* (London: Routledge & Kegan Paul, 1987); Michael MacDonald, *Mystical Bedlam: Madness, Anxiety and Healing in Seventeenth-Century England* (Cambridge: Cambridge University Press, 1981); Mary E. Fissell, *Patients, Power, and the Poor in Eighteenth-Century Bristol* (Cambridge: Cambridge University Press, 1991); Barbara Duden, *Geschichte unter der Haut: Ein Eisenacher Arzt und seine Patientinnen um 1730* (Stuttgart: Klett-Cotta, 1987); Edna H. Lemay, "Thomas Hérrier: A Country Surgeon Outside Angoulême at the End of the Eighteenth Century," *JSH* 10 (1976–77): 524–37; Ute Künzer, *Medizinisches Briefwechsel von Caroline von Humboldt und Friederike Bruhn* (Düsseldorf: Triltsch, 1976). Robert Jütte, however, exploits a range of archival materials in his description of the everyday life of patients and healers in Cologne in the late sixteenth and seventeenth centuries in *Ärzte, Heiler und Patienten: Medizinischer Alltag in der frühen Neuzeit* (Munich: Artemis & Winkler, 1991) and also in his "A Seventeenth Century Barber-Surgeon and His Patients," *MH* 33 (1989): 184–98.

4. Apparently some physicians kept case books, at least sporadically. In the preface to his *Bemerkungen und Beobachtungen über die Pocken in der Epidemie des Jahrs 1787* (Braunschweig: Schulbuchhandlung, 1788), Georg Friedrich Hildebrandt tells, for example, how he kept records on smallpox patients during the 1787 epidemic in Braunschweig.

5. StAWf, 9 Alt Hedwigsburg 16, 8, and 16 Apr. 1755.

6. Police report, 10 Dec. 1796, StAWf, 2 Alt 11490, fols. 46–7; payment from Prussia came eighteen months later, on 16 June 1798, ibid., fol. 55; for Lieb's case, see 2 Alt 11491, fols. 65, 72, 28 Apr. and 5 May 1801. Cf. similar instances from 1802–4 in 2 Alt 11492.

7. StAWf, 17 N 2315, fols. 2–3, 5, 17 Mar. and 3 Apr. 1750.

8. "Serenissimi gnädigste Verordnung, die Aufnahme und Verpflegung armer Kranken auf dem platten Lande betreffend," StAWf, 40 Slg. 10104, 7 June 1770; repeated 40 Slg. 11710, 22 May 1775, and ibid. 13030, 18 Feb. 1791; extended to include Jews on 4 Dec. 1776, Hinze, 122; provisions for payment of costs in "Serenissimi extendirte Verordnung die Aufnahme der sich erfindenden oder zugeführet werdenden armen Kranken auf dem platten Lande und in den Städten betreffend," 40 Slg 13399, 11 Aug. 1795. For cases in which the government was asked to pay for care and cure, see StAWf, 2 Alt 11488–93 (1760–1804). Similar provisions were made for those injured or wounded, "Verordnung, das Verfahren bey denen Curen der Verwundeten auf dem platten Lande betreffend," HAB Einbl. R2: 1327, 21 Apr. 1764; repeated ibid.: 2232, 4 Dec. 1783.

9. See, e.g., the cases in StAWf, 8 Alt Wolfenbüttel 132 (from 1630–1772); or the case of the "raving woman" in 1741, StAWf, 17 N 2314.

10. StAWf, 9 Alt Vechelde 89, 28 Oct. 1802.

11. StAWF, 2 Alt 11471, fols. 2–9, 19 Apr. 1755; StAWf, 17 N 2316, 4 Mar. 1755.

12. The fund was first established between 1749 and 1756. See StAWf, 2 Alt 11330, fols. 9–12, 18–19; ibid. 11492, fols. 39–41, report of 16 Feb. 1804.

13. See, e.g., Krünitz, s.v. "Bauer," where peasants are called not only "the oldest . . . but also the most useful and most indispensable" social group.

14. John Gagliardo, *From Pariah to Patriot: The Changing Image of the German Peasant, 1770–1840* (Lexington: University of Kentucky Press, 1969), 61.

15. Ibid., 69, 113–17, 139–40. For contemporary opinion in Braunschweig-Wolfenbüttel on popular enlightenment, see "Bedenklichkeit bei der Verfeinerung und Aufklärung des Landvolks, aus der wirklichen Welt, aus der Lage und dem Charakter des Landmanns abstrahirt; von einem Landprediger," *BM*, 3 Jan. 1789; C. H. F. Käufer, "Ueber die Aufklärung des Landmanns durch Bücher," *BM*, 28 June 1800.

16. See, e.g., Christian Ernst Fischer, *Versuch einer Anleitung zur medizinischen Armenpraxis* (Göttingen: Dieterich, 1799), 16.

17. "Erörterung der Frage: ob es für den Landmann nützlich und zuträglich sey, daß auf jedem Dorf sich ein Apotheker und ein Wundarzt befinde?" *Beiträge zum Archiv der medizinischen Polizei und der Volksarzneikunde* 4, no. 2 (1793): 134–35.

18. Fischer, *Versuch*, 29.

19. Letter from 1753, StAWf, 2 Alt 11331, fol. 10.

20. StAWf, 2 Alt 11453, fols. 18–19, 2 Sept. 1741.

21. StAWf, 111 Neu 3226, fols. 163–163a, 1 June 1761.

22. StAWf, 2 Alt 11472, fol. 32, 26 Mar. 1755.

23. Ibid. 11383, fol. 2, 17 July 1794.

24. StAWf, 111 Neu 3107, case 96, 8 Aug. 1814.

25. Report of Physicus Pini "wegen der angemerkten außerordentlichen mortalitaet in vorgangenen Jahr," StAWf, 2 Alt 11473, fols. 44–49, 30 May 1767.

26. StAWf, 2 Alt 11453, fols. 48, 52, 54, for 26 Sept. and 3 and 18 Oct. 1743.

27. "Verzeichnis in dieser Gemeinde, als in den Dorffe Heÿen kranckende Persohnen" (n.d. [Dec. 1757 or Jan. 1758]), StAWf, 111 Neu 3226, fol. 270.

28. StAWf, 111 Neu 3226, fol. 116, 6 Apr. 1761.

29. StAWf, 2 Alt 11484, fol. 28, 7 June 1761.

30. StAWf, 111 Neu 3234, fol. 166, 18 Aug. 1761.

31. Ibid. 3235, fol. 49, 30 Nov. 1793.

32. Ibid. 3228, fol. 149, n.d. (probably May/June 1771).

33. Report of Blum, 15 Feb. 1759, StAWf, 2 Alt 11482, fols. 6–7; response from Amt Gandersheim, 8 Mar. 1759, ibid., fols. 19–20.

34. StAWf, 111 Neu 3228, fols. 146–47, 21 May 1771.

35. StAWf, 2 Alt 11473, fol. 40, 29 May 1767.

36. Ibid. 11506, fols. 8–9, 14 Oct. 1791.

37. Edward Shorter, "The History of the Doctor-Patient Relationship," in *Companion Encyclopedia of the History of Medicine*, ed. William Bynum and Roy Porter (London: Routledge, 1993), 784. See also id., *Bedside Manners: The Troubled History of Doctors and Patients* (New York: Simon & Schuster, 1985, 1991).

38. Duden, *Geschichte*, 67–122; Duden points out (102) that Storch only touched patients in exceptional cases; MacDonald, *Mystical Bedlam*, 12–71; Ronald C. Sawyer, "Patients, Healers, and Disease in the Southeast Midlands, 1697–1634" (diss., Uni-

versity of Wisconsin, Madison, 1986), 243–56; N. D. Jewson, "The Disappearance of the Sick-Man from Medical Cosmology, 1770–1870," *Sociology* 10 (1976): 224–44.

39. Samuel August André Tissot, *Advice to the People in General with Regard to Their Health*, trans. J. Kirkpatrick (Boston: Mein & Fleeming, 1767), 1: 173–76; *Der Bauernfreund in Niedersachsen*, ed., Johann Lorenz Benzler (Lemgo: Meyer, 1755), 353–59, 369–82; Rudolf Becker, *Noth- und Hülfs-Büchlein für Bauersleute oder lehrreiche Freuden- und Trauer-Geschichte des Dorfs Mildheim: Für Jung und Alte beschrieben*, 8th ed. (Gotha and Leipzig: beym Verfasser, 1790), 1: 314–16.

40. Near the end of the century, however, more physicians advised evaluating the pulse by counting the number of beats per minute. For one example, see Tissot, *Advice*, 20–21.

41. Samuel Gottlieb Vogel, *Das Kranken-Examen: Oder allgemeine philosophische medicinische Untersuchung zur Erforschung der Krankheiten des menschlichen Körpers* (Stendal: bey D. C. Franze & Grosse, 1796). See also Roy Porter, "The Rise of Physical Examination," in *Medicine and the Five Senses*, ed. W. F. Bynum and Roy Porter (Cambridge: Cambridge University Press, 1993), 179–97.

42. Joseph Friedrich Gotthard, *Leitfaden für angehende Aerzte Kranke zu prüfen und Krankheiten zu erforschen mit einer Kranken- und Witterungsbeobachtungstabelle* (Erlangen: bey Johann Jakob Palm, 1793), 60, 170.

43. Tissot, *Advice*, 133–34.

44. Malcolm Nicolson, "The Art of Diagnosis: Medicine and the Five Senses," in *Companion*, ed. Bynum and Porter, 801–25; Porter, "Rise of Physical Examination"; S. J. Reiser, "The Decline of the Clinical Dialogue," *JMP* 3 (1978): 305–13.

45. Gotthard, *Leitfaden*, 61.

46. Ernst Gottfried Baldinger, *Artztneien, eine physicalisch-medicinische Monatschrift, zum Unterricht allen denen welche den Schaden des Quacksalbers nicht kennen* (Langensalza: Martini, 1766–67), 2: 13; Samuel August André Tissot, *Anleitung für das Landvolk in Absicht auf seine Gesundheit*, trans. H. C. Hirzel, 2d enlarged ed. (Augsburg and Innsbruck: Wolff, 1766), 29–32.

47. Gottfried Samuel Bäumler, *Mitleidiger Artzt, welcher überhaupt Alle Arme Krancke, insonderheit aber Die abgelegene Land-Leute gründlich und aufrichtig lehret / wie Sie mit Gemeinen Hauß-Mitteln und anderen nicht allzukostbaren Artzeneyen sich selbst curiren können*, 3d ed. (Strasbourg: Joh. Reinhold Dulßecker, der Aeltere, 1743), preface.

48. Heinrich Gottlieb Zerrenner, *Volksbuch: Ein faßlicher Unterricht in nüzlichen Erkenntnissen und Sachen mittelst einer zusammenhängenden Erzehlung für Landleute um sie verständig, gut, wohlhabend, zufriedener und für die Gesellschaft brauchbarer zu machen* (Magdeburg: Im Verlag der Scheidhauerschen Buchhandlung, 1787), 192–93.

49. For northwestern Germany, and especially for the duchy of Oldenburg, see Jonas Goldschmidt, *Volksmedicin im nordwestlichen Deutschland* (Bremen: J. G. Heyse, 1854; reprint, Leer: Schuster, 1978).

50. Johann Jakob Heinrich Bücking, *Versuch einer medicinischen und physikalischen Erklärung deutscher Sprichwörter und sprichwörtlicher Redensarten* (Stendal: Franzen & Grosse, 1797; reprint, Leipzig: Zentralantiquariat der Deutschen Demokratischen Republik, 1976); Johann Heinrich Helmuth, *Volksnaturlehre zur Dämpfung des Aberglaubens* (Braunschweig: Schulbuchhandlung, 1786); and several articles by Johann

Barthold Hoffmann in *BA*, e.g.: "Von dem herrlichen Nutzen des Birkensaftes wider die Krätze," 22 Sept. 1759; "Nachricht von einem besonderen Mittel wider die Wassersucht," 6 Jan. 1762; "Von dem Nutzen der Schaafgarbe, besonders wider die goldene Ader," 25 Aug. 1762.

51. Michael R Buck, *Medicinischer Volksglauben und Volksaberglauben aus Schwaben: Eine kulturgeschichtliche Skizze* (Ravensburg: Dorn, 1865); Victor Fossel, *Volksmedicin und medicinischer Aberglauben in Steiermark: Ein Beitrag zur Landeskunde* (Graz: Leuschner & Lubensky, 1885); Max Höfler, *Deutsches Krankheitsnamen-Buch* (Munich: Piloty & Loehle, 1899; reprint, Hildesheim: Georg Olms, 1970); id., *Volksmedizin und Aberglaube in Oberbayerns Gegenwart und Vergangenheit* (Munich: Otto Galler, 1893); Oskar von Hovorka and Adolf Kronfeld, *Vergleichende Volksmedizin* (Stuttgart: Strecker & Schröder, 1908–9).

52. Paul Diepgen, *Deutsche Volksmedizin: Wissenschaftliche Heilkunde und Kultur* (Stuttgart: Enke, 1935); Gustav Jungbauer, *Deutsche Volksmedizin: Ein Grundriß* (Berlin: Walter de Gruyter, 1934).

53. "Ethnomedicine" is defined as the study of healing outside that of academic medicine, whatever its ethnic origins, Joachim Strely, "Ethnomedizin: Entwurf einer Zeitschrift," *Ethnomedizin: Zeitschrift für Interdisziplinäre Forschung* 1 (1971): 8, cited in Elfriede Grabner, *Grundzüge einer ostalpinen Volksmedizin* (Vienna: Östereichischen Akademie der Wissenschaften, 1985). See also Rudolf Schenda, "Volksmedizin—was ist das heute?" *Zeitschrift für Volkskunde* 69 (1973): 189–210, and id., "Stadtmedizin—Landmedizin: Ein Versuch zur Erklärung subkulturalen medikalen Verhaltens," in *Stadt-Land-Beziehungen: Verhandlungen des 19. Deutschen Volkskundekongresses in Hamburg vom 1. bis 7. Oktober 1973* (Göttingen: Vandenhoeck & Ruprecht, 1975), 147–69.

54. Grabner, *Grundzüge*, 116–19; Ludwig Büttner, *Fränkische Volksmedizin: Ein Beitrag zur Volkskunde Ostfrankens* (Erlangen: Palm & Enke, 1935), 25.

55. See esp. Goldschmidt, *Volksmedicin*, 11–46, comments on "Allgemeine Pathologie" and "Diätetik." Although Oldenburg, with its close links to the Low Countries and its widespread use of plattdeutsch, is not identical to Braunschweig-Wolfenbüttel, Goldschmidt's observations are still useful.

56. Ibid., 136, 139.

57. Porter and Porter, *In Sickness and in Health*, 7; Beier, *Sufferers and Healers*, 31.

58. Françoise Loux, "Folk Medicine," in *Companion*, ed. Bynum and Porter, 664.

59. Thomas Broman, "Rethinking Professionalization: Theory, Practice and Professional Ideology in Eighteenth-Century German Medicine," *JMH* 67 (1995): 835–72; Mary Fissell, "Innocent and Honorable Bribes: Medical Manners in Eighteenth-Century Britain," in *The Codification of Medical Morality: Historical and Philosophical Studies of the Formalization of Western Medical Morality in the Eighteenth and Nineteenth Centuries*, vol. 1: *Medical Ethics and Etiquette in the Eighteenth Century*, ed. Robert Baker, Dorothy Porter, and Roy Porter (Dordrecht: Kluwer, 1993), 41–42.

60. And this interpretation is very much in line with what others have argued for the seventeenth and eighteenth centuries. See, e.g., Porter and Porter, *In Sickness and Health*; id., *Patient's Progress*; Roy Porter, *Health for Sale*; Beier, *Sufferers and Healers*; Fissell, *Patients*.

61. Baldinger, *Artztneien*, 2: 118–23, 152; Franz Peter Leopold Gennzinger,

Quaestio inauguralis medica an a fascino, et diabolo, hominibus morti? (Vienna: Joseph Kurzbock, 1765), quoted in ibid., 141–42.

62. Baldinger, *Artztneien,* 2: 106.

63. In his magnificent *Peasants into Frenchman: The Modernization of Rural France* (Stanford, Calif.: Stanford University Press, 1976), Eugen Weber looks at the most backward parts of the French countryside and tends to present them as norms. In *The Superstitious Mind: French Peasants and the Supernatural in the Nineteenth Century* (New Haven, Conn.: Yale University Press, 1987), Judith Devlin seems to have accepted the comments of unsympathetic observers at face value. *HDA*, a great compilation on superstitions, is similar in tone.

64. James Sheehan, *German History, 1770–1866* (Oxford: Oxford University Press, 1989), 149 n. 8.

65. In "Conflicting Attitudes Towards Inoculation in Enlightenment Germany," in, *Medicine in the Enlightenment,* ed. Roy Porter (Amsterdam: Rodopi, 1995), 208, Andreas-Holger Maehle argues that easy generalizations about "religious resistance" to inoculation cannot be made.

66. On the use of human fat, see *HDA*, 2: 1373–85, s.v. "Fett."

67. Nancy G. Siraisi, *Medieval and Early Renaissance Medicine: An Introduction to Knowledge and Practice* (Chicago: University of Chicago Press, 1990), 104–6, 115–23.

68. Krünitz, s.v. "Frühlings-Cur," asserts that such cures should not be taken automatically, but only when a person has determined that his body was clogged with the impurities accumulated over the winter.

69. Elfriede Grabner, "'Schnurziehen' und 'Fontanellensetzen': Künstliche Wunden als Krankheitsableitung im Wechselspiel von Schul-und Volksmedizin," *Schweizerisches Archiv für Volkskunde* 62 (1966): 133–50.

70. "Designatio der aus den Actis judicialibus des Amt Hessen, den Fuscher Mercker zu Pabstdorff betreffend, excerpirten unbefugten Curen," StAWf, 2 Alt 11609, fols. 52–54, n.d. (May 1750).

71. Bücking, *Versuch,* 66–68, 69–71, 86–88, 91–92, 251–53, 266–68, 422–23, 558–59.

72. Ibid., 558–59.

73. A number of articles investigating herbal remedies were published from the late 1750s through the early 1770s.

74. *HDA*, 2: 1211–15, s.v. "Farbe," and 7: 803, "Rote Farbe"; Michael Howard, *Traditional Folk Remedies: A Comprehensive Herbal* (London: Century, 1987), 44–51.

75. Howard, *Traditional Folk Remedies,* 44–51; Grabner, *Gründzuge,* 232–58; id., "Die 'transplantation morborum' als Heilmethode in der Volksmedizin," *Österreichische Zeitschrift für Volkskunde,* n.s., 21 (1967): 178–95; Tissot, *Advice,* 201–2.

76. Höfler, *Krankheitsnamen-Buch;* numerous entries in *HDA*.

77. Johann Heinrich Lange, *Tentamen medico-physicum de remediis Brunsuicensium domesticis* (Braunschweig: Schulbuchhandlung, 1765). I thank Mary Wessling for providing me with a photocopy of this work. I also used the parts translated by Leonhard Ludwig Finke, *Versuch einer allgemeinen medicinisch-praktischen Geographie worin der historische Theil der einheimischen Völker- und Staaten-Arzneykunde vorgetragen wird* (Leipzig: Weidmann, 1792–95), 2: 446–51.

78. Finke, *Versuch,* 446–51; Collegium medicum [Johann Bernhard Martini],

Dispensatoruium pharmacevticvum brvnsvicense (Braunschweig: Waisenhaus, 1777), in which the register of German names for medicines was especially useful.

79. "Actum Salder," StAWf, 111 Neu 3120, 28 Feb. 1778.

80. "Amt Hessen," 16 July 1798, and "Pro Memoria," 11 Aug. 1798, StAWf, 111 Neu 3115, case 206.

81. StAWf, 2 Alt 11200, fol. 53, 20 Jan. 1770.

82. On the treatment of rabies, see Samuel Tissot, *The Family Physician: or, Advice with Respect to Health including Directions for the Prevention and Cure of Acute Diseases, Extracted from Dr. Tissot, by the late Rev. John Wesley, A.M.*, 8th ed. (London: Thomas Cordeuz, 1810), 65–67, who recommended mercury, bleeding, emollient clysters, vomitives, and ointments applied locally. See also Klaus Burghard, *Die Tollwuttherapie im Jahrhundert vor Pasteur* (Frankfurt am Main: Peter Lang, Europäische Hochschulschriften, 1991), 55–66.

83. StadtH, B VII 11a Nr. 3, 4 May 1770.

84. StAWf, 111 Neu 3109, case 133, 9 Dec. 1816.

85. Ibid. 3114, case 181, n.d. (1815).

86. Except where otherwise noted, I have extracted these examples from the burial records of the communities of Bornum (StAWf, 1 Kb 193 [1748–1810]) and Walkenried (ibid. 1223–24 [1667–1814]). References are indicated in the text by year of death and place.

87. "Amt Stauffenberg," StAWf, 111 Neu 3107, case 85, 8 and 20 Sept. 1798.

88. "Amt Hessen," 16 July 1798, and "Pro Memoria" from 11 Aug. 1798, StAWf, 111 Neu 3115, case 206.

89. StadtB, C VII P7, fols. 249–64, 20 and 25 Feb., 8 Mar., 6 Apr. 1758.

90. "Verzeichniß derer Patienten, welche sich in District C befinden," StadtB, C VII P7, fols. 265–77, for 15, 22, and 29 Apr., 6, 13, 20 and 27 May, 3 and 17 June 1758 (the list for 10 June is missing).

91. Ibid. For chest complaints, eight patients saw a physician, four another healer, three used a home remedy, and sixteen used nothing; for fever, eighteen people saw physicians, four went to other healers, five turned to home remedies, and thirty-two reported using nothing.

92. Jan Brügelmann, *Der Blick des Arztes auf die Krankheit im Alltag 1779–1850: Medizinische Topographien als Quelle für die Sozialgeschichte der Gesundheitswesens* (Berlin: Freie Universität, 1982), 143.

93. Oswald Adolf Erich and Richard Beitl, *Wörterbuch der deutschen Volkskunde*, 2d rev. ed. (Stuttgart: Alfred Krüner, 1955), s.v. "Fieber."

94. The ten-year period ran from 1752 to 1761, and excluded 1757 and 1758, years for which no data are available. Meeting of medical society, 1 Apr. 1758, StAWf, 111 Neu 3249, fols. 41–42. The society met another two, perhaps three times during the late spring and summer of 1738. The four doctors practicing in Wolfenbüttel attended most meetings. During these sessions, the society considered a series of mortality reports for the period January through May, ultimately forwarding its findings on to the Collegium medicum. "Actum Wolfenbüttel d. 17 Mai In Societate medica," StAWf, 111 Neu 3249, fols. 58, 60–66; statistics are taken from "General-Liste der Gebohrenen und Gestorbenen zu Wolfenbüttel von 1752. bis 1765. incl.," StAWf, 34N Fb. 1 X 12.

95. "Actum Wolfenbüttel d. 17 Mai 1758 In Societate medica," ibid., fol. 56.

96. *Niedersächsisches Städtebuch,* ed. Erich Keyser (Stuttgart: W. Kohlhammer, 1952), 46.

97. According to the report of Physicus Schulze in Calvörde, StAWf, 111 Neu 3253, fol. 85, 8 Mar. 1769.

98. Ibid., fols. 90–92, report of Collegium medicum, 2 Mar. 1769.

99. Ibid., fols. 90, 125, 2 Mar. and 7 Apr. 1769.

100. StAWf, 2 Alt 11400, fols. 2–4, 2 Nov. 1772.

101. Ibid., fols. 5–15, "Actum auf dem Rathhause zu Blankenburg," 8 and 12 Oct. 1772.

102. Ibid. 11482, fols. 6–7, 15 Feb. 1759.

103. Ibid., fols. 12–17, for 8, 9, 18, 29, and 31 Jan., and 2, 3, 8, 12, and 15 Feb. 1759.

104. Ibid., fols. 19–20, 8 Mar. 1759.

105. Struve's report of 25 Aug. 1757, StAWf, 111 Neu 3226, fols. 222–28; "Verzeichnis in dieser Gemeinde, als in den Dorffe Heÿen kranckende Persohnen," ibid., fol. 270, n.d. (Aug. 1757).

106. StAWf, 2 Alt 11465, fols. 18–19, 29 May 1794.

107. Ibid. 11287, fol. 60, 18 Jan. 1788; StAWf, 8 Alt Lutter am Barenberg 31, fol. 16, 13 Apr. 1773. In the last case, the boy's stepfather refused to allow the boy to be circumcised, fearing that his weak child would not survive the surgery (ibid., fol. 19, 24 Apr. 1773).

108. Fragmentary reports are available for 1753–54, 1759, 1772, and 1773. A complete set of monthly reports exists only for 1774, in StAWf, 8 Alt Seesen 3 Nr. 8.

109. The number of healers consulted and home remedies used totals more than eighty-one because patients often consulted one or more practitioners, or used one or more remedies, serially or simultaneously. See StAWf, 10 Alt Hehlen 6–16.

110. Ibid., 8.

111. "Specificatio einiger Patienten welche ich binnen anderhalb biß zwei Jahre allhier in Braunschweig curiret," StAWf, 2 Alt 11293, fols. 21–27. We have only very few case books with which to work. The famous Dr. Ernst Heim, who practiced in Berlin in the late eighteenth and first third of the nineteenth century, recorded quite a large practice in his diary: 393 patients in 1784, about 1,000 in 1790, and 1,346 for 1795. In addition, he had a large practice among the sick poor, estimated at about 3,000–4,000 a year, but this should be taken to mean 3,000–4,000 visits rather than 3,000–4,000 individuals. Private patients were listed as individuals, and the number of visits in a day was huge. For instance, on 7 June 1790, Heim noted that he made 73 visits, and 20 other people sought advice from him in his home. See Georg Wilhelm Keßler, *Der alte Heim,* 2d ed. (Leipzig: Brockhaus, 1846), cited in Manfred Stürzenbecher, *Beiträge zur Berliner Medizingeschichte: Quellen und Studien zur Geschichte des Gesundheitswesens vom 17. bis zum 19. Jahrhundert* (Berlin: de Gruyter, 1966), 81–82.

Another practice that has been analyzed in some detail is that of Samuel Thomas Soemmerring. His case book, "Praxis in Frankfurt," remains in private possession—like, one suspects, many others yet to be discovered. In this volume, Soemmerring recorded 393 consultations; thirteen for 1785, twenty-two for 1793; the rest for the period from Nov. 1795 to the end of Dec. 1796. Analyzing the social makeup of the case book in "Nicht nur Hölderlin: Das ärztliche Besuchsbuch Soemmerrings als Quelle für sein soziales Umfeld in Frankfurt am Main," *MJ* 28 (1993): 123–24, 127–29, Franz Dumont has found that out of a total of 256 patients, 55 were from merchant families; 39, artisans; 17, bankers; 8, book dealers or bookbinders; 8, members of the upper, and 10 of the lower, civil bureaucracy; 7, members of the military; 5, lawyers; 6, servants; 4, clergymen; 4, members of the city council; 2, innkeepers; 2, tutors; 2, members of the municipal patriciate; 4, Jews; and 1, a foreign surgeon. Merchant families thus constituted the largest group among Soemmering's patients, followed by artisans. Noncitizens—day laborers and the like—are totally missing. Unlike Heim, Soemmerring rarely saw as many as a dozen patients a day.

112. Resolution forbidding Barthold the right to practice internal medicine, 7 May 1722, StAWf, 2 Alt 11294, fol. 4; "Responsum Juris Helmstadiense d. Doctoris Medicina Joh. Nicol. Barthold . . . betref.," 29 May and 1 June 1722, ibid., fols. 31–37.

113. StAWf, 2 Alt 11293, fols. 21–27, "Specificatio."

114. StAWf, 111 Neu 3103, "Nach den Listen der Gestorbenen von 1839. hat der Chirurgus Ahrberg in Wetteborn behandelt," case 2.

115. Ibid., "Actum Amt Greene," 17 July, 1801, case 5.

116. Ibid., 6 and 13 July 1816.

117. StAWf, 8 Alt Stauffenberg 641, "Actum Amt Stauffenberg," 14 Nov. 1782.

118. StAWf, 111 Neu 3106, 16 Feb. 1793, case 61[1].

119. StAWf, 111 Neu 3106, "Actum Gandersheim," 10 July 1802, case 63.

120. StAWf, 111 Neu 3106, 7 Sept. 1802, case 64.

121. Ibid. 3110, "Actum Braunschweig wegen des Gerichts," 17 Sept. 1800, case 140.

122. Ibid.

123. Ibid.

124. Geneviève Miller, *The Adoption of Inoculation for Smallpox in England and France* (Philadelphia: University of Pennsylvania Press, 1957); Claudia Huerkamp, "A History of Smallpox Vaccination in Germany: A First Step in the Medicalization of the General Public," *JCH* 20 (1985): 617–35; Ute Frevert, *Krankheit als politisches Problem, 1770–1880: Soziale Unterschichten in Preußen zwischen medizinischer Polizei und staatlicher Sozialversicherung* (Göttingen: Vandenhoeck & Ruprecht, 1984), 69–73; Eberhard Wolff, "Der 'Medizinische Kulturkampf'—Die Medikalisierung des Patienten durch die Pockenschutzimpfung im 19. Jahrhundert," in *Ergebnise und Perspektiven: Sozialhistorischer Forschung in der Medizingeschichte: Protokoll, Kolloquium zum 100. Geburtstag von Henry Ernst Sigerist*, ed. Susanne Hahn and Achim Thom (Leipzig: Karl-Sudhoff Institut, University of Leipzig, 1991), 89–103; Maehle, "Conflicting Attitudes." On smallpox vaccination in Braunschweig-Wolfenbüttel, see, too, Andreas Weißmann, "Die Schutzpockenimpfung im Herzogtum Braunschweig-Wolfenbüttel von 1800 bis zum Impfgesetz vom April 1833" (Magisterarbeit, Modern History, Technical University Braunschweig, 1993). Peter Albrecht has investigated smallpox inoculation in the city of Braunschweig, and what follows relies heavily on his work, "Versuche zur Popularisierung der Blatterninokulation in der Stadt Braunschweig von 1754 bis 1780" (manuscript).

125. Fifty-five pro-inoculation articles appeared in *BA* from 1766 through 1774 (Albrecht, "Versuche").

126. StAWf, 2 Alt 11467, 17 Nov. 1754, pp. 2–3 and passim. This included plans for establishing an *Inokulations-Anstalt*.

127. Maehle, "Conflicting Attitudes"; Frevert, *Krankheit*, 70–71; J. C. W. Juncker, *Gemeinnützige Vorschläge und Nachrichten über das beste Verhalten der Menschen in Rücksicht der Pockenkrankheit: Erster Versuch über die mittlern Stände nebst einem Anhange für Ärzte* (Halle: Schwetschke & Sohn, 1792), 60, cited in Albrecht, "Versuche."

128. Report of Collegium medicum "über die große Mortalität der Pocken und die Mittel dieselbe zu verhuten," StAWf, 2 Alt 11500, fol. 54, 18 Jan. 1788; Hildebrandt, *Bemerkungen*, 2.

129. August Ludwig Schlözer, *Briefwechsel meist historischen und politischen Inhalts* (Göttingen: Vandenhöck & Ruprecht, 1780–82), quoted in Friedrich Wilhelm Klärich, "Etwas über die Pockenepidemie zu Göttingen 1777, und über die Inoculation der Pocken," *HM*, 16 Feb. 1778.

130. StAWf, III Neu 3253, fol. 91, 2 Mar. 1769; report of Collegium medicum, ibid., fol. 126, 7 Apr. 1769; report from Dr. Brückmann, ibid., fol. 118, 5 Apr. 1769.

131. Ibid., fols. 122–23, 6 Apr. 1769.

132. StAWf, 2 Alt 11469, fol. 3, 1 May 1768; ibid., fols. 5–6, 2 May 1768.

133. Ibid. 11517, report of Collegium medicum, 30 June 1806, pp. 55–62.

134. The most important of these were [Christian Rudolf Wilhelm] Wiedemann, [Theodor Georg August] Roose, and [Ernst August Wilhelm] Himly, "Ueber die Kuhblatternimpfung," *BM*, 8 and 15 Nov. 1800; "Anfrage des Hrn. Stadtwundarztes Mayer, die Inokulation der Kuhpocken betreffend, nebst deren Beantwortung," *BM*, 25 Apr. 1801; Wiedemann, "Ueber den Fortgang der Kuhpocken in Paris," *BM*, 27 June and 4 July 1801; W.[ilhelm Hermann Georg] Remer, "Vertheidigung der Kuhblatternimpfung, gegen die ihr von Hrn. Dr. Markus Herz zu Wein, gemachten Vorwürfe," *BM*, 26 Sept., 3 and 10 Oct. 1801; [Georg Rudolph] Lichtenstein, "Nachricht von den mißlungenen Impfungen der Kuhpocken in Oebisfelde," *BM*, 27 Mar. and 3 Apr. 1802; [Georg August Heinrich] Mühlenbein, "Einige Regeln für ungeübtere Impfärzte bei den Schutzblattern," *BM*, 19 May and 5 June 1802; Vogler, "Etwas über die Schutzpocken," *BM*, 29 Oct. 1803; Wilhelm Harcke, "Einige Worte über die Impfung der Schutzblattern und über die Nothwendigkeit, diese Impfung zum Gesetze zu machen," *BM*, 31 May 1806; [Lorenz?] von Crell, "Nachricht von der Impfung mit der Materie von den natürlichen Blattern, bey acht Kindern, welche schon die Schutzblattern vorher überstanden hatten," *BM*, 18 Apr. 1807; Wilhelm Remer, "Nachricht an das Publikum von scheinbar ohne schützenden Erfolg in Helmstedt geschehen Impfungen der Schutzblattern," *BM*, 14 Feb. 1807; "Dringender Warnung für Eltern, die Wohlthätigkeit der Schutzpocken nicht länger zu verkennen; durch einen traurigen Vorfall veranlaßt," *BM*, 4 Apr. 1807.

135. Weißmann, "Schutzpockenimpfung," 39; StAWf, 8 Alt Campen Gr. 24 Nr. 4, fols. 1–3, 6, for 9, 20, and 27 May 1805.

136. StAWf, III Neu 3252, fols. 5–8, 6 May 1805.

137. StAWf, 8 Alt Neubrück 196, fol. 42, 27 May 1805, "Verzeichniß von denen Eltern im Fürstl. Amte Neubrück und Gerichte Veltenhof, welche ihren Kindern die Schutz-Blattern / Kuh-Pocken / wollen freywillig einimpfen laßen, gegen Bezahlung vor jedes Kindt 2 ggr. und einige welche sich geweigert haben."

138. StAWf, III Neu 3355, fols. 21–41, 27 Feb. 1802; list, fols. 36–41. For

another example, see the list of parents in village of Neubrück who were willing to have their children vaccinated, StAWf, 8 Alt Neubrück 196, fol. 42, "Verzeichniß von deren Eltern," 27 May 1805.

139. StAWf, 111 Neu 3350, fols. 23–24, 2 Dec. 1802.

140. Ibid. 3354, fols. 15–17, 15 Nov. 1802.

141. Ibid. 3361, report of Amt, 3 Nov. 1815, fols. 3–4; ibid., "Pro Memoria" to Collegium medicum, fols. 11–14, here fol. 13, 19 Feb. 1816.

142. Ibid., fol. 1, 20 Feb. 1815.

143. Ibid. 3362, reports of Spohr, 22 Nov. and 17 Dec. 1815, fols. 2–3, 8.

144. Irvine Loudon, "Leg Ulcers in the Eighteenth and Early Nineteenth Century," *JRCGP* 31 (1981): 263–73; 32 (1982): 301–9.

145. StAWf, 2 Alt 11630, fols. 49–50, 9 Aug. 1780. The concession was very cautiously worded and gave Dreyer the right to practice only when a physician recommended the use of his plaster in writing (ibid., fol. 61, 5 Oct. 1780).

146. Ibid. 11631, report of Collegium medicum, 22 Mar. 1791, fols. 20–22.

147. Ibid., fols. 50–51, 30 Dec. 1793; StadtB, C VII S20, vol. 8, fols. 15–24, 24 Jan. 1794.

148. StAWf, 2 Alt 11631, "Actum Neustadt Rathhaus Braunschweig," 17 Oct. 1780, fols. 9–11.

149. Ibid. 11628, fols. 24, 43–44, 4 July 1774 and 7 Sept. 1775.

150. Ibid., fol. 21, 1 July 1774; ibid., fol. 22, 16 Oct. 1772.

151. Ibid., fol. 27, 19 July 1775; ibid., fols. 38–39, 5 Sept. 1775.

152. Ibid. 11627, "Acta inquisitionalia," 25 Apr. 1774, fols. 58–60; ibid., "Actum Neustadt Rathhaus Braunschweig," 3 May 1774, fols. 61–62.

153. Ibid. 11628, fol. 29, 8 Feb. 1772.

154. *HDA*, 3: 760–66, 762–65, 804–5, s.v. "Geschwulst," "Geschwür," and "Gewächs."

155. Erika Håkansson, "Über Volksmedizin des 17. bis 19. Jahrhunderts im Aachener Raum" (diss., Technical University, Aachen, 1975), 87, 91.

156. Ibid., 88; *HDA*, 5: 455–58, s.v. "Krebs."

157. StAWf, 2 Alt 11628, fols. 30–31, from 1772.

158. Ibid. 11283, fols. 62, 68–72, for 2 and 21 Oct. and 2 Nov. 1751.

159. Ibid., fols. 64–67, 76, 81, for 20 Nov. and 16 Dec. 1751, 6 Feb. 1752.

160. Ibid., fol. 76, 16 Dec. 1751.

161. Ibid. 11628, fol. 32, 1 July 1772; see similar testimonial from the tithe collector Conrad Böckel on Busch's treatment of his wife in ibid., fol. 26, 18 July 1775.

162. Ibid., fol. 48, 21 Oct. 1775.

163. Ibid. 11367, fols. 24–25, 29–30, 4 and 27 Mar. 1775.

164. Håkansson, "Volksmedizin," 90; *HDA*, 1: 1685–86, 1757–61, s.v. "Brüste" and "Butter."

165. StAWf, 2 Alt 11628, fol. 40 "Actum in Geistl. Gericht Braunschweig,"; ibid., fol. 47, 21 Oct. 1775.

166. Ibid., fol. 42, 7 Sept. 1775.

167. Ibid., fol. 35, 20 July 1773; see also testimony of Christian Friedrich Westphal, whom Busch treated for blind hemorrhoids, ibid., fol. 43, 7 Sept. 1775.

168. Zedler, s.v. "Haemorrhoides"; also *HDA*, 1: 171–72, s.v. "Ader, goldene."

The spontaneous flow from the "golden vein" was considered "worth gold" because it made payment for the usual bloodletting unnecessary. Later in the century, there was growing disagreement. In *Die Hämorrhoiden: Den Freunden dauerhafter Gesundheit gewidmet* (Berlin and Stettin: auf Kosten des Publici, 1775), 5–6, Franz Anton May, for one, insisted that blood flow from hemorrhoids was not analogous to menstruation, although he did feel it indicated other, more serious problems brought on by constipation, as well a generally weak constitution.

169. StAWf, 111 Neu 3103, "Actum in curia Wolfenbüttel," 23 Nov. 1750, case 8.

170. Ibid., "Actum in Collegio med. Brschwg.," 8 July 1751, case 8.

171. Ibid. 3105, case 41, 4 June 1799.

172. Ibid. 3115, case 202, 11 and 14 Feb. 1809.

173. Ibid. 3118, 24 Nov. 1770; ibid. 3108, case 105, 25 Jan. and 1 Feb. 1796, 5 June 1799, 6 Sept. 1802.

174. StAWf, 2 Alt 11628, fols. 45–46, 19 Oct. 1775.

175. StAWf, 9 Alt Wendhausen 144, "Actum Wendhausen," 7 Aug. 1776.

176. StAWf, 111 Neu 3103, "Actum in curia Wolfenbüttel," case 8, 4 Dec. 1750; ibid., "Actum in Collegio med. Bschwg," 8 July 1751.

177. Ibid. 3113, "Actum Salder," case 171^I, 27 Mar. 1797; ibid., "Pro Memoria" to Amt Lichtenberg, case 171^{II}, 10 July 1802.

178. Ibid., "Actum Wolfenbüttel," 20 May 1797.

179. Ibid., case 171^I, 27 Apr. 1797.

180. "Liste der Geborenen, Kopulirten, Kranken und Todten, von Monat December 1794," 2 Jan. 1795; also StAWf, 111 Neu 3115, case 205, 18 May 1802.

181. Loudon, "Leg Ulcers."

182. In *Handwerkschirurgen: Sozialgeschichte einer verdrängten Berufsgruppe* (Göttingen: Vandenhoeck & Ruprecht, 1989), 105–6, Sabine Sander points out that major operations were probably exceptions in most surgical practices, and that surgeons were cautious about undertaking them.

183. Anthropologists have often referred to a special time of ritual, which includes healing rituals. See, e.g., the work of Victor W. Turner, particularly *The Ritual Process: Structure and Anti-Structure* (Chicago: Aldine, 1969), 1–43, and *Process, Performance and Pilgrimage: A Study in Comparative Sociology* (New Delhi: Concept, 1979), 60–93. And we should not forget that "modern, scientific medicine" itself is hardly free of ritualism (see, e.g., Roy Porter, "Introduction," in *Patients*, ed. Porter, 13–14). It seems to me that Jens Lachmund and Gunnar Stollberg accord rather more importance to the surrounding social world, to cultural expectations, and their roles within the medical encounter. Drawing on the autobiographies of laypeople and patients, as well as Georg Christian Gottlieb von Wedekind's *Ueber das Betragen des Arztes, den Heilungsweg, durch Gewinnung des Zutrauens und durch Ueberredung des Kranken* (Mainz: Andreä in Frankfurt, 1789), Lachmund and Stollberg seek to "understand the meaning and the problems" of the medical encounter. (54) "Typical of this drama," they conclude

was the flexibility of both the matrix of social relationships involved as well as the meaning of illness. What we have called dramaturgical authority went together with the symbolic shaping of illness. One mediated the other, problems arising on one dimension could be balanced by rearrangements on the other one. The audience held an important position in this plot. It was not always at odds with doctors, but always suspected the drama enacted on stage. And if time arrived, it did not hesitate to intervene; then it could turn from being an audience into becoming a powerful agent and spoil the doctor's game.

Jens Lachmund and Gunnar Stollberg, "The Doctor, His Audience, and the Meaning of Illness: The Drama of Medical Practice in the Late Eighteenth and Early Nineteenth Centuries," in *The Social Construction of Illness: Illness and Medical Knowledge in Past and Present*, ed. Lachmund and Stollberg (Stuttgart: Franz Steiner, 1992), 64–65.

184. StAWf, 111 Neu 3103, "Actum Wolfenbüttel," 30 Nov. 1778, case 11; ibid., "Actum in des Feder-Schützen Asmus Behausung auf das Kloster St. Laurenti," 21 Jan. 1779,; ibid., "Actum Wolfenbüttel von wegen des adel. Gerichts Sambleben," 18 Feb. 1779.

185. Ibid. 3104, "Actum Gericht Supplingenburg," 24 Sept. 1799, case 40.

186. Ibid., "Actum Braunschweig im Fürstl. Gerichte Vechelde," 10 Oct. 1804, case 23[1].

187. Ibid., 7 Nov. 1804.

188. Ibid. 3115, "Actum Amt Jerxheim," 19 July 1803, case 200.

189. StAWf, 2 Alt 11624, fols. 3–4, "Actum bey dem ordentl. Schliesstedt Gericht," 15 June 1771.

190. Ibid., 11623, fols. 24–25, 3 May 1771.

191. StAWf, 111 Neu 3115, "Actum Amt Jerxheim," 14 Aug. 1788, case 206.

192. Ibid. 3109, "Actum Gericht Destedt," 2 July 1803, and "Actum Wolfenbüttel im Fürstl. Amte Salzdahlum," 3 July 1801, case 121.

193. Ibid. 3112, case 151, 20 Oct. 1803.

194. StadtH, B VII 11a Nr. 3, 3 June 1755.

195. StAWf, 111 Neu 3100, case 2.

196. Ibid. 3110, "Actum Braunschweig wegen des Gerichts," 17 Sept. 1800, case 140.

197. Ibid., "Amt Gandersheim," 18 Sept. 1802, case 139.

198. Ibid. 3112, "Actum Braunschweig," 24 and 28 Jan. 1805, case 157.

199. Ibid. 3117, 10 Aug. 1765.

200. Ibid. 3108, case 102, 16 June 1800.

201. Ibid.,13 May 1800; ibid., case 103, 30 Dec. 1819.

202. Ibid. 3107, case 77, 17 Mar. 1810.

203. StAWf, 2 Alt 11287, investigation conducted by Amt Vorsfelde, 4 Jan. 1780, fols. 9–11.

204. Ibid. 11285, "General-Protocoll bey der Visitation im Harz District vom d. 7. Dec. bis d. 24 incl. 1767," 24 Dec. 1767, 26 Apr. 1768; and report of Amt Langelsheim, 28 June 1768, fols. 50–52, 54–55, 57.

205. Ibid. 11290, fol. 10–12, 9 June 1802; ibid., fol. 10, quoting Johann Heinrich Sternberg, *Erinnerungen und Zweifel gegen die Lehre der Aerzte von dem schweren Zahnen der Kinder* (Hannover: Helwing, 1802), 1: 879.

206. StAWf, 111 Neu 3108, case 106, 26 July 1803.

207. Ibid. 3113, "Actum Braunschweig im Krl. Amte Eich den 23[ten] July 1800," case 166.

208. The two testimonies were taken on 26 July 1800 (ibid.).

209. There has also, I think, been a tendency to generalize about the early modern period without sufficient regard to the differences between the sixteenth and the eighteenth centuries. Discussing "The Social Construction of Illness in the Early Modern Period," in *Social Construction*, ed. Lachmund and Stollberg, 31, Robert Jütte cautions readers, for example, to remember "the strong current of magico-causal thinking in a society which was, to a large extent, only superficially christianized and in which diseases were often associated with the action of evil ghosts and demons."

210. StAWf, 111 Neu 3111, case 150ᶦ, 16 Oct. 1797.

211. In *Vom Kranken zum Patienten: "Medikalisierung" und medizinische Vergesellschaftung am Beispiel Badens, 1750–1850* (Stuttgart: Franz Steiner, 1993), 322, Francisca Loetz observes that simply contrasting the costs of cure with incomes or the prices of food and other products probably tells us nothing at all about the way people calculated the price of health. Even if costs were "objectively high," she points out, we know little about "subjective" values, which would have been decisive.

Conclusion

1. See, e.g., Ute Frevert, *Krankheit als politisches Problem, 1770–1880: Soziale Unterschichten in Preußen zwischen medizinischer Polizei und staatlicher Sozialversicherung* (Göttingen: Vandenhoeck & Ruprecht, 1984); Claudia Huerkamp, "The History of Smallpox Vaccination in Germany: A First Step in the Medicalization of the General Public," *JCH* 20 (1985): 617–35; Alfons Labisch, "Doctors, Workers and the Scientific Cosmology of the Industrial World: The Social Construction of 'Health' and the 'Homo Hygienicus,'" ibid., 599–615. Labisch has described "health" and "health-conscious behavior" as "one aspect of the process by which the working class was integrated into the world of industrial society" (607).

2. As Francisca Loetz has done for Baden in *Vom Kranken zum Patienten: "Medikalisierung" und medizinische Vergesellschaftung am Beispiel Badens, 1750–1850* (Stuttgart: Franz Steiner, 1993), 73–87.

3. See, e.g., "Etwas über die medizinischen oder innerliche Praxis und das eigene Arzneyausgeben der Amtswundärzte auf dem Lande. Aus einem gutachtlichen Bericht," *Archiv der medizinischen Polizey und der gemeinnützligen Arzneikunde* 5 (1786): 266–81.

Major Holdings Consulted

Most of research for this book was done in the Niedersächsisches Staatsarchiv-Wolfenbüttel (StAWf), Stadtarchiv Braunschweig, Stadtarchiv Helmstedt, and in the Herzog August Bibliothek in Wolfenbüttel. I also worked more briefly in the Stadtarchiv Königslutter and in the Ratsarchiv Hornburg.

Most of the files and boxes in StAWf 2 Alt are consecutively paginated, and I have cited individual documents by date and folio number(s). This is also true for StAWf 111 Neu, with the exception of the files on Pfuscherey (111 Neu 3103–16), which I have prefered to cite by case (as they were organized in the late eighteenth and early nineteenth centuries) and by date. The individual files are arranged alphabetically by last name of the person investigated. Many files in StAWf 8 Alt, 9 Alt, and 10 Alt are unpaginated, and here I have refered to the document by date and, if available, by title or type of document (e.g., Pro memoria). I have also included titles for some other documents where I felt the title was useful for the reader to know. I have followed these conventions as well for documents in Stadtarchiv Braunschweig, Stadtarchiv Helmstedt, and Stadtarchiv Königslutter, as well as for the other holdings of the Staatsarchiv Wolfenbüttel. Occasionally, I refer to an entire file. I usually do this when my information or impression was gained from reading the whole file.

Niedersächsisches Staatsarchiv-Wolfenbüttel (StAWf)

40 Slg (Verordnungs-Sammlung ältere Teil, 1498–1813)

2 Alt (Kanzlei, [Geheime] Ratsstube)

2 Alt 11164	Collegium medicum, Obersanitätskollegium
2 Alt 11273–412	Hof-, Stadt- und Landmedici und -physici; Societates Medicae; Landchirurgen, Bader; Zahnärzte und Hühneraugenärzte
2 Alt 11413–48	Hebammen
2 Alt 11449–518	Krankheiten und Seuchen und deren Bekämpfung
2 Alt 11519–607	Pest
2 Alt 11608–34	Medizinische Pfuschereien
2 Alt 11635–709	Apotheken, Arzneien-Handel: In Allgemeinen
2 Alt 11873–902	Badestuben

111 Neu (Obersanitätskollegium und Landesmedizinalkollegium)

111 Neu 1–305	Medizinal-Kollegium, Obersanitäts-Kollegium, Landesmedizinal-Kollegium
111 Neu 450–536	Medizinalpersonal, allgemein

111 Neu 537–1036	Ärzte
111 Neu 1037–264	Physikate
111 Neu 1265–541	Chirurgen
111 Neu 1542–614	Bader, Barbiere
111 Neu 1615–77	Militärärzte und -Chirurgen
111 Neu 1651–77	Zahnärzte, Augenärzte, andere Heilkundige ("Marktschreier")
111 Neu 1723–99	Hebammenwesen
111 Neu 3098–134	Pfuschereien
111 Neu 3135–254	Infektionskrankheiten
111 Neu 3348–408	Impfwesen: Pockenerkrankungen; Pockenimpfung, Verfügungen, Bericht; Pockenimpfung in einzelnen Physikaten
111 Neu 3419–45	Medizinische Druckschriften, Verzeichnisse des Medizinalpersonals, Statistiken

1 N Schöppenstedt

6 Blg (Ämter): Blankenburg, Börnecke, Heimburg, Stiege

5 Blg (Stiftsamt Walkenried)

8 Alt (Ämter): Achim, Campe, Eich, Neubrück, Ottenstein, Rothenhof

9 Alt (Fürstliche Gerichte und Vogteien): Bettmar, Hedwigsburg, Vechelde, Wendhausen

10 Alt (Adelige Gerichte): Bodenberg, Bornhausen, Bornum (Wolfenbüttel), Bornum (Helmstedt), Brunkensen, Burgdorf, Deensen, Duttenstedt, Glentorf, Halchter, Hedwigsburg, Hehlen, Linden, Meinbrexen, Scheppau, Wendessen

20 Alt (Dorfbeschreibungen): various

1 Kb (Kirchenbücher der Gemeinde im Bereich der evangelisch-lutherischen braunschweigischen Landeskirche aus der Zeit vor 1815)

Stadtarchiv Braunschweig (StadtB)

B IV 13c: 1–18	Medizinalwesen
B IV 16	Personalia
C I 1: 1–41	Sammlung städtischer und herzoglicher Verordnungen
C II 1	Abdecker
C II 3	Apotheker und Ärzte
C II 4	Bader und Barbiere
C III 2: 16	Materialienpreisen
C III 2: 26	Gildeartikel für den Chirurgen
C III 8: 2	Barbiere
C VII A 8	Abdeckerei
C VII A 14	Accouchir-Anstalt
C VII B 7: I–VII	Barbier- und Baderamt
C VII P 7	Pest und andere epidemische Krankheiten

C VII S 20	Sanitätswesen
C VII S 32	Seelenlisten der hiesigen Einwohner
C VII S 42	Seiltanzer, Gaukler, Hermaphroditen
C VII V 11	Venerisch befundene Personen
C VII W 14	Wahnsinnige
C VII Z 7	Zahnärzte

Stadtarchiv Helmstedt (StadtH)

B V 21c	Ratsapotheke
B V 22 Nr. 1	Nachtrichter und Abdeckerei
B V 22 Nr. 3–4	Abdeckerei
B VII 11 Nr. 1	Ailhaudisches Pulver
B VII 11 Nr. 2	Augenärzte
B VII 11 Nr. 3	Annahme von Bademütter
B VII 11 Nr. 4	Bestellung Bademütter
B VII 11 Nr. 5	Verhaltungsregeln bei der Kinder Blattern
B VII 11 Nr. 8	Einzelschriftsstücke
B VII 11 N. 9, 10	Hebammen
B VII 11a Nr. 1–4	Collegium medicum
B VII 11c Nr. 1–6	Epidemien
B VII 11f Nr. 1	Physikat in Helmstedt
B VII 11k Nr. 1	Verpachtung der Baderei-Neustadt
B VII 11k Nr. 2	Annahme der Bademütter
B VII 17	Allerlei Concessionen des Rats
B VII 24 (2) Nr. 1–4	Bader Gilde
B VII 24 (3) Nr. 1–4	Barbiere Gilde
B VII 12 Nr. 2	Jahrmärkte, Hausieren

Stadtarchiv Königslutter (StadtK)

K II, 2	Die Hebammen zu Königslutter
St I, 1	Beschreibung der Stadt (1761)
St III, 5	Dr. Dedekinds Projekt, Anbau Zucker-Ahorn
St VIII, 1	Verpachtung der Baderei
St VIII, 2	Anstellung der Aerzten
St IX, 17	Liste der Geborenen, Getrauten, Begrabenen

Primary Literature

Ailhaud, Jean. *Kurzer Auszug der merkwürdigsten Genesungen so durch die Ailhaudschen Pulver gewirket worden, aus den dreien Theilen der deutschen Genesungs-Briefe gezogen.* Strasbourg: Lorenz, 1768.

———. *Médicine universelle ou traité de l'origine des maladies.* Carpentras: D. G. Quenin, 1764.

———. *Traité de l'origine des maladies et de l'usage de la poudre purgative. . . . Avec un recueil de plusieurs guérisons apérées par ce remède.* Avignon: J. Rousset, 1742.

————. *Universal-Arzney; oder Abhandlung von dem Ursprunge der Krankheiten und dem Gebrauche des abführenden Pulvers.* Strasbourg: Lorenz, 1765.

Ailhaud, Jean Gaspard. *Lettres de guerison opérées par le reméde universal, pour servir de suite à celles publiées, . . . 1755–1773.* 4 vols. Carpentras: D. G. Quenin, 1765–74.

Alphabethisches Verzeichniss der in dem Herzogthum Braunschweig-Lüneburg belegenen Städte, Flecken, Dörfer, Aemter, Stifter, Klöster, etc. Braunschweig: Vieweg, 1816.

Archiv der medizinischen Polizey und der gemeinnützigen Arzneikunde. Edited by Johann Christian Friedrich Scherf. 6 vols. Leipzig: Mengandchen, 1783–87.

Baldinger, Ernst Gottfried. *Artzeneien, eine physicalisch-medicinische Monatschrift, zum Unterricht allen denen welche den Schaden des Quacksalbers nicht kennen.* 2 vols. Leipzig: Martini, 1766–67.

————. *Biographien jetztlebender Ärzte und Naturforscher in und ausser Deutschland.* Jena: Hartung, 1772.

————. *Ueber Medizinal-Verfassung: Eine Rede.* Offenbach: Weiß & Brede, 1782.

Baldinger, Ernst Gottfried, and Friedrich Börner. *Nachrichten von den vornehmsten Lebensumständen und Schriften jetztlebender berühmter Aerzte und Naturforscher in und um Deutschland.* 3 vols. Wolfenbüttel: Johann Christoph Meissner, 1749–64.

Bartisch, Georg. *"Ophthalmodoyleia," das ist "Augendienst." Neuer und wohlgegründeter Bericht von Ursachen und Erkenntniss aller Gebrechen, Schäden und Mängel der Augen und des Gesichts.* Dresden: Stöckel, 1583. Reprint. Stuttgart: Medicina rara, 1977.

Bäumler, Gottfried Samuel. *Kurze Beschreibung des im Winter-Monat / MDCCXXXIV zu Germersheim und andern Orten am Rhein-Strohm herumgegangenen Hitzigen und Bösartigen Fiebers / Nebst denen dargegen gebrauchten / theils vorbauenden, theils helffenden Mitteln: Zum Nutzen des Ober-Amts Germersheim entworffen.* Strasbourg: Johnann Daniel Dulßecker, 1743.

————. *Mitleidiger Artzt, welcher überhaupt Alle Arme Krancke, insonderheit aber Die abgelegene Land-Leute gründlich und aufrichtig lehret / wie Sie mit Gemeinen Hauß-Mitteln und anderen nicht allzukostbaren Artzeneyen sich selbst curiren können.* 3d ed. Strasbourg: Joh. Reinhold Dulßecker, der Aeltere, 1743. 1st ed., slightly different title. Strasbourg: Joh. Reinhold Dulßecker, der Aeltere, 1736.

————. *Präservirender Artzt; oder gründliche Anweisung wie sich der Mensch durch eine ordentliche Diät, bey guter Gesundheit erhalten, und folglich zu einem hohen und geruhigen Alter gelangen könne.* Strasbourg: Johann Reinhold Dulßecker, der Aeltere, 1738.

Becher, Johann Joachim [?]. *Kluger Haus-Vater, verständige Haus-Mutter, vollkommener Land-Medicus.* Leipzig: Friedrich Groschuff, 1698.

Becker, Rudolf Zacharias. *Noth- und Hülfsbüchlein für Bauersleute, oder lehrreiche Freude- und Trauer-Geschichte des Dorfs Mildheim: Für Junge und Alte beschrieben.* Gotha and Leipzig: Göschen, 1788.

Behrens, Rudolph August. *Oratio de fortuna medicorum aucta in terris Brunsuicensibus quam in primo consessu Collegii Medicin d. XXIII. Mart. ann. MDCCXXXXVII gratulando recitavit.* Braunschweig: Meyer, 1748[?].

Benzler, Johann Lorenz, ed. *Der Bauernfreund in Niedersachsen* Lemgo: Meyer, 1755.

Bourgeois, Louise. *Observations diverses sur la stérilité, perte de fruict, foecondité, accouchements et maladies des femmes et enfants nouveaux naiz: Amplement traitees et heursement practiquées.* Paris: A. Saugrain, 1609.

Brawe, Gerhard Matthias Friedrich. *De coctionis atque criseos in febribus impendimentis variisque noxis inde oriundis*. Göttingen: n.p., 1768.

Brückmann, Urban Friedrich. *Abhandlungen von Edelsteinen*. 2d ed. Braunschweig: Schulbuchhandlung, 1773.

Brunner, J. D. F. *Entdeckung der Irrthümer und Bosheiten der Hebammen*. Solingen, 1740.

Buecking, Johann Jakob Heinrich. *Der Arzt und der Afterarzt*. Stendal: Franzen & Grosse, 1789.

———. *Versuch einer medicinischen und physikalischen Erklärung deutscher Sprichwörter und sprichwörtlicher Redensarten*. Stendal: Franzen & Grosse, 1797. Reprint. Leipzig: Zentralantiquariat der Deutschen Demokratischen Republik, 1976.

Callisen, Adolf Karl Peter. *Medizinisches Schriftsteller-Lexikon der jetztlebenden Ärzte, Wundärzte, Geburtshelfer, Apotheker und Naturforscher aller gebildeten Völker*. 33 vols. Copenhagen: Auf Kosten des Verfassers gedruckt im Königlichen Taubstummen Institut zu Schleswig, 1830–45.

du Coudray, Angélique Marguerite Le Bousier. *Abrégé de l'art des accouchements*. Paris: Widow of Delaguette, 1759. Reprint. Paris: Editions Roger Dacosta, 1976.

Daniel, Christian Friedrich. *Bibliothek der Staats-Arzneikunde oder der gerichtlichen Arzneikunde und medicinischen Polizey von ihrem Anfange bis auf das Iahr 1784*. Halle: Hemmerde, 1785.

Dedekind, Johann Julius Wilhelm. *Curart der Pocken*. Holzminden: Fleckeisen in Helmstedt, 1791.

Dehne, Johann Christian Konrad. *Versuch einer vollständigen Abhandlung von dem Maiwurme und dessen Anwendung in der Wuth und Wasserscheu: Nebst Anmerkungen über die Natur dieser Krankheit, ihrer ansteckenden Eigenschaften und Behandlung*. 2 vols. Leipzig: Weygand, 1788.

[Dietz, Johann]. *Master Johann Dietz: Surgeon in the Army of the Great Elector and Barber to the Royal Court*. New York: Dutton, 1923.

"Erörterung der Frage: ob es für den Landmann nützlich und zuträglich sey, daß auf jedem Dorf sich ein Apotheker und ein Wundarzt befinde?" *Beiträge zum Archiv der medizinischen Polizei und der Volksarzneikunde* 4, no. 2 (1793): 134–35.

Ettner, Johann Christoph von. *Des getreuen Eckarths Medicinischer Maul-Affe Oder der Entlarvte Markt-Schreyer*. Frankfurt and Leipzig: Bey Michael Rohrlachs seel. Wittib und Erben, 1720.

———. *Des getreuen Eckarths unvorsichtige Heb-Amme, in welcher wie eine Heb-Amme oder Kinder-Mutter, die ihr Gewissen wohl in acht nehmen will, beschaffen seyn, und wie sie nebenst dem erforderten Medico so wohl denen Unverheuratheten, als Verheuratheten und Kindern in ihren Kranckheiten und Zufällen getreulich beystehen und helffen soll*. Leipzig: J. F. Braun, 1715.

———. *Des getreuen Eckhardts unwürdiger Doctor, In welchem Wie ein Medicus, der rechtschaffen handeln will / beschaffen seyn soll; Hernach bewährteste Arzney-Mittel in allerhand Kranckheiten und Zufällen Menschlichen Leibes zu gebrauchen*. Ausburg and Leipzig: bey Lorentz und Gottlieb Göbels Seel. Erben Buchhändlung, 1697.

———. *Des getreuen Eckhardts verwegener Chirurgus, In welchem Wie ein rechtschaffener Chirurgus beschaffen seyn solle / was er für Tugenden an sich nehmen / und welcherley Laster er zu fliehen*. Ausburg and Leipzig: bey Lorentz und Gottlieb Göbels Seel. Erben Buchhändlung, 1698.

Faust, Bernhard Christoph. *Gedanken über Hebammen und Hebammenschulen auf dem Lande*. Frankfurt: Andreä, 1784.

———. *Gesundheits-Katechismus zum Gebrauche in den Schulen und beym häuslichen Unterrichte*. 2d ed. Bückeburg and Leipzig: Kummer, 1794.

Finke, Leonhard Ludwig. *Versuch einer allgemeinen medicinisch-praktischen Geographie worin der historische Theil der einheimischen Völker- und Staaten-Arzneykunde vorgetragen wird*. 3 vols. Leipzig: Weidmann, 1792–95.

Fischer, Christian Ernst. *Versuch einer Anleitung zur medizinischen Armenpraxis*. Göttingen: Dieterich, 1799.

Frank, Johann Peter. *System einer vollständigen medicinischen Polizey*. 9 vols. Mannheim: C. F. Schwan, 1779–1827.

Fredersdorff, Leopold Friedrich. *Anweisung für angehende Justizbeamter und Unterrichter*. 2 vols. Lemgo: Meyer, 1772.

———. *Practische Anleitung zur Land-Polizey aus allgemeinen Grundsätzen mit Hinweis auf die Fürstl. Braunschweigischen Wolfenbüttelschen Landes-Gesetze*. Pyrmont: Helwing, 1800.

Gesenius, Carl. *Das Meyerrecht, mit vorzüglicher Hinsicht auf den Wolfenbüttelschen Theils des Herzogthums Braunschweig-Lüneburg*. 2 vols. Wolfenbüttel: Albrecht, 1801, 1803.

Gesenius, Wilhelm. *Ueber das epidemische faulichte Gallenfieber in den Jahren 1785 und 1786*. Leipzig: Jacobäer, 1788.

———. *Versuch einer lepidopterologischen Encyklopadie oder Handbuch für angehende Schmetterlingssammler*. Erfurt: bey Georg Adam Keyser, 1786.

Goldschmidt, Jonas. *Volksmedizin im Nordwestlichen Deutschland*. Bremen: J. G. Heyse, 1854. Reprint. Leer: Schuster, 1978.

Gotthard, Joseph Friedrich. *Leitfaden für angehende Aerzte Kranke zu prüfen und Krankheiten zu erforschen mit einer Kranken- und Witterungsbeobachtungstabelle*. Erlangen: Bey Johann Jakob Palm, 1793.

Gruner, Christian Gottfried. *Almanach für Aerzte und Nichtaerzte*. Jena: Cuno, 1782–96.

———. *Gedanken von der Arzneiwissenschaft*. Breslau: Kora, 1772.

Hassel, Georg, and Karl Bege. *Geographisch-statische Beschreibung der Fürstenthümer Wolfenbüttel und Blanckenburg*. 2 vols. Braunschweig: Vieweg, 1802–3.

Helmuth, Johann Heinrich. *Volksnaturlehre zur Dämpfung des Aberglaubens*. Braunschweig: Waisenhausbuchhandlung, 1786.

Hildebrandt, Georg Friedrich. *Bemerkungen und Beobachtungen über die Pocken in der Epidemie des Jahres 1787*. Braunschweig: Schulbuchhandlung, 1788.

———. *Lehrbuch der Anatomie des Menschen*. 4 vols. Braunschweig: Schulbuchhandlung, 1789–92.

———. *Taschenbuch für die Gesundheit auf das Jahr 1801*. Erlangen: Heyder, 1801.

Hinze, August. *Lexicon aller Herzogl.[ichen] Braunschweigischen Verordnungen, welche die medicinische Policey betreffen*. Stendal: Franzen & Grosse, 1793.

Holdefreund, Johann Röttger Salomo. *Abhandlung von epidemischen Stickhusten der Kinder*. Helmstedt: Fleckeisen, 1775.

Hoorn, Johan von. *Die Zwo um ihrer Gottesfurcht und Treue willen von GOTT wohlbe-*

lohnte Weh-Mütter Siphra und Pua. 2d ed. Stockholm and Leipzig: bey Gottfried Kiesewettern, 1737.

Horenburg, Anne. *Wohlgemeynender und Nöhtiger Unterricht der Heeb-Amme.* Hannover and Wolfenbüttel, 1700.

Hoven, Friedrich Wilhelm von. *Lebenserinngerungen.* Edited by Hans-Günther Thalheim. Berlin: Rütten & Loening, 1984.

———. *Versuch über das Wechselfieber und seiner Heilung besonders durch die Chinarinde.* 2 vols. Winterthur: Heinrich Steiner, 1789–90.

Hufeland, Christoph Wilhelm. *Bemerkungen über die natürlichen und künstlichen Blattern zu Weimar im Jahr 1788.* Leipzig: Bey G. J. Göschen, 1789.

———. *Die Kunst das menschlichen Leben zu verlängern.* Jena: Gotthold Ludwig Fiedler, in der akademischen Buchhandlung, 1797.

Juncker, Johann Christian Wilhelm. *Gemeinnützige Vorschläge und Nachrichten über das beste Verhalten der Menschen in Rücksicht der Pockenkrankheit: Erster Versuch über die mittlern Stände nebst einem Anhange für Ärzte.* Halle: Schwetschke & Sohn, 1792

———. *Grundsätze der Volksarzneikunde: Zur bequemeren Benutzung des mündlichen Vortrages seinen Herren Zuhörern entworfen.* Halle: Waisenhaus, 1787.

Kerstner, Christian Wilhelm. *Medizinisches Gelehrtenlexikon: Darinnen die Leben der berühmtesten Aerzte, sammt deren wichtigsten Schriften, sonderbaresten Entdeckungen und merkwürdigsten Streitigkeiten etc.* Jena: n.p., 1740.

Klinge, J. W. G. "Einige physisch-medicinische Bemerkungen über die Gegend und das Klima der Kurhannoverischen freyen Bergstadt St. Andreasberg, so wie auch über die Lebensweise und Krankheiten der Bewohner derselben." *Journal der Arzneykunde und practischen Wundarzneykunst* 6 (1798): 880–904.

Koch, Heinrich Andreas. *Versuch einer pragmatischen Geschichte des Durchlauchtigsten Hauses Braunschweig und Luneburg.* Braunschweig: Waisenhaus, 1764.

Kortum, Carl Georg Theodor. *Beiträge zur praktischen Arzneiwissenschaft.* Göttingen: Vandenhoeck & Ruprecht, 1796.

"Kritischer Versuch über das Wort Aufklärung, zur endlichen Beylegung der darüber geführten Streitigkeiten." *Deutsche Monatschrift* 1790: 11–44, 205–33.

Krügelstein, Johann Friedrich. *Noth- und Hülfsbüchlein in der Ruhr und epidemischen Krankheiten überhaupt.* Ohrduff: n.p., 1803.

Krünitz, Johann Georg. *D. Johann Georg Krünitz's ökonomisch-technologische Encyklopädie oder allgemeines System der Staats-, Stadt-, Haus-, und Landwirthschaft und der Kunstgeschichte in alphabetischer Ordnung.* 242 vols. Berlin: J. Pauli, 1773–1858.

Kurzer Auszug des Systems der Herren von Ailhaud über den Ursprung der Krankheiten. Strasbourg: Christmann & Levrault, 1766.

Lange, Johann Heinrich. *Briefe über verschiedene Gegenstände der Naturgeschichte und Arzneykunst.* Lüneburg and Leipzig: Johann Friedrich Wilhelm Lemke, 1775.

———. *Tentamen medico-physicum de remediis Brunsuicensium domesticis.* Braunschweig: Schulbuchhandlung, 1765.

Lentin, Lebrecht Friedrich Benjamin. *Beobachtungen der epidemischen und einiger sporadischer Krankheyten am Oberharze vom Jahre 1777 bis incl. 1782.* Dessau and Leipzig: Buchhandlung der Gelehrten, 1783.

———. *Beobachtungen einiger Krankheiten.* Göttingen: Vandenhoeck, 1774.

———. *Denkwürdigkeiten, betreffend Luftbeschaffenheit, Lebensart, Gesundheit und Krankheit der Einwohner Clausthals, in den Jahren 1774 bis 1777*. Hannover: Hahn, 1800.

Loeber, Christian Joseph. *Anfangsgründe der Wundarzneykunst*. Langensalza: Schneider, 1770.

———. *Belustigungen in den Badern von Dresden: Eine Wochenschrift*. Dresden: n.p., 1778.

———. *De cordis fabrica et functione atque de sanguinis per cor et vasa sanguinea circulatione*. Erfurt: n.p., 1767.

———. *Freuden Hans Hubrig's: Ein 112jähr.[iger] Greis*. Dresden: n.p., 1778.

———. *Sendschreiben von einer glücklich geheilten Lungenentzundung Hans Hubrigs*. Friedrichstadt: n.p., 1767.

———. *Sendschreiben von wiedergekommenden Pocken nach der Einpfropfung*. Erfurt: n.p., 1767.

[Martini, Johann Bernhard]. *Dispensatoruium pharmacevticvum brvnsvicense*. Braunschweig: Waisenhaus, 1777.

May, Franz Anton. *Die Hämorrhoiden: Den Freunden dauerhafter Gesundheit gewidmet*. Berlin and Stettin: auf Kosten des Publici, 1775.

———. *Stolpertus: Ein junger Arzt am Krankenbette*. New ed. 5 vols. Mannheim: Schwan und Götz, 1800–1807. Vol. 4: *Stolpertus der Polizei-Arzt im Gerichtshof der medizinischen Polizeigesetzgebung von einem patriotischen Pfläzer*. 1802.

Metzger, Johann Daniel. *Beytrage zur Geschichte der Frühlings-Epidemie in Jahre 1782*. Königsberg und Leipzig: Hartung, 1782.

———. *Vermischte medicinische Schriften*. Königsberg: n.p., 1782.

Meusel, Johann. *Lexikon der vom Jahre 1750 bis 1800 verstorbenen teutschen Schriftsteller*. 4th ed. 15 vols. Leipzig: G. Fleischer, der Jungere, 1802–16.

Meyer, Johann Friedrich. *Verbesserter Schreib-Calender / Auf das Jahr nach Christi Geburt [. . .] Wobey der Julianische, Gregorianische und ein besondern Haus-Calender wie auch eine Genealogische Verzeichnis aller jetzt-lebenden Hochst- und Hohen Häuser in Europa: Mit Fleiß gestellet durch Johannem Meyerum. Quedl. Saxon. Mit herzogl. Braunschw. Lüneb. gnädigsten Privilegio*. Braunschweig: F. W. Meyer, 1720.

Nemnich, Philipp Andreas. *Lexicon nosologicum polyglotton omnium morborum, symptomatum vitiorumque et affectionum propria nomina decem diversis linguis explicata continens*. Hamburg: C. Müller, 1801.

Nolde, Adolph Friedrich. *Notizen zur Kultur-Geschichte der Geburtshilfe in dem Herzogthum Braunschweig*. Erfurt: Hennings, 1807.

Nootnagel, Daniel. "Vorschlag Aberglauben und Vorurtheile auszurotten." *Deutsches Museum* 1 (1778): 148–55.

Osterhausen, Johann Karl. *Ueber medicinische Aufklärung*. Zurich: Geßner, 1798.

Paullini, Christian Franz. *Die heylsame Dreck-Apotheke, Wie nemlich mit vielen verachteten Dingen, Fast alle, ja auch die schwerste, gifftigste Kranckheiten, und bezauberte Schäden von Haupt biss zun Fussen, inn- und äusserlich curiret worden*. Berlin: Georgi, 1714.

———. *Das Hoch-und-Wohl-gelahrte Teutsche Frauen-Zimmer Nochmals mit merckliche Zusatz vorgestellet*. Frankfurt and Leipzig: J. C. Stößel, 1705.

Richter, Benjamin. *Den grossen Unterschied zwischen rechtschaffener Medicorum und deren Quacksalber medicinischen Wissenschaften und Curen: Kurtz und deutlich beschrieben*. Görlitz: n.p., 1716.

Rinna von Sarenbach, Ernst. *Repertorium der vorzüglichsten Kurarten, Heilmittel, Opera-tionsmethoden etc. welche während der letzten vier Jahrzehnde angewendet oder empfohlen worden sind: Für Aerzte und Wundärzte als klinische Memorabilien aus der Literatur jenes Zeitraums zusammengetragen und alphabetisch geordnet.* Also appeared as *Klinisches Jahrbuch.* 4 vols. Vienna: Anton Strauß's sel. Witwe; Günz: Carl Reichard, 1833–36.

Rochow, Friedrich Eberhard von. *Der Kinderfreund: Ein Lesebuch zum Gebrauch in Landschulen.* Munich: J. B. Strobl, 1789.

Roose, Theodor Georg August. *Taschenbuch für gerichtliche Aerzte und Wundärzte bei gesetzmässigen Leichenöffnungen.* Bremen: Wilmans, 1800.

Rüling, Johann Philipp. *Physisch-medicinisch-ökonomisch Beschreibung der zum Fürsten-thum Göttingen gehörigen Stadt Northeim und ihrer umliegenden Gegend.* Göttingen: Vandenhök & Ruprecht, 1779.

Salzmann, Christian Gotthilf. *Moralisches Elementarbuch, nebst einer Anleitung zum nützlichen Gebrauch desselben.* Leipzig: Hubert Göbels, 1785.

Schlözer, August Ludwig. *Briefwechsel meist historischen und politischen Inhalts.* 3 vols. Göttingen: Vandenhöck & Ruprecht, 1780–82.

Schlüter, Friedrich. *Immerwährende Gesundheits-Kalender oder Hausbuch zur Kenntniß und Erhaltung der Gesundheit.* Braunschweig: Schulbuchhandlung, 1799.

———. *Pockenbuch oder höchstnöthiger und bewährter Unterricht an alle Eltern deren Kinder die Pocken noch nicht gehabt haben.* 2d enlarged ed. Braunschweig: Schulbuchhand-lung, 1798.

[Schrader, Catharina Geertruida]. *C. G. Schrader's Memoryboeck van de vrouwens: Het notitieboek van een Friese vroedvrouw, 1693–1745.* With an introduction by M. J. Lieburg and commentary by G. J. Kloostermann. 2d ed. Amsterdam: Rodophi, 1984.

———. *"Mother and Child Were Saved": The Memoirs (1693–1740) of the Frisian Midwife Catharina Schrader.* Translated and annotated by Hilary Marland. With introduc-tory essays by M. J. van Lieburg and G. J. Kloostermann. Amsterdam: Rodophi, 1987.

Schreger, Bernhard Nathan Gottlieb. *Kritisches Dispensatorium der geheimen, spezi-fischen und universellen Heilmittle die nach ihren Erfindern, ihren Wirkungen, oder nach denen Krankheiten, in denen sie empfohlen werden, benennt worden.* Leipzig: Weygand, 1795.

Schwabe, Ernst. *Anweisung zu den Pflichten und Geschäften eines Stadt- oder Land-Physikus.* 2 vols. Erfurt: Keyser, 1786–87.

Selle, Christian Gottlieb. *Medicina clinica oder Handbuch der medicinischen Praxis.* Berlin: C. F. Himburg, 1802.

———. *Rudimenta pyretologiae methodica.* [Mediolani]: B. Cominus, 1787.

Siegemund, Justine. *Die König.[lichen] Preußische und Chur-Brandenb.[urgischen] Hof-Wehe-Mutter.* Leipzig: Johann Friedrich Braun, 1715.

Stark, Johann Christian. *Versuch einer wahren und falschen Politik der Aerzte, zu Vorle-sungen bestimmt.* Jena: Voigt, 1784.

Sternberg, J. H. *Erinnerungen und Zweifel gegen die Lehre der Aerzte von dem schweren Zahnen der Kinder.* Hannover: Helwing, 1802.

Stoll, Johann. *Staatswissenschaftliche Untersuchungen und Erfahrungen über das Medicinal-*

wesen nach seiner Verfasssung, Gesetzgebung und Verwaltung. 3 vols. Zurich: Orell, 1812–14.

Stolle, Gottlieb. *Anleitung zur Historie der medizinischen Gelahrheit.* 3 vols. Jena: J. Meyers, seel. Wittwe, 1731.

Struve, Christian August. *Interessante Anekdoten für Aerzte und Nichtärzte: Zur Aufheiterung und belehrenden Unterhaltung.* Görliz: bei Hermsdorf und Anton, 1796.

Süssmilch, Johann Peter. *Die göttliche Ordnung in denen Veranderungen des menschlichen Geschlechts.* 4th enlarged ed. 3 vols. Berlin: Buchhandlung der Realschule, 1775–76.

Tissot, Samuel August André David. *Advice to the People in General with Regard to their Health.* Translated by J. Kirkpatrick. 2 vols. Boston: Mein & Fleeming, 1767.

———. "An Account of the Disease Called Ergot, in French, from Its Supposed Cause, viz., Vitiated Rye." *Philosophical Transactions* 1 (1765): 106–26.

———. *Anleitung für das Landvolk in Absicht auf seine Gesundheit.* Translated by H. C. Hirzel. 2d enlarged ed. Augsburg & Innsbruck: Wolff, 1766.

———. *Avis au peuple sur sa santé.* Lausanne: J. Zimmerli, 1761.

"Übersicht des Medizinalwesens der Herzogthums Braunschweig." *Medizinische National-Zeitung für Deutschland* 2, no. 15 (11 March 1799): 237–40.

Unzer, Johann August. *Der Arzt.* 12 vols. Hamburg: n.p., 1760–64.

———. *Medicinisches Handbuch.* Lüneburg and Hamburg: G. C. Berth, 1770.

———. *Ueber die Ansteckung besonders der Pocken: In einer Beurtheilung der neuen Hofmannischen Pockentheorien.* Leipzig: Johann Friedrich Junius, 1778.

Vogel, Samuel Gottlieb. *Das Kranken-Examen: Oder allgemeine philosophische medicinische Untersuchungen zur Erforschung der Krankheiten des menschlichen Körpers.* Stendal: Franzen & Grosse, 1796.

Wachsmuth, Johann Heinrich. *Panacea solaris, oder Universal-Gold-Balsam, wodurch Alle Krankheiten des Menschlichen Leibes, so wohl innerliche as äuserliche, besonders Schlag-Fluß, Jammer, Podagra, und alle Arten der Gicht, Stein, Krebs und verstopfte Monaths-Zeiten etc. glücklich durch göttlichen Seegen gehoben worden.* Nordhausen: n.p., 1733.

———. *Spiritus vitae catholicus, oder Universal-Lebens-Spiritus, wodurch in Alchymia alles was zum Universal nöthig ist, in Medicina aber in Curirung der Kranckheiten ein grosses kan ausgerichtet werden.* Nordhausen: n.p., n.d.

Weber, Friedrich August, ed. *Onomatologia medico-practica Encyklopädisches Handbuch für ausübende Aerzte in alphabetischer Ordnung ausgearbeitet von einer Gesellschaft von Aerzten.* 4 vols. Nuremburg: Raspe, 1783–86.

Weigel, Christoph. *Abbildung der gemein-nützlichen Haupt-Stände von denen Regenten und ihren so in Friedens- als Krieg-Zeiten zugeordneten Bedienten an biß auf alle Künstler und Handwercker nach jedes Ambts- und Beruffs-Verrichtungen weist nach dem Leben gezeichnet.* Regensburg: n.p., 1698.

Wichmann, Johann Ernst. *Beytrag zur Geschichte der Kriebelkrankheit im Jahre 1770.* Leipzig and Celle: Gsellius, 1771.

Zedler, Johann Heinrich. *Grosses vollständiges Universal-Lexikon, aller Wissenschaften und Künste.* 64 vols. Halle and Leipzig: Johann Heinrich Zedler, 1732–50.

Zerrenner, Heinrich Gottlieb. *Volksbuch: Ein faßlicher Unterricht in nüzlichen Erkenntnissen und Sachen mittelst einer zusammenhängenden Erzehlung für Landleute um sie verständig, gut, wohlhabend, zufriedener und für die Gesellschaft brauchbarer zu machen.* Magdeburg: Scheidhauerschen Buchhandlung, 1787.

Zimmermann, Johann George von. *Von der Ruhr unter dem Volke im Jahre 1765, und denen mit derselben eingedrungenen Vorurtheilen, nebst einigen allgemeinen Aussichten in die Heilung dieser Vorurtheile.* Zurich: Füeßli, 1767. New ed. Zurich: Füeßli, 1787.

Zückert, Johann Friedrich. *Medizinisches Tischbuch oder Cur und Präservation der Krankheiten durch diätetische Mittel.* Berlin: Mylius 1771.

———. *Von den wahren Mitteln, die Entvölkerung eines Landes in epidemischen Zeiten zu verhüten.* Berlin: Mylius, 1773.

Secondary Literature

Abel, Wilhelm. "Landwirtschaft, 1648–1800." In *Handbuch des deutschen Wirtschafts- und Sozialgeschichte*, edited by Hermann Aubin and Wolfgang Zorn, 1: 495–530. 2 vols. Stuttgart: Union, 1976–78.

Achilles, Walther. *Die steuerliche Belastung der braunschweigischen Landwirtschaft und ihr Beitrag zu den Staatseinnahmen im 17. und 18. Jahrhundert.* Hildesheim: August Lax, 1972.

———. *Vermögensverhältnisse braunschweigischer Bauernhöfe im 17. und 18. Jahrhundert.* Stuttgart: Gustav Fischer, 1965.

Ackerknecht, Erwin H. *Geschichte der Medizin.* 4th rev. ed. Stuttgart: Ferdinard Enke, 1979.

Ackermann, Evelyn Bernette. *Health Care in the Parisian Countryside, 1880–1914.* New Brunswick, N.J.: Rutgers University Press, 1990.

Adlung, Alfred, and Georg Urdang. *Grundriß der Geschichte der deutschen Pharmazie.* Berlin: J. Springer, 1935.

Agena, Carl-August. "Der Amtmann im 17. und 18. Jahrhundert—Ein Beitrag zur Geschichte des Richter- und Beamtentums." Diss., University of Göttingen, 1973.

Albrecht, Peter. *Die Förderung des Landesausbaues im Herzogtum Braunschweig-Wolfenbüttel im Spiegel der Verwaltungsakten des 18. Jahrhunderts (1671–1806).* Braunschweig: Waisenhaus, 1980.

———. "Versuche zur Popularisierung der Blatterninokulation in der Stadt Braunschweig von 1754 bis 1780." Manuscript.

Artelt, Walter. "Das medizinische Braunschweig um 1770." *Medizinhistorisches Journal* 1 (1966): 240–60.

Barthel, Christian. *Medizinische Polizey und medizinische Aufklärung: Aspekte des öffentlichen Gesundheitsdiskurses im 18. Jahrhundert.* Frankfurt: Campus, 1989.

Beier, Lucinda McCray. *Sufferers and Healers: The Experience of Illness in Seventeenth-Century England.* London: Routledge and Kegan Paul, 1987.

Beneke, Otto. *Von unehrlichen Leuten: Culturhistorische Studien und Geschichten aus vergangenen Tagen deutscher Gewerbe und Dienste, mit besonderer Rücksicht auf Hamburg.* 2d rev. ed. Berlin: Hertz, 1889.

Berkner, Lutz. "Inheritance, Land Tenure and Peasant Family Structure: A German Regional Comparison." In *Family and Inheritance: Rural Society in Western Europe, 1200–1800*, edited by Jack Goody and E. P. Thompson, 71–95. Cambridge: Cambridge University Press, 1976.

Biraben, Jean-Noël. "Histoire de classifications de causes de décès et de maladies aux XVII\u{e} et XIX\u{e} siècles." In *Mensch und Gesundheit in der Geschichte / Les Hommes et la santé dans lans l'histoire*, edited by Arthur E. Imhof, 23–34. Husum: Matthicsen, 1984.

Black, Anthony. *Guilds & Civic Society in European Political Thought from the Twelfth Century to the Present.* Ithaca, N.Y.: Cornell University Press, 1984.

Blackbourn, David, and Geoff Eley. *The Peculiarities of German History: Bourgeois Society and Politics in Nineteenth-Century Germany.* Oxford: Oxford University Press, 1984.

Blécourt, Willem de, Willem Frijhoff, and Marijke Gijswijt-Hofstra, eds. *Grenzen van genezing: Gezondheid, ziekte en genezen in Nederland, zestiende tot begin twintigste eeuw.* Hilversum: Verloren, 1993.

Blickle, Peter. *Studien zur geschichtlichen Bedeutung des deutschen Bauernstandes.* Stuttgart: Gustav Fischer, 1989.

———. "Untertanen der Frühneuzeit: Zur Rekonstruktion der politischen Kultur and der sozialen Wirklichkeit Deutschlands im 17. Jahrhundert." *Vierteljahrschrift für Sozial- und Wirtschaftsgeschichte* 70 (1983): 483–522.

Blickle, Renate. "Nahrung und Eigentum als Kategorien in der ständischen Gesellschaft." In *Ständische Gesellschaft und soziale Mobilität*, edited by Wilfried Schulze, 73–93. Munich: R. Oldenbourg, 1988.

Bornstedt, Wilhelm. *Chronik von Stöckheim: Siedlungsgeographie, Sozial- und Kulturgeschichte eines braunschweigischen Dorfes.* Stockheim bei Braunschweig: ACO, 1967.

———. *Geschichte des Braunschweigischen Bauerntums: Ein Beitrag zur Rechts-, Sozial- und Kulturalgeschichte der ländlichen Bevölkerung in Südostniedersachsen in der vorindustriellen Zeit.* Braunschweig: Landeskreisverwaltung, 1970.

Bourdieu, Pierre. *Outline of a Theory of Practice.* Cambridge: Cambridge University Press, 1977.

Bouvet, Maurice. *Histoire de la pharmacie en France des origines à nos jours.* Paris: Editions Occitania, 1937.

———. "Un Exempel de publicité médico-pharmaceutique par brochures au XVIIIᵉ siècle: Le remède universel au poudre d'Ailhaud." *La Pharmacie française* 26 (May 1922): 193–207.

Braun, Hans-Joachim. "Economic Theory and Policy in Germany, 1750–1800." *Journal of European Economic History* 4 (1975): 301–22.

Breuer, Stefan. "Sozialdisciplinierung: Problem and Problemverlagerungen eines Konzepts bei Max Weber, Gerhard Oestreich and Michel Foucault." In *Soziale Sicherheit und soziale Disziplinierung*, edited by Christoph Sachße and Florian Tennstedt, 45–49. Stuttgart: Suhrkamp, 1986.

Breuer, Stefan, Hubert Treiber, and Manfred Walther. "Entstehungsbedingungen des modernen Anstaltstaates." In *Entstehung und Strukturwandels des Staates*, edited by Stefan Breuer and Hubert Treiber, 75–153. Opladen: Westdeutscher, 1982.

Brewer, John, and Roy Porter, eds., *Consumption and the World of Goods.* London: Routledge, 1993.

Breyer, Harald. *Johann Peter Frank: "Fürst unter den Ärzten Europas".* Leipzig: S. Hirzel, 1983.

Broman, Thomas Hoyt. "Rethinking Professionalization: Theory, Practice and Professional Ideology in Eighteenth-Century German Medicine." *Journal of Modern History* 67 (1995): 835–72.

———. "The Transformation of Academic Medicine in Germany, 1780–1820." Diss., Princeton University, 1987.

Brown, Clive. *Louis Spohr: A Critical Biography*. Cambridge: Cambridge University Press, 1984.

Brown, P. S. "Medicines Advertised in Eighteenth-Century Bath Newspapers." *Medical History* 20 (1976): 152–68.

Brügelmann, Jan. *Der Blick des Arztes auf die Krankheit im Alltag, 1779–1850: Medizinische Topographien als Quelle für die Sozialgeschichte der Gesundheitswesens*. Berlin: Freie Universität, 1982.

Brunner, Otto. "Hausväterliteratur." In *Handwörterbuch der Sozialwissenschaften*. 5th ed. 12 vols. Stuttgart: Gustav Fischer, 1956–65.

Bubb, Werner. *Das Stadtarztamt zu Basel: Seine Entwicklungsgeschichte vom Jahre 1529 bis zur Gegenwart*. Zurich: Leemann, 1942.

Buchanan, James H. *Patient Encounters: The Experience of Disease*. Charlottesville, Va.: University Press of Virginia, 1989.

Buck, Michael R. *Medicinischer Volksglauben und Volksaberglauben aus Schwaben: Eine kulturgeschichtliche Skizze*. Ravensburg: Dorn, 1865.

Bulst, Niethard, and Robert Delort, eds. *Maladies et société (XIIᵉ–XVIIᵉ siècles): Actes du colloque de Bielefeld novembre 1986*. Paris: Editions du Centre nationale de la recherche scientifique, 1989.

Burghard, Klaus. *Die Tollwuttherapie im Jahrhundert vor Pasteur*. Frankfurt am Main: Peter Lang, Europäische Hochschulschriften, 1991.

Burke, Peter, and Roy Porter, eds. *The Social History of Language*. Cambridge, Eng. and New York: Cambridge University Press, 1987.

Burkhard, Georg. *Die deutschen Hebammenordnungen von ihren ersten Anfängen bis auf die Neuzeit*. Leipzig: W. Engelmann, 1912.

Büttner, Ludwig. *Fränkische Volksmedizin: Ein Beitrag zur Volkskunde Ostfrankens*. Erlangen: Palm & Enke, 1935.

Bynum, William F., and V. Nutton, eds. *Theories of Fever from Antiquity to the Enlightenment*. London: Wellcome Institute for the History of Medicine, 1981.

Bynum, William F., and Roy Porter, eds. *Companion Encyclopedia of the History of Medicine*. 2 vols. London: Routledge, 1993.

———. *Medical Fringe & Medical Orthodoxy, 1750–1850*. London: Croom Helm, 1987.

———. *Medicine and the Five Senses*. Cambridge: Cambridge University Press, 1993.

Camporesi, Pietro. *The Incorruptible Flesh: Bodily Mutation and Mortification in Religion and Folklore*. Translated by Tania Croft-Murray and Helen Elsom. Cambridge: Cambridge University Press, 1988.

Carmichael, Ann. *Plague and the Poor in Renaissance Florence*. Cambridge: Cambridge University Press, 1986.

Chartier, Roger. *Cultural History: Between Practices and Representations*. Ithaca, N.Y.: Cornell University Press, 1988.

Childers, Thomas. "Political Sociology and the 'Linguistic Turn.'" *Central European History* 22 (1989): 381–93.

Chisick, Harvey. *The Limits of Reform in the Enlightenment: Attitudes Toward the Education of the Lower Classes in Eighteenth-Century France*. Princeton, N.J.: Princeton University Press, 1981.

Coleman, William. "Health and Hygiene in the *Encyclopédie*: A Medical Doctrine for the Bourgeoisie." *Journal of the History of Medicine* 29 (1974): 399–421.

"Das Collegium Anatomico Chirurgicum und die Accouchir-Anstalt in Braunschweig" in *Zum Aufbau der Hebammenschulen in Niedersachsen im 18. und 19. Jahrhundert von Dokumenten, Darstellungen und Instrumenten in der Wandelhalle des Niedersächsischen Landtags vom 23. September - 16. Oktober 1981.* Exhibition catalog. Hannover: Niedersächsischens Sozialminister, 1981.

Cook, Harold J. *The Decline of the Old Medical Regime in London.* Ithaca, N.Y.: Cornell University Press, 1986.

———. *Trials of an Ordinary Doctor: James Groenevelt in Seventeenth Century London.* Baltimore: Johns Hopkins University Press, 1994.

Cook, Trevor. *Samuel Hahnemann: The Founder of Homeopathic Medicine.* Wellingborough, Northamptonshire: Thorsons, 1981.

Corsi, Pietro, and Paul Weindling, eds. *Information Sources in the History of Medicine and Science.* London: Butterworth Scientific, 1983.

Crew, David F. "*Alltagsgeschichte*: A New Social History 'From Below.' " *Central European History* 22 (1989): 394–407.

Cunningham, Andrew, and Roger French, eds. *The Medical Enlightenment of the Eighteenth Century.* Cambridge: Cambridge University Press, 1990.

Danckert, Werner. *Unehrliche Leute: Die verfemten Berufe.* Bern: Francke, 1963.

Darmon, Pierre. *La Longue Traque de la variole: Les Pionniers de la médicine preventive.* Paris: Libraire académique Perrin, 1986.

Darnton, Robert. "The History of Mentalities: Recent Writings on Revolution, Criminality, and Death in France." In *Structure, Consciousness and History*, edited by Richard H. Brown and Stanford M. Lyman, 106–36. Cambridge, Mass.: Harvard University Press, 1978.

———. *The Literary Underground of the Old Regime.* Cambridge, Mass.: Harvard University Press, 1982.

Davis, Natalie Zemon. *Fiction in the Archives: Pardon Tales and their Tellers in Sixteenth-Century France.* Stanford, Calif.: Stanford University Press, 1987.

Desaive, Jean-Paul, et al. *Médicins, climat et épidémies à la fin du XVIII siècle.* Paris: Mouton, 1971.

Devlin, Judith. *The Superstitious Mind: French Peasants and the Supernatural in the Nineteenth Century.* New Haven, Conn.: Yale University Press, 1987.

Diepgen, Paul. *Deutsche Volksmedizin: Wissenschaftliche Heilkunde und Kultur.* Stuttgart: Enke, 1935.

Döhnel, Karl-Rudolf. *Das Anatomisch-Chirurgische Institut in Braunschweig, 1750–1869.* Braunschweig: Waisenhaus, 1957.

Dornheim, Jutta. *Kranksein im dörflichen Alltag.* Tübingen: Vereinigung für Volkskunde, 1983.

Dorwart, Reinhold August. *The Prussian Welfare State Before 1740.* Cambridge, Mass.: Harvard University Press, 1971.

———. "The Royal College of Medicine and Public Health in Brandenburg-Prussia 1685–1740." *Medical History* 2 (1958): 13–23.

Ducret, Siegfried. *Fürstenberger Porzellan.* 3 vols. Vol. 1: *Geschichte der Fabrik.* Braunschweig: Klinkhard & Biermann, 1965.

Duden, Barbara. *Geschichte unter der Haut: Ein Eisenacher Arzt und seine Patientinnen um 1730.* Stuttgart: Klett-Cotta, 1987.

Dumont, Franz. "Nicht nur Hölderlin: Das ärztliche Besuchsbuch Soemmerrings als Quelle für sein soziales Umfeld in Frankfurt am Main." *Medizinhistorisches Journal* 28 (1993): 123–55.

Eckart, Wolfgang, and Johanna Geyer-Kordesch, eds. *Heilberufe und Kranke im 17. und 18. Jahrhundert.* Münster: Burg, 1982.

Elias, Norbert. *The Civilizing Process.* Translated by Edmund Jephcott. 2 vols. Oxford: Blackwell, 1978.

———. *The Court Society.* Translated by Edmund Jephcott. Oxford: Blackwell, 1983.

Eisenberg, Leon. "Disease and Illness: Distinctions Between Professional and Popular Ideas of Sickness." *Culture, Medicine and Psychiatry* 1 (1972): 9–23.

Emch-Dériaz, Antoinette. "The Non-Naturals Made Easy." In *The Popularization of Medicine, 1650–1850,* edited by Roy Porter, 134–59. London: Routledge, 1992.

———. *Tissot: Physician of the Enlightenment.* New York: P. Lang, 1992.

Erich, Oswald Adolf, and Richard Beitl. *Wörterbuch der deutschen Volkskunde.* 2d rev. ed. Stuttgart: Alfred Krüner, 1955.

Erlebtes, Erzähltes, Erforschtes: Festgabe für Hans Wohltmann. Stadte: Selbstverlag des Stadter Geschichts- und Heimatsvereins, 1964.

Ernst, Fritz. *Kleinjogg der Musterbauer in Bildern seiner Zeit.* Zurich: Atlantis, 1935.

Farr, James R. *Hands of Honor: Artisans and Their World in Dijon, 1550–1650.* Ithaca, N.Y.: Cornell University Press, 1988.

Fasbender, Heinrich. *Geschichte der Geburtshilfe.* Jena: Gustav Fischer, 1906. Reprint. Hildesheim: Georg Olms, 1964.

Fischer, Alfons. *Beiträge zur Kulturhygiene des 18. und zu Beginn des 19. Jahrhunderts im deutschen Reiche.* Leipzig: J. A Barth, 1928.

———. *Geschichte des deutschen Gesundheitswesens.* 2 vols. Berlin: Kommissionsverlag F. A. Herbig, 1933.

Fischer, Wolfram. *Handwerksrecht und Handwerkswirtschaft um 1800.* Berlin: Dunker & Humblot, 1955.

Fissell, Mary E. "Innocent and Honorable Bribes: Medical Manners in Eighteenth-Century Britain." In *The Codification of Medical Morality: Historical and Philosophical Studies of the Formalization of Western Medical Morality in the Eighteenth and Nineteenth Centuries,* vol. 1: *Medical Ethics and Etiquette in the Eighteenth Century,* edited by Robert Baker, Dorothy Porter, and Roy Porter, 19–45. Dordrecht: Kluwer, 1993.

———. *Patients, Power, and the Poor in Eighteenth-Century Bristol.* Cambridge: Cambridge University Press, 1991.

Forberger, Rudolf. "Zu den Begriffen 'Manufactur' und 'Fabrik' in technischer und technologischer Sicht." In *Technologischer Wandel im 18. Jahrhundert,* edited by Ulrich Troitzsch, 175–81. Wolfenbüttel: Herzog August Bibliothek, 1981.

Fossel, Victor. *Volksmedicin und medicinischer Aberglauben in Steiermark: Ein Beitrag zur Landeskunde.* Graz: Leuschner & Lubensky, 1885.

Foucault, Michel. *Discipline and Punish: The Birth of the Prison.* Translated by Alan Sheridan. New York: Pantheon Books, 1977.

François, Etienne. *Die unsichtbare Grenze: Protestanten und Katholiken in Augsburg 1648–1806.* Sigmaringen: Thorbecke, 1993.

Freidson, Eliot. *Professional Dominance: The Social Structure of Medical Care.* New York: Atherton Press, 1970.

——. *Profession of Medicine.* New York: Harper & Row, 1970.

French, Roger, and Andrew Wear, eds. *The Medical Revolution of the Seventeenth Century.* Cambridge: Cambridge University Press, 1989.

Frevert, Ute. *Krankheit als politisches Problem, 1770–1880: Soziale Unterschichten in Preußen zwischen medizinischer Polizei und staatlicher Sozialversicherung.* Göttingen: Vandenhoeck & Ruprecht, 1984.

Fuhse, Franz. "Die Bader und Barbiere in der Stadt Braunschweig während des 16. Jahrhunderts." In *Unsere Heimat Niedersachsen,* 30–36. Braunschweig, 1924.

Gagliardo, John G. *From Pariah to Patriot: The Changing Image of the German Peasant, 1770–1840.* Lexington: University of Kentucky Press, 1969.

Garrison, Fielding H. *An Introduction to the History of Medicine.* 4th revised and enlarged ed. Philadelphia: W. B. Saunders, 1929.

Gélis, Jacques. *La Sage-femme ou le médicin: Une Nouvelle Conception de la vie.* Paris: Fayard, 1988.

Gelfand, Toby. "A 'Monarchical Profession' in the Old Regime: Surgeons, Ordinary Practitioners, and Medical Professionalization in Eighteenth-Century France." In *Professions and the French State, 1700–1900,* edited by Gerald Geison, 149–180. Philadelphia: University of Pennsylvania Press, 1984.

——. *Professionalizing Modern Medicine: Paris Surgeons and Medical Science and Institutions in the Eighteenth Century.* Westport, Conn.: Greenwood Press, 1980.

Genschorek, Wolfgang. *Christoph Wilhelm Hufeland: Der Arzt, der das Leben verlängern half.* Leipzig: S. Hirzel, 1984.

——. *Ernst Ludwig Heim: Das Leben eines Volkarztes.* Leipzig: S. Hirzel, 1985.

Gerade, Adolf. "Blankenburg vom Mittelalter bis zum 18. Jahrhundert." *Braunschweigische Heimat* 50 (1964): 33–40.

Gerbert, Annelise. *Öffentliche Gesundheitspflege und staatliches Medizinalwesen in den Städten Braunschweig und Wolfenbüttel im 19. Jahrhundert.* Braunschweig: Selbstverlag des Braunschweigischen Geschichtsvereins, 1983.

Geyer-Kordesch, Johanna. "Fevers and Other Fundamentals: Dutch and German Medical Explanations, c. 1680–1730." In *Theories of Fever from Antiquity to the Enlightenment,* edited by W. F. Bynum and Vivian Nutton, 99–120. London: Wellcome Institute for the History of Medicine, 1981.

——. "'Der Galante Patient': Verhaltenserwartungen für Kranke im 18. Jahrhundert in Deutschland." In *Deutsch-Niederländische Bezieungen in der Medizin des 18. Jahrhunderts: Vorträge des Deutsch-Niederländischen Medizinhistorikertreffens 1982,* edited by Richard Toellner and Martin J. van Lieburg, 3–16. Amsterdam: Rodophi, 1985.

——. "Medizinische Fallbeschreibungen und ihre Bedeutung in der Wissensrefrom des 17. und 18. Jahrhunderts." *Medizin, Gesellschaft und Geschichte* 9 (1990): 7–19.

——. "Passions and the Ghost in the Machine: Or What Not to Ask about Science in Seventeenth- and Eighteenth-Century Germany." In *The Medical Revolution of the Seventeenth Century,* edited by Roger French and Andrew Wear, 145–63. Cambridge: Cambridge University Press, 1989.

Gleixner, Ulrike. "Hebammen als Amtsfrauen und Gutachterinnen auf dem Land: Eine Fallstudie (Altmark 18. Jahrhundert)." In *Frauen in der ländlichen Gesellschaft der Frühen Neuzeit*, edited by Heide Wunder and Christina Vanya. Forthcoming.

Göckejan, Gerd. *Kurieren und Staat machen: Gesundheit und Medizin in der bürgerlichen Welt.* Frankfurt am Main: Suhrkamp, 1985.

Goldberg, Ann. "An Analysis of Insanity in Nineteenth-Century Germany: Sexuality, Delinquency, and Anti-Semitism in the Records of the Eberbach Asylum." Diss., University of California, Los Angeles, 1992.

Goldstein, Jan. *Console and Classify: The French Psychiatric Profession in the Nineteenth Century.* Cambridge: Cambridge University Press, 1987.

———. "Foucault Among the Sociologists: The 'Disciplines' and the History of the Professions." *History and Theory* 23, no. 1 (1984): 170–92.

Goody, Jack, Joan Thirsk, and E. P. Thompson, eds. *Family and Inheritance: Rural Society in Western Europe, 1200–1800.* Cambridge: Cambridge University Press, 1976.

Görges, Wilhelm, Ferdinand Spehr, and Franz Fuhse. *Väterlandische Geschichten und Denkwürdigkeiten der Lande Braunschweig und Hannover: Ein Volksbuch.* 3d ed. 2 vols. Braunschweig: Appelhans, 1925–29.

Goubert, Jean-Pierre. *Malades et medicins en Bretagne, 1770–1790.* Paris: Librairie C. Klincksieck, 1974.

———, ed. *La Médicalisation de la société française, 1770–1830.* Waterloo, Ont.: Historical Reflections Press, 1982.

Grabner, Elfriede. *Grundzüge einer ostalpinen Volksmedizin.* Vienna: Östereichischen Akademie der Wissenschaften, 1985.

———, ed. *Volksmedizin: Probleme und Forschungsgeschichte.* Darmstadt: Wissenschaftliche Buchgesellschaft, 1967.

Graefe, Christa. *Forstleute: Von den Anfängen einer Behörde und ihren Beamten (Braunschweig-Wolfenbüttel, 1530–1607).* Wiesbaden: Harrassowitz in Kommission, 1989.

Green, Monica. "Women's Medical Practice and Health Care in Medieval Europe: Review Essay." *Signs: Journal of Women in Culture and Society* 14 (1989): 434–73.

Gyr, Ueli, ed. *Festschrift für Arnold Niederer zum 65. Geburtstag.* Basel: Schweizerische Gesellschaft für Volkskunde, 1980.

Haberling, Elseluise. *Beiträge zur Geschichte des Hebammenstands.* Osterwieck: Staude, 1940.

Hahn, Walter. *Handel und Handelspolitik im Herzogtum Braunschweig-Wolfenbüttel in der Regierungszeit der Herzöge Karl I. und Karl Wilhelm Ferdinand (1735–1806): Ein Beitrag zur Geschichte der deutschen Kleinstaaten des 18. Jahrhunderts.* Braunschweig: Appelhans, 1931.

Håkansson, Erika. "Über Volksmedizin des 17. bis 19. Jahrhunderts im Aachener Raum." Diss., Aachen Technical University, 1975.

Hartmann, Fritz. "Hausvater und Hausmutter als Hausarzt in der Frühen Neuzeit." In *Staat und Gesellschaft in Mittelalter und Früher Neuzeit: Gedenkschrift für Joachim Leuschner*, edited by Katharina Colberg, Hans-Heinrich Nolte, and Herbert Obenaus, 151–75. Göttingen: Vandenhoeck & Ruprecht, 1983.

Hauptmeyer, Carl-Hans. "Aufklärung und bäuerliche Oppositionen im zentralen Niedersachsen des ausgehenden 18. Jahrhunderts." In *Das Volk als Objekt obrigkeit-*

lichen Handelns, edited by Rudolf Vierhaus, 197–217. Tübingen: Max Niemeyer, 1992.

———. "Dorf und Territorialstaat im zentralen Niedersachsen." In *Landgemeinde und frühmoderner Staat: Beiträge zum Problem der gemeindlichen Selbstverwaltung in Dänemark, Schleswig-Holstein und Niedersachsen in der frühen Neuzeit,* edited by Ulrich Lange, 217–35. Sigmaringen: Jan Thorbecke, 1988.

Havemann, Wilhelm. *Geschichte der Lande Braunschweig und Lüneburg.* 3 vols. Göttingen: Dieterichsche Buchhandlung, 1853–57.

Heller, Robert. "'Priest-Doctors' as a Rural Health Service in the Age of Enlightenment." *Medical History* 19 (1975): 361–83.

Henning, Friedrich-Wilhelm. *Landwirtschaft und ländliche Gesellschaft in Deutschland.* 2d enlarged ed. 2 vols. Paderborn: Schöningh, 1985–88.

Henretta, James A. "Families and Farms: *Mentalité* in Pre-Industrial America." *William and Mary Quarterly,* 3d ser., 35 (1978): 3–32.

Herzlich, Claudia, and Janine Pierret. *Illness and Self in Society.* Translated by Elborg Forster. Baltimore: Johns Hopkins University Press, 1987.

Hickel, Erika. *Apotheken, Arzneimittel und Naturwissenschaften in Braunschweig, 1677–1977.* Braunschweig: Hagenmarkt Apotheke, 1977.

Hinrichs, Ernst, and Günther Wiegelmann, eds. *Sozialer und kultereller Wandel in der ländlichen Welt des 19. Jahrhunderts.* Wolfenbüttel: Herzog August Bibliothek, 1982.

Hirsch, August, Ernst Gurlt, and Albrecht Werner, eds. *Biographisches Lexikon der hervorragenden Ärzte aller Zeiten und Völker.* 6 vols. Berlin: Urban & Schwarzenberg, 1884–88.

Hirschberg, Julius. *Geschichte der Augenheilkunde im Mittelalter und in der Neuzeit.* Vol. 13 of *Handbuch der gesamten Augenheilkunde,* edited by Alfred Graefe und Theodor Saemisch. 2d rev. ed. Leipzig: W. Engelmann, 1898.

Höfler, Max. *Deutsches Krankheitsnamen-Buch.* Munich: Piloty & Loehle, 1899. Reprint. Hildesheim: Georg Olms, 1970.

———. *Volksmedizin und Aberglaube in Oberbayerns Gegenwart und Vergangenheit.* Munich: Otto Gallcr, 1893.

Hopkins, Donald. *Princes and Peasants: Smallpox in History.* Chicago: University of Chicago Press, 1983.

Hovorka, Oskar von, and Adolf Kronfeld. *Vergleichende Volksmedizin.* 2 vols. Stuttgart: Strecker & Schröder, 1908–9.

Howard, Michael. *Traditional Folk Remedies: A Comprehensive Herbal.* London: Century, 1987.

Hueg, Adolf. *Dorf und Bauerntum: Eine Fibel als Hilfsbuch zur Niedersächsischen Dorfgeschichtsforschung (Dorffibel).* Oldenburg: Gerhard Stalling, 1939.

Huerkamp, Claudia. *Der Aufstieg der Ärzte im 19. Jahrhundert: Vom gelehrten Stand zum professionellen Experten: Das Beispiel Preußens.* Göttingen: Vandenhoeck & Ruprecht, 1985.

———. "The History of Smallpox Vaccination in Germany: A First Step in the Medicalization of the General Public." *Journal of Contemporary History* 20 (1985): 617–35.

Hufton, Olwen H. *The Poor of Eighteenth-Century France, 1750–1789.* Oxford: Clarendon Press, 1974.

Huisman, Frank. "Itinerant Medical Practitioners in the Dutch Republic: The Case of Groningen." *Tractrix* 1 (1989): 63–83.

——. *Stadsbelang en standsbesef: Gezondheidszorg en medisch beroep in Groningen, 1500–1730*. Rotterdam: Erasmus, 1992.

Hunt, Lynn, ed. *The New Cultural History*. Berkeley: University of California Press, 1989.

Hutton, Patrick. "The History of Mentalities: The New Map of Cultural History." *History and Theory* 20, no. 3 (1981): 237–59.

Imhof, Arthur. *Die gewonnenen Jahre: Von der Zunahme unserer Lebensspanne seit dreihundert Jahren oder von der Notwendigkeit einer neuen Einstellung zu Leben und Sterben. Ein historischer Essay*. Munich: Beck, 1981.

——. "Methodological Problems in Modern Urban History Writing: Graphic Representations of Urban Mortality, 1750–1850." In *Problems and Methods in the History of Medicine*, edited by Roy Porter and Andrew Wear, 101–32. London: Croom Helm, 1987.

——. *Die verlorenen Welten: Alltagsbewältigung durch unsere Vorfahren—und weshalb wir uns heute so schwer damit tun*. Munich: Beck, 1984.

——, ed. *Biologie des Menschen in der Geschichte*. Munich: Beck, 1981.

——, ed. *Leib und Leben in der Geschichte der Neuzeit*. Berlin: Duncker & Humblot, 1983.

——, ed. *Mensch und Gesundheit in der Geschichte*. Husum: Matthiesen, 1980.

Ingrao, Charles. *The Hessian Mercenary State: Ideas, Institutions, and Reform under Frederick II, 1760–1785*. Cambridge: Cambridge University Press, 1987.

——. "The Problem of 'Enlightened Absolutism' and the German States." *Journal of Modern History* 58 (1986): S161–80.

Jäck, Karl, and Ernst Theodor Nauck. *Zur Geschichte des Sanitätswesen im Fürstenberg*. Allensbach-Bodensee: Boltze, 1951.

Jentsch, Irene. *Zur Geschichte des Zeitungslesens in Deutschland am Ende des 18. Jahrhunderts: Mit besonderer Berücksichtigung der gesellschaftlichen Formen des Zeitungslesens*. Leipzig: Stein, 1937.

Jewson, N. D. "The Disappearance of the Sick-Man from the Medical Cosmology." *Sociology* 10 (1976): 225–44.

——. "Medical Knowledge and the Patronage System in Eighteenth Century England." *Sociology* 8 (1974): 369–85.

Jones, Colin. *Charity and Bienfaisance: The Treatment of the Poor in the Montpellier Region, 1740–1815*. Cambridge: Cambridge University Press, 1982.

——. "Medicine, Madness and Mayhem from the 'Roi Soleil' to the Golden Age of Hysteria (17th to the late 19th Centuries)." *French History* 4 (1990): 378–88.

Jones, Colin, and Jonathan Barry, eds. *Medicine and Charity Before the Welfare State*. London: Routledge, 1991.

Jungbauer, Gustav. *Deutsche Volksmedizin: Ein Grundriß*. Berlin: Walter de Gruyter, 1934.

Jütte, Robert. *Ärzte, Heiler und Patienten: Medizinischer Alltag in der frühen Neuzeit*. Munich: Artemis & Winkler, 1991.

——. "A Seventeenth-Century Barber-Surgeon and His Patients." *Medical History* 33 (1989): 184–98.

——. "The Social Construction of Illness in the Early Modern Period." In *The Social Construction of Illness*, edited by Jens Lachmund and Gunnar Stollberg, 23–38. Stuttgart: Franz Steiner, 1992.

Kaiser, Wolfram, and Arina Völker. *Die Entwicklung von Medizinalorganisation und Bevölkerungsversorgung am territorialen Beispiel von Anhalt.* Halle-Wittenberg: Martin-Luther-Universität, 1987.

——. *Universität und Physikat in der Frühgeschichte des Amtsarztwesens.* Wissenschaftliche Beiträge der Martin-Luther-Universitäts Halle-Wittenberg, no. 53. Halle: Martin-Luther-Universität, 1980.

Kaplan, Steven. *Bread, Politics and Political Economy in the Reign of Louis XIV.* 2 vols. The Hague: M. Nijhoff, 1976.

Karcher, J. *Felix Platter: Lebensbild des Baseler Stadtarztes 1536–1614.* Basel: Helbing & Lichtenhahn, 1949.

Kellenbenz, Hermann. *Deutsche Wirtschaftsgeschichte.* Vol. 1, *Von den Anfängen bis zum Ende des 18. Jahrhunderts.* Munich: Beck, 1977.

Keller, Albrecht. *Der Scharfrichter in der deutschen Kulturgeschichte.* Bonn: K. Schroeder, 1921.

Keyser, Erich, ed. *Niedersächsisches Städtebuch.* Stuttgart: W. Kohlhammer, 1952.

King, Lester. *Medical Thinking: A Historical Preface.* Princeton, N.J.: Princeton University Press, 1982.

——. *The Medical World of the Eighteenth Century.* Chicago: University of Chicago Press, 1958.

——. *The Philosophy of Medicine: The Early Eighteenth Century.* Cambridge, Mass.: Harvard University Press, 1978.

——. *The Road to Medical Enlightenment, 1650–1695.* New York: American Elsevier, 1970.

——. "Stahl and Hoffmann: A Study in Eighteenth-Century Animism." *Journal of the History of Medicine and Allied Sciences* 19 (1964): 118–30.

Knodel, John E. *Demographic Behavior in the Past: A Study of Fourteen German Village Populations in the Eighteenth and Nineteenth Century.* Cambridge: Cambridge University Press, 1988.

Kocka, Jürgen. "Sozialgeschichte—Strukturgeschichte—Gesellschaftsgeschichte," *Archiv für Sozialgeschichte* 15 (1975): 43–50.

Kohl, Jill, and Mary Lindemann. "Augustus in tenebris." In *Barocker Lust-Spiegel: Studien zur Literatur des Barock. Festschrift für Blake Lee Spahr*, edited by Martin Bircher, Jörg-Ulrich Fechner, and Gerd Hillen, 187–204. Amsterdam: Rodopi, 1984.

Kondratowitz, Hans-Joachim von. "The Medicalization of Old Age: Continuity and Change in Germany from the Late Eighteenth to the Early Twentieth Century." In *Life, Death, and the Elderly: Historical Perspectives*, edited by Margaret Pelling and Richard Smith, 134–164. London: Routledge, 1991.

Kopitzsch, Franklin, ed. *Aufklärung, Absolutismus und Bürgertum in Deutschland: Zwölf Aufsätze.* Munich: Nymphenburger, 1976.

Kraus, Wilfried. "Untersuchungen zur Geschichte der Stadt Königslutter im 18. Jahrhundert." Hausarbeit, Braunschweig, 1967.

Küther, Carsten. *Menschen auf der Straße: Vagierende Unterschichten in Bayern, Franken und Schwaben in der zweiten Hälfte des 18. Jahrhunderts*. Göttingen: Vandenhoeck & Ruprecht, 1983.

Labisch, Alfons. "Doctors, Workers and the Scientific Cosmology of the Industrial World: The Social Construction of 'Health' and the 'Homo Hygienicus'." *Journal of Contemporary History* 20 (1985): 599–615.

———. "'Hygiene ist Moral—Moral is Hygiene—': Soziale Disziplinierung durch Ärzte und Medizin." In *Soziale Sicherheit und soziale Disziplinierung*, edited by Christoph Sachße and Florian Tennstedt, 286–303. Stuttgart: Suhrkamp, 1986.

Labisch, Alfons, and Reinhard Spree, eds. *Medizinische Deutungsmacht im sozialen Wandel des 19. und frühen 20. Jahrhunderts*. Bonn: Psychiatrie-Verlag, 1989.

Lacapra, Dominick. "Is Everyone a *Mentalité* Case? Transference and the Culture Concept." *History and Theory* 20, no. 3 (1984): 296–311.

Lachmund, Jens, and Gunnar Stollberg, "The Doctor, His Audience, and the Meaning of Illness: The Drama of Medical Practice in the Late 18th and Early 19th Centuries." In *The Social Construction of Illness*, edited by Lachmund and Stollberg, 53–66. Stuttgart: Franz Steiner, 1992.

———, eds. *The Social Construction of Illness*. Stuttgart: Franz Steiner, 1992.

Larsen, Magali Sarfatti. *The Rise of Professionalism: A Sociological Analysis*. Berkeley: University of California Press, 1977.

Larsen, Øivind. "Eighteenth Century Diseases, Diagnostic Trends and Mortality." *Scandinavian Population Studies* 5 (1979): 38–54.

———. "Die Krankheitsauffassung und ihre historische Interpretation: Ein Auswertungsmodell aufgrund von norwegischen Medizinalberichten aus dem 19. Jahrhundert." In *Mensch und Gesundheit in der Geschichte*, edited by Arthur Imhof, 45–58. Husum: Matthiesen, 1980.

La Vopa, Anthony. *Grace, Talent, and Merit: Poor Students, Clerical Careers, and Professional Ideology in Eighteenth-Century Germany*. Cambridge: Cambridge University Press, 1988.

Leavitt, Judith Walzer. "Medicine in Context: A Review Essay of the History of Medicine." *American Historical Review* 95 (1990): 1471–84.

Lebrun, François. *Les Hommes et la mort en Anjou aux 17ᵉ et 18ᵉ siècles: Essai de démographie et de psychologie historiques*. Paris: Mouton, 1971.

———. *Se soigner autrefois: Médicins, saints et sorciers aux 17ᵉ et 18ᵉ siècles*. Paris: Temps actuels, 1983.

Lee, W. R. "The Mechanism of Mortality Change in Germany, 1750–1850." *Medizinhistorisches Journal* 15 (1980): 244–68.

———. *Population Growth, Economic Development and Social Change in Bavaria, 1750–1850*. New York: Arno Press, 1977.

Lemay, Edna H. "Thomas Hérrier: A Country Surgeon Outside Angoulême at the End of the Eighteenth Century." *Journal of Social History* 10 (1976–77): 524–37.

Léonard, Jacques. *La Vie quotidienne du medicin de province au XIXᵉ siècle*. Paris: Hachette, 1977.

Lichtenberg, Heinz Otto. *Unterhaltsame Bauernaufklärung: Ein Kapital Volksbildungsgeschichte*. Tübingen: Tübinger Vereinigung für Volkskunde, 1970.

Lindemann, Mary. "'Aufklärung' and the Health of the People: 'Volksschriften' and Medical Advice in Braunschweig-Wolfenbüttel, 1756–1803." In *Das Volk als Ob-*

jekt obrigkeitlichen Handelns, edited by Rudolf Vierhaus, 101–20. Tübingen: Max Niemeyer, 1992.

———. "Confessions of an Archive Junkie." In *Theory, Method, and Practice in Social and Cultural History*, edited by Peter Karsten and John Modell, 152–80. New York: New York University Press, 1992.

———. "The Enlightenment Encountered: Medical Practice and Enlightenment in Northern Germany, 1750–1820." In *Medicine in the Enlightenment*, edited by Roy Porter, 181–97. Amsterdam: Rodopi, 1995.

Lipp, Carola, Wolfgang Kaschuba, and Eckart Frahm, eds., *Nehren: Eine Dorfchronik der Spataufklärung von F. A. Köhler*. Tübingen: Tübinger Vereinigung für Volkskunde, 1981.

Loetz, Francisca. "Histoire des mentalités und Medizingeschichte: Wege zu einer Sozialgeschichte der Medizin." *Medizinhistorisches Journal* 27 (1992): 272–91.

———. *Vom Kranken zum Patienten: "Medikalisierung" und medizinische Vergesellschaftung am Beispiel Badens, 1750–1850*. Stuttgart: Franz Steiner, 1993.

Loudon, Irvine. "Leg Ulcers in the Eighteenth and Early Nineteenth Century." *Journal of the Royal College of General Practitioners* 31 (1981): 263–73; 32 (1982): 301–9.

———. *Medical Care and the General Practitioner, 1750–1850*. Oxford: Oxford University Press, 1986.

———. "The Nature of Provincial Medical Practice in Eighteenth-Century England." *Medical History* 29 (1985): 1–32.

Loux, Françoise. *Le Jeune Enfant et son corps dans la médicine traditionelle*. Paris: Flammarion, 1978.

———. *Pierre-Martin de La Martinère: Un Médecin au XVIIᵉ siècle*. Paris: Imago, 1988.

———. *Sagesse du corps: La Santé et maladie dans les proverbs françaises*. Paris: Maisonneuve & Larouse, 1978.

Lüdtke, Alf. "Was ist und wer treibt Alltagsgeschichte?" In *Alltagsgeschichte: Zur Rekonstruktion historischer Erfahrung und Lebensweise*, edited by Alf Lüdtke, 9–47. Frankfurt: Campus, 1989.

Lütge, Friedrich. *Geschichte der deutschen Agrarverfassung bis zum 19. Jahrhundert*. 2d rev., improved, and enlarged ed. Stuttgart: Ulmer, 1967.

McClelland, Charles E. *The German Experience of Professionalization: Modern Learned Professions and Their Organizations from the Early Nineteenth Century to the Hitler Era*. Cambridge: Cambridge University Press, 1991.

MacDonald, Michael. *Mystical Bedlam: Madness, Anxiety and Healing in Seventeenth-Century England*. Cambridge: Cambridge University Press, 1981.

McGowen, Randall. "Identifying Themes in the Social History of Medicine." *Journal of Modern History* 63 (1991): 81–90.

McKendrick, Neil, John Brewer, and J. H. Plumb. *The Birth of Consumer Society in the Commercialization of Eighteenth-Century England*. Bloomington: Indiana University Press, 1982.

Marland, Hilary, *Medicine and Society in Wakefield and Huddersfield, 1780–1870*. Cambridge: Cambridge University Press, 1987.

———, ed. *The Art of Midwifery*. London: Routledge, 1993.

Matossian, Mary Kilbourne. *Poisons of the Past: Molds, Epidemics, and History.* New Haven, Conn.: Yale University Press, 1989.

La Médicalisation de la société française, 1770–1830. Special issue of *Historical Reflections / Réflexions historiques* 9, nos. 1–2 (1982).

La Médicalisation en France du XVIIIe au début du XXe siècle. Special issue of *Annales: Economies, Sociétés, Civilisations* 32 (1977).

Medicine, History and Society. Special Issue of *Journal of Contemporary History* 20 (1992).

Medick, Hans, and David W. Sabean, eds. *Emotionen und materielle Interessen: Sozialanthropologie und historische Beiträge zur Familienforschung.* Göttingen: Vandenhoeck & Ruprecht, 1984.

Menssen, Brigette, and A.-M. Taube. "Hebammen und Hebammenwesen in Oldenburg in der zweiten Hälfte des 18. und zu Beginn des 19. Jahrhunderts." In *Regionalgeschichte: Probleme und Beispiele,* edited by Ernst Hinrichs and W. Norden. Hildesheim: Lax, 1980.

Mergel, Thomas. *Zwischen Klasse und Konfession: Katholisches Bürgertum im Rheinland 1794–1914.* Göttingen: Vandenhoeck & Ruprecht, 1994.

Miller, Geneviève. *The Adoption of Inoculation for Smallpox in England and France.* Philadelphia: University of Pennsylvania Press, 1957.

———. "Airs, Waters, and Places in History." *Journal of the History of Medicine* 17 (1962): 129–38.

Moderhack, Richard, ed. *Braunschweigische Landesgeschichte im Überblick.* 3d ed. Braunschweig: Waisenhaus, 1979.

Mohrmann, Ruth-E. *Alltagswelt im Land Braunschweig: Stadtische und ländliche Wohnkultur vom 16. bis zum frühen 20. Jahrhundert.* 2 vols. Münster: F. Coppenrath, 1990.

Muir, Edward, and Guido Ruggiero, eds. *Microhistory and the Lost Peoples of Europe: Selections from Quaderni Storici.* Translated by Eren Branch. Baltimore: Johns Hopkins University Press, 1991.

Nagy, Doreen Evenden. *Popular Medicine in Seventeenth-Century England.* Bowling Green, Ohio: Bowling Green University Press, 1988.

Oehme, Johannes. "Gesundheitserziehung und Hausväterliteratur." *Mittheilungen der TU Braunschweig* 23, no. 1 (1988): 53–57.

Oestreich, Gerhard. *Geist und Gestalt des frühmodernen Staates: Ausgewählte Aufsätze.* Berlin: Duncker & Humblot, 1969.

———. "Policey und Prudentia civilis in der barocken Gesellschaft von Stadt und Staat." In *Barock-Symposium 1974: Stadt-Schule-Universität-Buchwesen und die deutsche Literatur im 17. Jahrhundert,* edited by Albrecht Schöne, 10–21. Munich: Beck, 1976.

Oppelt, Wolfgang. *Über die "Unehrlichkeit" des Scharfrichters: Unter bevorzugter Verwendung von Ansbacher Quellen.* Langfeld: Antiquariat Traute Gottschalk, 1976

Park, Katharine. *Doctors and Medicine in Early Renaissance Florence.* Princeton, N.J.: Princeton University Press, 1985.

Payne, Harry C. *The Philosophes and the People.* New Haven, Conn.: Yale University Press, 1976.

Peickert, Heinz. *Geheimmittel im deutschen Arzneiverkehr: Ein Beitrag zur Wirtschaftsgeschichte der Pharmazie und zur Arzneispezialitätenfrage.* Leipzig: Edelmann, 1931.

Pelling, Margaret. "Medical Practice in Early Modern England: Trade or Profession?" In *The Professions in Early Modern England*, edited by Wilfrid Prest, 90–128. London: Croom Helm, 1987.

Pelling, Margaret, and Richard Smith, eds. *Life, Death, and the Elderly: Historical Perspectives*. London: Routledge, 1991.

Penners, Theodor. "Bevölkerungsgeschichtliche Probleme der Land-Stadtwanderung—untersucht an der ländlichen Abwanderung in die Städte Braunschweig und Wolfenbüttel um die Mitte des 18. Jahrhunderts: Mit einer Übersichtskarte." *Braunschweigisches Jahrbuch* 47 (1966): 125–57.

Perkins, Wendy. "Midwives Versus Doctors: The Case of Louise Bourgeois." *The Seventeenth Century* 3 (1988): 135–57.

———. "The Relationship Between Midwife and Client in the Works of Louise Bourgeois." *Seventeenth-Century French Studies* 11 (1989): 28–45.

Peter, Jean-Pierre. "Disease and the Sick at the End of the Eighteenth Century." In *Biology of Man in History: Selections from the Annales: Economies, Sociétés, Civilisations*, edited by Robert Forster and Orest Ranum, translated by Elborg Forster and Patricia Ranum, 81–124. Baltimore: Johns Hopkins University Press, 1975.

———. "Kranke und Krankheiten am Ende des 18. Jahrhunderts (aufgrund einer Untersuchung der Königlich-Medizinischen-Gesellschaft, 1774–1794." In *Biologie des Menschen in der Geschichte*, edited by Arthur Imhof, 274–326. Munich: Beck, 1981.

Petersen, Walter. *Verzeichnis der Einblattdrucke und Handschriften aus dem Rechtsleben des Herzogtums Braunschweig-Lüneberg: Ergänzt um den Nachweis weiterer Quellen.* 2 vols. Wiesbaden: In Kommission bei Harrasowitz, 1984.

Pflanz, Manfred. "Der Entschluß, zum Arzt zu gehen." *Hippokrates* 35 (1964): 894–97.

Piechocki, Werner. "Das hallesche Physikat im 18. Jahrhundert." *Wissenschaftliche Beiträge der Martin-Luther-Universität Halle-Wittenberg* 36 (1977): 185–206.

Porter, Dorothy, and Roy Porter, *Patient's Progress: Doctors and Doctoring in Eighteenth-Century England*. Stanford, Calif.: Stanford University Press, 1989.

Porter, Roy. "Before the Fringe: 'Quackery' and the Eighteenth-Century Medical Market." In *Studies in the History of Alternative Medicine*, edited by Roger Cooter, 1–26. New York: St. Martin's Press, 1988.

———. *Doctor of Society: Thomas Beddoes and the Sick Trade in Late-Enlightenment England*. London: Routledge, 1992.

———. *Health for Sale: Quackery in England, 1660–1850*. Manchester: Manchester University Press, 1989.

———. "Lay Medical Knowledge in the Eighteenth Century: The Gentleman's Magazine." *Medical History* 29 (1985): 138–68.

———. "The Patient's View: Doing Medical History from Below." *Theory and Society* 14 (1985): 175–98.

———, ed. *Medicine in the Enlightenment*. Amsterdam: Rodopi, 1995.

———, ed. *Patients and Practitioners: Lay Perceptions of Medicine in Pre-Industrial Society*. Cambridge: Cambridge University Press, 1985.

———, ed. *The Popularization of Medicine, 1650–1850*. London: Routledge, 1992.

Porter, Roy, and Dorothy Porter. *In Sickness and in Health: The British Experience, 1650–1850*. New York: Basil Blackwell, 1988.

Porter, Roy, and Andrew Wear, eds. *Problems and Methods in the History of Medicine.* London: Croom Helm, 1987.

Prest, Wilfrid, ed. *The Professions in Early Modern England.* London: Croom Helm, 1987.

Raeff, Marc. *The Well-Ordered Police State: Social and Institutional Change Through Law in the Germanies and Russia, 1600–1800.* New Haven, Conn.: Yale University Press, 1983.

Ramsey, Matthew. *Professional and Popular Medicine in France, 1770–1830: The Social World of Medical Practice.* Cambridge: Cambridge University Press, 1988.

———. "Traditional Medicine and Medical Enlightenment: The Regulation of Secret Remedies in the Ancien Régime." *Historical Reflections / Refléxions historiques* 9 (1982): 215–32.

Rather, L. J. *Mind and Body in Eighteenth-Century Medicine: A Study Based on Jerome Gaub's De regimine mentis.* London: Wellcome Historical Library, 1965.

———. "The 'Six Things Non-Natural': A Note on the Origins and Fate of a Doctrine and a Phrase." *Clio Medica* 3 (1968): 337–47.

Reimann, F. K. *Ackerbau und Viehhaltung in vorindustriellen Deutschland.* Kitzingen-Main: Holzner, 1953.

Reininghaus, Wilfried. *Gewerbe in der Frühen Neuzeit.* Munich: R. Oldenbourg, 1990.

Rhamm, August. *Die Verfassungsgesetze des Herzogthums Braunschweig.* Braunschweig: Friedrich Vieweg & Sohn, 1900.

Richardson, Ruth. *Death, Dissection and the Destitute.* London: Routledge & Kegan Paul, 1987.

Riley, James C. *The Eighteenth-Century Campaign to Avoid Disease.* New York: St. Martin's Press, 1987.

———. "The Medicine of the Environment in Eighteenth-Century Germany." *Clio Medica* 18 (1963): 167–78.

———. *Sickness, Recovery and Death: A History and Forecast of Ill Health.* Iowa City: University of Iowa Press, 1989.

Risse, Guenter B. "Causes of Death as Historical Problem." Paper presented at a conference on the History of the Registration of Causes of Death, 11–14 November 1993, Indiana University, Bloomington.

———. "Epidemics and Medicine: The Influence of Disease on Medical Thought and Practice." *Bulletin of the History of Medicine* 53 (1979): 505–19.

———. "Hospital History: New Sources and Methods." In *Problems and Methods in the History of Medicine,* edited by Roy Porter and Andrew Wear, 175–203. London: Croom Helm, 1987.

———. *Hospital Life in Enlightenment Scotland: Care and Teaching at the Royal Infirmary of Edinburgh.* Cambridge: Cambridge University Press, 1986.

Robisheaux, Thomas. *Rural Society and the Search for Order in Early Modern Germany.* Cambridge: Cambridge University Press, 1989.

Rohner, Ludwig. *Kalendergeschichte und Kalender.* Wiesbaden: Athenaion, 1978.

Rohr, Heinz. *Geschichte der Stadt Königslutter am Elm.* Braunschweig: Hans Oeding, 1981.

Roi, Ludwig du. "Leben und Wirken des Leibarztes Johann Philipp du Roi, 1741–

1785." In *17. Jahresbericht des Vereins für Naturwissenschaft zu Braunschweig*. Braunschweig: Schulbuchhandlung, 1913.

Rosenberg, Charles E. *Explaining Epidemics and Other Studies in the History of Medicine*. Cambridge: Cambridge University Press, 1992.

———. "Medical Text and Social Context: William Buchan's *Domestic Medicine*." *Bulletin of the History of Medicine* 57 (1983): 22–42.

Rothenberg, Winifred B. "Explanation in History: In Defense of Operationalism." In *Theory, Method and Practice in Social and Cultural History*, edited by Peter Karsten and John Modell, 134–51. New York: New York University Press, 1992.

———. *From Market-Place to a Market Economy: The Transformation of Rural Massachusetts, 1750–1850*. Chicago: University of Chicago Press, 1992.

Rothschuh, Karl E. *Konzepte der Medizin in Vergangenheit und Gegenwart*. Stuttgart: Hippocrates, 1978.

Rousseau, G. S. "John Wesley's *Primitive Physic*." *Harvard Library Bulletin* 6 (1968): 242–56.

Russell, Andrew, ed. *The Town and State Physician in Europe from the Middle Ages to the Enlightenment*. Wolfenbüttel: Herzog August Bibliothek, 1981.

Sabean, David Warren. "Aspects of Kinship Behaviour and Property in Western Europe before 1800." In *Family and Inheritance: Rural Society in Western Europe, 1200–1800*, edited by Jack Goody, Joan Thirsk, and E. P. Thompson, 96–111. Cambridge: Cambridge University Press, 1976.

———. *Power in the Blood: Popular Culture and Village Discourse*. Cambridge: Cambridge University Press, 1984.

———. *Property, Production, and Family in Neckarhausen, 1700–1870*. Cambridge: Cambridge University Press, 1990.

Sachße, Christoph, and Florian Tennstedt, eds. *Soziale Sicherheit und soziale Disziplinierung*. Stuttgart: Suhrkamp, 1986.

Sander, Sabine. *Handwerkschirurgen: Sozialgeschichte einer verdrängten Berufsgruppe*. Göttingen: Vandenhoeck & Ruprecht, 1989.

Sawyer, Ronald. "Patients, Healers, and Disease in the Southwest Midlands, 1597–1634." Diss., University of Wisconsin, Madison, 1986.

Schaper, Robert. "Arzt und Apotheker—Das Physikat in Helmstedt." *Aus der Heimat —Für die Heimat*. Supplement to *Helmstedter Kreisblatt*, 10 September 1966.

———. "Krankenbehandlung der Armen—. . . und die Waisenkinder?" *Aus der Heimat—Für die Heimat*. Supplement to *Helmstedter Kreisblatt*, 24 September 1966.

Scheel, Günter. "Kurbraunschweig und die übrigen welfischen Lande." In *Deutsche Verwaltungsgeschichte*, vol. 1, *Vom Spätmittelalter bis zum Ende des Reiches*, edited by Kurt G. A. Jeserich, Hans Pohl, and Georg-Christoph von Unruh, 741–63. Stuttgart: Deutsche Verlagsanstalt, 1983.

Schenda, Rudolf. "Stadtmedizin—Landmedizin: Ein Versuch zur Erklärung subkulturalen medikalen Verhaltens." In *Stadt-Land-Beziehungen: Verhandlungen des 19. Deutschen Volkskongresses in Hamburg vom 1. bis 7. Oktober 1973*, 147–69. Göttingen: Vandenhoeck & Ruprecht, 1975.

———. *Volk ohne Buch: Studien zur Sozialgeschichte der populären Lesestoff, 1770–1910*. Frankfurt am Main: Vittorio Klostermann, 1970.

———. "Volksmedizin—was ist das heute?" *Zeitschrift für Volkskunde* 69 (1973): 189–210.

Schipperges, Heinrich. *Die Kranken im Mittelalter.* Munich: Beck, 1990.

Schlumbohm, Jürgen. "Bauern—Kötter—Heuerlinge. Bevölkerungsentwicklung und soziale Schichtung in einem Gebiet ländlichen Gewerbes: Das Kirchspiel Delin bei Osnabrück, 1650–1860," *Niedersächsisches Jahrbuch für Landesgeschichte* 58 (1986): 77–88.

Schmidt, Hanno. "Philanthropismus und Volksaufklärung im Herzogthum Braunschweig-Wolfenbüttel in der zweiten Hälfte des 18. Jahrhunderts." In *Das Volk als Objekt obrigkeitlichen Handelns,* edited by Rudolf Vierhaus, 171–95. Tübingen: Max Niemeyer, 1992.

Schmidt, Wilhelm. *Der braunschweigische Landtag von 1766–1770.* Göttingen: Angermann, 1912.

Schneider, Wolfgang. *Lexikon zur Arzneimittelgeschichte.* 7 vols. Frankfurt am Main: Govi, 1968–75. Vol. 4, *Geheimmittel und Spezialitäten.* 1969.

Schulze, Winfried. *Bäuerliche Widerstand und feudale Herrschaft in der frühen Neuzeit.* Stuttgart-Bad Cannstatt: Frommann-Holzboog, 1980.

———, ed. *Aufstände, Revolten, Prozesse: Beiträge zur bäuerlichen Widerstandsbewegungen im frühneuzeitlichen Europa.* Stuttgart: Klett-Cotta, 1983.

Sellin, Volker. "Mentalität und Mentalitätsgeschichte." *Historische Zeitschrift* 241 (1985): 555–98.

700 Jahre Blankenburg. Magdeburg: Städtisches Verkehrsamt [Blankenburg-Harz], 1937.

Sewell, William H., Jr. *Work and Revolution in France: The Language of Labor from the Old Regime to 1848.* Cambridge: Cambridge University Press, 1980.

Sheehan, James. *German History, 1770–1866.* Oxford: Oxford University Press, 1989.

Sheils, William, ed. *The Church and Healing.* Oxford: Oxford University Press, 1982.

Shorter, Edward. *Bedside Manners: The Troubled History of Doctors and Patients,* New York: Simon & Schuster, 1985. New ed. *Doctors and Their Patients: A Social History.* New Brunswick, N.J.: Transaction Publishers, 1991.

———. *Women's Bodies: A Social History of Women's Encounters with Health, Ill-Health, and Medicine.* New Brunswick, N.J.: Transaction Publishers, 1991.

Siegert, Reinhardt. "Aufklärung und Volkslekture: Exemplarisch dargestellt an Rudolph Zacharias Becker und seinem *Noth- und Hülfsbüchlein.*" *Archiv für Geschichte des Buchwesens* 19 (1978): cols. 1253–1348.

Siraisi, Nancy. *Medieval and Early Renaissance Medicine: An Introduction to Knowledge and Practice.* Chicago: University of Chicago Press, 1990.

Slack, Paul. "Mirrors of Health and Treasures of Poor Men: The Use of Vernacular Medical Literature in Tudor England." In *Health, Medicine and Mortality in the Sixteenth Century,* edited by Charles Webster, 237–73. Cambridge: Cambridge University Press, 1979.

Smith, Pamela H. *The Business of Alchemy: Science and Culture in the Holy Roman Empire.* Princeton, N.J.: Princeton University Press, 1994.

Spohr, Louis. *Lebenserinnerungen,* edited by Folker Göthel. Tutzing: Hans Schneider, 1968.

Starr, Paul. *The Social Transformation of American Medicine: The Rise of a Sovereign Profession and the Making of a Vast Industry*. New York: Basic Books, 1982.

Stolberg, Michael. "Gottesstrafe oder Diätsünde?: Zur Mentalitätsgeschichte der Cholera." *Medizin, Gesellschaft und Geschichte* 8 (1989): 9–25.

———. "Patientenschaft und Krankheitsspektrum in ländlichen Arztpraxen des 19. Jahrhunderts." *Medizinhistorisches Journal* 28 (1993): 3–27.

Stollberg, Gunnar. "Health and Illness in German Workers' Autobiographies from the Nineteenth and Early Twentieth Centuries." *Social History of Medicine* 6 (1993): 261–76.

Stroup, John Michael. *The Struggle for Identity in the Clerical Estate: Northwest German Protestant Opposition to Absolutist Policy in the Eighteenth Century*. Leiden: Brill, 1984.

Stürzbecher, Manfred. *Beiträge zur Berliner Medzingeschichte: Quellen und Studien zur Geschichte des Gesundheitswesens vom 17. bis zum 19. Jahrhundert*. Berlin: de Gruyter, 1966.

———. "Betrachtungen zur Historiographie der Medizinalordnungen." *Öffentlicher Gesundheitsdienst* 25 (1963): 282–88.

———. "Einige Bemerkungen zur Geschichte der Medizinalgesetzgebung im deutschen Sprachgebiet." *Veröffentlichungen der internationalen Gesellschaft für Geschichte der Pharmazie*, n.s., 24 (1964): 123–32.

———. "The Physici in German-speaking Countries from the Middle Ages to the Enlightenment." In *The Town and State Physician in Europe from the Middle Ages to the Enlightenment*, edited by Andrew W. Russell, 123–40. Wolfenbüttel: Herzog August Bibliothek, 1981.

———. "Zur Geschichte der brandenburgischen Medizinalgesetzgebung im 17. Jahrhundert." In *Beitrage zur Berliner Medizingeschichte*, edited by Manfred Stürzbecher, 1–66. Berlin: de Gruyter, 1966.

———. "Zur Geschichte der Medizinalgesetzgebung im Fürstbistum Münster im 17. und 18. Jahrhundert." *Westfälische Zeitschrift* 114 (1964): 165–91.

———. "Zur Geschichte des Berliner Stadtphysikus im 18. und 19. Jahrhundert." *Medizinische Welt* 1962: 1956–63.

Sührig, Hartmut. "Der Braunschweiger Volkskalender in der Zeit der Spätaufklärung." *Braunschweigisches Jahrbuch* 62 (1981): 87–112.

———. *Die Entwicklung der niedersächsischen Kalender im 17. Jahrhundert*. Göttingen: Buchhändler-Vereinigung, 1979.

Sussman, George D. "Enlightened Health Reform, Professional Medicine and Traditional Society: The Cantonal Physicians of the Bas-Rhin, 1810–1870." *Bulletin of the History of Medicine* 51 (1977): 565–84.

Temkin, Owsei. *Galenism: Rise and Decline of a Medical Philosophy*. Ithaca, N.Y.: Cornell University Press, 1973.

Theibault, John C. "Coping with the Thirty Years' War: Villages and Villagers in Hesse-Kassel, 1600–1680." Diss., Johns Hopkins University, 1986.

Thillaud, Pierre L. *Les Maladies et la médicine en pays basque nord à la fin de l'Ancien Régime, 1690–1789*. Geneva: Libraire Droz, 1983.

Thomas, Keith V. *Man and the Natural World: Changing Attitudes in England, 1500–1800*. London: Allen Lane, 1983.

————. *Religion and the Decline of Magic: Studies in Popular Beliefs in the Sixteenth and Seventeenth Centuries.* London: Weidenfeld & Nicolson, 1971.

Thompson, E. P. "The Moral Economy of the English Crowd in the Eighteenth Century." *Past and Present* 50 (February 1971): 76–136.

Titmuss, Richard H. *The Gift Relationship: From Human Blood to Social Polity.* London: Allen & Unwin, 1970.

Troßbach, Werner. *Sozialbewegung und politische Erfahrung: Bäuerliche Protest in hessischen Territorien, 1648–1806.* Weingarten: Drumlin, 1987.

Tuchman, Arleen Marcia. *Science, Medicine, and the State in Germany: The Case of Baden, 1815–1871.* Oxford: Oxford University Press, 1993.

Turner, Victor W. *Process, Performance and Pilgrimage: A Study in Comparative Sociology.* New Delhi: Concept, 1979.

————. *The Ritual Process: Structure and Anti-Structure.* Chicago: Aldine, 1969.

Tutzke, Dietrich. "Das Budissiner Landphysikat." *Sudhoffs Archiv* 47 (1963): 394–405.

————. *Christian August Struve (1767–1807): Leben und Werk eines Görlitzer Arztes im Dienste des Humanismus der Aufklärungszeit.* Görlitz: Rat der Stadt Görlitz, 1957.

————. "Die Entwicklung des Hebammenwesens in der Oberlausitz bis zum Beginn des 19. Jahrhunderts." *Oberlausitzer Forschung* (1961): 284–306.

————. "Über statistische Untersuchungen als Beitrag zur Geschichte des Hebammenwesens im ausgehenden 18. Jahrhundert." *Centaurus* 4 (1965): 351–59.

————. "Zur materiellen Lage der Niederlausitzer Hebammen im 18. Jahrhundert." *Sudhoffs Archiv* 45 (1961): 334–40.

Ulbricht, Otto. *Kindsmord und Aufklärung in Deutschland.* Munich: R. Oldenbourg, 1990.

Ulrich, Laurel Thatcher. *A Midwife's Tale: The Life of Martha Ballard, Based on Her Diary, 1785–1812.* New York: Knopf, 1990.

Vann, James Allen. *The Making of a State: Württemberg, 1593–1793.* Ithaca, N.Y.: Cornell University Press, 1984.

Vierhaus, Rudolf, ed. *Deutsche patriotische und gemeinnützige Gesellschaften.* Wolfenbüttel: Herzog August Bibliothek, 1980.

Waddington, Ivan. *Power and Control in the Doctor-Patient Relationship: A Developmental Approach.* Leicester: Leicester Faculty of Social Sciences, 1978.

Walker, Mack. *German Home-Towns: Community, State, and General Estate, 1648–1871.* Ithaca, N.Y.: Cornell University Press, 1971.

Weber, Eugen. *Peasants into Frenchmen: The Modernization of Rural France.* Stanford, Calif.: Stanford University Press, 1976.

Weber, Max. *Wirtschaft und Gesellschaft.* Tübingen: Mohr, 1922.

Webster, Charles, ed. *Health, Medicine and Mortality in the Sixteenth Century.* Cambridge: Cambridge University Press, 1976.

Wehler, Hans-Ulrich. *Deutsche Gesellschaftsgeschichte.* Vol. 1, *Vom Feudalismus des alten Reiches bis zur defensiven Modernisierung der Reformära, 1700–1815.* Munich: Beck, 1987.

Weis, Eberhard. "Enlightenment and Absolutism in the Holy Roman Empire: Thoughts on Enlightened Absolutism in Germany." *Journal of Modern History* 58 (1986): S181–97.

Weispfennig, H. "Die Hausväterliteratur in Barock und Aufklärung." *Medizinische*

Ökologie: Aspekte und Perspektiven, edited by Maria Blomke, Heinrich Schipperges, and Gustav Wagner. Heidelberg: Huthig, 1979.

Weißmann, Andreas. "Die Schutzpockenimpfung im Herzogtum Braunschweig-Wolfenbüttel von 1800 bis zum Impfgesetz vom April 1833." Magisterarbeit, Modern History, Technische Hochschule, Braunschweig, 1993.

Weisz, George. "The Politics of Medical Professionalization in France, 1845–1848." *Journal of Social History* 12 (1978): 3–30.

Wessling, Mary Nagle. "Medicine and Government in Early Modern Württemberg." Diss., University of Michigan, 1988.

———. "Official Medicine and Customary Medicine in Early Modern Württemberg: The Career of Christoph Friedrich Pichler." *Medizin, Gesellschaft und Geschichte* 9 (1990): 21–44.

Wiesner, Merry. "Early Modern Midwifery: A Case Study." *International Journal of Women's Studies* 6 (1983): 26–43.

Wille, Friedrich Carl. *Über Stand und Ausbildung der Hebammen im 17. und 18. Jahrhundert in Chur-Brandenburg.* Berlin: Ebering, 1934.

Wilson, Renate. "Die hallischen Waisenhausmedikamente und die 'Hochst nötige Erkenntnis' in Kolonialstaat Georgien, 1733–1765." *Schriftenreihe für Technik, Naturwissenschaften und Medizin* 28 (1991): 109–28.

Wilson, Renate, and Hans Joachim Poeckern, "Pietism and Medical Care in Colonial Georgia," *Medizin, Gesellschaft und Geschichte* 9 (1990): 99–126.

Winkle, Stefan. *Johann Friedrich Struensee: Arzt—Aufklärer—Staatsmann. Beitrag zur Kultur-, Medizin- und Seuchengeschichte der Aufklärungszeit.* Stuttgart: Gustav Fischer, 1983.

Wittich, Werner. *Die Grundherrschaft in Nordwestdeutschland.* Leipzig: Dunckert & Humblot, 1896.

———. *Ländliche Verfassung Niedersachsens und Organisation des Amts im 18. Jahrhundert.* Darmstadt: L. C. Wittich'sche Hofbuchdruckerei, 1891.

Woehlkens, Erich. *Pest und Ruhr im 16. und 17. Jahrhundert: Grundlagen einer statistisch-topographischen Beschreibung der großen Seuchen, insonder in der Stadt Uelzen.* Hannover: Niedersächsisches Heimatsbund, 1954.

Wohlwill, Adolf. *Hamburg während der Pestjahre 1712–1714.* Hamburg: L. Gräfe & Sillem, 1893.

Wolf, Eric R. *Peasants.* Englewood Cliffs, N.J.: Prentice-Hall, 1966.

Wunder, Heide. *Die bäuerliche Gemeinde in Deutschland.* Göttingen: Vandenhoeck & Ruprecht, 1986.

Young, J. Harvey. *The Toadstool Millionaires.* Princeton, N.J.: Princeton University Press, 1961.

Zaunick, Rudolph, with a contribution by Dietrich Tutzke. *Der Dresdener Stadtphysikus Friedrich August Röber, 1765–1827: Ein sächsischer Gesundheitswissenschaftler in der Nachfolge Johann Peter Franks.* Leipzig: Barth, 1966.

Zimmermann, Friedrich Wilhelm Rudolf. "Die Organisation der Verwaltung im Herzogtum Braunschweig nach ihrer geschichtlichen Entwicklung." *Beiträge zur Statistik des Herzogthums Braunschweig* 9 (1889).

Zimmermann, Heinz. *Arzneimittelwerbung in Deutschland vom Beginn des 16. bis Ende des 18. Jahrhunderts.* Würzburg: Jal, 1974.

abortion, 346
absolutism, 370
abuse, 59
accidents, 239, 243, 251–52, 257, 259, 314
Achilles, Walther, 40–41
Ackerleute, 40
Actuarius, 33
administration, 55
advertisements, 153, 158, 162, 362
Advice to the People on Their Health, 66
age: and health, 301; in Hehlen, 255; of those treated by physicians, 317
ague, 296
Ahlshausen, fever in, 321
Ahrberg (surgeon in Wetteborn), 325–28
Ahrens (bathmaster and barber-surgeon in Stauffenberg), 327–28
Ailhaud, Jean (father), 172–73, 270
Ailhaud, Jean (son), 172
Aix-en-Provence, 172
Albers (barber-surgeon in Wolfenbüttel), 345, 348, 366
Albers (bathmaster in Boistedt), 218
Aldefeldt, Johann (merchant in Braunschweig), 176–77, 180
Alltag, 107, 250
Alltagsgeschichte, 6, 16
almanacs, 262
Altenburg, J. F. (pastor in Bisperode), 95
Altona river, 285
Altvater, Christina (midwife in Braunschweig), 199–200
amenorrhea, 346
Amt, 10, 32–34
Amtmänner, 21, 33, 289, 370
amulets, 361–62
analogy, 309
Anatomical-Surgical Institute (Braunschweig), 79, 137, 186, 197
Anbauer, 40
anima, 263

Anton Ulrich, 29
Apfel, Heinrich (physicus in Stadtoldendorf and Blankenburg), 99, 101–2, 117, 125
apothecaries, 105, 162–63
army surgeons, 151; feldshers, 323
arthritis, 256
artisans: culture of, 43–44; distribution of, 37, 42–43; nonguilded, 46; polyfunctional world of, 44, 47–48; rural, 43
Asmus (widow), 232–33, 353
asthma, 240
August the Younger, 29, 153–55
Austria, 19, 369

Babenroth, Anton (surgeon in Helmstedt), 187
Bächtold-Stäubli, Hanns, 306, 310
Baldinger, Ernst, 263, 302, 305
baptisms, 203
barber-surgeons: and *Pfuscherey,* 218; practice of, 185–86; protection of rights, 170; with surgeons in guild, 184–85
Barber-Surgeons' Guild (Braunschweig), 169, 186
bargaining process, 25, 50, 102
Bartels, Johann (soldier), 218
Barthold, Johann (physician in Braunschweig), 148, 324–25
bathhouses, 185, 188, 192
bathmasters: appointment, 60–61, 185; conflicts with surgeons, 183–94; and encroachment, 182–83; medical practice, 185
Bathmasters' Guild, 186
Bathmasters' Ordinance (1580), 185
Bauermeister, 39
Baumgarten (pastor and his wife), 100
Bäumler, Gottfried, 263, 265–67, 270, 302
Bavaria, 20, 369
Becker (midwife in Braunschweig), 201

Becker, Rudolf, 66, 70
Behrend (medical student), 194
Behrens, Hans, 352–53
Behrens, Rudolf August (dean of Collegium medicum), 57, 160, 175
Beier, Lucinda, 304
Beierstedt (surgeon in Vechelde), 217, 354–55
Beireis, Gottfried (professor of medicine), 179, 283–84, 286
Beltz, Georg (physicus in Hasselfelde), 111–12
Berger, Johann (identically named brothers, bathmasters in Weser district), 146–47
Berlin powders, 297
Bettmar (*Amt*), 87
births/deaths, 237, 239, 274
Bismarck (physician), 88
Bisperode, 95
Blankenburg (district): industry, 36; medical practitioners, 146; physicate, 98, 101, 112; physicus's salary, 101; population, 31
Blankenburg (town): description, 29–30; *Honorationes* in, 112, 299; physician in, 92; physicus candidates, 99–102; plague in, 64; report on, 276–78; surgeon-bathmaster conflict, 191–92
Bleichrode, 3
blessings, 307
Blum (physician in Lutter am Barenberge), 100
Blum, Conrad (physicus in Blankenburg): appointment, 89; competition with, 177; conflict with *Amtmann*, 114–16; and dysentery in Bornumhausen, 297; and dysentery in Gandersheim, 246; and fever in Opperhausen, 298, 320
Blume (medical licentiate), 146
Blumen (physicus in Blankenburg), 3
Blumenberg (surgeon in Gandersheim), 115, 320
Böckel, Conrad (cottager), 13
Bockenum, 10, 63
Bode (surgeon in Seesen), 220
bonum publicum, 8–9, 188, 217
Borges, Wilhelm (physicus in Stadtoldendorf), 95
Bornum, 10, 251, 259–60
Bornumhausen, 10, 297
böse Hals, 241

Bosse, Johann (physicus in Helmstedt), 84
Bötticher (widow), 128
Bourdieu, Pierre, 23
Bourgeoise, Louise, 194
bowel obstruction, 311
Braess, Hermann, 69
Brandstedt, von (as medical practitioner), 355–56
Bräune, 241
Braunschweig: disease patterns, 260–62; epidemics, 315; guilds, 42–43; hospital, 293; medical practitioners, 145; municipal archive, 16; physicus in, 81–83; plague, 63–64; police, 32; smallpox deaths, 331–32
Braunschweig-Wolfenbüttel: administration, 26, 55; agriculture, 34–36, 38–42; archives, 369; bureaucracy, 17, 25, 108; commerce, 175; description, 29; districts, 30; economic structure, 34–42; estates, 31, 55, 188; forestry, 34, 36; general history, 29–31; government, 20, 31–34, 243; guilds, 42–47; industry, 36–37, 175; land distribution, 38–39; land survey, 32; local health measures, 283; medical ordinances, 59–65; "Middle House," 29; "New House," 29; popular medical enlightenment, 65–67; policy making, 49–59; population, 30; ruling house, 29–30; rural and urban life, 47–49; sick poor, 292; territorial fragmentation, 30; village government, 34; village society, 38–40
bread-thieves, 169, 171
breast-feeding, 277, 280–81
breast lumps and sores, 257, 343–45
Breithaupt, Johann (pastor and schoolmaster in Bornum), 252
Brincksitzer, 40
Brown, John, 264
Brückmann, Urban (member of Collegium medicum), 97, 137, 318, 333
Brügelmann, Jan, 240–41, 272
Brunonianism, 264
Brustkrankheit, 241, 255. *See also* diseases: of chest and throat
Bücking, Johann (physicus in Wolfenbüttel), 303, 309
Büdekken, Elenora (midwife in Twieflingen), 213

Bühring, Johann (physicus in Hasselfelde), 104, 136, 335–36
bullatis, 59
bureaucracy, medical, 51
Bürgerlichkeit, 134–35
burgher's livelihood, 44, 47. *See also* Nahrung
burgher-peasant, 48
Busch, Johann (paperhanger and healer in Vorsfelde): Collegium medicum on, 229; concession for, 229; cures of, 13, 342–45, 347–48, 351, 366; initial successes, 228; medical practice, 227–29, 339–41; objections to, 229; treatment of Martin Wendenberg, 340–41
Butterbrodt, Johann (surgeon in Helmstedt), 193

cachexia, 259, 312, 342
Cagliostro, Count, 173
Calvörde: health in, 278, physicate of, 111; physicus in, 100; smallpox in, 318
cameralism, 20
Campen, von (tramp), 361
cancers, 239, 257, 341–43
carnivalists, 151–52
case books, 76, 290
case histories, 301
Cassamata (Italian "eye-doctor"), 156
cataracts, 153. *See also* oculists
catarrh, 266
catholica, 172, 173
Catholic priest, 363
cattle plagues, 35
cause of death, 238, 251. *See also* mortality
Cellarius (Bürgermeister in Helmstedt), 113–14
Celle, 29
Centner, Johann (physicus in Schöningen), 88, 104, 258
chevalier d'industrie, 166, 171
chicory, 35
children, 257, 301, 313, 347–50, 367
Christine Louise, 146
civilizing process, 23
Claudius, Matthias, 69
Claudiz (miller), 354
Claus (bathmaster in Wolfenbüttel), 346
Clausthal (Hannover), 98
clysters, 313

Coblentz, Martin (executioner in Berlin), 223
codification, 25, 27, 79
Colditz (pastor in Zorge), 5
collegia medica, 75
Collegium medicum: on abortifacients, 347; as advisory body, 54–55, 96, 104; approval of medicines, 174; assessors of, 57; on causes of disease, 280–81; character, 32, 63, 140, 370; composition, 56–58; creation, 53; decisions, 104, 284–89; duties, 53, 140; effectiveness, 55; goals, 57; improvement of midwifery, 208; and inoculation, 331; licensing, 149; and medical reform, 281; membership, 58–59, 79, 332–33; as patron, 126; and peripatetic practitioners, 158; and physici, 111, 141, 143; and physici selection, 84, 100–101; and popular medical enlightenment, 70; and population decline, 280–81; and quackery, 61; and recalcitrant patients, 299; relationship with local authorities, 55–56; reports to, 3, 10–11; on smallpox, 318–19, 332–33. *See also* Privy Council
colporteurs, 162
commercial capitalism, 164–65
commercialization, 19, 43
commodities, 181
common good, 182, 371
communities, 221, 291
competition, medical, 372
congenital deformities, 322
constitution, 313
consultations: medical, 300–301; serial, 323, 327, 329–30, 340, 345, 355, 357–59, 365; simultaneous, 323. *See also* physicians: consultations with; surgeons: consultations with
consumerism: growth, 13, 19, 62, 171, 173; in medicine, 63, 158–59, 162–65, 372; mentality of, 14, 166, 182; studies of, 62
consumption, 259, 313. *See also* diseases: of chest and throat
convulsions, 240
cooperation, 54–55, 107
cordon sanitaire, 64
corn doctors, 64, 156
corporatism: and identity, 103; language of, 163, 167, 170, 370; meaning of, 9, 15,

corporatism (*cont.*)
  19, 17, 60–61, 63, 194, 371; mentality
  of, 170; and physicians, 170
Councilor von Köring, 153, 156
Cramer (*Amtmann* in Königslutter), 295
Cramer (surgeon in Walkenried), 112
Crusis (cloister), 79
Crusius (bathmaster in Hedwigsburg), 291
cures: combination of, 362 (*see also* consultations: serial; consultations: simultaneous); costs of, 345; dramaturgy of,
  359, 363; expectations of, 351; magical,
  305–7, 362; and ritual, 359; and show
  business, 359; spring, 307–8; superstitious, 305, 362; sympathetic, 290,
  306–7, 309, 359, 361–62; unsuccessful,
  349–50; for venereal disease, 173
custom, 27, 186

damp, 285
Daspe, 253, 323
deaths: in childbirth, 239; from protracted
  illnesses, 314; sudden, 314. *See also* mortality
debts, 133
Dedekind, Johann (physicus in Königslutter, Schöppenstedt, and Holzminden),
  123–26, 136
defensive modernization, 22
Dehne, Johann (physicus in Schöningen),
  106
Delligsen, 36
Delmer, Lt., 178
dental tools, 160–61
depopulation, 237
Dettum, 69
diarrhea, 242–43. *See also* dysentery
Diepgen, Paul, 303
Diez (captain), 230
disciplining, social, 22–24, 288, 373
diseases: attitudes toward, 236; causes of,
  265–70, 273–74, 313; of chest and
  throat, 240–41, 257–59; of children,
  238, 322; classification of, 238, 240–43;
  and local administration, 90; and environment, 243, 271; explanations of,
  262, 307; gastrointestinal, 241–42; inappropriate responses to, 294; interpretation of, 274; mysterious, 247; nonlethal,
  243; numerical importance of, 238; occurrence of, 238; outbreaks of, 299; pat-

terns of, 240, 242; scattered incidence of,
  244, 247; of skin, 271; statistics on, 272
  (*see also* morbidity); terms for, 240 (*see
  also* nosology); treatment of, 269; undiagnosed, 244; world of ten, 261–62
dissection, 130
Disziplin. See disciplining, social
divine interval, 261
doctrine of signs, 309
documentary record, 17, 49, 56, 236–37,
  369
domestic industry, 37, 49
Dorfgericht, 39
Dorotheenstadt (parish in Berlin), 240–41
drastionien, 174
Dreyer, Friedrich (cobbler), 229, 351, 366,
  337–39
dropsy, 240
Drüsen (midwife in Saustadt), 213
Du Coudray, Angelique le Boursier, 194
Dupuy de la Porcherie, 172
Du Roi, Johann (physicus in Braunschweig, secretary of Collegium medicum), 79, 137
dye plants, 35
dysentery: in Ammensen, 246; causes, 267–
  68; in Delligsen, 247; in Eil near
  Boffzen, 245–46; epidemics, 64–65, 81,
  242–47, 258, 261, 297, 321–22, 324; in
  Escherhausen, 249; experience of, 245;
  in Fürstenberg, 245; in Gandersheim,
  246; in Greene, 246; in Hamm Münden,
  245; in Naensen, 246; treatment of, 268;
  in Wensen, 246; in Weser district, 245–
  46
dysmenorrhea, 346

ecclesiastical authorities, 370
Eckermann (surgeon in Braunschweig),
  339, 348
economy of makeshifts, 228
Eggeling (surgeon in Neubrück), 334
Eggers (superintendent in Harzburg), 94–
  95, 296
Eicke (physician in Escherhausen), 95
Eicke, Friedrich (physicus in Gan-
  dersheim), 107, 124–25
Einen (midwife in Gittelde), 209
Elbe river, 29
elderly, 367
Elias, Norbert, 23–24

Elisabeth Ernestine Antoinette (abbess in Gandersheim), 106–7
elite culture, 19
elite/popular medicine, 290
Ellrich, 3, 5
emetics, 313
empiétement, 150
empirics, 166
encircling, 310
encroachment, 163–64, 166–67, 182–83, 204. *See also Pfuscher; Pfuscherey*
enemas, 313
Engelade, 10, 120
Enlightenment: character of, 47, 138–39, 371–72; as clique, 295; definition, 65; and education, 131; and government, 20, 22–23; medical, 14; of peasants, 294; and reforms, 371–72. *See also* physici: and Enlightenment; popular medical enlightenment
entrepreneurs, 164, 171–72, 182, 372. *See also* peddlers
environmentalism, 271–72
epidemics: evidence of, 243; experience of, 243–50, 256, 321; impact of, 248; legislation on, 63–65; and medical choice, 315–22; during Seven Years' War, 248–49
epilepsy, 302
ergot, 275
erysipelas, 302, 312
Eschershausen, 34, 205–6
ethnography, 307
ethnomedicine, 303
everyday life, 108, 129
evidence, 236, 285
executioner: income of, 223; as medical practitioner, 222–25, 307, 323–24; position of, 222–23

Fabricius, Johann (lithotomist), 159
Fabriken, 36. *See also* Braunschweig-Wolfenbüttel: industry
face-to-face relationships, 80
Fahner, J. C. (physicus in Hohenstein, Prussia), 99
Fahrenholtz, Johann (physicus in Königslutter and Wolfenbüttel), 111, 193–94
fair price, 44
Fasbender, Heinrich, 196

fatalism, 11–12, 306
Faust, Bernhard, 66
feldsher, 323
fevers: as diagnosis, 325; epidemics of, 244; inflammatory, 238, 269; intermittent, 241, 256; malignant, 247–48, 255, 310, 316, 320; names of, 244; nervous, 316; occurrence of, 241; putrid, 316, 321; scarlet, 296; seasoning, 241; types of, 238, 241, 247, 317; "vicious," 249–50
fiction, 7, 17
"Filth-Pharmacopoeia," 310
Fincci, Peter, 82
Fincke (surgeon in Seesen), 190–91, 219–20
Findler (*Pfuscher*), 215
Fischer (mining clerk in Walkenried), 5
Fischer (surgeon in Supplingenburg), 189
Fissell, Mary, 165, 307
fistulas, 239, 257, 340–41, 345
Flecken, 30
Flentge (shepherd in Hagen), 295, 323–24
Flögen, von (member of Privy Council), 55–56, 59, 106, 232
folk: disregard for health, 296; healers, 12, 166; medicine, 300, 302–15, 373; prejudices of, 296; responses to illness, 295; wisdom, 16
fontanelles, 308
Foucault, Michel, 22–24
fractures, 240
Frank, Johann Peter, 274, 279
Frankfurt, 43
Fredersdorf (police director in Braunschweig), 158
Freÿenburg, Clare (midwife in Eschershausen), 206
Freyer, Gottlieb (physicus in Holzminden), 220
Fridrich, Christian ("a baptized Jew"), 5
Friedrich (knacker in Calvörde), 219, 328–29
Friedrich Ulrich, 29
Friesel. See purples
Fröhlich (executioner in Ahlfeld), 329, 366
Funcke (commissioner in Schöppenstedt), 285–86
Funcke, Conrad (executioner in Braunschweig), 223
Fürstenberg, 104

Futtermenger, Johann (bathmaster in Seesen), 190

Gackens, Catharine (midwife in Alversdorf), 213
Gagliardo, John, 294
Galenism, 263–64
Gandersheim (*Amt*), 37
Gandersheim (town): abbey, 30, 106; artisans, 147; guilds, 43; hospital, 292; medical care in, 293; medical practitioners, 147; midwives, 207; physicus, 58, 115; plague, 63; report on, 278; smallpox in, 334; vaccination in, 334
Geheimer Rat. See Privy Council
Gellert, Christian Fürchtegott, 129
gemeine Mann, der, 293
Gennzinger, Franz, 305
"Georg and Maria" (fictional peasants), 271, 302
Georgi (subphysicus in Blankenburg), 98–99
Gercke (midwife in Neumarck), 209
Gericht, 32
Geröder districts (Prussia), 5–6
Gesenius, Wilhelm (physicus in Walkenried), 137
Gesundheits-Katechismus, 66
Girault (dentist), 156, 362
Giseler, Laurentius (physicus in Braunschweig), 82, 135
glass cutting, 121
Glauber salts, 174
Gnädigst Privilegierte Braunschweigische Zeitung für Städte, Flecken und Dörfer, 69
Goesche (*medicus practicus* in Bevern), 146
Goldschmidt, Jonas, 303–4
Goslar, 10, 127
Gotthard, Joseph, 301–2
Göttingen, inoculation in, 332
governance, 20, 243
Grabner, Elfriede, 307
Graf (apothecary in Schöningen), 104
Graham, 172
Granzien, Ludolf (*Amtmann* in Gandersheim), 115–16, 296
Gravenhorst brothers, 36, 174
Gregor, Viktor (physicus in Braunschweig), 82
Grimme (village headman in Hohegeiss), 5
grocers, 180

Großkotsassen, 40
Groß-Vahlberg (estate near Schöppenstedt), 285
Grotian (forester in Holzminden), 117
"ground rabbits" (*Bönhasen*), 166. *See also* guilds; *Pfuscher*
Grundherr, 39
Grünenplan, 112
Gruner, Christian, 72
Guelphs, 29
guilds: and consumerism, 182; control of, 45, 159, 234; economic rights of, 180; and economic rivalry, 167, 234; and health care, 291; "just" pricing by, 44; and livelihood, 161; and medical practitioners, 46; and medicine, 171; mentality of, 45; ordinances about, 45; and progress, 62

haemorrhagia cerebri, 259
Hagen (widow in Voightsdahlum), 357
Hagen, Christian von (physicus in Königslutter, Helmstedt, and Braunschweig), 57
Hahn (bathmaster in Gadenstedt), 311
Hahnemann, Samuel, 93, 134
Hainen, Catherine (midwife in Lelm), 209
Halbspänner, 40
Hamburg, 43
Hammer, Johann (bathmaster in Lutter am Barenberge), 231
Handdienst, 39
Handwörterbuch des deutschen Aberglaubens, 306, 310
Hannover, 29
Hantelmann (privy councilor and *Amtmann* in Holzminden), 56, 88
Happe, Ernestus (surgeon in Weser district), 146
Harke, August (physicus in Gandersheim and Calvörde), 334
Härtel (physician in Alfeld), 95
Harz (district), 29–31, 36, 88, 207
Harzburg (*Amt*), 10, 120, 213
Hasselfelde, 92–94, 336
Haupt (bathmaster in Blankenburg), 192
Hauptkirche parish (Wolfenbüttel), 316
Hausnotdurft, 47, 161, 165, 372
Hausväterliteratur, 263
healers: alternative, 12; peripatetic, 18, 151–52; popular, 12, 168; sedentary, 18;

sympathetic, 359, 361–62 (*see also* cures: sympathetic)

health: attitude toward, 236; definition of, 265, 290; desire for, 368, 373; and diet, 269–71, 308; in early modern Europe, 289; environment, 265, 271, 277; and equilibrium, 264, 307–8; and evacuations, 266, 301, 313; history of, 16; and humors, 308; indifference to, 305; and lifestyle, 265; and moderation, 308; and overexertion, 313–14; parables about, 302; and the passions, 264, 276; preservation of, 269–70; statistics on, 272; and wars, 314, 236–37

"health instruction for the people," 68, 70

health policy, 27, 50, 72

health *règlement*, 66

Hebel, Johann, 69

Hedwigsburg, 291–92

Hehlen: deaths in, 255–56; description, 253, 317, 323–24; morbidity in, 256; records on, 323–24

Hehn (magistrate in Königslutter), 188

Heidorn (midwife in Braunschweig), 201

Heiland (magistrate in Walkenried), 4–7, 9

Heim, Ernst, 80–81

Heine (horse doctor), 361

Heine, Elisabeth (midwife in Westendorf), 213

Heinmeyer, Anne (midwife in Hehlen), 209

Heinze (knacker in Neuwallmoden), 224

Heister (privy councilor), 56

Held, Rudolf (*Landmedicus*), 87

Hellwig (physicus in Fürstenberg), 103–4

Helmstedt: bathhouse, 186–88; city council, 114; description, 30, 32, 34, 42, 118; medical practitioners, 145–46; medical society, 59; municipal archive, 16; physicus, 83–84, 113–14; plague, 63; university of, 43, 48, 120

Helmuth, Johann (pastor), 69, 303

hemorrhoids, 345–46

Henrichs, Marie (midwife in Helmstedt-Neumarck), 209

Henser (schoolmaster in Wolfshagen), 120

Herrhausen, 10

Hertz (bathmaster in Braunschweig), 316

Hesse, 20

Heyen, 297

Heym (physician), 13

Hieronymi, Georg (physicus in Wolfenbüttel), 88, 248, 316

Hildebrandt, Georg (professor), 137, 265, 272–73

Hilmer (oculist), 153, 156

Himly, Karl (professor), 137

Hingstin, Ilsa (midwife in Seesen), 208

Hinze, August (physicus in Calvörde and Vorsfelde), 77, 253, 273

Hippocratism, 264, 272

Hirsch (journeyman surgeon in Seesen), 191

Hirsch, August, 123, 129, 137

historiam epidemia, 120–21. *See also* epidemics

Hoerstal (pastor in Schöningen), 179

Höfer (physicus in Braunschweig), 57

Höfer, Josua (apothecary in Gandersheim), 147

Hoffman, Friedrich, 173

Hoffmann, Johann (physicus in Calvörde and Stadtoldendorf): as botanist, 309; in Calvörde, 111; on cause of disease, 275, 279, 287; on herbal remedies, 303; and *Pfuscherey*, 295

Höfler, Max, 310

Hofmeister, 136

Hohegeiss, 4, 6

Hohenstein, 5

Hohmann (apothecary in Stadtoldendorf), 105

Holdefreund, Johann (physicus in Königslutter), 105–6, 110, 123, 137

Holtensen, 206

Holzminden: dysentery in, 320–21; guilds, 43; industry, 36; malignant fever in, 295; physicate, 103, 124; physicians, 104; physicus, 115–16; plague, 63

Holzmindisches Wochenblatt, 69

home doctoring, 14

homeopathy, 93

home remedies: Lange on, 137; types of, 296–97, 305, 310; uses of, 307, 316, 329, 339, 345–46

home towns, 43, 45, 47, 161

Honorationes, 26, 81, 253

hopeless cases, 342

Hoorn, Johann von, 197

Horenburg, Anne (midwife in Braunschweig), 195–97

Hornburg, municipal archive in, 16

hospitals, 292
Hotopp (widow), 296
Hoven, Friedrich von, 80
Höxter, 104
Hubrig, Hans, 129, 132
Hufeland, Christoph, 133, 242, 263–65
Hufton, Olwen, 228
Hummel (physician in Blankenburg), 146
humoralism, 264
humors, 243, 308
Hundemarck (medical practitioner in Braunschweig), 316
hygienic literature, 65
hysteria, 302

identity, 203, 289
ignorance, 305
iliac passion, 311
illness: asthenic, 264; attitudes toward, 236; description, 307; definition, 253, 290; experience of, 243, 262, 327–28; fatalism in, 11–12, 306; and imagination, 264, 314–15; language of, 311; narratives of, 290, 300–301, 312, 337, 353; nonlethal, 256, 322–31; perceptions of, 365; and poverty, 275; religion, 20, 306; sthenic, 264. *See also* diseases
Immerwährende Gesundheits-Kalender, 66
imperial free cities, 45
Imperial Trade Edict (1731), 44–45
incantations, 307
"Increase and Decrease of the Inhabitants," 11, 237, 273–74, 276
industry, 37
influenza, 257, 261
information, 239
infringement, 166–67. *See also Pfuscherey*
Ingrao, Charles, 22
inoculation: acceptance of, 306, 333; articles about, 138; attitudes toward, 367; in Königslutter, 333; large-scale, 332; and medical decisions, 290; opposition to, 306, 331, 333; reaction to, 109; success of, 332, 373; support for, 331
insiders/outsiders, 26, 109, 221, 370
in spe succedendi, 199, 202
interloper, 166, 171
interloping, 14, 233, 372
internal/external cures, 348–49, 351, 356
Ittershagen (medical student), 174

Jammer, 242
Jerze, 10
Jordan (physician), 135
Joseph, Seligman (Jew in Hildesheim), 342–43
Joseyli (surgeon in Vorsfelde), 340
journeymen, 291. *See also* guilds
Julian (actor and dentist), 160–61
Julius Hospital (Würzburg), 80
Juncker, Johann, 263, 265–66
Jungbauer, Gustav, 303
Junker, von (*Amtmann* in Schöppenstedt), 127
Jürgens (feldsher), 341
Jürgens, August (veterinarian in Helmstedt), 146
Jürgens, Zacharias (administrator of saltpeter works), 231–32, 317–38
jus nominendi, 88
Justiarius, 33

Kahle (physician), 92
Karl's School (Würzburg), 80
Käseberg (miller in Bettmar), 359
Kästner, Nicolaus (physician in Walkenried), 6
Kayser (physician in Wolfenbüttel), 248
Keck (body-physician), 146
Kelling, Heinrich (sympathetic healer in Salder), 361
Kinderfreund, Der, 66
Kleinjogg, 69
Kleinkotsassen, 40
Klein-Rhüden, 10, 251
Klein Vahlberg, 335
knackers, 218, 223–24
Knackschmidt (feldsher in Braunschweig), 316
Knieriem (soldier's wife), 346–47
Knopp, August (bathmaster in Stadtoldendorf), 147
Knupf, Ferdinand (medicine peddler and carnivalist), 156–57
Köhler (medicine peddler), 216
Königslutter (town): bathhouse, 187–90; description, 43, 87, 123; municipal archive, 16; plague, 64
Könnecker, Maria (midwife in Gandersheim), 147
Kraps, Heinrich Valentin (bathmaster in Helmstedt), 186–87

Kraps, Johann Heinrich (bathmaster in Helmstedt), 187
Kratzenstein (physician), 93
Krätzer (physician in Calvörde), 226
Krätzer, Georg (executioner in Calvörde), 226
Krätzer, Peter (executioner in Calvörde), 225–26
Krebs, Friedrich (physicus in Blankenburg and Walkenried), 99, 112
Kreyenburg, Just (physicus in Helmstedt), 84, 113
Kriebel (cantor in Langelsheim), 120
Krügelstein, Johann, 66
Krüger, Margaretha (midwife in Holzminden and Braunschweig), 202–3, 205
Krünitz, Johann Georg, 167, 307
Küchingen, 298–99
Kunst, 159
Kunze (pastor in Wolfenbüttel), 252
Küster, Ferdinand (physicus in Calvörde), 101

Ladius (pastor in Opperhausen), 298
landowners, 21
Landphysicus, 79
Landtagsabschiede, 31
Lange (soldier), 230–31, 330, 356–57
Lange, Johann (physicus in Helmstedt), 97, 137, 268, 310
Langelsheim (*Amt*), 10, 120, 250
language: of artisans, 175; of illness, 311–13; of labor, 7; of livelihood, 205; of quackery, 14
Langwell (surgeon in Lutter am Barenberge), 220–21
Lattman (physician), 174
Laue (feldsher in Braunschweig), 316
Laurentius (apothecary in Bisperdoe), 95
laxatives, 270–71, 313
legislation, medical, 50, 62–63
leg ulcers, 229, 239, 257, 269, 314, 337, 339
Lehnert, David (oil peddler), 170
Lentin, Friedrich, 273
licensing, 159
Lichtenberger (Ailhaud's agent in Strasbourg), 176
Liebenberg, 13
Liebrecht, Johann (physician in Gandersheim), 147, 327
lifestyle, 110, 371

Lindemann, Johann (physicus in Königslutter), 205
lists: of inoculees, 333; of patients, 324–25; of products, 163–64
lithotomists, 156
livelihood: appropriate, 165; citizen's (*bürgerliche Nahrung*), 161; definition, 161–62; disruption of, 166; language of, 175, 190, 205; loss of, 15, 171, 223; and midwives, 203; protection of, 62–63, 170; questions of, 10, 186; responsibility for, 170. *See also Nahrung*
local authorities, 292, 299
Loeber, Christian (physicus in Calvörde and Vorsfelde), 99, 129–33, 136
Loux, Françoise, 304
Löwendleinen, 37
Lower Saxony, 29
Lucas, Johann (dentist and medicine peddler), 158
Lüneburg, 29, 97
Lungensucht, 240–41, 257–59
Lütge (bathmaster in Langelsheim), 219
Lutter am Barenberge (*Amt*): description, 29; medical practitioners in, 148; peasant holding in, 41; reports from, 120; smallpox in, 335
lying-in facility (Braunschweig), 197

Macholdus, Antonius (physicus in Braunschweig), 82
macrobiotics, 263
madder, 37
Magdeburg, 113
magic: decline of, 306; and disease causation, 11; and healing, 20, 290, 359–65. *See also* cures: magical; cures: sympathetic; thaumaturgy
magistrates, 278, 370
Mahlum, 257–58
malpractice, 59, 169
manufactories: definition, 36; Küblingen, 127; size, 36; workers in, 37, 43
Marcard (physician in Thedinghausen), 268
market culture, 182
market demand, 15
market economy, 62, 166
marketing: changes in, 177, 372–73; disputes over, 176–77; strategies of, 173
marketplace, 13, 62
market towns, 30

Markt-Flecken, 30
Martini, Johann (dean of Collegium medicum), 55, 57, 79, 101, 124, 204, 298–99
Martini, Ludwig (Jr.) (surgeon in Gandersheim), 147
Martini, Ludwig (Sr.) (surgeon in Gandersheim), 147
mastectomy, 344
maternity care, 67
Mattenberg (*Amtmann* in Walkenried), 4, 9
Mävern (midwife in Badenhausen, Neu-
 und Oberhütte), 209
Maxmilian (doctor), 92
May, Friedrich (physicus in Schöningen
 and Schöppenstedt), 99, 101, 104–6
measles, 238
mechanism, 263–64
Meder (physicus in Walkenried), 6
mediating authorities, 31–32
medical advice: as commodity, 165, 357,
 364; as gift, 165
medical alternatives, 290
medical care: as advice, 356–57; costs, 217,
 292, 356–57, 367; payments for, 296,
 319–20; for the poor, 117–18, 291–92;
 provision for, 293
medical choice. *See* medical decisions
medical competence, 160
medical decisions: concepts of, 13; cultural
 values and, 221–22; logic of, 34, 71, 108,
 133, 289–91, 329, 337, 356–57, 365; and
 moral economy, 181–82; unwise, 293
medical encounter: boundaries of, 354–55;
 character of, 290, 363–65; complexity
 of, 366; and larger world, 337, 358–59,
 364; participants in, 300–301, 358–59
medical hierarchies, 149
medicalization: process, 168–69, 288, 369,
 373; theories, 18, 373
medical landscape, 144
Medical Ordinance (Prussia, 1685), 5
Medical Ordinance (1721), 51–53, 59–60,
 82, 149–50, 156, 162
Medical Ordinance (1747), 51–54, 58–61,
 88, 150, 162
medical pluralism, 233–34. *See also* medical
 decisions
medical police, 81, 89
medical practice: boundaries of legitimate,
 59, 159, 255; and communities, 234–35;

concessions for, 157, 159–60, 221; il-
 licit/licit, 18
medical practitioners: distribution, 300;
 economic viability, 159; examination of,
 60; livelihood, 149; medical students as,
 192–93; names for, 74; numbers of, 144,
 147–48, 165; peripetatic, 74, 153, 162;
 privileges, 151; sedentary, 74; self-image,
 149; variety, 13, 21, 144, 151, 222, 290–
 91, 300, 350–51. *See also* bathmasters;
 executioner; feldsher; midwives; physicians; surgeons
medical promiscuity, 305
medical reform, 11, 22, 74, 81, 216, 288,
 305, 373
medical societies, 53, 59, 248
medical topographies, 21, 272–73, 279, 283
Medicamenten-Expedition (Halle), 172
medicastris, 59
medicine: academic, 373; alternative, 168;
 as business, 180; effect of, 367; in eighteenth century, 263; foreign, 180; fringe,
 12, 168; and governing, 283–88; herbal,
 303, 309; history of, 15–16, 168; internal, 151; manufacture, 162; marketing,
 176; monitoring, 173–74; ortho-
 dox/unorthodox, 73; panaceas, 173;
 peddling, 162, 373; popular/elite, 73,
 262, 303–4 (*see also* professions); proprietary, 165, 171, 173, 182; as science,
 180; specifics, 171, 173; systems of, 264–
 65, 366; vendors, 162
medici practici. See medical practitioners: variety of
medicus forensis, 77
medicus provincialus, 85
Meibom, Johann von (dean of Collegium
 medicum), 55, 57, 127, 174
Meierrecht, 39
Meierzins, 39
Meisterei. See executioner
melancholy, 267
Menschenfresser, 150
Menschenschlachter, 171
Menschensterben. See mortality
menses, 301, 346
mental disorders, 292–93
mentalities, 6, 16
Mercker (medical practitioner), 308
Mesmer, Anton, 172

Meßing (executioner in Halle), 297, 324, 393

Metzler, F. X., 316

Meyer (councilor in Braunschweig), 316

Meyer, Branden (wholesaler), 176

Meyer, Friedrich (physicus in Helmstedt), 96–97, 118

Meyer, Hermann (*Medicus & Chymicus*), 159

Meÿer, Rosine (midwife in Seesen), 208

Meyer, Thadaeus (operator and oculist), 156

miasmas, 243

Michaels (bathmaster in Wolfenbüttel), 231–32

midwifery, 194–205, 207. *See also* midwives; rural midwives

midwives: ages of, 199; conduct, 211; conflict with warming-women, 204–5; desirable attributes, 209; earnings, 207; entitlements, 117; examination of, 202; instruction of, 197; investigation of, 205; literacy, 197; lives, 194; as medical practitioners, 205; and *Pfuscherey*, 194; as professionals, 195; quality of, 281; as "sisters," 195. *See also* midwives (in Braunschweig); rural midwives

midwives (in Braunschweig): backgrounds, 197; earnings, 198–99, 201; husbands' occupation, 199; instructional costs for, 200–201; life histories, 197; numbers of, 197, 203–4; oaths of, 206; and *Pfuscherey*, 202–3; relationships among, 202; salary, 198–99; selection and training, 197–98, 200–202; size of practice, 198–99; supernumerary, 202. *See also* rural midwives

Mihle, Clara Catrina von der (midwife in Braunschweig), 197

military surgeons, 61, 169, 192–93; feldshers, 323

millers, 307

mining, 34, 36

Misch, Johanna (midwife in Gandersheim), 147

Mittelbacksche woman (medical practitioner), 358

mobility, 289

modernity, 23

modernization, 22–23, 25, 48

monopoly, medical, 51

moral cost accounting, 15

moral economy, 47, 61, 175, 181–82

moral judgments, 313

morbidity: causes, 239; data on, 236, 253

Möricke (blacksmith in Braunschweig), 329–30

mortality: age distribution, 242, 259; causes, 239–50; child, 259, 281; data on, 236, 238; of the elderly, 259; excessive, 275; infant, 274; listings of, 297–98; in prime of life, 259; records of, 253, 297–98. *See also* deaths

mortification, 239

mountebanks, 60

Mühlenbein, Georg (physicus in Schöningen), 138, 150, 355

Müller, Jacob (physicus in Seesen): Collegium medicum's dissatisfaction with, 119–21; conflicts with local community, 119–23, 219–20; education of, 135; and *Pfuscherey*, 222, 297; as physicus candidate, 106–7; reports of, 10, 13–14, 207

Münchehof, 118

Nahrung, 61, 161–62, 175, 223, 372

Nahrungs-Störerey, 166. *See also* breadthieves

Nahrungs-Verderber, 167. *See also* breadthieves

Neckerhausen (Württemburg), 48

"Neighbor Heinrich," 69

neighborliness, 14, 62

Neubrück, 334

Neues Hannöversches Magazin, 168

Neuhofer (midwife in Zorge), 4

Neustadt, 94

new cultural history, 16

Nezel, Siegfried (surgeon in Walkenried), 3, 9

Nicolai (surgeon in Harzburg), 214–17, 366

Nienstedt (physician in Braunschweig), 312

non-naturals, 249, 265–66

Nordhausen, 3

nosology, 238, 240, 302

notables, 21. *See also Honorationes*

Noth- und Hülfsbüchlein in der Ruhr und epidemischen Krankheiten, 66

Nußbaum, Dorothea (midwife in Braunschweig), 201

obstetrical instruments, 302
obstructionism, 119
Ochersleben, 105
oculists, 153, 156
Oestreich, Gerhard, 22–23
Oettinger (hospital administrator in Braunschweig), 169–71
old age, 239
onera publica, 161, 191, 223
operateurs, 150–51
Opperhausen, 207, 298, 320
ordinances, 27, 75
Örlhausen, 206
Orxhausen, 207
Othmer (physician), 166
Otte (midwife in Zorge), 207, 210–11

pain, 368
pamphlets, 64–65, 268–69
panaceas, 172
Pape (bathmaster in Harzburg), 177, 214
Papen (surgeon in Seesen), 190, 219
parish registers, 250–53, 313
pastors: and administration of public health, 21, 289; criticism of physicians, 179; involvement in inoculation and vaccination, 77; and medical care, 179, 299; as medical practitioners, 70, 76–77; and parish registers, 237, 239, 313; and *Pfuscherey,* 296; and popular medical enlightenment, 70, 179; and *poudre purgative,* 179; and reporting of disease, 299
patent remedies, 151–52
patients: and consultations, serial, 222 (*see also* consultations: serial); disregard for physicians, 297; expectations, 290, 351–52, 365; narratives, 301 (*see also* illness: narratives of); process of becoming, 21; questions for, 300–301; response to illness, 297
patria, 84
patriotism, 277
patronage: and enlightenment, 138–39 (*see also* Enlightenment: as clique); in government, 26, 33, 75; networks of, 58; and physici, 102, 135, 142; and physicians, 79–80, 372; in towns, 188

Paulus (physician), 346
peasants: attitudes toward, 293; disregard for health, 295; economic condition, 41; ignorance, 295–97; mentality, 38; political, 31; reevaluation of, 293–94; types of, 40; underclass (*unterbäuerliche*), 40, 48
Peasants' War (1525), 31
peddlers: medicine, 216; oil, 162–63
pediatrics, 67
Pelling, Margaret, 12
Pestalozzi, Johann, 66
Peter, Jean-Pierre, 240
Peters (joiner in Bortfeld), 358
Petsch (physician in Braunschweig), 316
Petzold, Martin (medicine peddler), 159
Pfannenschmidt, Julianne (midwife-designate in Zorge), 210–11
Pfuscher: definition, 61, 150, 166–67; economics, 215–16, 218; in guilds, 46, 171; and local authorities, 220; local support for, 219–21; rivalry among, 215, 221; variety, 222, 227. *See also* quacks
Pfuscherey: casual, 230; conditions fostering, 219; defense of, 216–17; definition, 14, 61, 166; and guilds, 15, 166–67, 170–71; of medical students, 192–94; toleration of, 168; use of term, 150, 167, 214. *See also* quackery
pharmacopoeia, 173, 311
philosophes, 10
physical examination, 300–301
physicates: conditions in, 111; expansion of, 91–92; history of, 81
physici: age, 142; and agronomy, 136–37; *Alltag* of, 107; and *Amtmänner,* 90; applicants for, 96, 105, 126; appointment of, 95–96, 103, 141–42; arrival in district, 110; aspirations, 135–36; attributes, 96–97; as authors, 137; as bureaucrats, 83, 108; in cities and towns, 53, 91; as clients, 73, 75, 142; and Collegium medicum, 110, 123; community position, 114, 289, 370–71; competition among, 102, 125; conflicts over, 89; contracts with, 82; data analysis, 237; duties, 58, 72, 75, 77; and Enlightenment, 73, 75, 133, 136; entitlements, 110, 117; family backgrounds, 136; forensic duties, 7, 117; in Gandersheim, 73; history, 75, 77, 81; instructions for, 89; lifestyle, 100,

108, 135–36, 143; and local authorities, 89, 113–14, 119–20; and locals, 110, 123; and medical policy, 140–41; multiple roles, 79, 108; network of, 85; objections to, 87, 104–6, 109–10, 124, 142; patronage of, 73; payments for, 87, 90, 117, 119, 142; and the poor, 117–19; private practice, 125; and Privy Council, 87; and public health, 107–8; regulation of, 90; reports of, 75; reputation, 100, 114; salaries, 58, 103, 110, 112–13, 141; selection, 92, 100, 102; self-image, 73; 1696 plan for, 85; social mobility, 135; transfer of, 124, 126, 135, 142; transportation, 89–90

physicians: consultations with, 321–23, 336–39, 365–66; and corporatism, 166; education of, 304–5; and folk medicine, 303; learnedness of, 304; lifestyle, 304; objections to, 298; problems of, 8; and professionalization, 17; as professionals, 372; right to practice, 125; self-image, 373

Pini, Ernst (physicus in Wolfenbüttel and Schöppenstedt), 111, 126–29, 286–88, 296

plague: doctors for, 77; edicts about, 64; hospital for, 293; occurrence of, 63, 65, 81, 236, 242–44

pneumonia, 257. *See also* diseases: of chest and throat

poaching, 15, 190, 233

police ordinances (*Polizey-Ordnungen*), 27, 32

policy: implementation, 18; making, 49–51, 56, 139–40, 237, 243, 371; medical, 20, 70

political culture, 32

Pollitz, Johann (apothecary in Thedinghausen), 177

popular culture, 18

popular/elite, 74, 165

popular medical enlightenment: agents of, 66–67, 70, 279; audience for, 263; debate over, 66, 294–95; definition, 63; and peasants, 66; physician involvement, 262; publications, 262–63, 295

popular religiosity, 20, 306

population growth, 48, 289

populationism, 63, 67

"populuxe" items, 182

porcelain works (in Fürstenburg), 79

Porter, Dorothy, 16, 304

Porter, Roy, 13, 15–16, 62, 158, 164–65, 304

possession, demonic, 305–6

potatoes, 35, 284–86

Pott, Johann (secretary and dean of Collegium medicum), 57, 79, 99, 144–45, 175, 232, 333

poudre d'Ailhaud, la. See poudre purgative

poudre purgative: analysis of, 173; Collegium medicum and, 179–80; condemnation of, 172; effects of, 173; manufacture of, 176; physici and, 179; sale of, 175–76; support for, 178; Tissot on, 172; uses of, 173, 178

poultice, 337, 341, 344

Praesun, Johann (medicine peddler), 180

prayers, 307

pregnancy, 346

privileges. *See* medical practice: concessions for

Privy Council (*Geheimer Rat*): and Collegium medicum, 54, 104, 370; on commerce and industry, 174, 181; composition of, 32; decisions of, 289; and guilds, 46, 181; and health policies, 27; and physici, 116; responsibilities of, 32

professional identity, 9, 103

professionalization, 18, 75, 140, 164, 168–70, 372–73

professions: female, 195; history of, 74; in medicine, 167, 373

professors, 79, 83

prognosticon, 67

property, 62

protectionism, 36, 180. *See also* Braunschweig-Wolfenbüttel: commerce; Braunschweig-Wolfenbüttel: industry

proto-industrialization, 37

proverbs, 16

provision, 175

Prümann (tanner's apprentice in Wiede), 5

Prussia, 5, 19–20, 45, 51, 369

publication, medical, 137–38

public health, 58, 68

public interest, 182

pulse, 301–2

purgatives. *See* laxatives
purples, 115, 238, 241, 257

quackery: cases of, 169; charges of, 169;
   and consumerism, 158; definition, 61–
   63, 168–69; investigations of, 291, 365;
   perceptions of, 165; in Seesen, 121; use
   of term, 14, 167
quacks: description, 10, 12, 150, 164–71;
   definition, 151; numbers of, 214; use of
   term, 171
Quacksalberey. See quackery; quacks

Raabe, August, 69
rabies, 257, 259, 311, 313
Raebcke, 38
Raeff, Marc, 22–25, 139
Ragolosche powder, 173
Ralwes (physician), 345
Ramsey, Matthew, 12, 73, 166
reason, 371
reciprocity, 357
Reck (councilor in Braunschweig), 316
Reck (pastor in Ahlshausen), 321
Reese, Georg (physicus in Königslutter),
   99, 101
refining, 36
regimental surgeons, 323
Reichmann (apothecary in Braunschweig),
   316
Reichsdeputationshauptschluß, 30
Reinbeck (physician), 100
Reitenmeyer (physician in Braunschweig),
   339
rèmede universel, 172. *See also poudre purgative*
Reser (clothes peddler in Eich), 362–64
retail trade, 177
Rheinischer Hausfreund, 69
rheumatism, 256, 269
rheums, 239, 315
Richter, Benjamin, 167
Richter, Christian (physicus in Helmstedt),
   83
Riddagshausen (cloister), 79
Riedt, Georg (bathmaster in Stadtolden-
   dorf), 147
Riley, James, 261–62, 271–72
Rochow, Friedrich Eberhard von, 66
Röhle (apothecary), 99, 214–15
Roose, Theodor, 137

rootedness, 289
Rörhand, Carl, 81, 117, 335
Rose (knacker in Schöppenstedt), 224
Rosenstern, von (*Amtmann* in Wickensen),
   117
Rote Zeitung, 69
Rudelstaedter (physician in Gandersheim),
   100
Rudolph August, 29
Rüland (surgeon in Königslutter), 189–90,
   348–49
rural midwives: and community, 214; complaints about, 210; conditions of, 208,
   212; earnings, 208, 212; education, 213;
   entitlements, 207–8; husbands, 213; and
   infant deaths, 213; livelihood, 212; and
   local authorities, 213; low standard of,
   205; and maternal deaths, 213; oath, 214;
   opinion of physicus, 214; satisfaction
   with, 207, 213–14; selection, 209–11;
   status, 208–9; training, 207
rural/urban, 74
Russia, 102

Sabean, David, 18, 48
Sachsa, 5
St. Leonhard hospital (Braunschweig), 292
St. Ludgeri (cloister), 30
St. Petersburg, 101, 113, 137
sal ammoniaco, 174
sal seignette, 174
Salzgitter, 10
Salzmann, Christian, 66
Sambleben (*Amt*), 117
Sandart, Philip, 99
Sander, Sabine, 12–13, 18
Sandorfÿ, 220
Saxony, 20, 369
scarletina, 258
Schamler, Gottlieb (dentist), 157–58
Schartzfeld, 97–98
Schatzkollegium, 31
Schäuerchen, 242, 259
Scheer's Essence, 180
Scheermesser, Johann (executioner in
   Helmstedt), 224–25
Scheibe, Ernst (bathmaster in Stadtolden-
   dorf), 147
Scheibner, Georg (physicus in
   Schöningen), 11, 105, 279

Schiller, Friedrich von, 80
Schiller, J. (physician in Quedlinburg), 99, 101
Schindler, Christian (draper in Braunschweig), 157
Schlagel (student), 193
Schlegel (pastor in Hohegeiss), 5
Schlemme (surgeon in Blankenburg), 192
Schlewecke, 10
Schlözer, August, 332
Schlüter, Friedrich, 66
Schmidt (forester in Langelsheim), 120
Schmidt (physician in Neustadt), 312
Schmidt, Ernest (surgeon in Weser district), 146
Schmidt, Heinrich (charcoal-burner in Harzburg), 100, 214–15, 220
Schmidt, Jochimb (oculist), 153
Schmidt, Joseph, 94
Schönejahn, Johann, 188–89
Schöningen (district), 30–31, 34, 43, 87–88
Schöningen (town): physicus in, 87, 97–98; plague in, 63
schoolmasters: and administration of public health, 21; *Pfuscherey* of, 231; statistics collection, 237, 239, 298
Schöppenstedt (*Amt*), 30, 43, 104
Schöppenstedt (town): beer, 284; description, 87, 283–84; diet, 284; fertility, 287; mortality rates, 283–84; reports on, 283–88; smallpox in, 297; water, 284–85
Schrader, Anna (midwife in Braunschweig), 200
Schramm, 186–87
Schreeden, Hans (executioner in Helmstedt), 225
Schreger, Bernhard, 173
Schroll, Johann, 101
Schrott (physician), 94–95
Schüler (*Amtmann* in Schöppenstedt), 127, 284
Schulze, Jason (substitute physicus in Walkenried), 276–78
Schulze, Johann (physicus in Calvörde), 98, 133, 278
Schuster (surgeon in Blankenburg), 191
Schwabe, Johann, 77
Schwancke (surgeon in Blankenburg), 191–92, 319–20
Schwartze (executioner in Seesen), 13

Schwindsucht, 240–41, 257–59
Seebode, Christian (member of Collegium medicum), 57, 97, 342
Seehausen, Dorothea (midwife in Braunschweig), 200
Seesen (*Amt* and town): artisans, 43; ironworks, 36; midwifery, 205–8; physicus, 58, 95; quackery in, 13; report on, 280
Seiffart (physician in Sambleben), 117
Seiffert (oculist in Braunschweig), 153
Seitz (apothecary in Gandersheim), 116
Seven Years' War, 35, 236–38, 255, 287, 289, 314
Sewell, William, 7, 170
sextons, 237, 239, 289, 300, 313
sick poor, 293
Siegemund, Justine, 194
Siegesbeck, Johann (physicus in Helmstedt), 113–14, 137
Siegreich, Christoph (dentist), 160–61
Sievers (physicus in Stadtoldendorf and Holzminden), 103–4
silk, 36
Sintdorf (physician in Goslar), 366–67
Siphra und Pua, 197
smallpox: in Braunschweig, 318; cause of, 269; as childhood disease, 238, 258, 322; as epidemic, 64, 244, 272, 321; in Hehlen, 253; and mortality, 238–39, 242, 259, 261; in parish registers, 251; as postnatal birth control, 331; treatments for, 296, 309, 367. *See also* inoculation; vaccination
snake-charmers, 60
Société royale de médicine, 240, 272
solar microscope, 121
soldiers, 193. *See also Pfuscher; Pfuscherey*
Sommer, Johann (professor and member of Collegium medicum), 137, 201, 203, 212, 330, 364
Spanndienst, 39
Spangenberg (physician in Einbeck), 321
Spangenberg, Georg (physicus in Walkenried), 3, 7–9, 14, 17, 54, 146, 207, 222, 258, 279
Spiess, Friedrich (physicus in Braunschweig), 82
Spohr, Carl Friderich (physicus in Wolfenbüttel, Blankenburg, and Calvörde), 81

Spohr, Carl Heinrich (physicus in Seesen and Gandersheim): complaints about *Pfuscher*, 215, 222; in Gandersheim, 147; life history, 134–35; on mortality lists, 297–98; and music, 134–35; as physicus candidate, 104–5; in Seesen, 250; and smallpox in Münchehof, 118–19; as vaccinator, 336
Spohr, Christoph (surgeon in Alfeld), 134
Spohr, Louis, 134–35
Stadtoldendorf: artisans, 43; growth, 294; medical practitioners, 147; physicus's salary, 58; plague, 63–64; reports on, 275–76, 278–79
Stadtphysicus, 53, 91
Stahl, Georg, 173
state: absolute, 73; bureaucratic, 22, 25–26; character of, 370–71; models, 22; modern, 22; role of, 22–24, 139; seventeenth- and eighteenth-century, 24; Weberian, 22; "well-ordered police," 22–23
State Archive of Lower Saxony (Wolfenbüttel), 16
statistics: collection, 21; evaluation, 237; use of, 243, 286, 288; vital, 21, 236
Stauffenberg (*Amt*), 118
Sternberg, J. H., 361–62
stillbirths, 239. *See also* mortality: infant
Stolle (apothecary in Astfeld), 215
Stolze (physicus in Stadtoldendorf), 96
Stoughton's Stomach Tonic, 180
Strasbourg, 176
Streuberg (physician in Goslar), 13
stroke, 256, 266–67, 367
Strukturgeschichte, 6
Struve, Carl (physicus in Holzminden), 91–92, 117, 255, 275–76, 297, 321
Stüber, Johann (surgeon in Helmstedt), 193
subsistence crisis, 35
Subsistenz, 177. *See also* livelihood; *Nahrung*
sudorifics, 313
sugar beets, 123
superstition: extent of, 305–6; popular, 11–12, 305, 373; practices, 302–3
suppressione menstruorum, 346
surgeons: appointment of, 185; conflicts with bathmasters, 183–94; consultations with, 323 (*see also* consultations); and corporatism, 60–61; education, 191–92;

encroachment and, 182–83; examination of, 186; franchises for, 185–86; limits on practice, 151; medical practice of, 185; numerus clausus, 192; ordinances concerning, 185; protection of rights, 170; rural, 218–19; in Württemburg, 13
Surgeons' Guild (Braunschweig), 169, 229
surgery, 339, 343–44, 351, 366
Süssmilch, Johann, 274, 279
swamps, 285

Tailors' Guild (Braunschweig), 324–35
taverners, 177
taxes, 39, 42, 244, 246
teething, 301, 361–62
temperaments, 264, 301
territoriality, 15, 161. *See also* encroachment
textiles, 37
thaumaturgy, 11, 362
Thedinghausen (*Amt*), 30–31
theft, 191
therapeutic experience, 15
therapies, 311
thermometer, 301
Thiele, Hans (horse doctor), 361
Thiéry, François, 172
Thilo, Otto (surgeon in Gandersheim), 147
Thirty Years' War, 236–37, 293
Thomasonians, 168
Thompson, E. P., 24, 47, 61, 181
three-field system, 41
Tiemann (Bürgermeister in Seesen), 56
tinctura macrocosmi, 224
Tissot, Samuel, 14, 66–67, 70, 262–67, 269–70, 300, 302, 310
tithe-holders, 21
tobacco, 35, 273–74
Topp, Friedrich (physicus in Wolfenbüttel), 274–76, 331
Tracht (surgeon in Lutter am Barenberge), 220–21
trade fairs, 43
transference, 307, 309–10
Traub (journeymen feldsher in Jerxheim), 355
Traut (official in Helmstedt), 187
traveling apothecary chest, 85
treatment, 290, 351–52, 366

troops, 294
trust, 299–300, 357
tumors, 239, 341

Uhlenhorst, Anton (bathmaster), 188
Unger's Digestive Powder, 180
Universal-Lexikon, 166
Unkermann, Georg (knacker in Braun-
    schweig), 224
Unzer, Johann August, 173, 263–64, 266
Uphoff, Johann (schoolmaster and sexton
    in Hehlen and Daspe), 252–57, 273, 323
uroscopy, 303

vaccination: articles on, 138; introduction
    of, 290, 331, 334; opposition to, 335–36;
    spread of, 333–36; support for, 334; in
    Veltenhof, 334
Vallstedt, 296
Vann, James, 25, 370
Varges (surgeon in Benneckenstein), 349–
    50
Vechelde, 293
Velteim, 131
Verbesserter Schreib-Calender, 67–68
Vibrans, Johann (physicus in Calvörde,
    Walkenried, Vorsfelde, Königslutter),
    93, 112, 126, 193, 226
villages: artisans in, 41 (*see also* artisans;
    guilds); character of, 108; descriptions
    of, 18; government of, 20; society of, 34,
    38–40, 42
violence symbolique, 23
Vogel, Samuel, 301
Vögler (surgeon in Hessen), 311
Vögler (surgeon in Jerxheim), 356
Volk, das, 293
Volkersheim, 10
Von der Ruhr unter dem Volke, 66
Vorsfelde, 279
Voß, Johann (physicus in Helmstedt), 83–
    84, 114

Wachsmuth, Johann (physicus in Holz-
    minden), 88, 91–92, 115–16, 146, 173,
    205, 295
Wageler, Carl (professor and member of
    Collegium medicum), 106, 137, 200
Walkenried (*Amt*): cloister, 29; deaths in,
    258; description, 30; diseases in, 258;

hospital, 314; medical conditions, 3–5;
    midwives, 4, 207; parish registers, 251,
    258; physicus, 112, 258–59; report on,
    279
Walker, Mack, 43, 47, 161
Wallmann (surgeon in Helmstedt), 311–12
Wandsbecker Bote, 69
Warburg (*Amt*), 29, 38
warming-women: as apprentice midwives,
    195; duties, 198; earnings, 200, 204;
    Pfuscherey of, 201, 204; privileges, 198;
    resentment of, 200; selection, 198; train-
    ing, 198. *See also* midwifery; midwives
    (Braunschweig)
wasting. *See* cachexia
Weber, Max, 24
Webster, Charles, 12
Weeks, Christoph (soldier), 218
Wehler, Hans-Ulrich, 22, 25
Welge, Johann (physicus in Harzburg), 95,
    334–35
Weltschopp, J. H. (monitor in Braun-
    schweig), 315–16
Weser (district): description, 30–31; indus-
    try, 37; medical practitioners, 146; physi-
    cate, 91–92; physicus, 88
wholesale trade, 177
whooping cough, 238, 258. *See also* dis-
    eases: of chest and throat
Wickensen (*Amt*), 37, 117
Widemann, Heinrich (professor and secre-
    tary of Collegium medicum), 69
Wiede, 4
Wilcke (*Amtmann* in Stadtoldendorf), 92
wills, 18
Winckelmann (physician in Campen), 334
Winsil (operator), 5
witchcraft, 306
Witte, Johann (feldsher), 159
Wochenblatt, der Wirth und die Wirthin, 69
Woemper, G. L., 168
Wolfenbüttel (city): description, 43, 48;
    disease patterns, 260; guilds in, 42; phys-
    icus in, 83; plague in, 63; police in, 32;
    report on, 274–75; smallpox in, 298
Wolfenbüttel (district): agriculture in, 34;
    description, 30–31; physicate, 87–88
Wolfshagen, 250
women, 277
worms, 301

Württemburg, 13, 18, 25
Würzburg, University of, 80

Zachariä, Just (editor of *Braunschwegische Anzeigen*), 178
Zedler, Johann, 166–67
Zehntherr, 39

Zerrenner, Heinrich, 269–70, 302
Ziegenbein (shepherd in Amselsen), 295, 297
Ziegler, Christian (physicus in Walkenried), 100
Zimmermann, Johann, 66
Zorge, 3–4, 6